New Insights into Parvovirus Research

New Insights into Parvovirus Research

Special Issue Editor

Giorgio Gallinella

MDPI • Basel • Beijing • Wuhan • Barcelona • Belgrade • Manchester • Tokyo • Cluj • Tianjin

Special Issue Editor
Giorgio Gallinella
University of Bologna
Italy

Editorial Office
MDPI
St. Alban-Anlage 66
4052 Basel, Switzerland

This is a reprint of articles from the Special Issue published online in the open access journal *Viruses* (ISSN 1999-4915) (available at: https://www.mdpi.com/journal/viruses/special_issues/Parvovirus).

For citation purposes, cite each article independently as indicated on the article page online and as indicated below:

LastName, A.A.; LastName, B.B.; LastName, C.C. Article Title. *Journal Name* **Year**, *Article Number*, Page Range.

ISBN 978-3-03928-310-1 (Pbk)
ISBN 978-3-03928-311-8 (PDF)

Contents

About the Special Issue Editor ix

Giorgio Gallinella
New Insights into Parvovirus Research
Reprinted from: *Viruses* **2019**, *11*, 1053, doi:10.3390/v11111053 1

Mario Mietzsch, Judit J. Pénzes and Mavis Agbandje-McKenna
Twenty-Five Years of Structural Parvovirology
Reprinted from: *Viruses* **2019**, *11*, 362, doi:10.3390/v11040362 7

Justin J. Kurian, Renuk Lakshmanan, William M. Chmely, Joshua A. Hull, Jennifer C. Yu, Antonette Bennett, Robert McKenna and Mavis Agbandje-McKenna
Adeno-Associated Virus VP1u Exhibits Protease Activity
Reprinted from: *Viruses* **2019**, *11*, 399, doi:10.3390/v11050399 41

Judit J. Pénzes, William Marciel de Souza, Mavis Agbandje-McKenna and Robert J. Gifford
An Ancient Lineage of Highly Divergent Parvoviruses Infects both Vertebrate and Invertebrate Hosts
Reprinted from: *Viruses* **2019**, *11*, 525, doi:10.3390/v11060525 57

Elizabeth Fahsbender, Eda Altan, M. Alexis Seguin, Pauline Young, Marko Estrada, Christian Leutenegger and Eric Delwart
Chapparvovirus DNA Found in 4% of Dogs with Diarrhea
Reprinted from: *Viruses* **2019**, *11*, 398, doi:10.3390/v11050398 79

Francesco Mira, Marta Canuti, Giuseppa Purpari, Vincenza Cannella, Santina Di Bella, Leonardo Occhiogrosso, Giorgia Schirò, Gabriele Chiaramonte, Santino Barreca, Patrizia Pisano, Antonio Lastra, Nicola Decaro and Annalisa Guercio
Molecular Characterization and Evolutionary Analyses of *Carnivore Protoparvovirus 1 NS1* Gene
Reprinted from: *Viruses* **2019**, *11*, 308, doi:10.3390/v11040308 87

Deepak Kumar, Suman Chaudhary, Nanyan Lu, Michael Duff, Mathew Heffel, Caroline A. McKinney, Daniela Bedenice and Douglas Marthaler
Metagenomic Next-Generation Sequencing Reveal Presence of a Novel Ungulate *Bocaparvovirus* in Alpacas
Reprinted from: *Viruses* **2019**, *11*, 701, doi:10.3390/v11080701 107

Toni Luise Meister, Birthe Tegtmeyer, Alexander Postel, Jessika-M.V. Cavalleri, Daniel Todt, Alexander Stang and Eike Steinmann
Equine Parvovirus-Hepatitis Frequently Detectable in Commercial Equine Serum Pools
Reprinted from: *Viruses* **2019**, *11*, 461, doi:10.3390/v11050461 115

Renáta Tóth, István Mészáros, Daniela Hüser, Barbara Forró, Szilvia Marton, Ferenc Olasz, Krisztián Bányai, Regine Heilbronn and Zoltán Zádori
Methylation Status of the Adeno-Associated Virus Type 2 (AAV2)
Reprinted from: *Viruses* **2019**, *11*, 38, doi:10.3390/v11010038 125

Wei Zou, Min Xiong, Xuefeng Deng, John F. Engelhardt, Ziying Yan and Jianming Qiu
A Comprehensive RNA-seq Analysis of Human Bocavirus 1 Transcripts in Infected Human Airway Epithelium
Reprinted from: *Viruses* **2019**, *11*, 33, doi:10.3390/v11010033 135

Oliver Caliaro, Andrea Marti, Nico Ruprecht, Remo Leisi, Suriyasri Subramanian, Susan Hafenstein and Carlos Ros
Parvovirus B19 Uncoating Occurs in the Cytoplasm without Capsid Disassembly and It Is Facilitated by Depletion of Capsid-Associated Divalent Cations
Reprinted from: *Viruses* **2019**, *11*, 430, doi:10.3390/v11050430 . . . . **149**

Elisabetta Manaresi and Giorgio Gallinella
Advances in the Development of Antiviral Strategies against Parvovirus B19
Reprinted from: *Viruses* **2019**, *11*, 659, doi:10.3390/v11070659 . . . . **171**

Thomas Zobel, C.-Thomas Bock, Uwe Kühl, Maria Rohde, Dirk Lassner, Heinz-Peter Schultheiss and Caroline Schmidt-Lucke
Telbivudine Reduces Parvovirus B19-Induced Apoptosis in Circulating Angiogenic Cells
Reprinted from: *Viruses* **2019**, *11*, 227, doi:10.3390/v11030227 . . . . **193**

Angelos G. Rigopoulos, Bianca Klutt, Marios Matiakis, Athanasios Apostolou, Sophie Mavrogeni and Michel Noutsias
Systematic Review of PCR Proof of Parvovirus B19 Genomes in Endomyocardial Biopsies of Patients Presenting with Myocarditis or Dilated Cardiomyopathy
Reprinted from: *Viruses* **2019**, *11*, 566, doi:10.3390/v11060566 . . . . **203**

Zaiga Nora-Krukle, Anda Vilmane, Man Xu, Santa Rasa, Inga Ziemele, Elina Silina, Maria Söderlund-Venermo, Dace Gardovska and Modra Murovska
Human Bocavirus Infection Markers in Peripheral Blood and Stool Samples of Children with Acute Gastroenteritis
Reprinted from: *Viruses* **2018**, *10*, 639, doi:10.3390/v10110639 . . . . **219**

Peng Xu, Xiaomei Wang, Yi Li and Jianming Qiu
Establishment of a Parvovirus B19 NS1-Expressing Recombinant Adenoviral Vector for Killing Megakaryocytic Leukemia Cells
Reprinted from: *Viruses* **2019**, *11*, 820, doi:10.3390/v11090820 . . . . **229**

Clemens Bretscher and Antonio Marchini
H-1 Parvovirus as a Cancer-Killing Agent: Past, Present, and Future
Reprinted from: *Viruses* **2019**, *11*, 562, doi:10.3390/v11060562 . . . . **241**

Assia Angelova and Jean Rommelaere
Immune System Stimulation by Oncolytic Rodent Protoparvoviruses
Reprinted from: *Viruses* **2019**, *11*, 415, doi:10.3390/v11050415 . . . . **261**

Sarah François, Doriane Mutuel, Alison B. Duncan, Leonor R. Rodrigues, Celya Danzelle, Sophie Lefevre, Inês Santos, Marie Frayssinet, Emmanuel Fernandez, Denis Filloux, Philippe Roumagnac, Rémy Froissart and Mylène Ogliastro
A New Prevalent Densovirus Discovered in *Acari*. Insight from Metagenomics in Viral Communities Associated with Two-Spotted Mite (*Tetranychus urticae*) Populations
Reprinted from: *Viruses* **2019**, *11*, 233, doi:10.3390/v11030233 . . . . **273**

Rui Li, Pengfei Chang, Peng Lü, Zhaoyang Hu, Keping Chen, Qin Yao and Qian Yu
Characterization of the RNA Transcription Profile of *Bombyx mori* Bidensovirus
Reprinted from: *Viruses* **2019**, *11*, 325, doi:10.3390/v11040325 . . . . **297**

About the Special Issue Editor

Giorgio Gallinella, MD, Ph.D., is an Associate Professor of Microbiology at the Department of Pharmacy and Biotechnology at the University of Bologna, Italy. He conducts research in the field of virology with a special interest in Parvovirus B19. He obtained a degree in Medicine and Surgery at the University of Bologna (1989), a Ph.D. in Microbiological Sciences at the University of Genova (1994), and a Medical Specialization Degree in Microbiology and Virology from the University of Bologna (1997). Since then, he has conducted scientific and didactic activity at the University of Bologna, Microbiology Section - Department of Pharmacy and Biotechnology.

viruses

MDPI

Editorial

New Insights into Parvovirus Research

Giorgio Gallinella

Department of Pharmacy and Biotechnology University of Bologna, 40138 Bologna, Italy; giorgio.gallinella@unibo.it; Tel.: +39-051-4290900

Received: 6 November 2019; Accepted: 11 November 2019; Published: 13 November 2019

Abstract: The family Parvoviridae includes an ample and most diverse collection of viruses. Exploring the biological diversity and the inherent complexity in these apparently simple viruses has been a continuous commitment for the scientific community since their first discovery more than fifty years ago. The Special Issue of 'Viruses' dedicated to the 'New Insights into Parvovirus Research' aimed at presenting a 'state of the art' in many aspects of research in the field, at collecting the newest contributions on unresolved issues, and at presenting new approaches exploiting systemic (-omic) methodologies.

Keywords: parvovirus; structural biology; genetics; oncolytic viruses; antivirals

1. Introduction

The family Parvoviridae includes an ample and most diverse collection of viruses. According to formal taxonomy [1], viruses in the family are all characterised by a linear ssDNA genome, 5–6 kb, and a small icosahedral capsid, 20–25 nm. The host range comprise both invertebrate and vertebrate hosts, giving rise to the main division into the two subfamilies, respectively Densovirinae and Parvovirinae. Further, different genera are recognised within these subfamilies, based on sequence homologies, reflective of evolutionary relationships. In fact, apart from the more general shared properties, a prominent feature is the ample diversity that can be observed between the members of the different genera regarding structure, genome organization and expression, virus–cell interaction, and impact on the host.

Exploring the biological diversity and the inherent complexity in these apparently simple viruses has been a continuous commitment for the scientific community since their first discovery more than fifty years ago. In addition, the translational implications of research on parvoviruses are relevant. Within the family, some viruses are important human and veterinary pathogens, in need of reliable diagnostic methods and efficient therapeutic, antiviral strategies. Rodent parvoviruses have long been studied not only as model systems, but also as tools for oncolytic therapy. Adeno-associated viruses (AAV) have found their way as sophisticated gene delivery vectors and begin now to display successfully their wide and expanding applicative potential.

The Special Issue of 'Viruses' dedicated to the 'New Insights into Parvovirus Research' aimed at presenting a 'state of the art' in many aspects of research in the field, at collecting the newest contributions on unresolved issues, and at presenting new approaches exploiting systemic (-omic) methodologies. Evolution, structural biology, viral replication, virus–host interaction, pathogenesis and immunity, gene therapy, and viral oncotherapy are a selection of topics that have been addressed in articles collected in this Special Issue.

2. The Articles in the Special Issue

Studies on the structural biology of viruses in the family can now collect the results of more than twenty-five years of active research, and about 100 structures resolved at high-resolution level are deposited and available. In this Special Issue, all related information is summarised and discussed in a landmark review paper [2]. Presently, the structures of representative viruses of all the different genera in the family are known, and information on capsid–receptor and capsid–antibodies interactions is accumulating. The importance of knowing at atomic level the topology of the capsid shells of these viruses allows for structure–function studies and has critical implications in several instances. First, when considering the tropism of viruses, this allows studying in detail the virus–host cell interactions, also, as a basis for a rational engineering of viruses as oncolytic agents or transduction vectors. Then, such information allows dissecting the capacity of the immune system to recognise and neutralise viruses, a protective effect against viral diseases but a potential problem when considering the use of virus-derived biologics. The common limitation to these studies is the still-unresolved structure of the VP1 unique region, a fractional moiety in the capsid, with a likely flexible and disordered structure, critical for viral infectivity because of the associated phospholipase activity. A novel enzymatic activity associated with this moiety in AAV2 is now presented in a paper in this collection [3].

Next-generation sequencing (NGS) technologies are now frequently in use and contribute effectively to the discovery of novel viruses in the family, as well as to the definition of their evolutionary relationships. Actually, the family picture of viruses in the family is continuously expanding, and new contributions are presented in this issue too. A most intriguing topic is the growing identification of members in the *Chappaparvovirus* genus, and chiefly the resulting inference of an ancient evolutionary divergence of members of this genus from other genera in the family, based both on genomic and structural comparative data [4]. A taxonomic reassessment of subdivisions in the family will be required to incorporate this novel information, and more upcoming work will certainly elucidate the characteristics of this group of viruses. Additionally, metagenomics sequencing led to the identification of a novel bocavirus in ungulates [5], a chappaparvovirus species in dogs [6] and a densovirus infecting acari [7]. On the other hand, molecular phylodynamics continues to yield valuable information, as in the study on spread and evolution of Carnivore protoparvovirus 1 reconstructed based on NS1/NS2 protein sequences [8]. As is always the case, metagenomics identification of viral sequences in biological samples tells us little about the ecology and potential pathogenetic role of a newly discovered virus, so that epidemiological and correlation studies should be required. In this issue, such a question has been addressed about the recently identified equine parvovirus-hepatitis, raising a concern about its possible transmission through contaminated human and veterinary medical products [9].

Novel technologies also allow a deeper and systemic inspection of the genetics and expression profile of viruses within infected cells. The methylation status of the AAV2 genome is presented in [10], showing a difference between packaged or integrated genomes and an inverse correlation with the capability of integrated genomes to be rescued. Epigenetic regulation of parvoviruses is a topic only rarely addressed, but that possibly would merit more attention when considering the long-term relationship of these viruses to their hosts. The transcription map of *Bombyx mori* bidensovirus has been thoroughly investigated and presented [11]. The transcriptome of Human Bocavirus 1 in polarised airway epithelial cells [12] has been analysed by comprehensive RNAseq, and, in this case, the use of NGS and combination of transcript mapping and quantitative analysis could yield a full insight into viral replication dynamics and expression. The aim now at hand by the application of next generation techniques is to obtain comprehensive paradigms to characterize a viral lifecycle and to interpret the effects of the virus within infected cells, possibly at single-cell level.

The initial phases of virus–cell interaction are a relevant matter of investigation. The interaction of *Junonia coenia* densovirus with the midgut barriers of caterpillars has been analysed in detail, to yield a picture of the initial phases of infection that involve binding to host glycans and later disruption of the peritrophic matrix, as presented in [13]. Concerning the human pathogenic parvovirus B19, its very selective tropism for erythroid progenitor cells critically depends on the presence of a specific receptor for the VP1 unique region, but the subsequent steps that are also critical to the outcome of infection still need to be further characterised. The contribution in this issue [14] provides evidence for a coordinated translocation of viral nucleocapsids and genome uncoating in the nucleus of infected cells.

Regarding translational issues, in addition to the engineering of AAVs as very successful gene transduction vectors, there is a long record of studies on the use of protoparvoviruses as oncolytic agents. Two excellent reviews summarise and address the complex issues [15,16] of the potential of protoparvoviruses as oncolytic viruses, describing their characteristics, the known mechanisms of oncolytic and oncosuppressive activity and in particular, how the interplay and cooperation with the host immune system can affect the control of tumours. After so many years of basic research, the first clinical applications of oncolytic parvovirus begin to yield promising results, this in turn prompting for further research to improve the anticancer profile of these agents. A different experimental approach is presented in [17], where the cytolytic properties of parvovirus B19 NS1 protein towards erythroid progenitor cells are exploited in a context of an Adenovirus-derived transduction vector, to obtain a selective oncolytic activity against megakaryocytic leukaemia cells.

The pathogenetic role and clinical implications of human parvoviruses are addressed in two studies presented in this collection, about the role of human bocaviruses and parvovirus B19. In an observational study [18], a significant association of human bocaviruses to gastroenteritis is reported, thus further expanding their clinical involvement in addition to the established association with respiratory tract infections. In a systematic review and meta-analysis study [19], the significance of the detection of parvovirus B19 genomes in endomyocardial biopsies of patients presenting with myocarditis or dilated cardiomyopathy is discussed. This review should be regarded as a very useful contribution to a long debated and far from settled issue. From such meta-analysis, the conclusion is that the mere detection of viral genomes is just indicative of the propensity of B19 to establish long-term persistence in tissues [20], and that implication as a causative agent in cardiomyopathies needs to be supported by some reliable evidence of biological activity of the virus.

Furthermore, concerning a role of parvovirus B19 in the development of cardiomyopathies, the possible effect of telbivudine in reducing the damage to endothelial progenitor cells caused by the presence of B19 is presented [21]. Telbivudine is an RT-enzyme inhibitor used as an antiviral in treating HBV, thus the protective effect against B19-derived cell damage is an unexpected, cell-targeted, and non-selective activity, a result prompting for further research in this field. More in general, parvovirus B19 is the most pathogenic virus to humans, responsible for a wide spectrum of clinical manifestations whose outcomes depend on a close interaction between the virus and the physiological and immunological condition of the infected individuals. Apart from the need for reliable diagnostics [22], there is an urgent need for antiviral treatments that might go beyond simple supportive or replacement strategies. The review in this issue [23] presents the recent results in this field, that led to the first identification of compounds with antiviral activity against parvovirus B19. These comprise retargeted drugs such as hydroxyurea, broad range antivirals such as cidofovir or its derivative brincidofovir, and novel compounds identified in drug-discovery screening experiments, such as some coumarin or flavonoid derivatives. This research, aimed at closing the gap with respect to antivirals available against other DNA viruses, thus, begins to yield interesting results, prompting for further discoveries meeting clinical needs.

3. Conclusions

As a conclusive remark, the collection of articles in this Special Issue devoted to 'New Insights into Parvovirus Research' and contributed by distinguished researchers should be regarded as significant for two main reasons, among others. First, some of the articles effectively present a 'state-of-the-art' overview in some main topics. Then, many articles show how the application of new methodologies, including but not limited to NGS, can be functional to the establishment of novel and more general paradigms in the field. In the near future, research on parvoviruses will certainly yield more answers to still-unresolved issues.

Funding: This research received no external funding.

Conflicts of Interest: The author declares no conflict of interest.

References

1. Cotmore, S.F.; Agbandje-McKenna, M.; Chiorini, J.A.; Mukha, D.V.; Pintel, D.J.; Qiu, J.; Soderlund-Venermo, M.; Tattersall, P.; Tijssen, P.; Gatherer, D.; et al. The family Parvoviridae. *Arch. Virol.* **2014**, *159*, 1239–1247. [CrossRef] [PubMed]
2. Mietzsch, M.; Penzes, J.J.; Agbandje-McKenna, M. Twenty-Five Years of Structural Parvovirology. *Viruses* **2019**, *11*, 362. [CrossRef] [PubMed]
3. Kurian, J.J.; Lakshmanan, R.; Chmely, W.M.; Hull, J.A.; Yu, J.C.; Bennett, A.; McKenna, R.; Agbandje-McKenna, M. Adeno-Associated Virus VP1u Exhibits Protease Activity. *Viruses* **2019**, *11*, 399. [CrossRef] [PubMed]
4. Penzes, J.J.; de Souza, W.M.; Agbandje-McKenna, M.; Gifford, R.J. An Ancient Lineage of Highly Divergent Parvoviruses Infects both Vertebrate and Invertebrate Hosts. *Viruses* **2019**, *11*, 525. [CrossRef] [PubMed]
5. Kumar, D.; Chaudhary, S.; Lu, N.; Duff, M.; Heffel, M.; McKinney, C.A.; Bedenice, D.; Marthaler, D. Metagenomic Next-Generation Sequencing Reveal Presence of a Novel Ungulate Bocaparvovirus in Alpacas. *Viruses* **2019**, *11*, 701. [CrossRef] [PubMed]
6. Fahsbender, E.; Altan, E.; Seguin, M.A.; Young, P.; Estrada, M.; Leutenegger, C.; Delwart, E. Chapparvovirus DNA Found in 4% of Dogs with Diarrhea. *Viruses* **2019**, *11*, 398. [CrossRef] [PubMed]
7. Francois, S.; Mutuel, D.; Duncan, A.B.; Rodrigues, L.R.; Danzelle, C.; Lefevre, S.; Santos, I.; Frayssinet, M.; Fernandez, E.; Filloux, D.; et al. A New Prevalent Densovirus Discovered in Acari. Insight from Metagenomics in Viral Communities Associated with Two-Spotted Mite (*Tetranychus urticae*) Populations. *Viruses* **2019**, *11*, 233. [CrossRef]
8. Mira, F.; Canuti, M.; Purpari, G.; Cannella, V.; Di Bella, S.; Occhiogrosso, L.; Schiro, G.; Chiaramonte, G.; Barreca, S.; Pisano, P.; et al. Molecular Characterization and Evolutionary Analyses of Carnivore Protoparvovirus 1 NS1 Gene. *Viruses* **2019**, *11*, 308. [CrossRef]
9. Meister, T.L.; Tegtmeyer, B.; Postel, A.; Cavalleri, J.V.; Todt, D.; Stang, A.; Steinmann, E. Equine Parvovirus-Hepatitis Frequently Detectable in Commercial Equine Serum Pools. *Viruses* **2019**, *11*, 461. [CrossRef]
10. Toth, R.; Meszaros, I.; Huser, D.; Forro, B.; Marton, S.; Olasz, F.; Banyai, K.; Heilbronn, R.; Zadori, Z. Methylation Status of the Adeno-Associated Virus Type 2 (AAV2). *Viruses* **2019**, *11*, 38. [CrossRef]
11. Li, R.; Chang, P.; Lu, P.; Hu, Z.; Chen, K.; Yao, Q.; Yu, Q. Characterization of the RNA Transcription Profile of Bombyx mori Bidensovirus. *Viruses* **2019**, *11*, 325. [CrossRef] [PubMed]
12. Zou, W.; Xiong, M.; Deng, X.; Engelhardt, J.F.; Yan, Z.; Qiu, J. A Comprehensive RNA-seq Analysis of Human Bocavirus 1 Transcripts in Infected Human Airway Epithelium. *Viruses* **2019**, *11*, 33. [CrossRef] [PubMed]
13. Pigeyre, L.; Schatz, M.; Ravallec, M.; Gasmi, L.; Negre, N.; Clouet, C.; Seveno, M.; El Koulali, K.; Decourcelle, M.; Guerardel, Y.; et al. Interaction of a Densovirus with Glycans of the Peritrophic Matrix Mediates Oral Infection of the Lepidopteran Pest Spodoptera frugiperda. *Viruses* **2019**, *11*, 870. [CrossRef] [PubMed]
14. Caliaro, O.; Marti, A.; Ruprecht, N.; Leisi, R.; Subramanian, S.; Hafenstein, S.; Ros, C. Parvovirus B19 Uncoating Occurs in the Cytoplasm without Capsid Disassembly and It Is Facilitated by Depletion of Capsid-Associated Divalent Cations. *Viruses* **2019**, *11*, 430. [CrossRef]
15. Angelova, A.; Rommelaere, J. Immune System Stimulation by Oncolytic Rodent Protoparvoviruses. *Viruses* **2019**, *11*, 415. [CrossRef]
16. Bretscher, C.; Marchini, A. H-1 Parvovirus as a Cancer-Killing Agent: Past, Present, and Future. *Viruses* **2019**, *11*, 562. [CrossRef]
17. Xu, P.; Wang, X.; Li, Y.; Qiu, J. Establishment of a Parvovirus B19 NS1-Expressing Recombinant Adenoviral Vector for Killing Megakaryocytic Leukemia Cells. *Viruses* **2019**, *11*, 820. [CrossRef]
18. Nora-Krukle, Z.; Vilmane, A.; Xu, M.; Rasa, S.; Ziemele, I.; Silina, E.; Soderlund-Venermo, M.; Gardovska, D.; Murovska, M. Human Bocavirus Infection Markers in Peripheral Blood and Stool Samples of Children with Acute Gastroenteritis. *Viruses* **2018**, *10*, 639. [CrossRef]
19. Rigopoulos, A.G.; Klutt, B.; Matiakis, M.; Apostolou, A.; Mavrogeni, S.; Noutsias, M. Systematic Review of PCR Proof of Parvovirus B19 Genomes in Endomyocardial Biopsies of Patients Presenting with Myocarditis or Dilated Cardiomyopathy. *Viruses* **2019**, *11*, 566. [CrossRef]

20. Bua, G.; Gallinella, G. How does parvovirus B19 DNA achieve lifelong persistence in human cells? *Future Virol.* **2017**, *12*, 549–553. [CrossRef]
21. Zobel, T.; Bock, C.T.; Kuhl, U.; Rohde, M.; Lassner, D.; Schultheiss, H.P.; Schmidt-Lucke, C. Telbivudine Reduces Parvovirus B19-Induced Apoptosis in Circulating Angiogenic Cells. *Viruses* **2019**, *11*, 227. [CrossRef] [PubMed]
22. Gallinella, G. The clinical use of parvovirus B19 assays: Recent advances. *Expert Rev. Mol. Diagn.* **2018**, *18*, 821–832. [CrossRef] [PubMed]
23. Manaresi, E.; Gallinella, G. Advances in the Development of Antiviral Strategies against Parvovirus B19. *Viruses* **2019**, *11*, 659. [CrossRef] [PubMed]

viruses

MDPI

Review

Twenty-Five Years of Structural Parvovirology

Mario Mietzsch †, Judit J. Pénzes † and Mavis Agbandje-McKenna *

Department of Biochemistry and Molecular Biology, Center for Structural Biology, The McKnight Brain Institute, University of Florida, Gainesville, FL 32610, USA; mario.mietzsch@ufl.edu (M.M.); judit.penzes@ufl.edu (J.J.P.)
* Correspondence: mckenna@ufl.edu; Tel.: +1-352-294-8393
† These authors contributed equally to this work.

Received: 19 March 2019; Accepted: 11 April 2019; Published: 20 April 2019

Abstract: Parvoviruses, infecting vertebrates and invertebrates, are a family of single-stranded DNA viruses with small, non-enveloped capsids with T = 1 icosahedral symmetry. A quarter of a century after the first parvovirus capsid structure was published, approximately 100 additional structures have been analyzed. This first structure was that of Canine Parvovirus, and it initiated the practice of structure-to-function correlation for the family. Despite high diversity in the capsid viral protein (VP) sequence, the structural topologies of all parvoviral capsids are conserved. However, surface loops inserted between the core secondary structure elements vary in conformation that enables the assembly of unique capsid surface morphologies within individual genera. These variations enable each virus to establish host niches by allowing host receptor attachment, specific tissue tropism, and antigenic diversity. This review focuses on the diversity among the parvoviruses with respect to the transcriptional strategy of the encoded VPs, the advances in capsid structure-function annotation, and therapeutic developments facilitated by the available structures.

Keywords: parvovirus; densovirus; single stranded DNA virus; X-ray crystallography; Cryo-EM; antibody interactions; receptor interactions

1. Introduction

The *Parvoviridae* are linear, single-stranded DNA packaging viruses with genomes of ~4 to 6 kb. They have a large host spectrum, spanning members of the phylum Cnidaria to amniote vertebrates. Currently the *Parvoviridae* is divided into two subfamilies based on their ability to infect either vertebrates or invertebrates [1]. Viruses infecting vertebrate and invertebrate hosts are assigned to *Parvovirinae* and *Densovirinae* subfamilies, respectively, although the monophyly of the latter is questioned due to the diversity of members, and new emerging vertebrate viruses close to the *Densovirinae* may require a new subfamily (Figure 1).

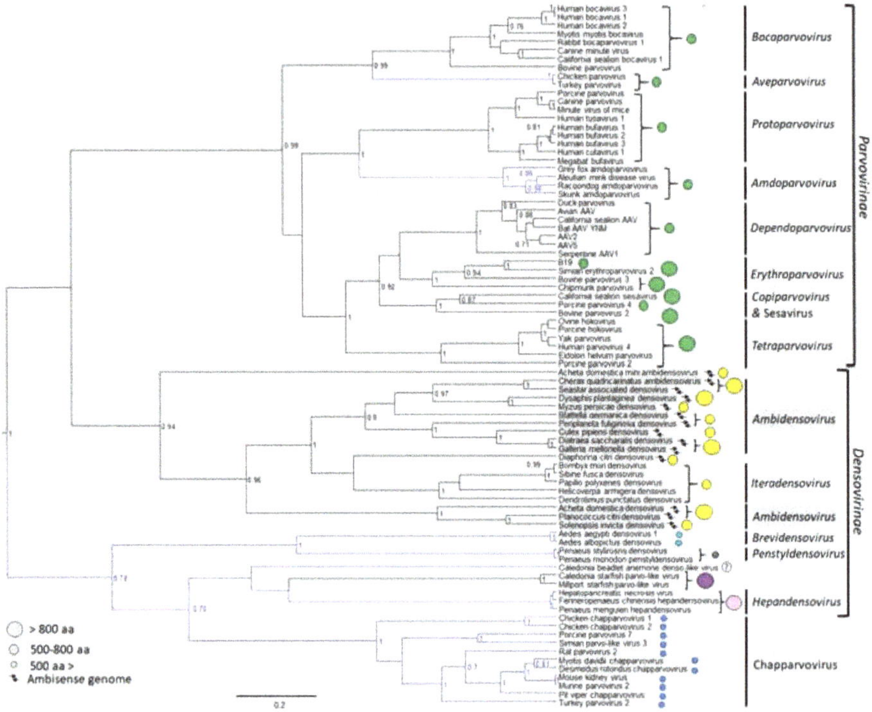

Figure 1. Evolutionary relationships of members of family *Parvoviridae* based on the conserved NS1 tripartite helicase domain. Branches of lineages highlighted in blue indicate the absence of a phospholipase A_2 (PLA_2) domain in the minor capsid viral protein, VP1. Capsid protein encoding gene homology is mapped as circles of different colors, where same colored circles indicate homologous genes (homology search defined, without the incorporation of the PLA_2 sequence, as whether a protein sequence gives a hit out of targeted 5000 sequences at an expectation value of 100 by the BlastP algorithm of the NCBI Blast application [2]). The size of the circle indicates the size of VP1 based on the scale to the left.

Parvovirus virions possess small non-enveloped capsids with a diameter of 200 to 280 Å [3–9]. Their T = 1 icosahedral capsids are assembled from 60 viral proteins (VPs) encoded from the right-hand side open reading frame (ORF) (Figures 2 and 3). This ORF, also known as *cap*, encodes up to four different VPs, depending on genus, of varying length, which all share a common C-terminal region [1]. Generally, the smallest VP, which comprises the common C-terminal region, is expressed at a higher rate compared to the larger VP forms and is, therefore, considered the major VP. The larger, less abundant VPs are N-terminal extended forms that contain regions important for the viral life cycle. Among these are a phospholipase A_2 (PLA_2) domain, a calcium-binding domain, and nuclear localization signals that are highly conserved in some genera [10–13]. The larger VPs are also incorporated into the capsid, albeit at low copy number, with the common C-terminus responsible for assembling the parvoviral capsid. In the different parvoviruses, the shared VP region varies between ~40 to 70 kDa in size (Figures 2 and 3). This review focuses on the transcription mechanism, and the sequence- and structure-based homology of the parvovirus VPs, as well as the characteristic features of the parvoviral capsids. We also discuss structure-function annotation and the use of structure to guide the development of gene delivery vectors.

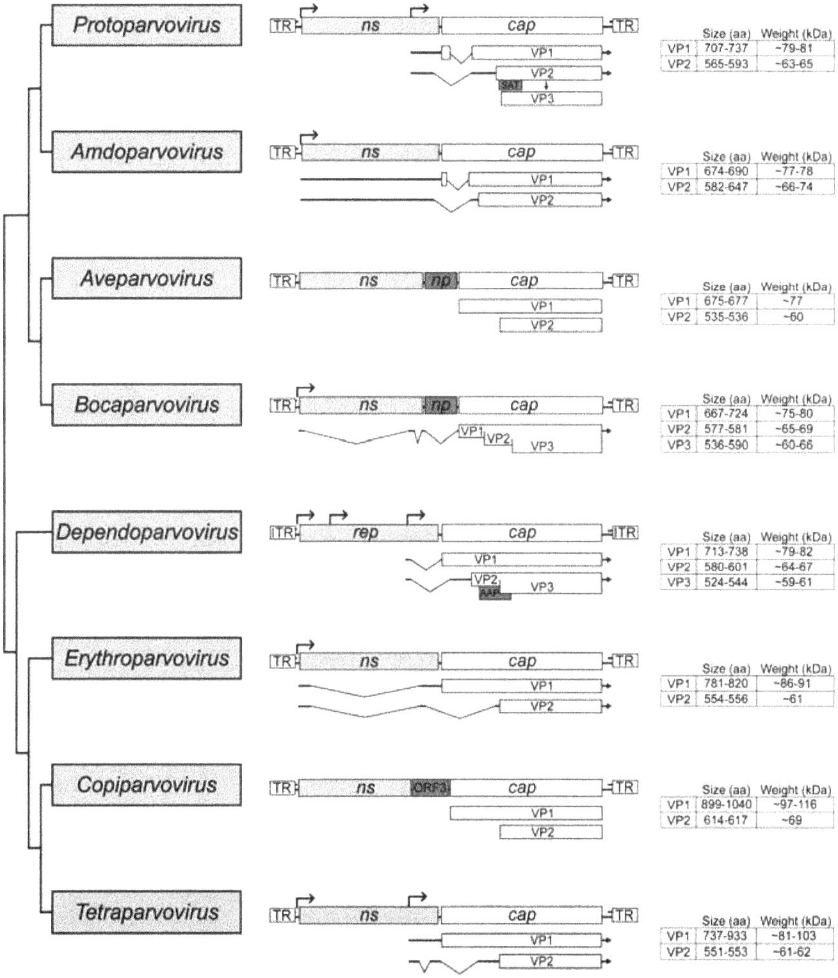

Figure 2. Cladogram of the subfamily *Parvovirinae*. The eight genera are shown. The general genome organization of each genus is shown in the middle with their ORF. The non-structural (NS) protein expressing genes *ns* or *rep* are simplified and only the ORF is shown. Below the *cap* ORF the transcripts for the expression of the individual VP are shown. On the right side the size and weight of the VPs are given. Note that the transcription profiles of the Aveparvovirus and Copiparvovirus genera have not been determined, and thus the sizes of the VPs are based on in silico predictions.

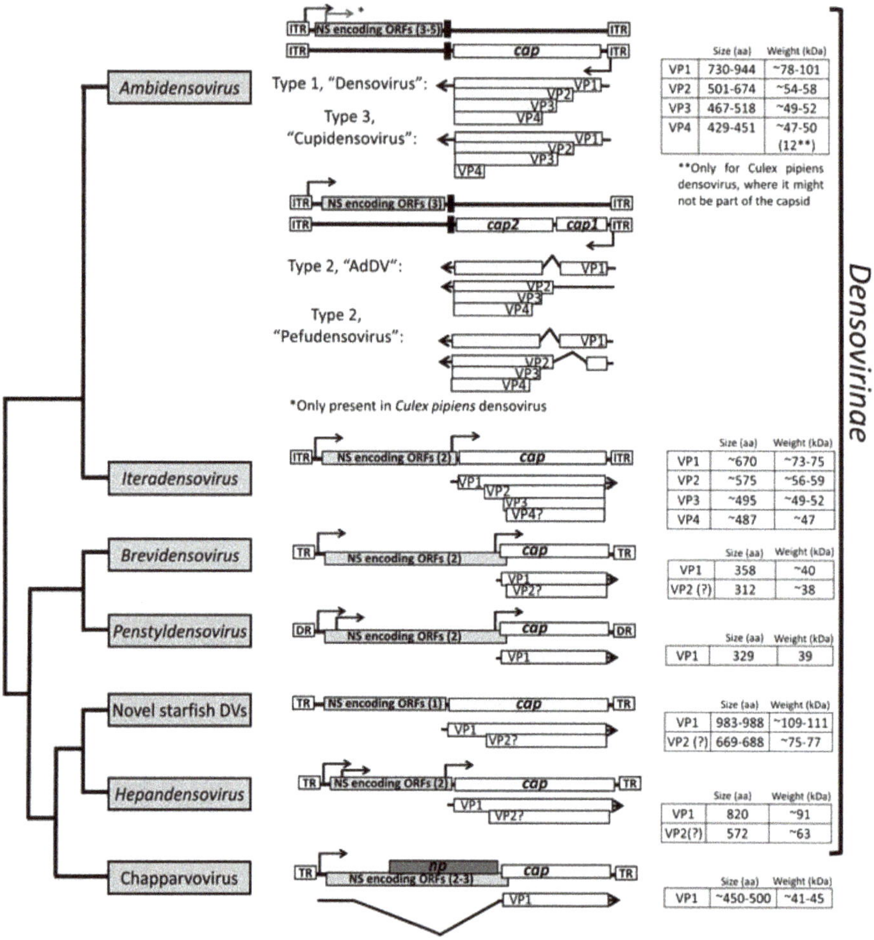

Figure 3. Cladogram of denso- and chapparvoviruses. The general genome organization and capsid protein expression strategy are shown. The *ns* genes are simplified and only the ORF is shown. The transcription strategy of members of genus *Hepandensovirus*, as well as of the new, unclassified starfish densoviruses, have not been determined, thus the sizes of the VPs are based on in silico predictions.

2. Parvovirinae

The Parvovirinae is subdivided into eight genera: *Amdoparvovirus*, *Aveparvovirus*, *Bocaparvovirus*, *Dependoparvovirus*, *Erythroparvovirus*, *Copiparvovirus*, *Protoparvovirus*, and *Tetraparvovirus* (Figures 1 and 2) [1]. As the genus name suggests, the dependoparvoviruses require helper virus functions for replication [14–18]. All other genera contain members capable of autonomous replication. The *Parvovirinae* viral genomes contain two or three ORFs (Figure 2). The left ORF, the ns or rep gene, encodes a series of regulatory proteins that are indispensable for viral replication. Due to its higher level of conservation, this gene is used for the classification of parvoviruses into different genera (Figure 1). The right ORF, the cap gene, encodes up to three VPs that assemble the capsid (Figure 2) [1]. In addition, multiple genera express smaller regulatory proteins, such as nucleoprotein 1 (NP1) by the *Aveparvovirus* and *Bocaparvovirus* encoded near the middle of their genome, or the assembly activating protein (AAP) by the *Dependoparvovirus*, and the small alternatively translated (SAT) and non-structural protein 2 (NS2) by the *Protoparvovirus*, encoded within alternative reading frames of the main ORFs.

2.1. Expression of the Parvovirinae VPs Utilizes Different Transcription Strategies

The VPs of the *Parvovirinae* are encoded in the same orientation as the *ns* or *rep* gene. Members of the *Amdoparvovirus*, *Bocaparvovirus*, and *Erythroparvovirus* use the same promoter for the expression of the NSs and VPs (Figure 2). The *Dependoparvovirus*, *Protoparvovirus*, and *Tetraparvovirus* utilize an additional promoter located at the 3′ end of the *ns/rep* gene for the expression of the *cap* ORF [19,20]. The transcription profiles for *Aveparvovirus* and *Copiparvovirus* are unknown. For the expression of the different VPs, most *Parvovirinae* members perform alternative splicing of their transcripts or utilize alternative start codons (Figure 2) [19–25]. Differences in splicing efficiency and leaky scanning during translation initiation, as well as the utilization of non-canonical start codons, result in the higher expression of the smallest VP form over the larger N-terminal extended forms (Figure 2) [20–25]. The translated VPs are translocated to the nucleus, where they assemble into the 60 mer capsid [26,27]. Based on their expression levels, the minor and major capsid VPs are reported to be incorporated at ratios of 1:10 for VP1:VP2 in capsids containing two VPs, for example, human parvovirus B19, and 1:1:10 for VP1:VP2:VP3 in capsids with three VPs, such as the Adeno-associated viruses (AAVs) [28–31]. For some *Parvovirinae* members this process is assisted by additional proteins, such as the AAP of the *dependoparvoviruses* or NS2 of the *protoparvoviruses* [27,32]. The viral genome is reportedly translocated into pre-assembled empty capsids utilizing the helicase function of NS/Rep proteins [33]. For some protoparvoviruses, proteolytic cleavage of VP2 following DNA packaging removes ~20 to 25 amino acids from the N-terminus to create VP3 (Figure 2) [34–37].

2.2. Parvovirinae Genera Display Distinct Capsid Surface Morphologies

The first structure of a parvovirus, that of wild type (wt) canine parvovirus (CPV), a member of *Protoparvovirus*, was published in 1991, with the VP structure coordinates deposited in 1993, a quarter of a century ago [6,38]. Since then numerous other capsid structures, >100, have been determined for the protoparvoviruses, as well as members of three other (of the eight) *Parvovirinae* genera, including complexes with receptors or antibodies (Table 1, Section 2.5, and Section 2.6). The structures of capsids alone include those of wt as well as variants. The studies have primarily utilized X-ray crystallography, and in recent years increasingly cryo-electron microscopy and 3-dimensional image reconstruction (cryo-EM) as the method began to generate atomic resolution structures. The most capsid (no ligand) structures determined have been for the dependoparvoviruses and protoparvoviruses, for which more than 20 structures are available, followed by four for the bocaparvoviruses, and one for *Erythroparvovirus* (Table 1).

Table 1. Summary of deposited *Parvovirinae* capsid structures.

Virus	Empty/Full	Structure Determination Method	Year	Resolution in Å	PDB-ID	Reference
			Protoparvovirus			
BuV1	Empty	Cryo-EM	2018	2.8	6BWX	Ilyas et al. [39]
BuV2	Empty	Cryo-EM	2018	3.8	6BX0	Ilyas et al. [39]
BuV3	Empty	Cryo-EM	2018	3.3	6BX1	Ilyas et al. [39]
CPV	Empty	X-Ray Crystallography	1993	3.0	2CAS	Wu et al. [38]
CPV	Full	X-Ray Crystallography	1996	2.9	4DPV	Xie et al. [40]
CPV-N93D	Full	X-Ray Crystallography	2003	3.3	1P5Y	Govindasamy et al. [41]
CPV-N93R	Full	X-Ray Crystallography	2003	3.3	1P5W	Govindasamy et al. [41]
CPV-d-A300D	Empty	X-Ray Crystallography	2000	3.3	1C8D	Simpson et al. [42]
CPV-d-A300D	Full	X-Ray Crystallography	1996	3.3	1IJS	Llamas-Saiz et al. [43]
CPV-d pH5.5	Empty	X-Ray Crystallography	2000	3.5	1C8H	Simpson et al. [42]
CPV2a	Full	X-Ray Crystallography	2014	3.3	4QYK	Organtini et al. [44]
FPV	Empty	X-Ray Crystallography	1993	3.3	1FPV	Agbandje et al. [45]
FPV	Empty	X-Ray Crystallography	2000	3.0	1C8F	Simpson et al. [42]
FPV low pH	Empty	X-Ray Crystallography	2000	3.0	1C8G	Simpson et al. [42]
FPV no $CaCl_2$	Empty	X-Ray Crystallography	2000	3.0	1C8E	Simpson et al. [42]
H-1PV	Full	X-Ray Crystallography	2013	2.7	4G0R	Halder et al. [46]
H-1PV	Empty	X-Ray Crystallography	2013	3.2	4GBT	Halder et al. [46]
LuIII	Empty	Cryo-EM	2017	3.2	6B9Q	Pittman et al. [47]
M. Spretus EVE	Empty	Cryo-EM	2018	3.9	6NF9	Callaway et al. [48]
MVMi	Full	X-Ray Crystallography	1997	3.5	1MVM	Llamas-Saiz et al. [49]
MVMi	Empty	X-Ray Crystallography	2005	3.5	1Z1C	Kontou et al. [50]
MVMi-L172W	Empty	X-Ray Crystallography	2011	4.2	2XGK	Plevka et al. [51]
MVMp	Full	X-Ray Crystallography	2005	3.3	1Z14	Kontou et al. [50]
MVMp-N170A	Empty	X-Ray Crystallography	2015	3.8	4ZPY	Guerra et al. [52]
PPV	Empty	X-Ray Crystallography	2001	3.5	1K3V	Simpson et al. [53]
			Bocaparvovirus			
BPV	Empty	X-Ray Crystallography	2015	3.2	4QC8	Kailasan et al. [5]
HBoV1	Empty	Cryo-EM	2017	2.9	5URF	Mietzsch et al. [54]
HBoV3	Empty	Cryo-EM	2017	2.8	5US7	Mietzsch et al. [54]
HBoV4	Empty	Cryo-EM	2017	3.0	5US9	Mietzsch et al. [54]

Table 1. *Cont.*

Virus	Empty/Full	Structure Determination Method	Year	Resolution in Å	PDB-ID	Reference
			Dependoparvovirus			
AAV1	Full	X-Ray Crystallography	2011	2.5	3NG9	Ng et al. [55]
AAV2	Full	X-Ray Crystallography	2002	3.0	1LP3	Xie et al. [3]
AAV2	Empty	Cryo-EM	2016	3.8	5IPI	Drouin et al. [56]
AAV2-L336C	Empty	Cryo-EM	2018	1.9	6E9D	Tan et al. [57]
AAV2-R432A	Empty	Cryo-EM	2016	3.7	5IPK	Drouin et al. [56]
AAV2.5	Full	Cryo-EM	2018	2.8	6CBE	Burg et al. [58]
AAV3	Full	X-Ray Crystallography	2010	2.6	3KIC	Lerch et al. [59]
AAV4	Full	X-Ray Crystallography	2007	3.2	2G8G	Govindasamy et al. [60]
AAV5	Empty	X-Ray Crystallography	2010	3.5	3NTT	Govindasamy et al. [61]
AAV6	Empty	X-Ray Crystallography	2010	3.0	3OAH	Ng et al. [55]
AAV6	Full	X-Ray Crystallography	2011	3.0	4V86	Xie et al. [62]
AAV8	Empty	X-Ray Crystallography	2007	2.6	2QA0	Nam et al. [63]
AAV8 pH7.5	Full	X-Ray Crystallography	2011	2.7	3RA4	Nam et al. [64]
AAV8 pH6.0	Full	X-Ray Crystallography	2011	2.7	3RA9	Nam et al. [64]
AAV8 pH5.5	Full	X-Ray Crystallography	2011	2.7	3RA8	Nam et al. [64]
AAV8 pH4.0	Full	X-Ray Crystallography	2011	2.7	3RA2	Nam et al. [64]
AAV8 pH4/7.5	Full	X-Ray Crystallography	2011	3.2	3RAA	Nam et al. [64]
AAV9	Empty	X-Ray Crystallography	2011	2.8	3UX1	Dimattia et al. [65]
AAV9-L001	Full	Cryo-EM	2019	3.2	6NXE	Guenther et al. [66]
AAV-DJ	Empty	Cryo-EM	2012	4.5	3J1Q	Lerch et al. [67]
AAVrh.8	Full	X-Ray Crystallography	2014	3.5	4RSO	Halder et al. [68]
AAVrh.32.33	Full	X-Ray Crystallography	2013	3.5	4IOV	Mikals et al. [69]
			Erythroparvovirus			
B19	Empty	X-Ray Crystallography	2004	3.5	1S58	Kaufmann et al. [4]

In all the structures, the N-terminal regions of the larger VP (e.g., VP1u), as well as the N-terminal 20-40 amino acids of the major VP, are not resolved. The N-termini of the larger VPs are believed to be located on the inside of the capsid and were shown not to affect the overall capsid structure [70]. The inability to determine the structure of these N-termini is likely due to their flexibility and their low copy numbers within the capsid. The exception to this was human parvovirus B19, for which low resolution cryo-EM maps showed density interpreted as the VP2 N-termini [71]. The flexibility resulting in the N-termini disorder arises from a glycine-rich N-terminal region present in most *Parvovirinae* (Figure 4). Furthermore, the low copy number of the minor VPs or a different positioning of the N-terminus of the different VPs is incompatible with the icosahedral averaging applied during structure determination. A disorder prediction indicates that the glycine-rich stretch is highly disordered in all analyzed *Parvovirinae*, while the VP1u and the overlapping C-terminal VP region are generally more ordered (Figure 5).

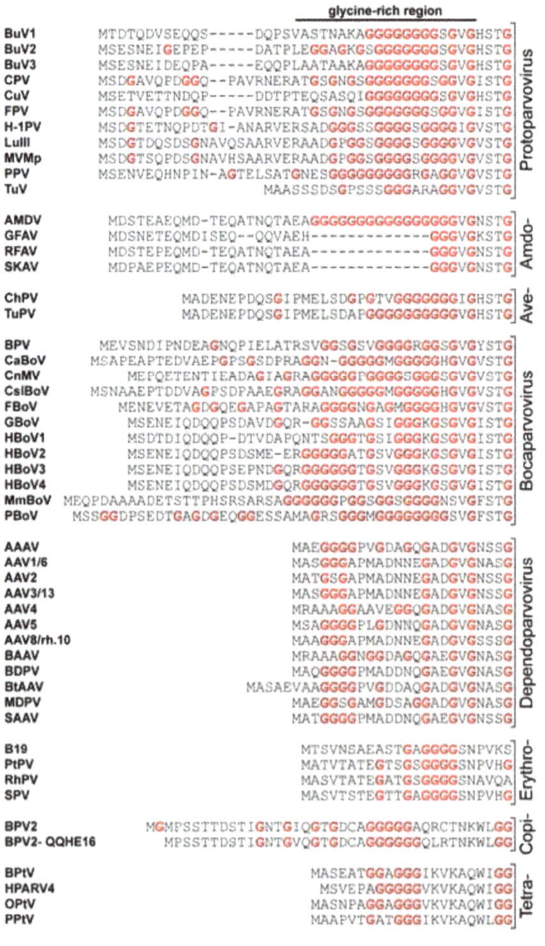

Figure 4. The N-termini of the major VPs of the *Parvovirinae*. For each genus a selection of available VP sequences are shown for the N-terminal 20–50 amino acids. All glycine residues are shown in red.

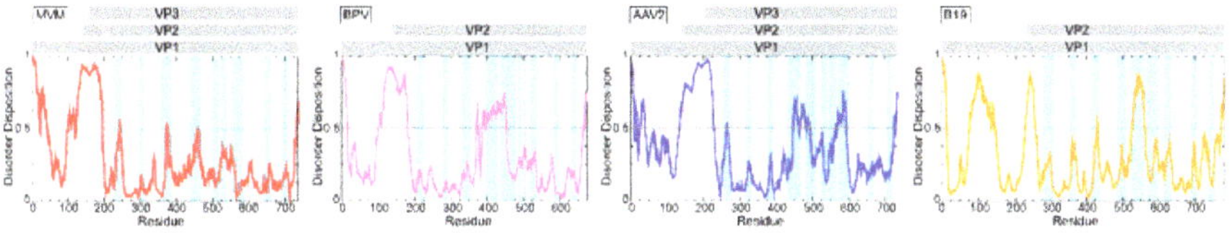

Figure 5. Disorder prediction for type members MVMp (red), BPV (pink), AAV2 (blue), and Parvovirus B19 (orange) VP1 by the PONDR_fit application [72]. Regions above 0.5 on the Y-axis are predicted to be disordered. Gray line drawings above the images indicate the approximate positions of the VPs. The regions highlighted in light blue indicate the locations of the surface exposed loops, the tops of which are defined as variable regions.

The cluster of glycines and associated flexibility likely serve to enable the externalization of VP1u for the PLA_2 function contained within [10]. Consistently, in reported *Parvovirinae* structures, the first ordered N-terminal residue of the overlapping VP region is located after the glycine-rich region, and inside the capsid under the only channel in the capsid. This channel, located at the icosahedral 5-fold axis, connects the inside and outside of the capsid (see below) [38,39,47,73,74]. The remainder of the VP is ordered to the C-terminus in all *Parvovirinae* structures determined to date.

The CPV structure confirmed the icosahedral nature of the parvovirus capsids with sixty VPs assembling one capsid via 2-, 3-, and 5-fold symmetry related interactions [6,38,75]. The *Parvovirinae* VP structures display significant similarity despite low sequence identities (Table 2). The ordered VP monomer region consists of a core eight-stranded (βB to βI) anti-parallel β-barrel motif, also known as a jelly roll motif, with a BIDG sheet that forms the inner surface of the capsid (Figure 6) [76]. This β-barrel is conserved in all parvoviral capsid structures determined to date, as has been reported for many other viruses. In addition, a βA strand that runs anti-parallel to the βB strand of the BIDG sheet, and a conserved helix, αA, located between strands βC and βD, are also part of conserved *Parvovirinae* core structure (Figure 6). Loops inserted between the β-strands of the β-barrel form the surface of the capsid. These loops are named after the β-strands that they connect, for example, the DE loop connects the βD and βE strands. The GH loop that connects the βG and βH strands is the largest surface loop consisting of multiple sub-loops (Figure 6). The surface loops contain the highest amino acid sequence and structural diversity among members of the same genus and between different parvoviruses in general (Figure 7). Differences at the apexes of these loops are termed variable regions (VRs), defined as two or more amino acids with Cα positions greater than 1 Å apart (for the dependoparvoviruses) [60] or 2 Å apart (for the other *Parvovirinae*) [46] when their VPs are superposed. For the VPs of protoparvoviruses, bocaparvoviruses, and dependoparvoviruses nine to ten VRs have been defined (Figure 7).

Table 2. Sequence identity and structural similarity among *Parvovirinae* type members.

	MVMp	BPV	AAV2	B19	
MVMp		46.8	54.1	41.5	Structural similarity [in %]
BPV	18.6		61.4	49.9	
AAV2	17.4	22.9		62.8	
B19	14.5	20.1	23.7		
	VP2/VP3 sequence identity [in %]				

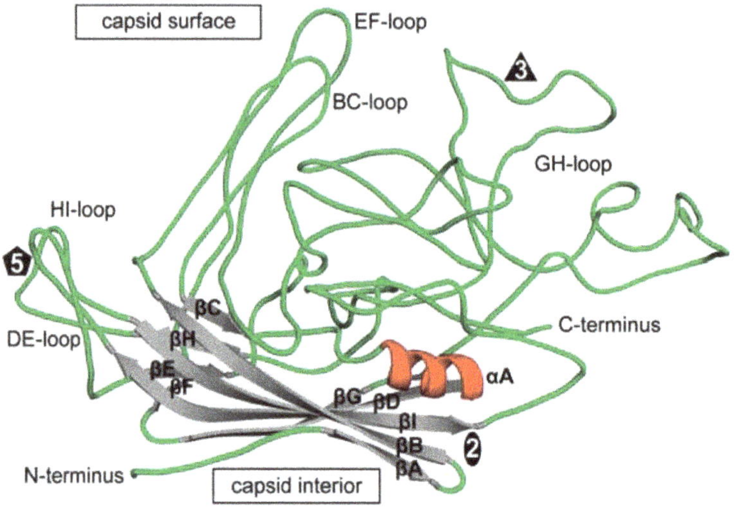

Figure 6. The structure of a VP monomer of CPV (PDB-ID: 2CAS). A cartoon ribbon diagram is shown. The beta strands (βA to βI, gray), α-helix A (red), interconnecting surface loops (with all secondary structure elements removed, green), and the N- and C-terminus are indicated. The approximate icosahedral 2-fold, 3-fold, and 5-fold axis are indicated by an oval, triangle, and pentagon, respectively. This image was generated using PyMOL [77].

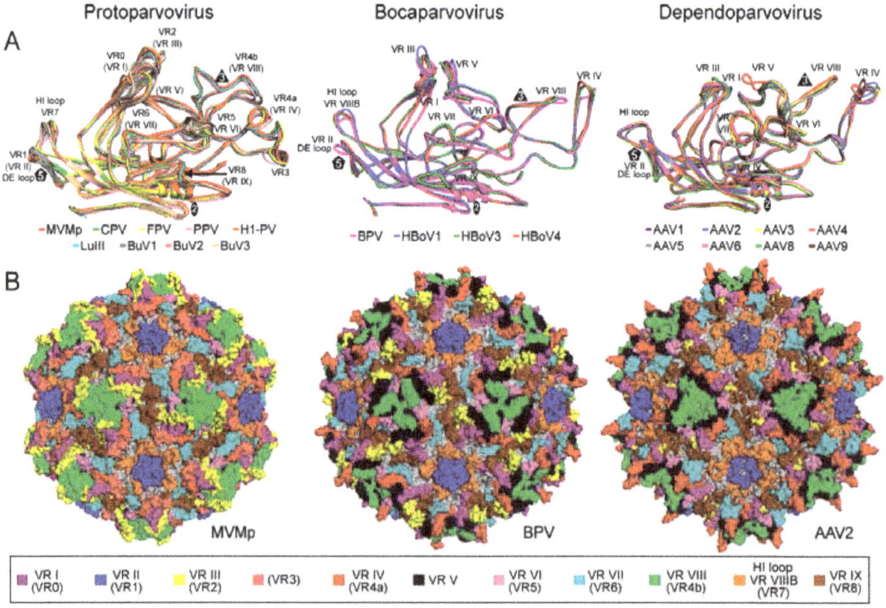

Figure 7. The VRs of the *Parvovirinae*. (**A**) Structural superposition of VP monomers from different members of *Protoparvovirus* (left), *Bocaparvovirus* (center), and *Dependoparvovirus*. Individual colors for the ribbons are as indicated. The VRs: VR-I to VR-IX (or VR0 to VR8 for the protoparvoviruses), the DE, and HI loops are shown. (**B**) Location of the VRs, colored as indicated, on the capsid surface of MVMp as an example for *Protoparvovirus* (left), BPV for *Bocaparvovirus* (center), and AAV2 for *Dependoparvovirus* (right). The figures were generated using PyMOL [77].

The locations of the VRs as well as the overall structure of the VP monomer within each genus and among the *Parvovirinae* are similar despite sequence identities as low as 15% (Table 2, Figure 7). The different VR conformations create distinct genus level morphologies for the capsids, although the capsids have the same overall characteristic features (Figure 8). These include a channel at the icosahedral 5-fold symmetry axes, assembled by five DE loops, surrounded by a depression, described as canyon-like, lined by the HI loop located above the neighboring VP's βCHEF strands. The channel at the 5-fold axes connects the interior of the capsid to the exterior and is believed to play an important role in most parvoviruses during the viral replication cycle by serving as the route of viral genome packaging, genome release, and the externalization of VP1u for its PLA_2 function [70,73]. Secondly, protrusions are located at or surrounding the icosahedral 3-fold axes assembled by loop/VR contributions from two or three VP monomers depending on genus (Figure 8). Variable regions IV, VR-V, and VR-VIII from two 3-fold related VP monomers contribute to the three separate protrusions of the dependoparvoviruses (Figures 7 and 8). Similarly, VR-IV, VR-V, and VR-VIII contribute to the 3-fold protrusions in the bocaparvoviruses, along with VR-I generating several dispersed peaks. In B19, two separate protrusions surround the icosahedral 3-fold axes (Figure 8). One of these protrusions is formed by VR-I and VR-III, the other by VR-VIII. However, the B19 structure lacks 13 residues within VR-V, which is located between both protrusions [4]. This region (aa 528–540, VP1 numbering) is predicted to be highly disordered (Figure 5) and could potentially merge both protrusions. In the animal protoparvoviruses, where the VRs are defined by Arabic numerals, VR0 (VR-I in the dependoparvoviruses), VR2 (VR-III), and VR4b (VR-VIII) form the single pinwheel 3-fold protrusions (Figures 7 and 8) [46,50,60]. In contrast, a deletion in VR4b near the 3-fold symmetry axis results in separated 3-fold protrusions for the bufaviruses (BuVs) (Figures 7 and 8) [39]. Within and among genera, the shape and size of the 3-fold protrusions vary because of sequence length and conformational loop differences. The variable surface loops at the 3-fold are reported to mediate the interactions of parvoviruses with different host factors, including receptors and antibodies (see Sections 2.6 and 2.7) [74]. Thirdly, a second depression is located at the 2-fold symmetry axes of the capsid (Figure 8). The floor of the depression is lined by a conserved (within genus) stretch of residues C-terminus of the βI strand. The shape of the depression, however, is variable in depth and width within and between genera (Figure 8) due to differences in side-chain orientations. The 2- and 5-fold depressions are separated by a raised capsid region, termed the 2-/5-fold wall, which displays structural variability among the *Parvovirinae* due to conformational differences in VR-VII and VR-IX. The 2-fold depression serves as a site for glycan receptor interaction for members of the protoparvoviruses, while the 2-/5-fold wall serves to bind receptors as well as antibodies for different genera (see Sections 2.6 and 2.7) [74].

Unique to the structure of bocaviruses is a "basket-like" feature underneath the 5-fold axis that extends the channel further into the interior of the capsid [5,54]. The basket arises from density located at the N-terminus of the observable VP structure and includes parts of the glycine-rich region [54]. This ordered density under the 5-fold channel poses a problem with the proposed infection mechanism. The hypothesis is that at low pH conditions, similar to the environment in the late endosome, structural rearrangements of the basket occur that open up the 5-fold channel for VP1u externalization for its PLA_2 function. Interestingly, the structures of AAV8, CPV, and feline panleukopenia virus (FPV) determined at low pH conditions show structural changes at residues and capsid surface loops, although the 5-fold channel was not reported to be altered [42,64].

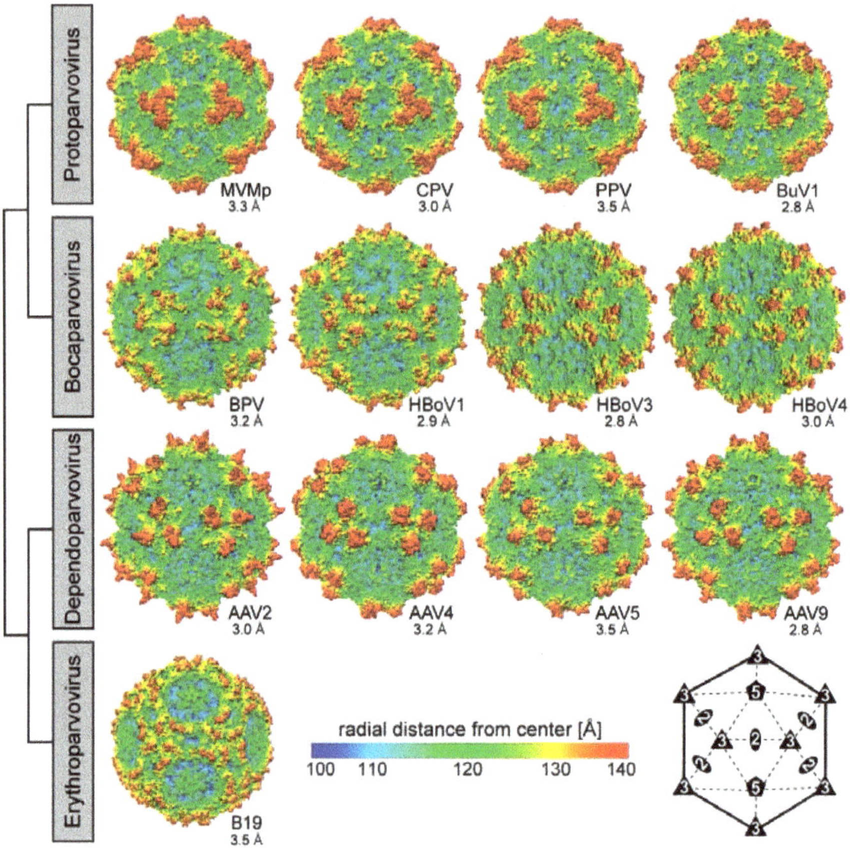

Figure 8. Capsid structures of the *Parvovirinae* subfamily. A selection of capsid structures is shown for *Protoparvovirus*, *Bocaparvovirus*, *Dependoparvovirus*, and *Erythroparvovirus*. The capsid surfaces are viewed down the icosahedral 2-fold axes and are colored according to radial distance from the particle center (blue to red), as indicated by the scale bar. The capsid images were generated using Chimera [78]. In the lower right hand side, a symmetry diagram illustrating the positions of the icosahedral symmetry axes on the capsid surfaces is shown.

2.3. *Nucleotides Are Ordered Inside Parvovirinae Capsids Despite Lack of Icosahedral Symmetry*

The ordering of nucleotides (nts) inside the capsids of some *Parvovirinae* is observed despite the lack of adherence of the single copy of the packaged genome or reporter gene to icosahedral symmetry. This has been observed for virus-like particles (VLPs) and DNA packaged (full) members of the dependoparvoviruses and full protoparvoviruses. A conserved pocket under the 3-fold symmetry axis shows the ordering of one or two nts for multiple AAV serotypes [59,60,63,64,68,69]. Low pH conditions reduced the ordered DNA density [64]. The loss of the nt density at pH 4.0 suggested loss of capsid-DNA interaction that serves as one of the steps leading to release of the genome from the capsid following endosomal trafficking during infection [64]. The ordering of an nt in VLPs in absence of Rep protein suggests that capsid assembly may require nucleation by an nt for the dependoparvoviruses [63]. For the protoparvoviruses, large stretches of ordered DNA, 11 nt in CPV [6], 19 nt in minute virus of mice strain i (MVMi) [49,50], and 10 nt in H-1PV [46], have been reported. The ordering of more nt compared to the dependoparvoviruses may be due to the packaging of only the negative sense genome in the protoparvoviruses, while the AAV packaging both polarities. The ordered protoparvoviruses nts are located within a pocket inside the capsid adjacent to the icosahedral 2-fold axes in all the viruses. This was suggestive of a recognition motif, but a search through the wt genome of CPV identified matches only when 2–3 nt mismatches were allowed [79]. Thus, the role of this organized DNA beyond a common binding site in the *Parvovirinae* is yet to be determined.

2.4. The Structure of Capsid Variants Provide Insight into Function

As listed in Table 1, the structures of several variants have been determined for the *Parvovirinae*. The aims of these studies were structure-function understanding of observed biological phenotypes. The majority of variant structures studied are for AAV2, CPV, and MVM, which are among the best functionally characterized members of this subfamily. Currently, the highest resolution virus structure is that of an AAV2 variant with the leucine at position 336 (VP1 numbering) mutated to a cysteine, AAV2-L336C, at 1.9 Å, obtained by cryo-EM [57]. This mutant has a genome packaging defect and altered VP1u externalization properties [80]. A comparison of this structure to wt AAV2 identified a destabilization of the VP N-terminus inside the capsid and the widening of the base of the 5-fold channel in the variant [57]. This observation supports previous claims that the 5-fold region functions as a portal of genome packaging and VP1u externalization, and that the correct arrangement of the residues in the channel plays a crucial role in these functions. The structure of a similar variant with the equivalent leucine mutated to a tryptophan, was analyzed for MVM, MVM-L172W (VP2 numbering), by X-ray crystallography (Table 1) [51]. This variant was also reported to have a DNA packaging defect and altered VP1u externalization dynamics phenotype [81]. In the MVM-L172W structure, the tryptophan blocked the channel and also induced a reorganization of the N-terminus of VP2 [51]. This suggests that different perturbations in the same structural location can result in a similar inhibitory phenotype. A second AAV2 variant, AAV2-R432A, also characterized the determinant of another genome packaging defective virus resulting from a single residue change [82]. In the wt AAV2 structure, this residue is located within the capsid, neither on the inside nor the outside surface, and at the 3-fold axes. Its side-chain interacts with the main-chain of a surface loop [56]. The AAV2-R432A structure, also determined by cryo-EM, detailed the propagation of capsid destabilization to distant sites from R432, including the rearrangement of the βA strand and movement of residue side-chains at the base of the 5-fold channel inside the capsid. The capsid was also less thermally stable than wt AAV2 [56]. Together, the data suggested that the structure rearrangements and destabilization resulted in packaging incompetence. The crystal structures of CPV variants, CPV-N93D, CPV-N93R, and CPV-A300D (VP2 numbering) in Table 1 were studied to understand the juxtaposition of amino acids controlling tissue tropism and antigenicity [41–43]. These residues form the footprint of the transferrin receptor and several antibody epitopes [43,83,84]. Furthermore, these studies showed that amino acid determinants could be localized far apart but function together [41,85].

2.5. Capsid-Receptor Complex Structures

The role of the parvoviral capsid is to protect the packaged genome and to deliver it to the nucleus of the target cells for the next replication cycle. For the *Parvovirinae*, glycan receptors, for example terminal sialic acid (SIA), galactoses, heparan sulfate proteoglycans, P-antigen, and various proteins, including AAVR, transferrin, laminin, fibroblast growth factor receptor, hepatocyte growth factor receptor, and epidermal growth factor receptor, serve as receptors [83,86–94]. The structures of several of the ligands bound to their capsids have been determined. Presently, the number of published capsid-receptor complex structures at atomic resolution is low (Table 3), but due the recent advancement of cryo-EM this number will increase. In capsid-glycan complex structures, the receptors are bound at or around the 3-fold protrusion (AAV2:heparin, AAV-DJ:heparin) [95–97], at the center of the 3-fold symmetry axis (AAV3:sucrose octasulfate, AAV5:SIA) [98,99], at the base of the 3-fold protrusion (AAV1:SIA) [100], and in a pocket near the 2-fold symmetry axis (MVM:SIA) [101]. The MVM-SIA structure was the first to be determined for a receptor complex. Similar to glycans, cellular protein receptors can bind symmetrical to the capsid, as has been shown recently for the PKD2 domain of AAVR to the capsid of AAV2 that interacts with the 3-fold protrusion and the 2-/5-fold wall [102]. However, larger protein receptors might bind with lower copy number to the capsid surface as observed for the transferrin receptor to CPV capsids [83]. The CPV-transferrin complex was the first structure determined for a protein receptor on a parvovirus capsid. The transferrin footprint is located on the 2-/5-fold wall and includes residues 93, 299, and 301 [83,85].

Table 3. Summary of published *Parvovirinae* capsid-receptor complex structures.

Virus	Receptor	Structure Determination Method	Year	Resolution in Å	Reference
AAV2	AAVR	Cryo-EM	2019	2.8	Zhang et al. [102]
AAV-DJ	heparinoid pentasaccharide	Cryo-EM	2017	2.8	Xie et al. [97]
AAV1	SIA	X-Ray Crystallography	2016	3.0	Huang et al. [100]
AAV5	SIA	X-Ray Crystallography	2015	3.5	Afione et al. [98]
AAV3	sucrose octasulfate	X-Ray Crystallography	2012	6.5	Lerch et al. [99]
AAV2	heparin	Cryo-EM	2009	8.3	O'Donnell et al. [95]
AAV2	heparin	Cryo-EM	2009	18.0	Levy et al. [96]
CPV	transferrin receptor	Cryo-EM	2007	25.0	Hafenstein et al. [83]
MVMp	SIA	X-Ray Crystallography	2006	3.5	López-Bueno et al. [101]

2.6. Capsid-Antibody Complex Structures

The infection by members of the *Parvovirinae* elicits the host immune response, resulting in both neutralizing and non-neutralizing antibodies raised against their capsids. In the human population, the seroprevalence against different members of the *Parvovirinae* can be high. For example, while the seroprevalence varies in different regions of the world, up to 80% of adults have antibodies against B19 [103]. Similar percentages of positivity exist against capsids of different AAV serotypes [104], up to 70% against the human bocaviruses [105], up to 85% against the different BuVs [106], and up to 40% against human parvovirus 4 [107]. In order to understand the antigenicity of these viruses, the structures of capsid antibodies (whole IgG or FAb) have been determined using cryo-EM (Table 4, Figure 9). The resolutions of these structures range from 23 to 3.1 Å (Table 4). The lower resolution structures are sufficient for the identification of epitopes on the capsid surface to confirm by mutagenesis. The higher resolution structures, e.g., AAV5-HL2476 and B19-human antibody complex, enables analysis of the capsid–antibody interaction for direct identification of contact residues on both sides, namely the capsid surface and residues in the CDRs of the antibody if the antibody sequence is available [108]. The complex structures have shown that almost the entire surface of these capsids can be bound by antibodies, with epitopes across the 2-fold, the 2-/5-fold wall, 3-fold protrusions, and around the 5-fold channel (Table 4, Figure 9). This information can inform the engineering of the capsids variants (Section 2.7), the development of vaccines against pathogenic members of the *Parvovirinae*, and for a better understanding of the viral life cycles, as some antibodies do not neutralize infection or can even further enhance their infection, as reported for B19 and for Aleutian mink disease parvovirus [109,110].

Table 4. Summary of published *Parvovirinae* capsid-antibody structures.

Virus	Antibody Name	Year	Binding Region	Neutralizing for Infection	Resolution in Å	Reference
			Protoparvovirus			
CPV	Fab-E	2012	side of 3-fold protrusions across 2-fold axis	Yes	4.1	Organtini et al. [111]
CPV	Fab-14	2009	3-fold protrusions	Yes	12.4	Hafenstein et al. [84]
FPV	Fab-6	2009	3-fold protrusions	Yes	18.0	Hafenstein et al. [84]
FPV	Fab-8	2009	2/5-fold wall	Yes	8.5	Hafenstein et al. [84]
FPV	Fab-15	2009	2/5-fold wall	Yes	10.5	Hafenstein et al. [84]
FPV	Fab-16	2009	2/5-fold wall	Yes	13.0	Hafenstein et al. [84]
FPV	Fab-B	2009	3-fold protrusions	Yes	14.0	Hafenstein et al. [84]
FPV	Fab-E	2009	side of 3-fold protrusions across 2-fold axis	Yes	12.0	Hafenstein et al. [84]
FPV	Fab-F	2009	side of 3-fold protrusions across 2-fold axis	Yes	14.0	Hafenstein et al. [84]
MVMi	B7	2007	center of 3-fold symmetry axis	Yes	7.0	Kaufmann et al. [112]
			Bocaparvovirus			
HBoV1	4C2	2016	3-fold protrusions	unknown	16.0	Kailasan et al. [113]
HBoV1	9G12	2016	3-fold protrusions	unknown	8.5	Kailasan et al. [113]
HBoV1	12C1	2016	3-fold protrusions	unknown	11.9	Kailasan et al. [113]
HBoV1	15C6	2016	around 5-fold symmetry axis	unknown	18.6	Kailasan et al. [113]
HBoV2	15C6	2016	around 5-fold symmetry axis	unknown	17.8	Kailasan et al. [113]
HBoV4	15C6	2016	around 5-fold symmetry axis	unknown	9.5	Kailasan et al. [113]

Table 4. *Cont.*

Virus	Antibody Name	Year	Binding Region	Neutralizing for Infection	Resolution in Å	Reference
			Dependoparvovirus			
AAV1	ADK1a	2015	3-fold protrusions	Yes	11.0	Tseng et al. [114]
AAV1	ADK1b	2015	2/5-fold wall	Yes	11.0	Tseng et al. [114]
AAV1	4E4	2013	side of 3-fold protrusions across 2-fold axis	Yes	12.0	Gurda et al. [115]
AAV1	5H7	2013	center of 3-fold symmetry axis	Yes	23.0	Gurda et al. [115]
AAV2	C37-B	2013	3-fold protrusions	Yes	11.0	Gurda et al. [115]
AAV2	A20	2012	2/5-fold wall	Yes	8.5	McCraw et al. [116]
AAV5	ADK5a	2015	2/5-fold wall	Yes	11.0	Tseng et al. [114]
AAV5	ADK5b	2015	2/5-fold wall to 5-fold symmetry axis	Yes	12.0	Tseng et al. [114]
AAV5	HL2476	2018	3-fold protrusions	Yes	3.1	Jose et al. [108]
AAV5	3C5	2013	2/5-fold wall in a tangential orientation	No	16.0	Gurda et al. [115]
AAV6	5H7	2013	center of 3-fold symmetry axis	unknown	15.0	Gurda et al. [115]
AAV6	ADK6	2018	3-fold protrusions & 2/5-fold wall	Yes	13.0	Bennett et al. [117]
AAV8	ADK8	2011	3-fold protrusions	Yes	18.7	Gurda et al. [118]
AAV9	PAV9.1	2018	center of 3-fold symmetry axis	Yes	4.2	Giles et al. [119]
			Erythroparvovirus			
B19	human Fab	2018	around 5-fold symmetry axis	Yes	3.2	Sun et al. [120]

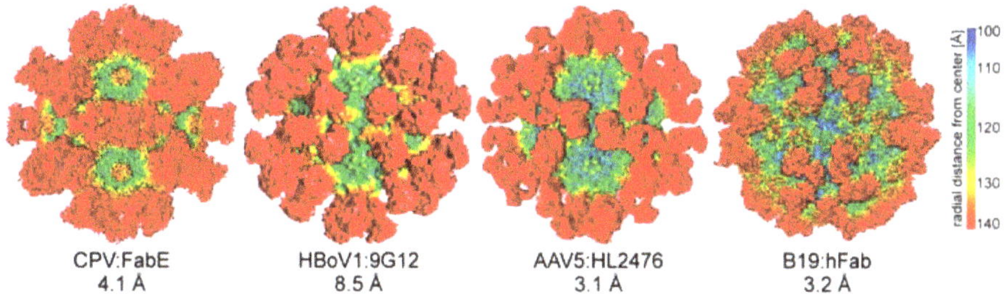

Figure 9. *Parvovirinae*-antibody complex structures. The highest resolution complex structures available for *Protoparvovirus*, *Bocaparvovirus*, *Dependoparvovirus*, and *Erythroparvovirus* are shown. The cryo-EM density maps are viewed down the icosahedral 2-fold axis and are colored according to radial distance from the particle center (blue to red), as indicated by the scale bar. The FAbs decorating the capsid surface are in red. The FAbs bind across the icosahedral 2-fold (e.g., CPV:FAbE), the 2-/5-fold wall (HBoV1:9G12), the 3-fold (AAV5:HL2476), and 5-fold depression (B19:hFab). The images were generated using Chimera [78]. (CPV: EMD-6629, B19: EMD-9110).

2.7. Engineering of Parvovirus Capsids to Create Biologics

The development of *Parvovirinae* members as biologics is primarily focused on the engineering of capsids of members that can be used as viral vectors in gene delivery applications, such as the AAVs [121], or more recently also bocaviral vectors [122]. For such vectors, a transgene expression cassette is packaged into the capsids instead of the wt viral genome [123]. These vectors are used to infect a desired target tissue to achieve long-term expression of the transgene to correct monogenetic diseases.

Following the discovery that AAV capsids become phosphorylated at tyrosine residues after cell entry subsequently leading to their degradation following lysine ubiquitination, reducing the transgene expression [124,125], the structural information of the AAV capsids was used to identify surface exposed tyrosines for modification [126]. Mutational analysis of these tyrosine residues to phenylalanine led to the development of engineered capsids that showed improved transduction efficiencies compared to vectors packaged into wt capsids [126]. Subsequent mutation of capsid surface serine, threonine, and lysines further improved transduction efficiency [127,128]. Another application of structure information for vector engineering is the modification of AAV capsids to escape pre-existing neutralizing antibodies utilizing the footprints mapped by cryo-EM. As mentioned above, a large percentage of the human population possesses anti-capsid antibodies against one or more AAV serotype due to natural exposures. These pre-existing antibodies bind to the capsids of administered AAV vectors and disrupt multiple steps required for successful transgene delivery, including receptor attachment, post-entry trafficking, and capsid uncoating events [129]. To circumvent these inhibitory events, different strategies have been developed, including the utilization of immunosuppressants [130–133], the utilization of alternative natural AAV capsids that are not detected by the pre-existing human antibodies [68], the use of empty capsids as decoys [134], and the structure-guided modification of the antigenic sites on the surface of the capsids [135]. For the latter strategy, the antigenic sites are identified using monoclonal antibodies, as mentioned in Section 2.6. By rational design or directed evolution, these sites can be changed to obtain new variants with escape phenotypes while maintaining infectivity [108,135,136]. While the majority of capsid engineering has been with AAVs, because of their high seroprevalence, vectors based on bocaviruses will face similar obstacles and require solutions to escape pre-existing immunity in the human population.

Another purpose for capsid engineering is the retargeting of vectors to specific receptors or tissues to restrict the broad tissue tropism of some AAV serotypes [137,138]. This can be achieved by insertion of specific targeting peptides into capsid surface loops, especially in the apexes of VR-IV and VR-VIII (Figure 7), e.g., for AAV2 variants 7m8 or r1c3 [138–140], directed evolution for a specific cell type [141], or structure guided approaches [142]. For some of these engineered AAVs, the structures of the modified capsids have been determined, e.g., AAV2.5, the first structure-guided in silico designed AAV gene delivery vector [58], AAV-DJ, a chimera created through random homologous recombination followed by directed evolution [67], and AAV9-L001, an AAV9 variant with a peptide lock to prevent off-target delivery [66].

3. Densovirinae

The *Densovirinae* encompasses members infecting exclusively invertebrates [143]. Currently, the subfamily consists of five genera, clustering into two separate lineages; *Ambi-* and *Iteradensovirus* infecting arthropods and echinoderms in the first, and *Brevi-*, *Hepan-*, and *Penstyldensovirus* infecting various arthropods, e.g., decapod crustaceans and insects in the second lineage (Figure 1) [1]. However, as the number of invertebrate-infecting parvoviruses from diverse host species has increased, the heterogeneity of the subfamily has become apparent, questioning the monophyly of prior genera, such as *Ambidensovirus* [1,13] (Figure 1). The second lineage includes additional, yet unclassified virus species. These viruses comprise the recently discovered starfish densoviruses of the species *Aster rubens* and a vertebrate-infecting parvovirus clade named Chapparvovirus after the Chiroptera-Aves-Porcine acronym based on the host species where these viruses were first discovered (Figure 1) [144]. Densoviral genomes vary in organization, unlike the subfamily *Parvovirinae*, and have a wider size range at between 3.9 and 6.3 kb. They also have either ambisense or monosense transcription. The left-hand side ORF contains the *ns* gene and expresses up to five proteins [145]. The right-hand side ORF is *cap* and encodes up to four VPs (Figure 3). All densoviruses discovered to date are capable of autonomous replication and pathogenic [1].

3.1. *The Densovirinae Utilize Diverse Strategies for VP Expression*

Densoviruses, like their vertebrate counterparts, have evolved diverse expression strategies to overcome the limitation of the coding capacity imposed by their small genome size (Figure 3) [146]. The transcription strategy has been determined for four of the five densovirus genera, and has not been experimentally derived for the *Hepandensovirus* or the new starfish densoviruses (GenBank accession numbers: MF190038 and MF190039). Overall, densoviral transcription relies more on leaky scanning than the alternative splicing utilized by the *Parvovirinae* (compare Figure 2 to Figure 3) [143]. This difference is an adaption to the host because invertebrates possess a lower percentage of alternatively spliced genes compared to vertebrates [147]. Consistently, the chapparvoviruses mentioned above (Figures 1 and 3) utilize alternative splicing as the major strategy to express their VPs [148]. As for the *Parvovirinae*, the smallest VP is the one with the largest incorporation into the capsid for densoviruses.

The *Ambidensovirus* display the most variable VP expression strategies, likely because the genus currently also contains the most members. Because of their unique ambisense genome organization, the *cap* gene is located on the opposite strand relative to the *ns* gene, both driven by the furthest upstream promoter embedded in the partially double-stranded region of the ITRs (Figure 3). There are three different VP expression strategies established for this genus [1]. Members of the first group, e.g., *Galleria mellonella* densovirus (GmDV), express a minor capsid VP1 from an unspliced transcript of the p93 promoter. Three additional VPs, VP2, VP3, and VP4 (major capsid VP), are expressed by leaky scanning [7,149]. These are reported to be incorporated into the capsid at a 1:9:9:41 ratio [7]. The second group, including *Periplaneta fulliginosa* densovirus (PfDV) and *Acheta domestica* densovirus (AdDV), has a split *cap* ORF for the minor capsid VPs joined by splicing of transcripts, with VP2, VP3, and VP4 expressed from leaky scanning of the unspliced transcript in case of AdDV. This results in both VP1 and VP2 having unique N-terminal regions. These VPs are reportedly incorporated into the AdDV capsid at a 1:11:18:30 ratio. In comparison, both VP1 and VP2 are translated from spliced transcripts in PfDV (Figure 3) [8,150,151]. The third group, represented by *Culex pipiens* densovirus of *Dipteran ambidensovirus 1*, has four VPs expressed from one unspliced transcript by leaky scanning, giving rise to a VP1, VP2, VP3, and a small 12 kDa VP4, which is a minor capsid protein with approximately the same incorporation as VP1. VP2 and VP3 are reportedly equally abundant in the capsid [145].

The *Iteradensoviruses* are related to the ambidensoviruses and have a similar VP expression strategy despite packaging monosense genomes. Although the exact number of VPs expressed is unknown, they use leaky scanning from the same unspliced transcript (Figure 3) [152]. SDS-PAGE analysis of *Bombyx mori* densovirus 1 (BmDV1) show three VPs, VP1, VP2, and VP3 [153]. *Penstyl-* and *Brevidensovirus* transcribe only a single unspliced VP transcript resulting in a single VP that is among the smallest in the *Parvoviridae* at 329 aa and 358 aa, respectively [154,155]. In contrast, the *Hepandensovirus cap* ORF encodes a large VP1, e.g., with hepatopancreatic necrosis virus having a VP1 of 830 aa from the largest *Parvoviridae* genome of 6.3 kb [146,156]. The two recently discovered densoviruses from the starfish species *Aster rubens*, closely related to the *Hepandensovirus* (Figure 3), both encode the largest VPs of the family, with 983 and 988 aa (GenBank accession numbers: MF190038 and MF190039).

3.2. *Densovirinae Capsid Structures Display Distinct Surface Morphology*

In contrast to the *Parvovirinae*, for which numerous capsid structures have been determined (Table 1), only four crystal structures are available for *Densovirinae* (Table 5). In addition, two low resolution structures have been determined using cryo-EM (Table 5). The high-resolution structures are for *Ambidensovirus* members GmDV at 3.7 Å [7] and AdDV 3.5 Å resolution [8]; *Iteradensovirus* member BmDV1 at 3.1 Å resolution [9]; and *Penstyldensovirus* member Penaeus stylirostris densovirus (PstDV) at 2.5 Å [157]. Two of these structures, GmDV and AdDV, were determined for DNA packaged (full) infectious virions. AdDV showed three pyrimindine bases ordered within the luminal surface at the 3-fold symmetry axis [8]. As previously stated, this ordering is unexpected given the lack of icosahedral symmetry for the single copy of the packaged genome. The cryo-EM structures are for *Ambidensovirus* member *Junonia coenia* densovirus (JcDV) at 8.7 Å resolution [158] and *Brevidensovirus* member *Aedes albopictus* densovirus (AalDV2) at 15.6 Å resolution [159].

Table 5. Capsid structures of *Densovirinae* determined to date.

Virus	Empty / Full	Structure Determination Method	Year	Resolution in Å	PDB-ID	Reference
			Ambidensovirus			
AdDV	Full	X-Ray Crystallography	2013	3.5	4MGU	Meng et al. [8]
GmDV	Full	X-Ray Crystallography	1998	3.6	1DNV	Simpson et al. [7]
JcDV	Empty	Cryo-EM	2005	8.7	N/A	Bruemmer et al. [158]
			Brevidensovirus			
AalDV2	Full	Cryo-EM	2004	15.6	N/A	Chen et al. [159]
			Iteradensovirus			
BmDV1	Empty	X-Ray Crystallography	2011	3.1	3P0S	Kaufmann et al. [9]
			Penstyldensovirus			
PstDV	Empty	X-Ray Crystallography	2010	2.5	3N7X	Kaufmann et al. [157]

Similarly to the *Parvovirinae* VP structures, a significant portion of the N-terminal region of the major capsid VP is also disordered in the densoviruses, e.g., 23 aa in GmDV and AdDV, 10 31 aa in PstDV, and 42 in BmDV1 [7–9,157]. Again, as for the *Parvovirinae*, disorder predictions for these viruses show disorder between the N and C-terminus at the glycine-rich region (Figures 10 and 11). The glycine-rich region is significantly shorter in the densoviruses, e.g., 6 aa in GmDV and 7 aa in AdDV compared to 12 aa in CPV, but still results in a lack of structure order (Figures 10 and 11). Interestingly, the BmDV1 structure currently represents the only parvoviral VP structure, where the last

40 C-terminal residues are also disordered. The C-terminal residue of densoviral VP structures, with the exception of BmDV1, are positioned near the 2-fold symmetry axis, similarly to the VP structures of the *Parvovirinae*, and exposed on the capsid surface [7–9,157].

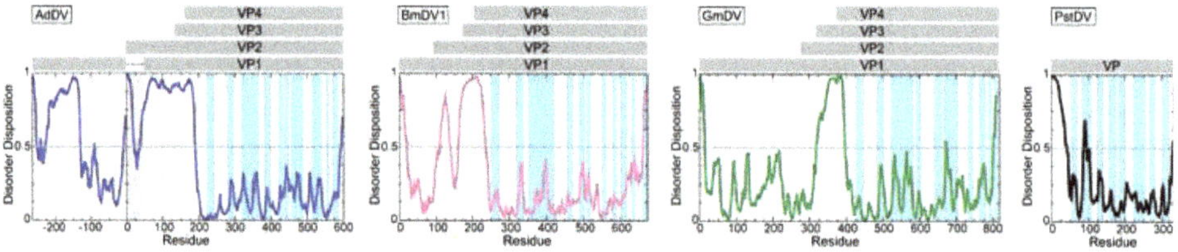

Figure 10. Disorder prediction for densoviruses. AdDV (blue), BmDV1 (pink), GmDV (green), and PstDV (black) VP1. The PONDR_fit application was utilized [72]. Regions above 0.5 on the Y-axis are predicted to be disordered. The approximate locations of the VPs are indicated in the grey bars above. In case of AdDV, both VP1 and VP2 have unique N-terminal regions. The regions highlighted in light blue in the disorder plot indicate the locations of the surface exposed loops, their apexes are VRs.

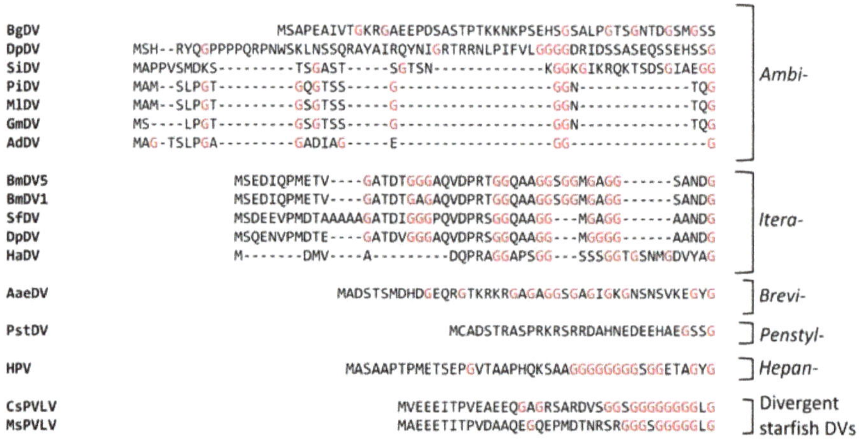

Figure 11. The N-termini of the major VPs of the *Densovirinae*. For each genus a selection of available VP sequences are shown for the N-terminal 20–50 amino acids. All glycine residues are in red.

The core of the densoviral VP is an eight-stranded jelly roll fold with an additional N-terminal strand, βA, and with large loops connecting the strands, as described above for the *Parvovirinae* (Figure 12). In the GmDV VP structure, considered the *Densovirinae* prototype, the EF and GH loops are further divided into five and four sub-loops, respectively (Figure 12). While the GH loop is the longest and forms most of the surface features, its length is significantly shorter compared to the corresponding loop in the *Parvovirinae* at 97 aa compared to 226 aa in CPV. Similar to the *Parvovirinae*, the GH loop is the most variable among ambidensoviruses, although VRs have not been defined, as has been done for the former viruses [7]. At the 2-fold symmetry axis, similarly to vertebrate parvovirus VPs, the densovirus structures have an alpha helix (αA). As a common feature for these viruses, a second α-helix is contained within the EF loop, with PstDV containing a third helix in the CD loop (Figure 12) [7–9,157].

An important and differentiating feature of the densoviral VP is the domain swapping observed at their N-terminus [7–9,157] (Figure 13). The βA strand of the swapped domain interacts with the 2-fold symmetry related VP's βB strand rather than the intra VP βA and βB interaction observed in the *Parvovirinae* (Figure 13). Thus, the luminal βBIDG sheet of the jelly roll core is still extended into a βABIDG sheet, as in the *Parvovirinae*, and the first observed N-terminal residue is also positioned underneath the 5-fold axis, but in this case, under that of the neighboring VP subunit (Figure 13). In the case of the GmDV VPs, the domain swapping is proposed to create additional hydrogen bonds with the 2-fold related VP's βB imparting increased stability [7]. A re-arrangement into an unswapped conformation is proposed to be required for VP1u externalization, although there is no experimental proof that this occurs [7]. In contrast to GmDV, in PstDV the distance between the swapped N-terminus and the βB of the neighboring VP is too large to form hydrogen bonds [157], while in AdDV, the βA contains three proline substitutions compared to GmDV, P24, P26, and P28, which makes such interactions impossible. In these two viruses, divalent cations observed at the N-terminus are hypothesized to confer stability [7,157].

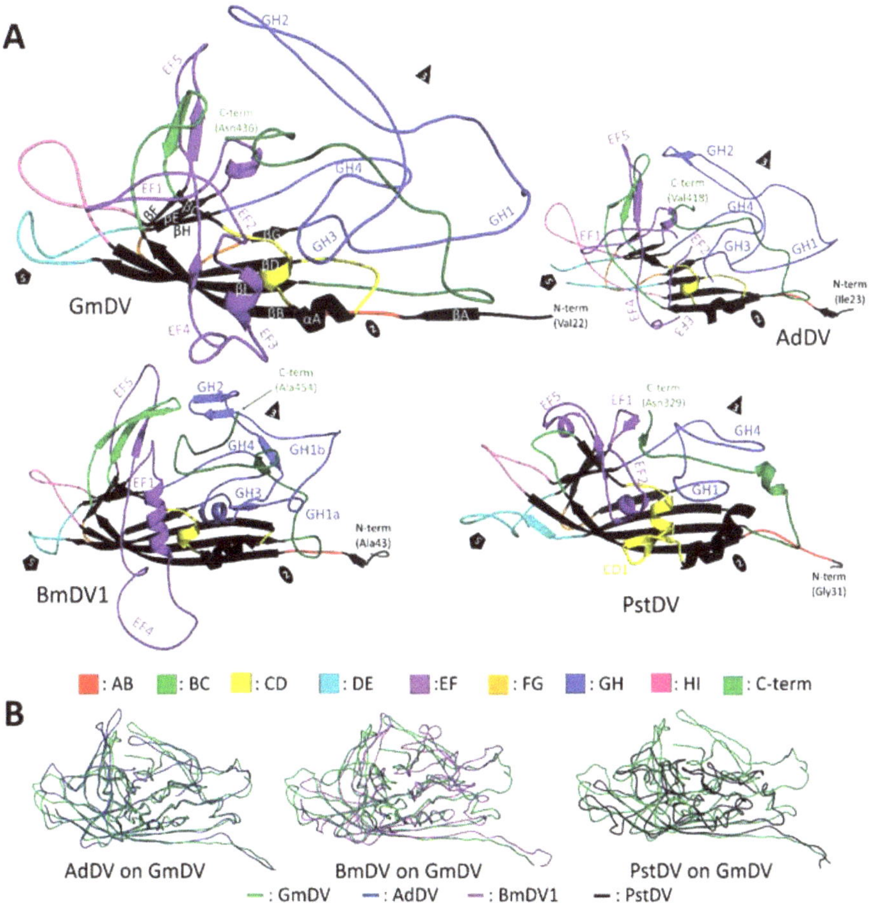

Figure 12. The densovirus VP structure. (**A**) Cartoon ribbon diagrams of the ordered common VP structures of GmDV and AdDV (top), BmDV1 and PstDV (bottom). The first ordered N-terminal residue and C-terminal residue are labeled. The conserved β-core and αA helix are colored in black and labeled in GmDV. Loops and subloops within the large loops are as colored in the key at the bottom and EF and GH sub-loops are labeled. The approximate 5-fold symmetry axis is marked by a pentagon, the 3-fold by a triangle, and the 2-fold by an ellipsoid. (**B**) A GmDV VP structure (*Ambidensovirus*) superimposed on the VPs of AdDV (left), BmDV1 (middle), and PstDV (right). Conformational diversity on the surface loops is evident, especially between GmDV and BmDV, and GmDV and PstDV.

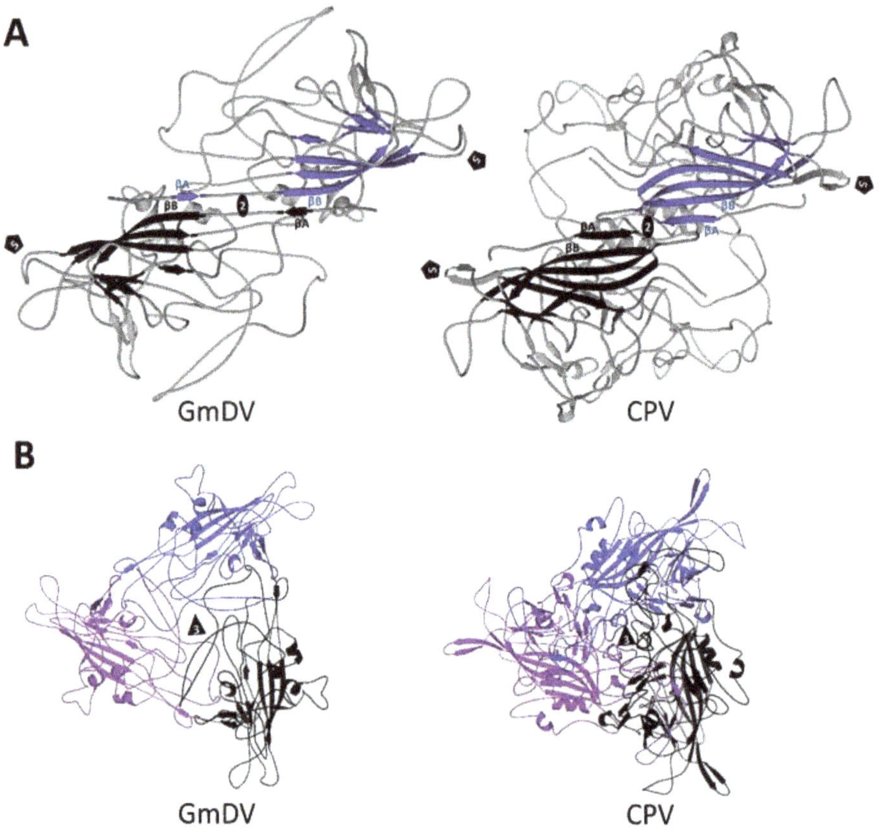

Figure 13. Multimeric interactions of densoviral and parvoviral VPs. (**A**) Ribbon cartoon diagrams of the interactions between βA and βB at the 2-fold symmetry axis of GmDV and CPV. The eight-stranded core, with the additional βA, which performs the domain swapping, are colored blue and black. (**B**) Interaction of three 3-fold symmetry related VPs for GmDV and CPV. The open annulus-like structure at the 3-fold axis of the densovirus trimer compared to the more closed arrangement in the vertebrate parvoviruses is evident. The triangle indicates the 3-fold axis and the pentagon the 5-fold axis.

The sequence identity among the VP monomers of the *Densovirinae* ranges from ~7% to 20% (Table 6). The structural similarity is higher and ranges from the value anticipated from the eight-stranded β-barrel core and αA helix at 20% to ~70% (calculated by DALI pairwise alignments [160]) between the PstDV and GmDV from different genera, and GmDV and AdDV from the same genus, respectively (Table 6). The structural diversity of densoviruses is mostly attributable to the CD, EF, and GH loops (Figure 12). In the PstDV VP structure, all loops are shorter than in the other three high-resolution structures due to the smaller size of the VP (Figures 3 and 12). When the GmDV VP structure is superimposed to that of CPV, up to 148 Cα atoms (36%) are similarly positioned (not shown). This is remarkable given the lower structure similarities between members of the subfamily (Table 6). The majority of the residues are located in the core [7].

Table 6. Sequence identity and structural similarity for densoviruses.

	Structural Similarity [%] Derived from DALI Z-Scores			
	GmDV	**AdDV**	**BmDV1**	**PstDV**
GmDV		68.2	45.6	20.4
AdDV	20		44.2	20
BmDV1	11	10		24.4
PstDV	9.2	9	7	
	Sequence identity on superposed C-alphas atoms [%]			

The overall capsid morphology of densoviruses can be divided into two types: One is a large, with diameter of ~235 to ~260 Å in the depressions and protrusions, respectively, while the other one is 215 to 250 Å, being the smallest capsids so far described for the *Parvoviridae* (Figure 14). For the larger capsids, including GmDV, AdDV, and BmDV1, the capsid surface is smooth with small spike-like protrusions surrounding the 5-fold axes. In GmDV the spikes, formed by the EF4 sub-loop, appear to be smaller compared to BmDV1 and AdDV, due to the protruding GH2 sub-loop filling up the depression surrounding them. In GmDV, a smaller second protrusion is formed by the BC loop. There is a depression at the 2-fold axes (Figure 14). In the second group, containing PstDV and AalDV2 (not shown), there are prominent protrusions surrounding the 5-fold axis, forming two rim-like concentric circles. The 2- and 3-fold symmetry axes have depressions (Figure 14). Approximating with capsid size, there is a variance among luminal volume and surface area of densovirus particles consistent with the range of packaged genome (Table 7).

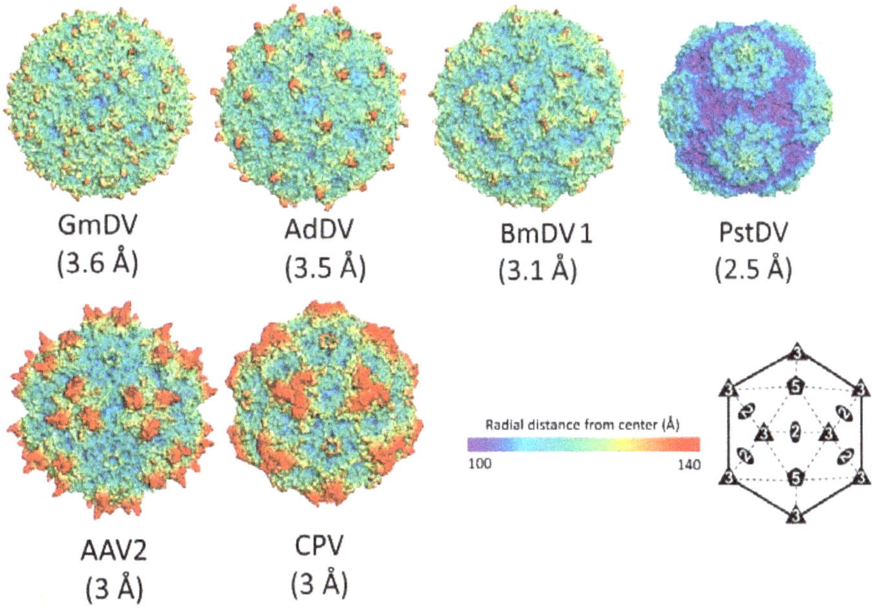

Figure 14. Densoviral capsid structures. The capsid surface images of GmDV, AdDV, BmDV1, and PstDV. The resolution of each structure is in parenthesis. The AAV2 and CPV capsid images are shown for comparison. The scale bar shows the radial distance (from the capsid center) used for the images. An icosahedral symmetry diagram indicating the positions of the visible symmetry axes on the capsid images are shown at the bottom right hand side.

Table 7. Dimensions, DNA content, and taxonomy of densovirus capsid structures.

	Inner Radius (Å)	Inner Surface Area (nm^2)	Inner Volume (nm^3)	Genome Size (nt)	Genus
GmDV	98.7	1223.2	4022.6	6039	*Ambidensovirus*
AdDV	91.7	1056.2	3227.8	5425	*Ambidensovirus*
BmDV1	98.7	1224	4027.5	5076	*Iteradensovirus*
PstDV	87.6	963.3	2811.5	3914	*Penstyldensovirus*
CPV	92.9	1084.8	3359.5	5323	*Protoparvovirus*
AAV2	89.9	1014.9	3040.4	4679	*Dependoparvovirus*

The 5-fold symmetry axis of the *Densovirinae*, similar to the *Parvovirinae*, contains a channel with a direct opening to the surface [7–9,157]. Its size is also similar, at 9 Å in diameter in GmDV, which is the same as for CPV. The inner wall of the channel is lined by large hydrophobic residues in all four structures, proposed to provide an interacting surface to the glycine-rich stretch of residues when the N-terminus is externalized. So far, the only densovirus for which PLA2 externalization has been investigated is AdDV. Meng et al. [8] found that heating of infectious AdDV particles to 70 °C resulted in increased PLA2 activity accompanied by genome ejection, while capsids remained intact. Both Simpson et al. and Meng et al. [7,8] speculated that the channel might also become occupied by stretches of VP2 and VP3 amino acids, although the role of these is currently unknown.

At the 3-fold symmetry axes, a β-annulus-like structure is present in densoviruses instead of the protrusions at or surrounding this region observed in the *Parvovirinae* (Figures 13 and 14). This is similar to the 3-fold region of (+)ssRNA viruses, such as Tomato Stunt Mosaic Virus of *Tomubusviridae* [161] and Southern Bean Mosaic Virus of *Solemoviridae* [162]. The annulus is formed by charged and flexible residues, with an ~10-Å wide opening in GmDV. This opening is less pronounced in BmDV1 and shows even less annulus-like appearance in the case of PstDV, where the shorter GH loops do not interdigitate between neighboring monomers [157].

3.3. Functions Associated with Densoviral Capsid Proteins

Compared to members of the *Parvovirinae*, little is known about the functions of densovirus VPs and the available information is mostly based on studies of members of *Ambidensovirus*. By comparing the VP4s of two closely related lepidopteran ambidensoviruses, GmDV and JcDV, eight variable, exposed regions were identified [158]. One of these was located at the 5-fold symmetry axis, in the DE loop, five in vicinity of the protrusions surrounding it, i.e., the EF1, EF2, and the GH1 sub-loops, one at the 3-fold axis, and one in the depression at the 2-fold axis. Attempts to mutate residues in JcDV to their counterpart in GmDV showed that mutated residues in the GH loop resulted in a decrease of the ability to cross the host midgut epithelium and a reduction of JcDV virulence if introduced through the natural, gastro-intestinal pathway [163]. When *ex vivo* infecting *Spodoptera frugiperda* hosts, the mutated virus became mis-targeted and accumulated in subcellular compartments of midgut epithelial cells instead of reaching their target receptors in the basal tight junctions [164].

Recent experiments on *Blattella germanica* densovirus 1 (BgDV1) of the genus ambidensovirus have shown that an in silico predicted, bipartite nuclear localization signal (NLS) in the C-terminus of all four VPs has an effect on the import of VP monomers to the assembly site located within the nucleus. In the same viral particles a nuclear export signal (NES) was also identified that is located in the VP2 unique N-terminal region (VP2u) and was proven to function during nuclear egress of assembled BgDV1 particles. These results imply that the ambidensoviral VP2u possesses an important function for intracellular trafficking of assembled progeny virions. For this purpose the VP2u domain likely needs to be externalized, similarly to VP1u [165]. Interestingly, a functional NLS has been described at the N-terminus of hepatopancreatic parvovirus (HPV) [166]. Recently the *Helicoverpa armigera* densovirus 2 (HaDV2) VPs were shown to enhance the structural promoter activity by 35-fold compared to the activation by NS [167]. A similar role in transcriptional regulation by capsids has been proposed for the AAVs of the *Parvovirinae* [168].

4. Summary

By the end of 2018, more than 100 capsid structures were published for the *Parvoviridae* (Figure 15). This includes lower resolution cryo-EM capsid structures alone or in complex with receptor or antibody molecules, and near-atomic and atomic resolution cryo-EM and crystal structures (Table 1, Table 3, Table 4, and Table 5). The VP coordinates for the first parvovirus capsid structure, CPV, was determined by X-ray crystallography [38]. In the following two decades, X-ray crystallography remained the method of choice to determine high-resolution capsid structures. The first parvoviral capsid structure determined by cryo-EM was for the Aleutian Mink Disease Virus (ADV) and displayed the general features of the surface of the parvoviral capsid at 22 Å resolution [169]. The first boost in the use of cryo-EM in structural parvovirology occurred after its utility for mapping the epitopes of monoclonal antibodies onto the capsid became evident. A second boost occurred with the development of direct electron detectors and their ability to record movie frames that can subsequently be aligned, which resulted in atomic resolution structures, for example, the structure of the AAV2-L336C variant at 1.86 Å resolution. This structure is currently the highest resolution parvovirus capsid structure, as well as all viruses (Figure 15). The most important aspect of the advances made in structural parvovirology is the ability to use the information obtained to functionally annotate the life cycle of these viruses. This ability provides the tools required to develop biologics in the form of vaccines or inhibitors for pathogenic members, for example, B19 and densoviruses, or gene delivery vehicles with improved efficacy for non-pathogenic members, such as the AAVs.

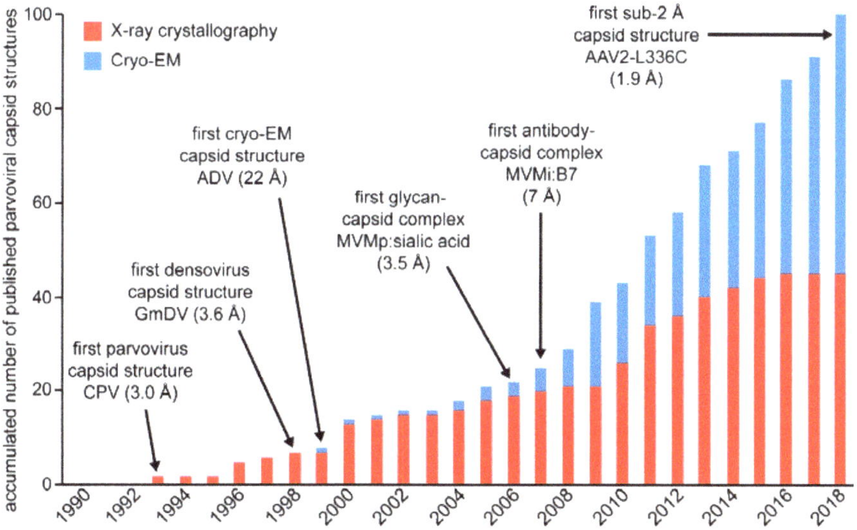

Figure 15. Overview of published parvoviral capsid structures since 1990. Structures determined by X-ray crystallography are shown in red and structures determined by cryo-EM in blue. Important milestones of structural parvovirology are indicated.

Funding: This work was supported by NIH R01 grants GM109524 and GM082946, and the University of Florida College of Medicine.

Conflicts of Interest: MAM is a SAB member for Voyager Therapeutics, Inc., and AGTC, has a sponsored research agreement with AGTC, Voyager Therapeutics, and Intima Biosciences, Inc., and is a consultant for Intima Biosciences, Inc. MAM is a co-founder of StrideBio, Inc. This is a biopharmaceutical company with interest in developing AAV vectors for gene delivery application. MAM and MM have IP in AAV technology, some licensed to Biotechnology companies.

References

1. Cotmore, S.F.; Agbandje-McKenna, M.; Canuti, M.; Chiorini, J.A.; Eis-Hubinger, A.M.; Hughes, J.; Mietzsch, M.; Modha, S.; Ogliastro, M.; Penzes, J.J.; et al. ICTV virus taxonomy profile: Parvoviridae. *J. Gen. Virol.* **2019**, *100*, 367–368. [CrossRef] [PubMed]
2. Camacho, C.; Coulouris, G.; Avagyan, V.; Ma, N.; Papadopoulos, J.; Bealer, K.; Madden, T.L. BLAST+: Architecture and applications. *BMC Bioinform.* **2009**, *10*, 421. [CrossRef] [PubMed]
3. Xie, Q.; Bu, W.; Bhatia, S.; Hare, J.; Somasundaram, T.; Azzi, A.; Chapman, M.S. The atomic structure of adeno-associated virus (AAV-2), a vector for human gene therapy. *Proc. Natl. Acad. Sci. USA* **2002**, *99*, 10405–10410. [CrossRef] [PubMed]
4. Kaufmann, B.; Simpson, A.A.; Rossmann, M.G. The structure of human parvovirus B19. *Proc. Natl. Acad. Sci. USA* **2004**, *101*, 11628–11633. [CrossRef]
5. Kailasan, S.; Halder, S.; Gurda, B.; Bladek, H.; Chipman, P.R.; McKenna, R.; Brown, K.; Agbandje-McKenna, M. Structure of an enteric pathogen, bovine parvovirus. *J. Virol.* **2015**, *89*, 2603–2614. [CrossRef] [PubMed]
6. Tsao, J.; Chapman, M.S.; Agbandje, M.; Keller, W.; Smith, K.; Wu, H.; Luo, M.; Smith, T.J.; Rossmann, M.G.; Compans, R.W.; et al. The three-dimensional structure of canine parvovirus and its functional implications. *Science* **1991**, *251*, 1456–1464. [CrossRef]
7. Simpson, A.A.; Chipman, P.R.; Baker, T.S.; Tijssen, P.; Rossmann, M.G. The structure of an insect parvovirus (Galleria mellonella densovirus) at 3.7 A resolution. *Structure* **1998**, *6*, 1355–1367. [CrossRef]
8. Meng, G.; Zhang, X.; Plevka, P.; Yu, Q.; Tijssen, P.; Rossmann, M.G. The structure and host entry of an invertebrate parvovirus. *J. Virol.* **2013**, *87*, 12523–12530. [CrossRef] [PubMed]
9. Kaufmann, B.; El-Far, M.; Plevka, P.; Bowman, V.D.; Li, Y.; Tijssen, P.; Rossmann, M.G. Structure of Bombyx mori densovirus 1, a silkworm pathogen. *J. Virol.* **2011**, *85*, 4691–4697. [CrossRef] [PubMed]
10. Zadori, Z.; Szelei, J.; Lacoste, M.C.; Li, Y.; Gariepy, S.; Raymond, P.; Allaire, M.; Nabi, I.R.; Tijssen, P. A viral phospholipase A2 is required for parvovirus infectivity. *Dev. Cell* **2001**, *1*, 291–302. [CrossRef]
11. Popa-Wagner, R.; Sonntag, F.; Schmidt, K.; King, J.; Kleinschmidt, J.A. Nuclear translocation of adeno-associated virus type 2 capsid proteins for virion assembly. *J. Gen. Virol.* **2012**, *93*, 1887–1898. [CrossRef]
12. Popa-Wagner, R.; Porwal, M.; Kann, M.; Reuss, M.; Weimer, M.; Florin, L.; Kleinschmidt, J.A. Impact of vp1-specific protein sequence motifs on adeno-associated virus type 2 intracellular trafficking and nuclear entry. *J. Virol.* **2012**, *86*, 9163–9174. [CrossRef] [PubMed]
13. Qu, X.W.; Liu, W.P.; Qi, Z.Y.; Duan, Z.J.; Zheng, L.S.; Kuang, Z.Z.; Zhang, W.J.; Hou, Y.D. Phospholipase A2-like activity of human bocavirus VP1 unique region. *Biochem. Biophys. Res Commun.* **2008**, *365*, 158–163. [CrossRef]
14. Buller, R.M.; Janik, J.E.; Sebring, E.D.; Rose, J.A. Herpes simplex virus types 1 and 2 completely help adenovirus-associated virus replication. *J. Virol.* **1981**, *40*, 241–247. [PubMed]
15. McPherson, R.A.; Rosenthal, L.J.; Rose, J.A. Human cytomegalovirus completely helps adeno-associated virus replication. *Virology* **1985**, *147*, 217–222. [CrossRef]
16. Weindler, F.W.; Heilbronn, R. A subset of herpes simplex virus replication genes provides helper functions for productive adeno-associated virus replication. *J. Virol.* **1991**, *65*, 2476–2483. [PubMed]
17. Chang, L.S.; Shi, Y.; Shenk, T. Adeno-associated virus P5 promoter contains an adenovirus E1A-inducible element and a binding site for the major late transcription factor. *J. Virol.* **1989**, *63*, 3479–3488.
18. Weitzman, M.D.; Linden, R.M. Adeno-associated virus biology. *Methods Mol. Biol.* **2011**, *807*, 1–23. [PubMed]
19. Laughlin, C.A.; Westphal, H.; Carter, B.J. Spliced adenovirus-associated virus rna. *Proc. Natl. Acad. Sci. USA* **1979**, *76*, 5567–5571. [CrossRef]
20. Qiu, J.; Soderlund-Venermo, M.; Young, N.S. Human parvoviruses. *Clin. Microbiol. Rev.* **2017**, *30*, 43–113.
21. Becerra, S.P.; Rose, J.A.; Hardy, M.; Baroudy, B.M.; Anderson, C.W. Direct mapping of adeno-associated virus capsid proteins b and c: A possible ACG initiation codon. *Proc. Natl. Acad. Sci. USA* **1985**, *82*, 7919–7923. [CrossRef]

22. Becerra, S.P.; Koczot, F.; Fabisch, P.; Rose, J.A. Synthesis of adeno-associated virus structural proteins requires both alternative mrna splicing and alternative initiations from a single transcript. *J. Virol.* **1988**, *62*, 2745–2754.
23. Trempe, J.P.; Carter, B.J. Alternate mrna splicing is required for synthesis of adeno-associated virus Vp1 capsid protein. *J. Virol.* **1988**, *62*, 3356–3363. [PubMed]
24. Qiu, J.; Pintel, D. Processing of adeno-associated virus rna. *Front. Biosci.* **2008**, *13*, 3101–3115. [CrossRef] [PubMed]
25. Qiu, J.; Yoto, Y.; Tullis, G.E.; Pintel, D. Parvovirus RNA processing strategies. In *Parvoviruses*; Edward Arnold, Ltd.: London, UK, 2006; pp. 253–274.
26. Wistuba, A.; Kern, A.; Weger, S.; Grimm, D.; Kleinschmidt, J.A. Subcellular compartmentalization of adeno-associated virus type 2 assembly. *J. Virol.* **1997**, *71*, 1341–1352.
27. Cotmore, S.F.; D'Abramo, A.M., Jr.; Carbonell, L.F.; Bratton, J.; Tattersall, P. The NS2 polypeptide of parvovirus MVM is required for capsid assembly in murine cells. *Virology* **1997**, *231*, 267–280. [CrossRef] [PubMed]
28. Cotmore, S.F.; McKie, V.C.; Anderson, L.J.; Astell, C.R.; Tattersall, P. Identification of the major structural and nonstructural proteins encoded by human parvovirus B19 and mapping of their genes by procaryotic expression of isolated genomic fragments. *J. Virol.* **1986**, *60*, 548–557.
29. Buller, R.M.; Rose, J.A. Characterization of adenovirus-associated virus-induced polypeptides in KB cells. *J. Virol.* **1978**, *25*, 331–338. [PubMed]
30. Snijder, J.; van de Waterbeemd, M.; Damoc, E.; Denisov, E.; Grinfeld, D.; Bennett, A.; Agbandje-McKenna, M.; Makarov, A.; Heck, A.J. Defining the stoichiometry and cargo load of viral and bacterial nanoparticles by orbitrap mass spectrometry. *J. Am. Chem. Soc.* **2014**, *136*, 7295–7299. [CrossRef] [PubMed]
31. Rose, J.A.; Maizel, J.V., Jr.; Inman, J.K.; Shatkin, A.J. Structural proteins of adenovirus-associated viruses. *J. Virol.* **1971**, *8*, 766–770.
32. Sonntag, F.; Schmidt, K.; Kleinschmidt, J.A. A viral assembly factor promotes AAV2 capsid formation in the nucleolus. *Proc. Natl. Acad. Sci. USA* **2010**, *107*, 10220–10225. [CrossRef]
33. Bleker, S.; Pawlita, M.; Kleinschmidt, J.A. Impact of capsid conformation and rep-capsid interactions on adeno-associated virus type 2 genome packaging. *J. Virol.* **2006**, *80*, 810–820. [CrossRef]
34. Clinton, G.M.; Hayashi, M. The parovivirus MVM: Particles with altered structural proteins. *Virology* **1975**, *66*, 261–267. [CrossRef]
35. Weichert, W.S.; Parker, J.S.; Wahid, A.T.; Chang, S.F.; Meier, E.; Parrish, C.R. Assaying for structural variation in the parvovirus capsid and its role in infection. *Virology* **1998**, *250*, 106–117. [CrossRef] [PubMed]
36. Paradiso, P.R. Infectious process of the parvovirus h-1: Correlation of protein content, particle density, and viral infectivity. *J. Virol.* **1981**, *39*, 800–807. [PubMed]
37. Farr, G.A.; Cotmore, S.F.; Tattersall, P. Vp2 cleavage and the leucine ring at the base of the fivefold cylinder control ph-dependent externalization of both the Vp1 N terminus and the genome of minute virus of mice. *J. Virol.* **2006**, *80*, 161–171. [CrossRef]
38. Wu, H.; Rossmann, M.G. The canine parvovirus empty capsid structure. *J. Mol. Biol.* **1993**, *233*, 231–244. [CrossRef] [PubMed]
39. Ilyas, M.; Mietzsch, M.; Kailasan, S.; Vaisanen, E.; Luo, M.; Chipman, P.; Smith, J.K.; Kurian, J.; Sousa, D.; McKenna, R.; et al. Atomic resolution structures of human bufaviruses determined by Cryo-electron microscopy. *Viruses* **2018**, *10*, 22. [CrossRef]
40. Xie, Q.; Chapman, M.S. Canine parvovirus capsid structure, analyzed at 2.9 A resolution. *J. Mol. Biol.* **1996**, *264*, 497–520. [CrossRef]
41. Govindasamy, L.; Hueffer, K.; Parrish, C.R.; Agbandje-McKenna, M. Structures of host range-controlling regions of the capsids of canine and feline parvoviruses and mutants. *J. Virol.* **2003**, *77*, 12211–12221. [CrossRef]
42. Simpson, A.A.; Chandrasekar, V.; Hebert, B.; Sullivan, G.M.; Rossmann, M.G.; Parrish, C.R. Host range and variability of calcium binding by surface loops in the capsids of canine and feline parvoviruses. *J. Mol. Biol.* **2000**, *300*, 597–610. [CrossRef]
43. Llamas-Saiz, A.L.; Agbandje-McKenna, M.; Parker, J.S.; Wahid, A.T.; Parrish, C.R.; Rossmann, M.G. Structural analysis of a mutation in canine parvovirus which controls antigenicity and host range. *Virology* **1996**, *225*, 65–71. [CrossRef] [PubMed]

44. Organtini, L.J.; Allison, A.B.; Lukk, T.; Parrish, C.R.; Hafenstein, S. Global displacement of canine parvovirus by a host-adapted variant: Structural comparison between pandemic viruses with distinct host ranges. *J. Virol.* **2015**, *89*, 1909–1912. [CrossRef] [PubMed]
45. Agbandje, M.; McKenna, R.; Rossmann, M.G.; Strassheim, M.L.; Parrish, C.R. Structure determination of feline Panleukopenia virus empty particles. *Proteins* **1993**, *16*, 155–171. [CrossRef] [PubMed]
46. Halder, S.; Nam, H.J.; Govindasamy, L.; Vogel, M.; Dinsart, C.; Salome, N.; McKenna, R.; Agbandje-McKenna, M. Structural characterization of H-1 parvovirus: Comparison of infectious virions to empty capsids. *J. Virol.* **2013**, *87*, 5128–5140. [CrossRef]
47. Pittman, N.; Misseldine, A.; Geilen, L.; Halder, S.; Smith, J.K.; Kurian, J.; Chipman, P.; Janssen, M.; McKenna, R.; Baker, T.S.; et al. Atomic resolution structure of the oncolytic parvovirus luiii by electron microscopy and 3d image reconstruction. *Viruses* **2017**, *9*, 321. [CrossRef] [PubMed]
48. Callaway, H.M.; Subramanian, S.; Urbina, C.; Barnard, K.; Dick, R.; Bator, C.M.; Hafentein, S.L.; Gifford, R.J.; Parrish, C.R. Examination and reconstruction of three ancient endogenous parvovirus capsid protein gene remnants found in rodent genomes. *J. Virol.* **2019**, *93*, e01542-18. [CrossRef]
49. Llamas-Saiz, A.L.; Agbandje-McKenna, M.; Wikoff, W.R.; Bratton, J.; Tattersall, P.; Rossmann, M.G. Structure determination of minute virus of mice. *Acta Crystallogr. Sect. D Biol. Crystallogr.* **1997**, *53*, 93–102. [CrossRef]
50. Kontou, M.; Govindasamy, L.; Nam, H.J.; Bryant, N.; Llamas-Saiz, A.L.; Foces-Foces, C.; Hernando, E.; Rubio, M.P.; McKenna, R.; Almendral, J.M.; et al. Structural determinants of tissue tropism and in vivo pathogenicity for the parvovirus minute virus of mice. *J. Virol.* **2005**, *79*, 10931–10943. [CrossRef]
51. Plevka, P.; Hafenstein, S.; Li, L.; D'Abrgamo, A., Jr.; Cotmore, S.F.; Rossmann, M.G.; Tattersall, P. Structure of a packaging-defective mutant of minute virus of mice indicates that the genome is packaged via a pore at a 5-fold axis. *J. Virol.* **2011**, *85*, 4822–4827. [CrossRef]
52. Guerra, P.; Valbuena, A.; Querol-Audi, J.; Silva, C.; Castellanos, M.; Rodriguez-Huete, A.; Garriga, D.; Mateu, M.G.; Verdaguer, N. Structural basis for biologically relevant mechanical stiffening of a virus capsid by cavity-creating or spacefilling mutations. *Sci. Rep.* **2017**, *7*, 4101. [CrossRef] [PubMed]
53. Simpson, A.A.; Hebert, B.; Sullivan, G.M.; Parrish, C.R.; Zadori, Z.; Tijssen, P.; Rossmann, M.G. The structure of porcine parvovirus: Comparison with related viruses. *J. Mol. Biol.* **2002**, *315*, 1189–1198. [CrossRef] [PubMed]
54. Mietzsch, M.; Kailasan, S.; Garrison, J.; Ilyas, M.; Chipman, P.; Kantola, K.; Janssen, M.E.; Spear, J.; Sousa, D.; McKenna, R.; et al. Structural insights into human bocaparvoviruses. *J. Virol.* **2017**, *91*, e00261-17. [CrossRef] [PubMed]
55. Ng, R.; Govindasamy, L.; Gurda, B.L.; McKenna, R.; Kozyreva, O.G.; Samulski, R.J.; Parent, K.N.; Baker, T.S.; Agbandje-McKenna, M. Structural characterization of the dual glycan binding adeno-associated virus serotype 6. *J. Virol.* **2010**, *84*, 12945–12957. [CrossRef] [PubMed]
56. Drouin, L.M.; Lins, B.; Janssen, M.; Bennett, A.; Chipman, P.; McKenna, R.; Chen, W.; Muzyczka, N.; Cardone, G.; Baker, T.S.; et al. Cryo-electron microscopy reconstruction and stability studies of the wild type and the R432A variant of adeno-associated virus type 2 reveal that capsid structural stability is a major factor in genome packaging. *J. Virol.* **2016**, *90*, 8542–8551. [CrossRef]
57. Tan, Y.Z.; Aiyer, S.; Mietzsch, M.; Hull, J.A.; McKenna, R.; Grieger, J.; Samulski, R.J.; Baker, T.S.; Agbandje-McKenna, M.; Lyumkis, D. Sub-2 A Ewald curvature corrected structure of an AAV2 capsid variant. *Nat. Commun.* **2018**, *9*, 3628. [CrossRef] [PubMed]
58. Burg, M.; Rosebrough, C.; Drouin, L.M.; Bennett, A.; Mietzsch, M.; Chipman, P.; McKenna, R.; Sousa, D.; Potter, M.; Byrne, B.; et al. Atomic structure of a rationally engineered gene delivery vector, aav2.5. *J. Struct. Biol.* **2018**, *203*, 236–241. [CrossRef]
59. Lerch, T.F.; Xie, Q.; Chapman, M.S. The structure of adeno-associated virus serotype 3b (aav-3b): Insights into receptor binding and immune evasion. *Virology* **2010**, *403*, 26–36. [CrossRef]
60. Govindasamy, L.; Padron, E.; McKenna, R.; Muzyczka, N.; Kaludov, N.; Chiorini, J.A.; Agbandje-McKenna, M. Structurally mapping the diverse phenotype of adeno-associated virus serotype 4. *J. Virol.* **2006**, *80*, 11556–11570. [CrossRef]
61. Govindasamy, L.; Dimattia, M.A.; Gurda, B.L.; Halder, S.; McKenna, R.; Chiorini, J.A.; Muzyczka, N.; Zolotukhin, S.; Agbandje-McKenna, M. Structural insights into adeno-associated virus serotype 5. *J. Virol.* **2013**, *87*, 11187–11199. [CrossRef]

62. Xie, Q.; Lerch, T.F.; Meyer, N.L.; Chapman, M.S. Structure-function analysis of receptor-binding in adeno-associated virus serotype 6 (AAV-6). *Virology* **2011**, *420*, 10–19. [CrossRef] [PubMed]
63. Nam, H.J.; Lane, M.D.; Padron, E.; Gurda, B.; McKenna, R.; Kohlbrenner, E.; Aslanidi, G.; Byrne, B.; Muzyczka, N.; Zolotukhin, S.; et al. Structure of adeno-associated virus serotype 8, a gene therapy vector. *J. Virol.* **2007**, *81*, 12260–12271. [CrossRef]
64. Nam, H.J.; Gurda, B.L.; McKenna, R.; Potter, M.; Byrne, B.; Salganik, M.; Muzyczka, N.; Agbandje-McKenna, M. Structural studies of adeno-associated virus serotype 8 capsid transitions associated with endosomal trafficking. *J. Virol.* **2011**, *85*, 11791–11799. [CrossRef] [PubMed]
65. DiMattia, M.A.; Nam, H.J.; Van Vliet, K.; Mitchell, M.; Bennett, A.; Gurda, B.L.; McKenna, R.; Olson, N.H.; Sinkovits, R.S.; Potter, M.; et al. Structural insight into the unique properties of adeno-associated virus serotype 9. *J. Virol.* **2012**, *86*, 6947–6958. [CrossRef]
66. Guenther, C.M.; Brun, M.J.; Bennett, A.D.; Ho, M.L.; Chen, W.; Zhu, B.; Lam, M.; Yamagami, M.; Kwon, S.; Bhattacharya, N.; et al. Protease-activatable adeno-associated virus vector for gene delivery to damaged heart tissue. *Mol. Ther.* **2019**, *27*, 611–622. [CrossRef] [PubMed]
67. Lerch, T.F.; O'Donnell, J.K.; Meyer, N.L.; Xie, Q.; Taylor, K.A.; Stagg, S.M.; Chapman, M.S. Structure of AAV-dj, a retargeted gene therapy vector: Cryo-electron microscopy at 4.5 A resolution. *Structure* **2012**, *20*, 1310–1320. [CrossRef] [PubMed]
68. Halder, S.; Van Vliet, K.; Smith, J.K.; Duong, T.T.; McKenna, R.; Wilson, J.M.; Agbandje-McKenna, M. Structure of neurotropic adeno-associated virus AAVrh.8. *J. Struct. Biol.* **2015**, *192*, 21–36. [CrossRef] [PubMed]
69. Mikals, K.; Nam, H.J.; Van Vliet, K.; Vandenberghe, L.H.; Mays, L.E.; McKenna, R.; Wilson, J.M.; Agbandje-McKenna, M. The structure of AAVrh32.33, a novel gene delivery vector. *J. Struct. Biol.* **2014**, *186*, 308–317. [CrossRef]
70. Kronenberg, S.; Bottcher, B.; von der Lieth, C.W.; Bleker, S.; Kleinschmidt, J.A. A conformational change in the adeno-associated virus type 2 capsid leads to the exposure of hidden Vp1 N termini. *J. Virol.* **2005**, *79*, 5296–5303. [CrossRef] [PubMed]
71. Kaufmann, B.; Chipman, P.R.; Kostyuchenko, V.A.; Modrow, S.; Rossmann, M.G. Visualization of the externalized Vp2 N termini of infectious human parvovirus B19. *J. Virol.* **2008**, *82*, 7306–7312. [CrossRef]
72. Xue, B.; Dunbrack, R.L.; Williams, R.W.; Dunker, A.K.; Uversky, V.N. Pondr-fit: A meta-predictor of intrinsically disordered amino acids. *Biochim. Biophys. Acta* **2010**, *1804*, 996–1010. [CrossRef] [PubMed]
73. Venkatakrishnan, B.; Yarbrough, J.; Domsic, J.; Bennett, A.; Bothner, B.; Kozyreva, O.G.; Samulski, R.J.; Muzyczka, N.; McKenna, R.; Agbandje-McKenna, M. Structure and dynamics of adeno-associated virus serotype 1 Vp1-unique n-terminal domain and its role in capsid trafficking. *J. Virol.* **2013**, *87*, 4974–4984. [CrossRef] [PubMed]
74. Agbandje-McKenna, M.; Kleinschmidt, J. Aav capsid structure and cell interactions. *Methods Mol. Biol.* **2011**, *807*, 47–92. [PubMed]
75. Bennett, A.; Mietzsch, M.; Agbandje-McKenna, M. Understanding capsid assembly and genome packaging for adeno-associated viruses. *Future Virol.* **2017**, *12*, 283–297. [CrossRef]
76. Chapman, M.S.; Agbandje-McKenna, M. Atomic structure of viral particles. In *Parvoviruses*; Bloom, M.E., Cotmore, S.F., Linden, R.M., Parrish, C.R., Kerr, J.R., Eds.; Edward Arnold, Ltd.: London, UK, 2006; pp. 109–123.
77. DeLano, W.L. *The Pymol Molecular Graphics Syste*; DeLano Scientific: San Carlos, CA, USA, 2002.
78. Pettersen, E.F.; Goddard, T.D.; Huang, C.C.; Couch, G.S.; Greenblatt, D.M.; Meng, E.C.; Ferrin, T.E. Ucsf chimera—A visualization system for exploratory research and analysis. *J. Comput. Chem.* **2004**, *25*, 1605–1612. [CrossRef]
79. Chapman, M.S.; Rossmann, M.G. Single-stranded DNA-protein interactions in canine parvovirus. *Structure* **1995**, *3*, 151–162. [CrossRef]
80. Grieger, J.C.; Johnson, J.S.; Gurda-Whitaker, B.; Agbandje-McKenna, M.; Samulski, R.J. Surface-exposed adeno-associated virus Vp1-NLS capsid fusion protein rescues infectivity of noninfectious wild-type Vp2/Vp3 and Vp3-only capsids but not that of fivefold pore mutant virions. *J. Virol.* **2007**, *81*, 7833–7843. [CrossRef] [PubMed]
81. Farr, G.A.; Tattersall, P. A conserved leucine that constricts the pore through the capsid fivefold cylinder plays a central role in parvoviral infection. *Virology* **2004**, *323*, 243–256. [CrossRef] [PubMed]

82. Wu, P.; Xiao, W.; Conlon, T.; Hughes, J.; Agbandje-McKenna, M.; Ferkol, T.; Flotte, T.; Muzyczka, N. Mutational analysis of the adeno-associated virus type 2 (AAV2) capsid gene and construction of aav2 vectors with altered tropism. *J. Virol.* **2000**, *74*, 8635–8647. [CrossRef]
83. Hafenstein, S.; Palermo, L.M.; Kostyuchenko, V.A.; Xiao, C.; Morais, M.C.; Nelson, C.D.; Bowman, V.D.; Battisti, A.J.; Chipman, P.R.; Parrish, C.R.; et al. Asymmetric binding of transferrin receptor to parvovirus capsids. *Proc. Natl. Acad. Sci. USA* **2007**, *104*, 6585–6589. [CrossRef] [PubMed]
84. Hafenstein, S.; Bowman, V.D.; Sun, T.; Nelson, C.D.; Palermo, L.M.; Chipman, P.R.; Battisti, A.J.; Parrish, C.R.; Rossmann, M.G. Structural comparison of different antibodies interacting with parvovirus capsids. *J. Virol.* **2009**, *83*, 5556–5566. [CrossRef] [PubMed]
85. Hueffer, K.; Govindasamy, L.; Agbandje-McKenna, M.; Parrish, C.R. Combinations of two capsid regions controlling canine host range determine canine transferrin receptor binding by canine and feline parvoviruses. *J. Virol.* **2003**, *77*, 10099–10105. [CrossRef] [PubMed]
86. Huang, L.Y.; Halder, S.; Agbandje-McKenna, M. Parvovirus glycan interactions. *Curr. Opin. Virol.* **2014**, *7*, 108–118. [CrossRef] [PubMed]
87. Pillay, S.; Meyer, N.L.; Puschnik, A.S.; Davulcu, O.; Diep, J.; Ishikawa, Y.; Jae, L.T.; Wosen, J.E.; Nagamine, C.M.; Chapman, M.S.; et al. An essential receptor for adeno-associated virus infection. *Nature* **2016**, *530*, 108–112. [CrossRef] [PubMed]
88. Mietzsch, M.; Broecker, F.; Reinhardt, A.; Seeberger, P.H.; Heilbronn, R. Differential adeno-associated virus serotype-specific interaction patterns with synthetic heparins and other glycans. *J. Virol.* **2014**, *88*, 2991–3003. [CrossRef] [PubMed]
89. Akache, B.; Grimm, D.; Pandey, K.; Yant, S.R.; Xu, H.; Kay, M.A. The 37/67-kilodalton laminin receptor is a receptor for adeno-associated virus serotypes 8, 2, 3, and 9. *J. Virol.* **2006**, *80*, 9831–9836. [CrossRef]
90. Qing, K.; Mah, C.; Hansen, J.; Zhou, S.; Dwarki, V.; Srivastava, A. Human fibroblast growth factor receptor 1 is a co-receptor for infection by adeno-associated virus 2. *Nat. Med.* **1999**, *5*, 71–77. [CrossRef]
91. Kashiwakura, Y.; Tamayose, K.; Iwabuchi, K.; Hirai, Y.; Shimada, T.; Matsumoto, K.; Nakamura, T.; Watanabe, M.; Oshimi, K.; Daida, H. Hepatocyte growth factor receptor is a coreceptor for adeno-associated virus type 2 infection. *J. Virol.* **2005**, *79*, 609–614. [CrossRef] [PubMed]
92. Weller, M.L.; Amornphimoltham, P.; Schmidt, M.; Wilson, P.A.; Gutkind, J.S.; Chiorini, J.A. Epidermal growth factor receptor is a co-receptor for adeno-associated virus serotype 6. *Nat. Med.* **2010**, *16*, 662–664. [CrossRef] [PubMed]
93. Wu, Z.; Miller, E.; Agbandje-McKenna, M.; Samulski, R.J. Alpha2,3 and alpha2,6 n-linked sialic acids facilitate efficient binding and transduction by adeno-associated virus types 1 and 6. *J. Virol.* **2006**, *80*, 9093–9103. [CrossRef] [PubMed]
94. Di Pasquale, G.; Kaludov, N.; Agbandje-McKenna, M.; Chiorini, J.A. Baav transcytosis requires an interaction with Beta-1-4 linked- glucosamine and gp96. *PLoS ONE* **2010**, *5*, e9336. [CrossRef] [PubMed]
95. O'Donnell, J.; Taylor, K.A.; Chapman, M.S. Adeno-associated virus-2 and its primary cellular receptor–cryo-em structure of a heparin complex. *Virology* **2009**, *385*, 434–443. [CrossRef] [PubMed]
96. Levy, H.C.; Bowman, V.D.; Govindasamy, L.; McKenna, R.; Nash, K.; Warrington, K.; Chen, W.; Muzyczka, N.; Yan, X.; Baker, T.S.; et al. Heparin binding induces conformational changes in adeno-associated virus serotype 2. *J. Struct. Biol.* **2009**, *165*, 146–156. [CrossRef] [PubMed]
97. Xie, Q.; Spear, J.M.; Noble, A.J.; Sousa, D.R.; Meyer, N.L.; Davulcu, O.; Zhang, F.; Linhardt, R.J.; Stagg, S.M.; Chapman, M.S. The 2.8 A electron microscopy structure of adeno-associated virus-dj bound by a heparinoid pentasaccharide. *Mol. Ther. Methods Clin. Dev.* **2017**, *5*, 1–12. [CrossRef]
98. Afione, S.; DiMattia, M.A.; Halder, S.; Di Pasquale, G.; Agbandje-McKenna, M.; Chiorini, J.A. Identification and mutagenesis of the adeno-associated virus 5 sialic acid binding region. *J. Virol.* **2015**, *89*, 1660–1672. [CrossRef]
99. Lerch, T.F.; Chapman, M.S. Identification of the heparin binding site on adeno-associated virus serotype 3B (AAV-3B). *Virology* **2012**, *423*, 6–13. [CrossRef]
100. Huang, L.Y.; Patel, A.; Ng, R.; Miller, E.B.; Halder, S.; McKenna, R.; Asokan, A.; Agbandje-McKenna, M. Characterization of the adeno-associated virus 1 and 6 sialic acid binding site. *J. Virol.* **2016**, *90*, 5219–5230. [CrossRef] [PubMed]

101. Lopez-Bueno, A.; Rubio, M.P.; Bryant, N.; McKenna, R.; Agbandje-McKenna, M.; Almendral, J.M. Host-selected amino acid changes at the sialic acid binding pocket of the parvovirus capsid modulate cell binding affinity and determine virulence. *J. Virol.* **2006**, *80*, 1563–1573. [CrossRef]
102. Zhang, R.; Cao, L.; Cui, M.; Sun, Z.; Hu, M.; Zhang, R.; Stuart, W.; Zhao, X.; Yang, Z.; Li, X.; et al. Adeno-associated virus 2 bound to its cellular receptor AAVR. *Nat. Microbiol.* **2019**, *4*, 675–682. [CrossRef]
103. Rohrer, C.; Gartner, B.; Sauerbrei, A.; Bohm, S.; Hottentrager, B.; Raab, U.; Thierfelder, W.; Wutzler, P.; Modrow, S. Seroprevalence of parvovirus B19 in the german population. *Epidemiol. Infect.* **2008**, *136*, 1564–1575. [CrossRef]
104. Boutin, S.; Monteilhet, V.; Veron, P.; Leborgne, C.; Benveniste, O.; Montus, M.F.; Masurier, C. Prevalence of serum igg and neutralizing factors against adeno-associated virus (AAV) types 1, 2, 5, 6, 8, and 9 in the healthy population: Implications for gene therapy using AAV vectors. *Hum. Gene Ther.* **2010**, *21*, 704–712. [CrossRef]
105. Guo, L.; Wang, Y.; Zhou, H.; Wu, C.; Song, J.; Li, J.; Paranhos-Baccala, G.; Vernet, G.; Wang, J.; Hung, T. Differential seroprevalence of human bocavirus species 1-4 in Beijing, China. *PLoS ONE* **2012**, *7*, e39644. [CrossRef] [PubMed]
106. Vaisanen, E.; Mohanraj, U.; Kinnunen, P.M.; Jokelainen, P.; Al-Hello, H.; Barakat, A.M.; Sadeghi, M.; Jalilian, F.A.; Majlesi, A.; Masika, M.; et al. Global distribution of human protoparvoviruses. *Emerg. Infect. Dis.* **2018**, *24*, 1292–1299. [CrossRef] [PubMed]
107. Sharp, C.P.; Vermeulen, M.; Nebie, Y.; Djoko, C.F.; LeBreton, M.; Tamoufe, U.; Rimoin, A.W.; Kayembe, P.K.; Carr, J.K.; Servant-Delmas, A.; et al. Changing epidemiology of human parvovirus 4 infection in sub-Saharan Africa. *Emerg. Infect. Dis.* **2010**, *16*, 1605–1607. [CrossRef]
108. Jose, A.; Mietzsch, M.; Smith, K.; Kurian, J.; Chipman, P.; McKenna, R.; Chiorini, J.; Agbandje-McKenna, M. High resolution structural characterization of a new aav5 antibody epitope toward engineering antibody resistant recombinant gene delivery vectors. *J. Virol.* **2018**, *93*, e01394-18. [CrossRef]
109. von Kietzell, K.; Pozzuto, T.; Heilbronn, R.; Grossl, T.; Fechner, H.; Weger, S. Antibody-mediated enhancement of parvovirus B19 uptake into endothelial cells mediated by a receptor for complement factor C1Q. *J. Virol.* **2014**, *88*, 8102–8115. [CrossRef]
110. Kanno, H.; Wolfinbarger, J.B.; Bloom, M.E. Aleutian mink disease parvovirus infection of mink macrophages and human macrophage cell line u937: Demonstration of antibody-dependent enhancement of infection. *J. Virol.* **1993**, *67*, 7017–7024. [PubMed]
111. Organtini, L.J.; Lee, H.; Iketani, S.; Huang, K.; Ashley, R.E.; Makhov, A.M.; Conway, J.F.; Parrish, C.R.; Hafenstein, S. Near-atomic resolution structure of a highly neutralizing Fab bound to canine parvovirus. *J. Virol.* **2016**, *90*, 9733–9742. [CrossRef] [PubMed]
112. Kaufmann, B.; Lopez-Bueno, A.; Mateu, M.G.; Chipman, P.R.; Nelson, C.D.; Parrish, C.R.; Almendral, J.M.; Rossmann, M.G. Minute virus of mice, a parvovirus, in complex with the fab fragment of a neutralizing monoclonal antibody. *J. Virol.* **2007**, *81*, 9851–9858. [CrossRef]
113. Kailasan, S.; Garrison, J.; Ilyas, M.; Chipman, P.; McKenna, R.; Kantola, K.; Soderlund-Venermo, M.; Kucinskaite-Kodze, I.; Zvirbliene, A.; Agbandje-McKenna, M. Mapping antigenic epitopes on the human bocavirus capsid. *J. Virol.* **2016**, *90*, 4670–4680. [CrossRef]
114. Tseng, Y.S.; Gurda, B.L.; Chipman, P.; McKenna, R.; Afione, S.; Chiorini, J.A.; Muzyczka, N.; Olson, N.H.; Baker, T.S.; Kleinschmidt, J.; et al. Adeno-associated virus serotype 1 (AAV1)- and AAV5-antibody complex structures reveal evolutionary commonalities in parvovirus antigenic reactivity. *J. Virol.* **2015**, *89*, 1794–1808. [CrossRef] [PubMed]
115. Gurda, B.L.; DiMattia, M.A.; Miller, E.B.; Bennett, A.; McKenna, R.; Weichert, W.S.; Nelson, C.D.; Chen, W.J.; Muzyczka, N.; Olson, N.H.; et al. Capsid antibodies to different adeno-associated virus serotypes bind common regions. *J. Virol.* **2013**, *87*, 9111–9124. [CrossRef]
116. McCraw, D.M.; O'Donnell, J.K.; Taylor, K.A.; Stagg, S.M.; Chapman, M.S. Structure of adeno-associated virus-2 in complex with neutralizing monoclonal antibody A20. *Virology* **2012**, *431*, 40–49. [CrossRef] [PubMed]
117. Bennett, A.D.; Wong, K.; Lewis, J.; Tseng, Y.S.; Smith, J.K.; Chipman, P.; McKenna, R.; Samulski, R.J.; Kleinschmidt, J.; Agbandje-McKenna, M. AAV6 K531 serves a dual function in selective receptor and antibody ADK6 recognition. *Virology* **2018**, *518*, 369–376. [CrossRef] [PubMed]

118. Gurda, B.L.; Raupp, C.; Popa-Wagner, R.; Naumer, M.; Olson, N.H.; Ng, R.; McKenna, R.; Baker, T.S.; Kleinschmidt, J.A.; Agbandje-McKenna, M. Mapping a neutralizing epitope onto the capsid of adeno-associated virus serotype 8. *J. Virol.* **2012**, *86*, 7739–7751. [CrossRef] [PubMed]
119. Giles, A.R.; Govindasamy, L.; Somanathan, S.; Wilson, J.M. Mapping an adeno-associated virus 9-specific neutralizing epitope to develop next-generation gene delivery vectors. *J. Virol.* **2018**, *92*. [CrossRef]
120. Sun, Y.; Klose, T.; Liu, Y.; Modrow, S.; Rossmann, M.G. Structure of parvovirus B19 decorated by Fabs from a human antibody. *J. Virol.* **2019**. [CrossRef]
121. Daya, S.; Berns, K.I. Gene therapy using adeno-associated virus vectors. *Clin. Microbiol. Rev.* **2008**, *21*, 583–593. [CrossRef]
122. Fakhiri, J.; Schneider, M.A.; Puschhof, J.; Stanifer, M.; Schildgen, V.; Holderbach, S.; Voss, Y.; El Andari, J.; Schildgen, O.; Boulant, S.; et al. Novel chimeric gene therapy vectors based on adeno-associated virus (AAV) and four different mammalian bocaviruses (BOV). *Mol. Ther. Methods Clin. Dev.* **2019**, *12*, 202–222. [CrossRef]
123. Gray, J.T.; Zolotukhin, S. Design and construction of functional AAV vectors. *Methods Mol. Biol.* **2011**, *807*, 25–46. [PubMed]
124. Zhong, L.; Li, B.; Jayandharan, G.; Mah, C.S.; Govindasamy, L.; Agbandje-McKenna, M.; Herzog, R.W.; Weigel-Van Aken, K.A.; Hobbs, J.A.; Zolotukhin, S.; et al. Tyrosine-phosphorylation of AAV2 vectors and its consequences on viral intracellular trafficking and transgene expression. *Virology* **2008**, *381*, 194–202. [CrossRef] [PubMed]
125. Zhong, L.; Zhao, W.; Wu, J.; Li, B.; Zolotukhin, S.; Govindasamy, L.; Agbandje-McKenna, M.; Srivastava, A. A dual role of EGFR protein tyrosine kinase signaling in ubiquitination of AAV2 capsids and viral second-strand DNA synthesis. *Mol. Ther.* **2007**, *15*, 1323–1330. [CrossRef] [PubMed]
126. Zhong, L.; Li, B.; Mah, C.S.; Govindasamy, L.; Agbandje-McKenna, M.; Cooper, M.; Herzog, R.W.; Zolotukhin, I.; Warrington, K.H., Jr.; Weigel-Van Aken, K.A.; et al. Next generation of adeno-associated virus 2 vectors: Point mutations in tyrosines lead to high-efficiency transduction at lower doses. *Proc. Natl. Acad. Sci. USA* **2008**, *105*, 7827–7832. [CrossRef] [PubMed]
127. Aslanidi, G.V.; Rivers, A.E.; Ortiz, L.; Song, L.; Ling, C.; Govindasamy, L.; Van Vliet, K.; Tan, M.; Agbandje-McKenna, M.; Srivastava, A. Optimization of the capsid of recombinant adeno-associated virus 2 (AAV2) vectors: The final threshold? *PLoS ONE* **2013**, *8*, e59142. [CrossRef]
128. Gabriel, N.; Hareendran, S.; Sen, D.; Gadkari, R.A.; Sudha, G.; Selot, R.; Hussain, M.; Dhaksnamoorthy, R.; Samuel, R.; Srinivasan, N.; et al. Bioengineering of AAV2 capsid at specific serine, threonine, or lysine residues improves its transduction efficiency in vitro and in vivo. *Hum. Gene Ther. Methods* **2013**, *24*, 80–93. [CrossRef] [PubMed]
129. Hurlbut, G.D.; Ziegler, R.J.; Nietupski, J.B.; Foley, J.W.; Woodworth, L.A.; Meyers, E.; Bercury, S.D.; Pande, N.N.; Souza, D.W.; Bree, M.P.; et al. Preexisting immunity and low expression in primates highlight translational challenges for liver-directed AAV8-mediated gene therapy. *Mol. Ther.* **2010**, *18*, 1983–1994. [CrossRef]
130. Velazquez, V.M.; Meadows, A.S.; Pineda, R.J.; Camboni, M.; McCarty, D.M.; Fu, H. Effective depletion of pre-existing anti-aav antibodies requires broad immune targeting. *Mol. Ther. Methods Clin. Dev.* **2017**, *4*, 159–168. [CrossRef] [PubMed]
131. Mingozzi, F.; High, K.A. Immune responses to AAV vectors: Overcoming barriers to successful gene therapy. *Blood* **2013**, *122*, 23–36. [CrossRef] [PubMed]
132. Arruda, V.R.; Favaro, P.; Finn, J.D. Strategies to modulate immune responses: A new frontier for gene therapy. *Mol. Ther.* **2009**, *17*, 1492–1503. [CrossRef]
133. Wang, Z.; Storb, R.; Halbert, C.L.; Banks, G.B.; Butts, T.M.; Finn, E.E.; Allen, J.M.; Miller, A.D.; Chamberlain, J.S.; Tapscott, S.J. Successful regional delivery and long-term expression of a dystrophin gene in canine muscular dystrophy: A preclinical model for human therapies. *Mol. Ther.* **2012**, *20*, 1501–1507. [CrossRef]
134. Mingozzi, F.; Anguela, X.M.; Pavani, G.; Chen, Y.; Davidson, R.J.; Hui, D.J.; Yazicioglu, M.; Elkouby, L.; Hinderer, C.J.; Faella, A.; et al. Overcoming preexisting humoral immunity to aav using capsid decoys. *Sci. Transl. Med.* **2013**, *5*, 194ra192. [CrossRef] [PubMed]
135. Tse, L.V.; Klinc, K.A.; Madigan, V.J.; Castellanos Rivera, R.M.; Wells, L.F.; Havlik, L.P.; Smith, J.K.; Agbandje-McKenna, M.; Asokan, A. Structure-guided evolution of antigenically distinct adeno-associated virus variants for immune evasion. *Proc. Natl. Acad. Sci. USA* **2017**, *114*, E4812–E4821. [CrossRef]

136. Tseng, Y.S.; Agbandje-McKenna, M. Mapping the aav capsid host antibody response toward the development of second generation gene delivery vectors. *Front. Immunol.* **2014**, *5*, 9. [CrossRef] [PubMed]
137. Buning, H.; Ried, M.U.; Perabo, L.; Gerner, F.M.; Huttner, N.A.; Enssle, J.; Hallek, M. Receptor targeting of adeno-associated virus vectors. *Gene Ther.* **2003**, *10*, 1142–1151. [CrossRef]
138. Yu, C.Y.; Yuan, Z.; Cao, Z.; Wang, B.; Qiao, C.; Li, J.; Xiao, X. A muscle-targeting peptide displayed on AAV2 improves muscle tropism on systemic delivery. *Gene Ther.* **2009**, *16*, 953–962. [CrossRef] [PubMed]
139. Dalkara, D.; Byrne, L.C.; Klimczak, R.R.; Visel, M.; Yin, L.; Merigan, W.H.; Flannery, J.G.; Schaffer, D.V. In vivo-directed evolution of a new adeno-associated virus for therapeutic outer retinal gene delivery from the vitreous. *Sci. Transl. Med.* **2013**, *5*, 189ra176. [CrossRef]
140. Judd, J.; Wei, F.; Nguyen, P.Q.; Tartaglia, L.J.; Agbandje-McKenna, M.; Silberg, J.J.; Suh, J. Random insertion of mcherry into vp3 domain of adeno-associated virus yields fluorescent capsids with no loss of infectivity. *Mol. Ther. Nucleic Acids* **2012**, *1*, e54. [CrossRef] [PubMed]
141. Asuri, P.; Bartel, M.A.; Vazin, T.; Jang, J.H.; Wong, T.B.; Schaffer, D.V. Directed evolution of adeno-associated virus for enhanced gene delivery and gene targeting in human pluripotent stem cells. *Mol. Ther.* **2012**, *20*, 329–338. [CrossRef]
142. Bowles, D.E.; McPhee, S.W.; Li, C.; Gray, S.J.; Samulski, J.J.; Camp, A.S.; Li, J.; Wang, B.; Monahan, P.E.; Rabinowitz, J.E.; et al. Phase 1 gene therapy for Duchenne muscular dystrophy using a translational optimized aav vector. *Mol. Ther.* **2012**, *20*, 443–455. [CrossRef]
143. Bergoin, M.; Tijssen, P. Densoviruses: A highly diverse group of arthropod parvoviruses. In *Insect Virology*; Asgari, S., Johnson, K.N., Eds.; Horizon Scientific Press: Norfolk, UK, 2010; pp. 59–82.
144. Palinski, R.M.; Mitra, N.; Hause, B.M. Discovery of a novel parvovirinae virus, porcine parvovirus 7, by metagenomic sequencing of porcine rectal swabs. *Virus Genes* **2016**, *52*, 564–567. [CrossRef] [PubMed]
145. Baquerizo-Audiot, E.; Abd-Alla, A.; Jousset, F.X.; Cousserans, F.; Tijssen, P.; Bergoin, M. Structure and expression strategy of the genome of Culex pipiens densovirus, a mosquito densovirus with an ambisense organization. *J. Virol.* **2009**, *83*, 6863–6873. [CrossRef]
146. Tijssen, P.; Penzes, J.J.; Yu, Q.; Pham, H.T.; Bergoin, M. Diversity of small, single-stranded DNA viruses of invertebrates and their chaotic evolutionary past. *J. Invertebr. Pathol.* **2016**, *140*, 83–96. [CrossRef]
147. Kim, E.; Magen, A.; Ast, G. Different levels of alternative splicing among eukaryotes. *Nucleic Acids Res.* **2007**, *35*, 125–131. [CrossRef] [PubMed]
148. Roediger, B.; Lee, Q.; Tikoo, S.; Cobbin, J.C.A.; Henderson, J.M.; Jormakka, M.; O'Rourke, M.B.; Padula, M.P.; Pinello, N.; Henry, M.; et al. An atypical parvovirus drives chronic tubulointerstitial nephropathy and kidney fibrosis. *Cell* **2018**, *175*, 530–543.e524. [CrossRef] [PubMed]
149. Tijssen, P.; Li, Y.; El-Far, M.; Szelei, J.; Letarte, M.; Zadori, Z. Organization and expression strategy of the ambisense genome of densonucleosis virus of Galleria mellonella. *J. Virol.* **2003**, *77*, 10357–10365. [CrossRef]
150. Yang, B.; Dong, X.; Cai, D.; Wang, X.; Liu, Z.; Hu, Z.; Wang, H.; Cao, X.; Zhang, J.; Hu, Y. Characterization of the promoter elements and transcription profile of Periplaneta fuliginosa densovirus nonstructural genes. *Virus Res.* **2008**, *133*, 149–156. [CrossRef]
151. Liu, K.; Li, Y.; Jousset, F.X.; Zadori, Z.; Szelei, J.; Yu, Q.; Pham, H.T.; Lepine, F.; Bergoin, M.; Tijssen, P. The Acheta domesticus densovirus, isolated from the european house cricket, has evolved an expression strategy unique among parvoviruses. *J. Virol.* **2011**, *85*, 10069–10078. [CrossRef] [PubMed]
152. Yu, Q.; Tijssen, P. Gene expression of five different iteradensoviruses: Bombyx mori densovirus, Casphalia extranea densovirus, Papilio polyxenes densovirus, Sibine fusca densovirus, and Danaus plexippus densovirus. *J. Virol.* **2014**, *88*, 12152–12157. [CrossRef] [PubMed]
153. Li, Y.; Zadori, Z.; Bando, H.; Dubuc, R.; Fediere, G.; Szelei, J.; Tijssen, P. Genome organization of the densovirus from Bombyx mori (BmDNV-1) and enzyme activity of its capsid. *J. Gen. Virol.* **2001**, *82*, 2821–2825. [CrossRef]
154. Pham, H.T.; Jousset, F.X.; Perreault, J.; Shike, H.; Szelei, J.; Bergoin, M.; Tijssen, P. Expression strategy of Aedes albopictus densovirus. *J. Virol.* **2013**, *87*, 9928–9932. [CrossRef] [PubMed]
155. Pham, H.T. Molecular Biology of Single-Stranded DNA Viruses in Shrimps and Crickets. Ph.D. Thesis, Université du Québec, Quebec City, QC, Canada, 2015.
156. Sukhumsirichart, W.; Attasart, P.; Boonsaeng, V.; Panyim, S. Complete nucleotide sequence and genomic organization of hepatopancreatic parvovirus (HPV) of penaeus monodon. *Virology* **2006**, *346*, 266–277. [CrossRef]

157. Kaufmann, B.; Bowman, V.D.; Li, Y.; Szelei, J.; Waddell, P.J.; Tijssen, P.; Rossmann, M.G. Structure of Penaeus stylirostris densovirus, a shrimp pathogen. *J. Virol.* **2010**, *84*, 11289–11296. [CrossRef]
158. Bruemmer, A.; Scholari, F.; Lopez-Ferber, M.; Conway, J.F.; Hewat, E.A. Structure of an insect parvovirus (Junonia coenia Densovirus) determined by cryo-electron microscopy. *J. Mol. Biol.* **2005**, *347*, 791–801. [CrossRef]
159. Chen, S.; Cheng, L.; Zhang, Q.; Lin, W.; Lu, X.; Brannan, J.; Zhou, Z.H.; Zhang, J. Genetic, biochemical, and structural characterization of a new densovirus isolated from a chronically infected aedes albopictus C6/36 cell line. *Virology* **2004**, *318*, 123–133. [CrossRef]
160. Holm, L.; Rosenstrom, P. Dali server: Conservation mapping in 3d. *Nucleic Acids Res.* **2010**, *38*, W545–W549. [CrossRef]
161. Harrison, S.C.; Olson, A.J.; Schutt, C.E.; Winkler, F.K.; Bricogne, G. Tomato bushy stunt virus at 2.9 a resolution. *Nature* **1978**, *276*, 368–373. [CrossRef] [PubMed]
162. Rossmann, M.G.; Abad-Zapatero, C.; Hermodson, M.A.; Erickson, J.W. Subunit interactions in southern bean mosaic virus. *J. Mol. Biol.* **1983**, *166*, 37–73. [CrossRef]
163. Multeau, C.; Froissart, R.; Perrin, A.; Castelli, I.; Casartelli, M.; Ogliastro, M. Four amino acids of an insect Densovirus capsid determine midgut tropism and virulence. *J. Virol.* **2012**, *86*, 5937–5941. [CrossRef] [PubMed]
164. Wang, Y.; Gosselin Grenet, A.S.; Castelli, I.; Cermenati, G.; Ravallec, M.; Fiandra, L.; Debaisieux, S.; Multeau, C.; Lautredou, N.; Dupressoir, T.; et al. Densovirus crosses the insect midgut by transcytosis and disturbs the epithelial barrier function. *J. Virol.* **2013**, *87*, 12380–12391. [CrossRef] [PubMed]
165. Kozlov, E.N.; Martynova, E.U.; Popenko, V.I.; Schal, C.; Mukha, D.V. Intracellular localization of blattella germanica Densovirus (BgDV1) capsid proteins. *Viruses* **2018**, *10*, 370. [CrossRef]
166. Owens, L. Bioinformatical analysis of nuclear localisation sequences in penaeid densoviruses. *Mar. Genomics* **2013**, *12*, 9–15. [CrossRef] [PubMed]
167. Xu, P.; Yuan, H.; Yang, X.; Graham, R.I.; Liu, K.; Wu, K. Structural proteins of helicoverpa armigera Densovirus 2 enhance transcription of viral genes through transactivation. *Arch. Virol.* **2017**, *162*, 1745–1750. [CrossRef] [PubMed]
168. Aydemir, F.; Salganik, M.; Resztak, J.; Singh, J.; Bennett, A.; Agbandje-McKenna, M.; Muzyczka, N. Mutants at the 2-fold interface of adeno-associated virus type 2 (AAV2) structural proteins suggest a role in viral transcription for aav capsids. *J. Virol.* **2016**, *90*, 7196–7204. [CrossRef] [PubMed]
169. McKenna, R.; Olson, N.H.; Chipman, P.R.; Baker, T.S.; Booth, T.F.; Christensen, J.; Aasted, B.; Fox, J.M.; Bloom, M.E.; Wolfinbarger, J.B.; et al. Three-dimensional structure of aleutian mink disease parvovirus: Implications for disease pathogenicity. *J. Virol.* **1999**, *73*, 6882–6891.

viruses

MDPI

Article

Adeno-Associated Virus VP1u Exhibits Protease Activity

Justin J. Kurian, Renuk Lakshmanan, William M. Chmely, Joshua A. Hull, Jennifer C. Yu, Antonette Bennett, Robert McKenna and Mavis Agbandje-McKenna *

Department of Biochemistry and Molecular Biology, Center for Structural Biology, The McKnight Brain Institute, University of Florida, Gainesville, FL 32610, USA; justinkurian@ufl.edu (J.J.K.); renuk@ufl.edu (R.L.); wchmely0812@ufl.edu (W.M.C.); the.hegemon@ufl.edu (J.A.H.); jennifer.yu@ufl.edu (J.C.Y.); dendena@ufl.edu (A.B.); rmckenna@ufl.edu (R.M.)

* Correspondence: mckenna@ufl.edu; Tel.: +1-352-294-8393

Received: 27 March 2019; Accepted: 19 April 2019; Published: 29 April 2019

Abstract: Adeno-associated viruses (AAVs) are being developed for gene delivery applications, with more than 100 ongoing clinical trials aimed at the treatment of monogenic diseases. In this study, the unique N-terminus of AAV capsid viral protein 1 (VP1u), containing a canonical group XIII PLA_2 enzyme domain, was observed to also exhibit proteolytic activity. This protease activity can target casein and gelatin, two standard substrates used for testing protease function but does not self-cleave in the context of the capsid or target globular proteins, for example, bovine serum albumin (BSA). However, heated BSA is susceptible to VP1u-mediated cleavage, suggesting that disordered proteins are substrates for this protease function. The protease activity is partially inhibited by divalent cation chelators ethylenediaminetetraacetic acid (EDTA) and ethylene-bis(oxyethylenenitrilo)tetraacetic acid (EGTA), and human alpha-2-macroglobulin (A2M), a non-specific protease inhibitor. Interestingly, both the bovine pancreatic (group VIIA) and bee venom (group III) PLA_2 enzymes also exhibit protease function against casein. This indicates that PLA_2 groups, including VP1u, have a protease function. Amino acid substitution of the PLA_2 catalytic motif (^{76}HD/AN) in the AAV2 VP1u resulted in attenuation of protease activity, suggesting that the protease and PLA_2 active sites are related. However, the amino acid substitution of histidine H38, which is not involved in PLA_2 function, to alanine, also affects protease activity, suggesting that the active site/mechanism of the PLA_2 and protease function are not identical.

Keywords: Adeno-associated virus; AAV; protease; phospholipase-A_2; PLA_2

1. Introduction

Adeno-associated viruses (AAVs) are members of the non-enveloped, single-stranded DNA packaging *Parvoviridae*. There are 13 non-human primate AAV serotypes, which range from 54 to 99% in capsid protein sequence identity [1,2]. In 2012, the European Medicines Agency approved "Glybera," an AAV1 based capsid for the treatment of lipoprotein lipase deficiency [3] and in 2017 the United States Food and Drug Administration approved "Luxturna", an AAV2 based vector for the treatment of Leber's congenital amaurosis [4]. Currently, there are more than 100 clinical trials using AAV for the treatment of monogenic diseases. The cell/tissue binding and entry properties of the different AAVs guide the choice of serotype used in treatment applications. The AAV capsid is built from three viral proteins (VPs): VP1, VP2 and VP3, which assemble in a 1:1:10 ratio to form the T = 1 capsid consisting of 60 VPs (with approximately 5 VP1, 5 VP2 and 50 VP3) [5]. These VPs are overlapping in sequence, with VP1 containing a unique N-terminus referred to as the VP1-unique (VP1u) region. This VP1u region contains a group XIII phospholipase-A_2 (PLA_2) domain [6] shown to be essential for virus escape from endosomal/lysosomal compartments during trafficking to the nucleus [7,8].

Additional to the PLA_2 activity, protease activity has also been associated with AAV capsids [9]. These studies showed that this protease activity was optimal at pH 7.4, attenuated at the lower pH of 5.5 and inhibited in the presence of a protease inhibitor cocktail. Protease function is common in many DNA and RNA viruses but these enzymatic domains are typically encoded separately from the viral structural proteins [10]. However, a few viral capsids have been shown to exhibit protease function, for example, Sindbis virus, which harbors a chymotrypsin-like serine protease motif [11].

In this study, AAV2 and AAV5 were used to identify the VP region responsible for the protease function, identify inhibitors/substrates and map residues associated with this function. The protease function was shown to reside within the VP1u region of the capsid and to be partially inhibited by metal chelators and the protein inhibitor alpha-2-macroglobulin (A2M). Additionally, the AAV2 protease was observed to have a preference for disordered protein substrates. Significantly, known PLA_2 enzymes, for example, the bovine pancreatic and bee venom PLA_2 enzymes also possess protease function, indicating that PLA_2 domains have additional functional roles not previously reported. Amino acid substitution for residues in the VP1u domain associated with PLA_2 catalysis resulted in impaired protease function and a corresponding decrease in virus transduction, suggesting a mechanistic link between PLA_2 domains and protease activity.

2. Materials and Methods

2.1. AAV2 Plasmid Mutagenesis

The QuikChange Lightning PCR site-directed mutagenesis kit (Agilent, Santa Clara, CA, USA) was utilized to make mutations onto an AAV2 template plasmid conferring ampicillin resistance (pXR2) [12]. Following digestion of template DNA by Dpn-1 enzyme, One Shot™ TOP10 Chemically Competent *E. coli* (Thermo Fisher Scientific, Waltham, MA, USA) were transformed using the PCR mix and incubated for 1 h in an orbital shaker set at 37 °C after the addition of Super Optimal Broth with Catabolite repression (S.O.C.) medium (Thermo Fisher Scientific). The *E. coli* cultures were plated onto LB-Agar containing ampicillin at a concentration of 50 µg/mL and incubated at 37 °C for a minimum of 12 h, followed by selection of individual bacterial colonies for a minimum of 12 h growth at 37 °C in lysogeny broth (LB) medium containing ampicillin at a concentration of 50 µg/mL. Plasmid DNA from these cultures was purified using a QIAprep Spin Miniprep Kit (Qiagen, Hilden, North Rhine-Westphalia, Germany) and mutations were confirmed by Sanger sequencing (Genewiz, South Plainfield, NJ, USA). Larger quantities of plasmid were produced by inoculating 500 mL of LB medium containing ampicillin at a concentration of 50 µg/mL with bacterial glycerol stocks containing plasmids with the desired mutations and growing cultures for a minimum of 12 h at 37 °C. Plasmid DNA for transfection was purified using a PureLink™ HiPure Plasmid Filter Maxiprep Kit (ThermoFisher Scientific). The rAAV2 variants made were ^{76}HD/AN, H95A, H38A, D69A and D97A. AAV2 VP variant VLPs were generated by site directed mutagenesis (Agilent) of the AAV2 plasmid pFBDVPm11 as previously reported [13]. Briefly, the VP1 and VP2 start codons were mutated to GCG to generate AAV2-VP13, AAV2-VP23 and AAV2-VP3 only constructs. The wild-type AAV2, AAV5 and mutant plasmids were used to generate recombinant VLPs in *Sf9* cells via the Bac-to-Bac expression system (Thermo Fisher Scientific) according to the manufacturer's protocol as previously reported [14].

2.2. Production and Purification of rAAV Capsids

HEK293 cells were grown on 15 cm plates in Dulbecco's Modified Eagle's Medium (Sigma-Aldrich, St. Louis, MO, USA) containing 10% *v/v* fetal bovine serum (Sigma-Aldrich) and 1% Antibiotic-Antimycotic (Thermo Fisher Scientific) to a confluency of 80%, followed by transient transfection using the pXR2 or pXR5, pHelper and pTR-UF3-Luc plasmids in an equimolar ratio [15–17], with polyethylamine (PEI) utilized as the transfection reagent. Transfected cells were incubated at 37 °C and 5% CO_2 for 72 h and subsequently harvested. Cells were pelleted by centrifugation at 1590× *g* for 30 min and resuspended in 1× TD buffer (1× PBS with 1 mM $MgCl_2$ and 2.5 mM KCl). Ten percent *w/v* PEG 8000 was added to the supernatant from the cell harvest and incubated at 4 °C for 12 h with mechanical stirring to precipitate virus. The PEG 8000-supernatant mix was centrifuged at 14,300× *g* for 90 min to pellet precipitated virus. The resulting supernatant was discarded, and the pellet was resuspended in 1× TD. The concentration of NaCl in the resuspended cell pellet was adjusted to 1 M and the cell pellet was lysed by a series of three freeze-thaw cycles in a liquid nitrogen bath. Following the final freeze cycle, 250 U of Benzonase nuclease (MilliporeSigma, Burlington, MA, USA) was added to both the lysed cell pellet and the resuspended pellet from PEG 8000 precipitation and incubated at 37 °C for 30 min in order to remove any unpackaged DNA on the capsid surface. The pellets were combined and clarified by centrifugation at 12,100× *g*. The supernatant was loaded onto a discontinuous iodixanol (Optiprep–Sigma-Aldrich) density gradient with layers at 15, 25, 40 and 60% as previously described [18] and centrifuged at 350,000× *g* for 1 h at 12 °C. Each gradient tube was collected in 1 mL fractions and analyzed for the presence of packaged DNA by qPCR. Combined fractions of either full (DNA containing) or empty (no DNA) particles were diluted by 10-fold in 1× TD buffer and loaded onto AVB Sepharose columns (GE Healthcare Life Sciences, Marlborough, MA, USA) at a rate of 1 mL/min. Columns were washed with 10 mL of 1× TD buffer at a rate of 1 mL/min, followed by elution with 0.1 M Glycine-HCl at pH 2.7 fractionated into 500 µL fractions. Each fraction was immediately combined with 100 µL of 1 M Tris buffer at pH 10.0 to neutralize the acidic elution buffer conditions. Peak fractions, as indicated by UV absorbance at 280 nm, were combined and buffer exchanged three times into buffer containing 20 mM HEPES, 20 mM MES, 20 mM NaAc, 150 mM NaCl using an Apollo 7 mL 150 kDa molecular weight cutoff centrifugal concentrator (Orbital Biosciences, Topsfield, MA, USA). The final buffer exchange cycle used 20 mM HEPES, 20 mM MES, 20 mM NaAc, 150 mM NaCl and 5 mM $CaCl_2$ (Universal Buffer) [19] and stored at 4 °C after assessing concentration and purity via sodium dodecyl sulfate–polyacrylamide gel electrophoresis (SDS-PAGE).

2.3. Production and Purification of AAV Virus-Like Particles (VLPs)

Infected cells were harvested at 72 h, resuspended in 1× TD, lysed by three freeze-thaw cycles with Benzonase nuclease (MilliporeSigma) treatment after the third freeze-thaw cycle as described above for rAAV2 samples. The supernatant was treated with 10% PEG 8000 and precipitated VLPs were harvested by centrifugation of the PEG-supernatant mixture at 14,300× *g* and the precipitate resuspended in 1× TD, followed by Benzonase treatment as above. The lysed cells and resuspended PEG precipitated capsids from the supernatant were combined and clarified via centrifugation at 12,100× *g*. The clarified lysate was loaded onto a discontinuous iodixanol gradient (15, 25, 40 and 60%) and centrifuged at 350,000× *g* for 1 h at 12 °C. Following ultracentrifugation, the 40 and 40/25 interface (containing the VLPs) were collected and diluted in a 20 mM Tris, 15 mM NaCl buffer (pH 8.5). The combined fractions were loaded onto a HiTrap Q XL column (GE Healthcare Life Sciences) and eluted with buffer containing 20 mM Tris-HCl, 500 mM NaCl (pH 8.5). Peak fractions were combined and concentrated using an Apollo 150 kDa MW cutoff centrifugal concentrator (Orbital Biosciences) and buffer-exchanged into Universal Buffer. Samples of wild type (wt) AAV2 and AAV5 empty capsids produced in HEK293 cells were also purified by iodixanol centrifugation, the 40 and 40/25 interface collected, further purified by ion-exchange chromatography and dialyzed into Universal Buffer at pH 7.4, as per the protocol described for the VLPs. All samples were stored at 4 °C prior to use.

2.4. Negative-Stain Transmission Electron Microscopy

The integrity of all purified virus samples was confirmed using transmission electron microscopy. For each sample, 2 µL of purified virus was applied to carbon-coated copper grids (Electron Microscopy Sciences, Hatfield, PA, USA) for 2 min followed by wicking of excess buffer with filter paper (GE Healthcare Life Sciences). Grids were washed with 10 µL of filtered water, excess liquid wicked off and then stained with 10 µL 1% uranyl acetate for 10 s. Stain was removed with filter paper and grids were imaged on a 120 keV Tecnai Spirit (Thermo Fisher Scientific).

2.5. Substrate Preparation and Protease Assays

Casein substrate (Sigma-Aldrich) was prepared by dissolving 50 mg of casein powder in 5 mL 1 M NaOH and dilution of the mixture with filtered dH_2O to a final volume of 50 mL. Following complete solubilization, the casein was dialyzed against 4 L of Universal Buffer prepared at pH 7.4. Following the final dialysis step, the casein was filtered using a 2 μm filter and stored at 4 °C until used. Gelatin substrate (Sigma-Aldrich) was prepared by reconstitution in filtered deionized water and mixing at 37 °C until solubilized, followed by storage at 4 °C. Several protein samples were purchased and reconstituted in filtered dH_2O prior to use in protease assays: bee venom PLA_2, bovine pancreatic PLA_2, A2M (Sigma-Aldrich) and trypsin (Thermo Fisher Scientific). Bovine serum albumin (BSA) was also purchased (Thermo Fisher Scientific), reconstituted in filtered dH_2O and incubated at 4 °C (native BSA) or at 100 °C for 30 min (heated BSA), followed by incubation at 4 °C for at least 1 h prior to further use. Protease assays were conducted by measuring breakdown of a substrate by SDS-PAGE analysis of samples incubated at 37 °C for specified time points. Protease inhibition studies used either an inhibitor cocktail (Pierce Protease Mini Tablets with and without EDTA), EDTA/EGTA or A2M that was added prior to assay initiation. Metal chelation inhibition assays used EDTA or EGTA at concentrations of either 4 mM or 100 mM EDTA in presence of AAV2 capsids at a concentration of 46 nM and 5 μg total amount of casein substrate. A2M inhibition studies used A2M at a concentration of 460 nM, AAV2 capsids at 46 nM and 5 μg total amount of casein substrate. Protease assays with BSA used 5 μg of native BSA (N-BSA) or heated BSA (H-BSA) in conjunction with AAV2 capsids at 15 nM or a trypsin control at 22 μM. In protease assays comparing different PLA_2 enzymes, bee venom PLA_2, bovine pancreatic PLA_2 and bovine serum albumin (BSA) were at a concentration of 5 μM and AAV2 capsids were at a concentration of 15 nM. 2.5 μg of casein substrate was present in each reaction. Protease assays comparing wt AAV2 to VP1u variant capsids utilized virus samples at 15 nM and total of 2.5 μg casein per reaction. Quantitation of substrate degradation was performed using gel densitometry with the Image Studio Lite software (Li-COR Biosciences, Lincoln, Nebraska, USA) and statistical significance was determined via single factor ANOVA analysis, with annotation conventions assigned per the following: ns ($p > 0.05$), * ($p \leq 0.05$), ** ($p \leq 0.01$), *** ($p \leq 0.001$), **** ($p \leq 0.0001$). Error bars on all figures represent standard error of the mean. Protease assays with AAV5 samples (at a concentration of 80 nM) were conducted using the Pierce Colorimetric Protease Assay Kit (Thermo Fisher Scientific) in accordance with manufacturer protocols; the lyophilized succinylated casein substrate was reconstituted in Universal Buffer at pH 7.4 or 5.5, instead of the supplied borate assay buffer. All experiments with quantification and statistical analysis applied were performed in triplicate.

2.6. PLA_2 Assays

PLA_2 activity of wt AAV2 and variant viruses (30 nM) were assessed using a $sPLA_2$ assay kit (Cayman Chemical, Ann Arbor, MI, USA) in accordance with the manufacturer's protocol. The assay plate was incubated at 37 °C for 72 h and absorbance readings at 414 nm were recorded and statistical significance was determined via single factor ANOVA analysis, with annotation conventions assigned per the following: ns ($p > 0.05$), * ($p \leq 0.05$), ** ($p \leq 0.01$), *** ($p \leq 0.001$), **** ($p \leq 0.0001$). Error bars on all graphs represent standard error of the mean. This assay was conducted at pH 8.0, the condition provided in the kit.

2.7. Cellular Transduction Assays

HEK293 cells were seeded in a 96-well plate and grown to 50% confluency (2.5×10^4 cells/well) at 37 °C and 5% CO_2. Media was removed from wells and virus added at a multiplicity of infection (MOI) of 10^4 in a volume of 30 μL (containing virus sample plus serum-free DMEM). Virus sample titer was determined by quantitative PCR as previously described [20]. For assays with A2M, 10 μg of A2M was incubated with 2.5×10^8 viral genomes (vg) of AAV2 for 24 h at either 4 or 37 °C. Plate was incubated for 30 min at 37 °C and 5% CO_2, followed by addition of 70 µL of DMEM containing 10% fetal bovine serum and 1% Antibiotic-Antimycotic. Plate was further incubated at 37 °C and 5% CO_2 for 48 h and luciferase expression was determined using a Luciferase Assay System (Promega, Madison, WI, USA). Prior to acquisition of luciferase activity, each well on the plate was gently washed three times with 50 µL of 1× PBS followed by cell lysis with 50 µL of a 1× preparation of the supplied 5× lysis buffer. Cell lysis proceeded for 20 min at room temperature, followed by transfer of 30 µL of lysate from each well into a new 96-well plate with opaque housing between individual wells (suitable for the determination of sample luminescence). Thirty microliters of luciferase assay reagent was added to each well and luminescence from each sample was acquired with a Synergy HTX Multi-Mode plate reader (BioTek, Winooski, VT, USA), and statistical significance was determined via single factor ANOVA analysis, with annotation conventions assigned per the following: ns ($p > 0.05$), * ($p \leq 0.05$), ** ($p \leq 0.01$), *** ($p \leq 0.001$), **** ($p \leq 0.0001$). Error bars on all graphs represent standard error of the mean.

2.8. Structural Modeling and Sequence Alignments

Structural models of the AAV2 VP1u (137 amino acids) and AAV5 VP1u (136 amino acids) domain were generated using the RaptorX protein prediction server [21]. Crystal structures of bee venom PLA_2, bovine PLA_2 and human $sPLA_2$ were accessed and downloaded from RCSB PDB (PDB IDs: 1POC, 1UNE and 1KQU, respectively). Images were rendered using UCSF Chimera [22] and RMSD values calculated using PyMOL [23]. Sequence alignments were performed using the Clustal Omega webserver [24].

3. Results and Discussion

3.1. AAV Protease Function Is VP1u Dependent, Active at Physiological pH, Calcium Enhanced and Inhibited by a Protein Protease Inhibitor

The protease activity associated with AAV serotypes has been previously reported [9]. Thus, a primary goal of this study was to locate and confirm the region within the VPs or capsid responsible for this function. Protease assays with wt AAV5 capsids containing all three VPs, VP1, VP2 and VP3 or only VP2 and VP3 showed that capsids missing VP1 had no protease activity at pH 7.4 (Figure 1A). In addition, protease activity was negligible for VP1, VP3 and VP3 containing capsids at pH 5.5 as previously reported [9] (Figure 1B).

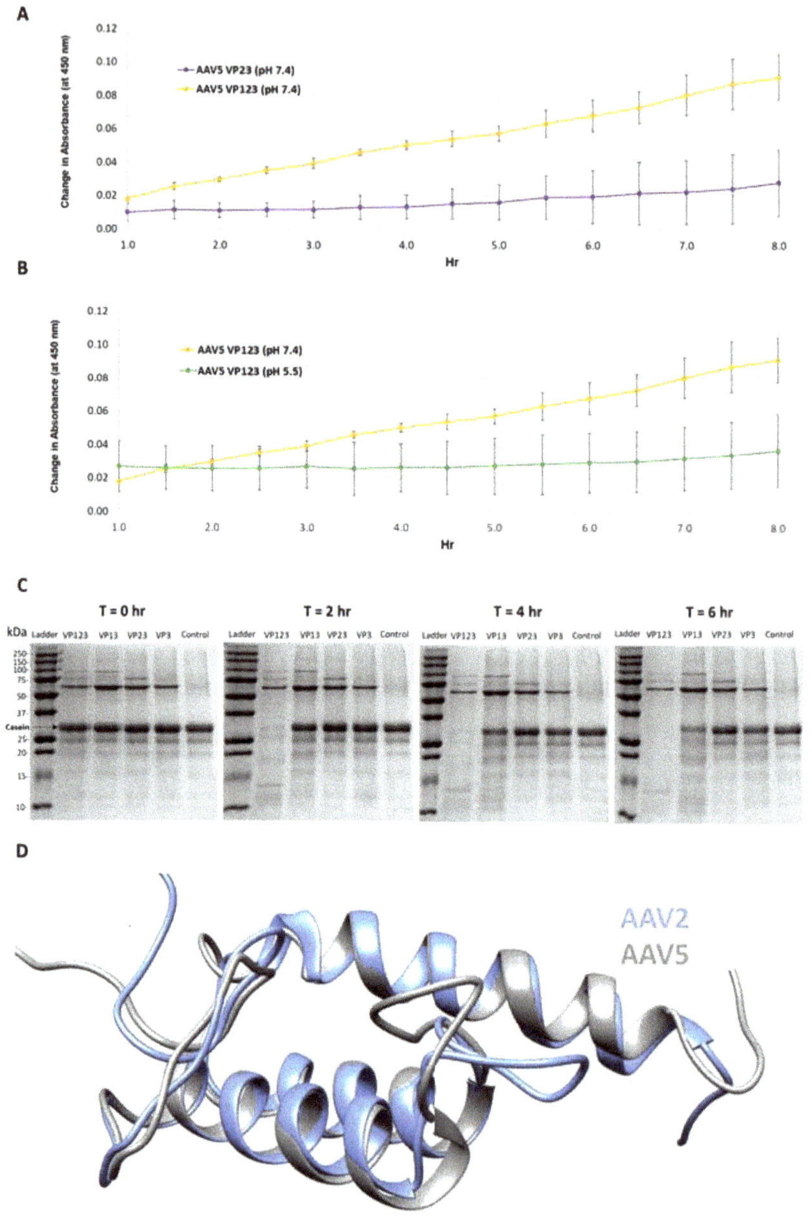

Figure 1. Protease activity is VP1 and neutral pH dependent. (**A**) Colorimetric readout (*y*-axis) over time (hr, *x*-axis) for a casein substrate degradation by AAV5 capsids assembled from VP1, VP2 and VP3 or only VP2 and VP3. (**B**) Same as in (**A**) but for AAV5 VP1, VP2 and VP3 capsids at pH 7.4 and 5.5. (**C**) SDS-PAGE of AAV2 VLPs, containing the VPs shown, incubated with a casein substrate at 37 °C for 2, 4 and 6 h. Observations confirm the need to have VP1 and physiological pH for activity. (**D**) Superposition of AAV2 (blue) and AAV5 (gray) VP1u models. *N*-terminal domains of models with predicted disorder not shown.

Protease assays with AAV2 VLP variants containing different combinations of VP: VP1, VP2 and VP3; VP1 and VP3; VP2 and VP3; and VP3 only, confirmed the need for VP1 for proteolytic activity (Figure 1C). Only the VLPs containing VP1 (lanes 1 and 2 after the molecular weight marker lane) showed the degradation of the casein substrate. The requirement of VP1 and hence VP1u in both AAV2 and AAV5 for the observed protease activity suggests that this domain shares sequence and structure similarity between the viruses (Figure 1D). Consistently, they share 68% amino acid identity and the 3D models predicted for ordered regions (residues 48–137 in AAV2 and 47–136 in AAV5), imply a three-helix bundle, with a calculated Cα RMSD of 0.6 Å (Figure 1D). These observations indicate that the VP1u region has a second enzymatic function in addition to the previously described PLA_2 activity [8]. However, the requirement of physiological and not acidic conditions for protease activity (Figure 1B) is in contrast to the PLA_2 activity that requires acidic conditions [25]. This protease function does not appear to act on other capsids or other VP1us in the context of the capsid, because there is no observable reduction in the abundance of the three VPs at the end of the reaction (Figure 1C). This is contrary to the characteristics of other proteases, for example, trypsin, in which the enzyme also eventually becomes its own substrate [26,27]. The current thinking is that VP1u is located in the capsid interior and becomes externalized during the endo/lysosomal pathway to enable the PLA_2 function required for capsid escape en route to the nucleus for genome replication. Significantly, the protease activity within the VP1u occurs without applying an external treatment, for example, heat, to the capsid to "externalize" this VP region as reported to be required for PLA_2 activity in assays outside a cell [28]. This suggests that the VP1u domain is dynamic in its capsid positioning and able to partially externalize for function in the absence of external treatments, including acidic pH and/or increased temperature conditions proposed to induce structural rearrangement of the capsid resulting in VP1u externalization [29–32].

A protease inhibitor cocktail with the divalent cation chelator EDTA was required to inhibit the AAV2 protease function, in addition to the observation that EDTA or EGTA alone reduced activity (Figure 2A,B). Assays with an excess of either of these chelators (100 mM, 10^7-fold molar excess to capsids) only inhibited ~50% of activity after 24 h (Figure 2B). This observation suggests that the catalytic activity can proceed independent of divalent cations. The VP1u of parvoviruses is predicted to have a calcium binding region that is located within residues 45–65 in AAV2 and is essential for PLA_2 activity [8]. A VP1u model predicts calcium bound in a loop adjacent to the PLA_2 active site HDXXY motif (Figure 2C). The prediction is that calcium binding plays a stabilization role for VP1u and therefore its PLA_2 and protease domain, because it lacks the disulfide bond interactions present in other PLA_2 domains [6]. The results suggest that the proteolytic function of the AAV2 VP1u differs in mechanism from its calcium-dependent PLA_2 activity.

The test of the general protease inhibitor, A2M, against AAV2 also resulted in ~50% loss in activity (Figure 3A). For these studies, the A2M was present at a 10-fold molar excess to the AAV2 capsid and achieved levels of inhibition comparable to EDTA/EGTA at 10^7-fold molar excess (Figure 2B). A2M contains a bait region into which enzymes are captured and their function inhibited [33]. A cellular transduction assay, conducted to determine if the inhibition of the proteolytic activity of AAV2 coincides with an effect on infectivity, showed a 5.5- to 7-fold increase in luciferase gene expression level for sample preincubated for 24 h at 37 and 4 °C, respectively (Figure 3B). The 37 and 4 °C treatments recapitulate protease assay and storage conditions, respectively. It is possible that improved cellular internalization of A2M via endocytosis by selective cell surface receptors [34,35] may be responsible for this increase in AAV2 transduction. Alternatively, this increase in transduction may be attributable to enhanced cellular growth by usage of A2M as an energy source similar to the effects of fetal bovine serum [36], thus also resulting in an improved luciferase gene expression. Significantly, the interaction between the serum protein human serum albumin (HSA) and AAVs was reported to increase cell binding and transduction [37]. A similar mechanism may be in effect for the observed increase in transduction for the AAV samples incubated with A2M.

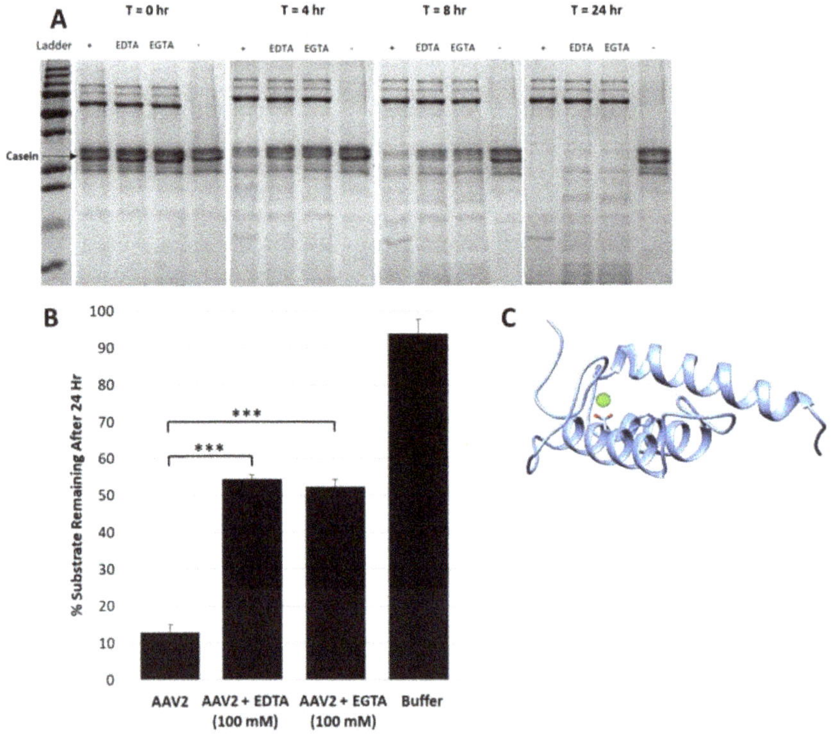

Figure 2. Metal chelators EDTA and EGTA reduce protease activity. (**A**) SDS-PAGE showing casein proteolysis by AAV2 in presence of 4 mM EDTA or EGTA. "+" indicates control with no inhibitor and "-" indicates control with no AAV2, that is, casein alone. The lane with AAV2 only ("+") shows fastest decrease in casein with time. (**B**) Quantification of casein proteolysis by AAV2 in presence of either 100 mM EDTA or 100 mM EGTA. The *y*-axis indicates the amount of remaining protein after 24 h. (**C**) Predicted RaptorX structure model of AAV2 VP1u. PLA_2 catalytic residues H75 and D76 are in orange colored sticks, the predicted site of bound calcium is denoted by a green sphere next to D76. A predicted disordered portion of AAV2 VP1u N-terminal residues is not shown. Statistical significance as indicated by asterisk annotations (*) are described in Material and Methods section.

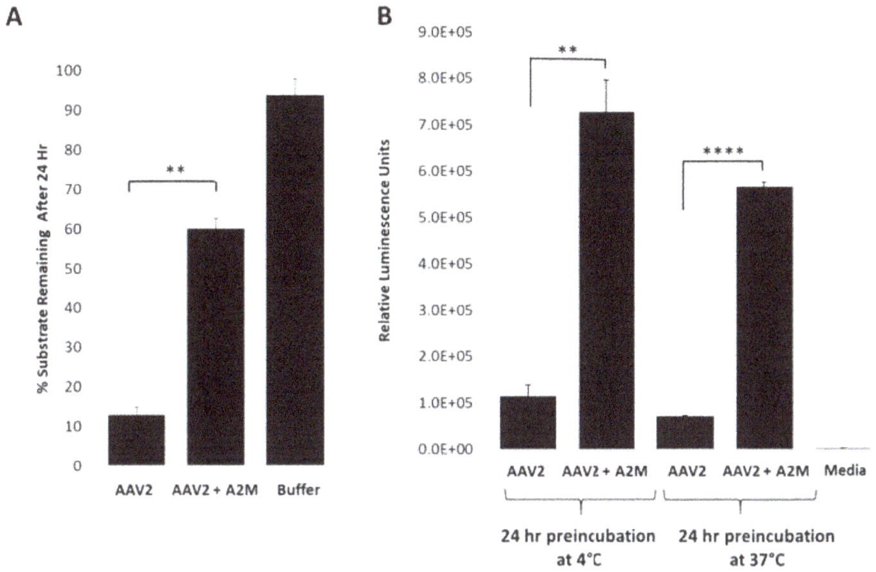

Figure 3. Alpha-2-macroglobulin inhibits protease function and correlates with increased cellular transduction. (**A**) AAV2 protease function inhibition in presence of A2M. The *y*-axis shows the amount of casein substrate remaining after 24 h at the conditions indicated (*x*-axis). (**B**) Luciferase gene expression (*y*-axis in relative luminescence units) for AAV2 with or without A2M (*x*-axis) prior to cell infection. Statistical significance as indicated by asterisk annotations (*) are described in Material and Methods section.

3.2. *The Targets for AAV2 Protease Activity Are Disordered or Unfolded Proteins*

Casein and gelatin substrates used in the protease assays have no defined tertiary structure and are disordered in nature. Casein is micellar in solution [38] and gelatin is a mix of heterogenous peptides generated from collagen hydrolysis [39]. Protease assays with both native and heat-treated BSA were conducted to test the possibility that disordered proteins are the target for the AAV2 VP1u protease function. The heat-treated BSA was degraded by AAV2 VP1u while native BSA was not (Figure 4A,B). In contrast, trypsin, used as a positive control protease, showed equivalent degradation of both the native and heat-treated BSA samples (Figure 4A,B). Prior studies have shown that heating of BSA results in an increase in the percentage of disordered secondary structure elements [40]. Thus, combined with the casein and gelatin substrate data showing degradation (Figures 1 and 4C), these observations suggest that the cellular targets for AAV2 protease activity are either intrinsically disordered proteins and/or proteins that possess unstructured regions.

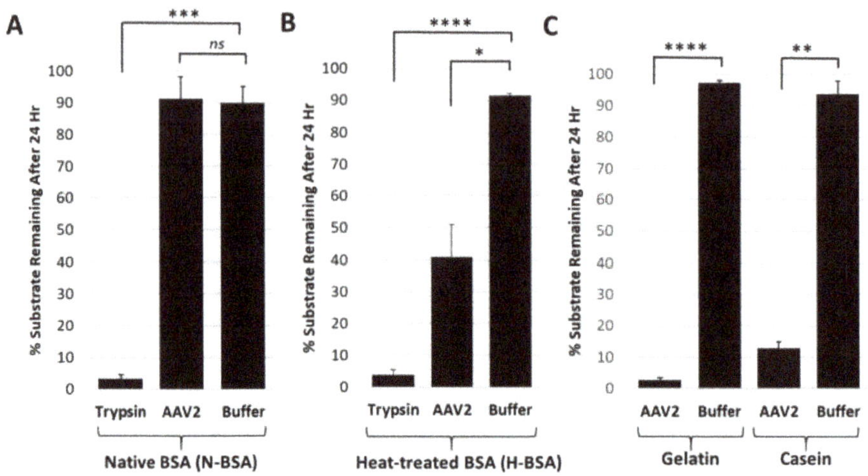

Figure 4. The AAV2 VP1u protease preferentially degrades disordered proteins. (**A**) Quantification of trypsin or AAV2 protease activity against native BSA (N-BSA). The *y*-axis shows the percentage of substrate remaining after 24 h under the conditions indicated in the *x*-axis. (**B**) Quantification of trypsin or AAV2 activity against heated BSA (H-BSA). Axes are as defined in (A). (**C**) Quantification of AAV2 activity against casein and gelatin. Axes are as defined in (A). Data for casein was shown in Figure 2. Statistical significance as indicated by asterisk annotations (*) are described in Material and Methods section.

Many cellular proteins fit the criteria of being intrinsically disordered or containing disordered regions, including transcription factors, cellular signaling proteins and nucleoporins [41]. Nucleoporins possess disordered phenylalanine-glycine repeats [42] and are major components of the nuclear pore complex (NPC). The parvoviruses traffic to the nucleus for genome replication and are predicted to interact with the NPC to facilitate entry [43]. Thus, it is possible that disordered proteins within the NPC are a target of the AAV2 protease function. While regions of the AAV2 VP1u are predicted to be disordered (Figure 2C) [30], as already stated above, self-degradation of VP1 in the context of the capsid is not evident during the 24 h time scale of the assays, possibly because the assembled capsid stabilizes the VP1u domain into a more ordered state compared to the 3D model generated (Figure 2C). In addition, it is possible that the ~5 individual VP1 monomers in the capsid and hence their VP1u, may be too distantly spaced and therefore incapable of inter-monomer cleavage.

3.3. *Protease Function May Be a General Activity for PLA_2 Enzymes*

The AAV protease activity resides within VP1u (Figure 1) that also contains a PLA_2 domain, thus known non-viral PLA_2 enzymes were tested for their ability to degrade proteins. The protease activity assay for two PLA_2 enzymes commonly used as positive controls, bee venom and bovine pancreatic, showed degradation of a casein substrate, albeit at a reduced level, 5- and 2-fold, respectively, compared to AAV2 (Figure 5A). This reduced activity was despite the use of a 50 molar higher concentration of the non-viral enzymes compared to AAV2, suggesting an enhanced activity with a functional yet to be described role in the virus. Interestingly, previous studies performed with human $sPLA_2$ and porcine PLA_2 indicated that these and other PLA_2 enzymes have the ability to cleave apolipoprotein A-1 when the substrate was not bound to lipids [44]. The authors of this study proposed that the proteolytic function observed may also be PLA_2 independent, because metal chelation inhibited PLA_2 function but was not enough to eliminate protease activity, as was also observed for the AAV2 VP1u (Figure 2). The VP1u of AAV2 shares sequence and structural homology with non-viral PLA_2s despite a lack of disulfide bonds (Figure 5B,C). This includes the residues required for PLA_2 activity and calcium binding. The structures include a 3-helix bundle with connecting loops, including the calcium binding loop (Figure 5B). These observations suggest convergent evolution in structure to aid function for these enzymes.

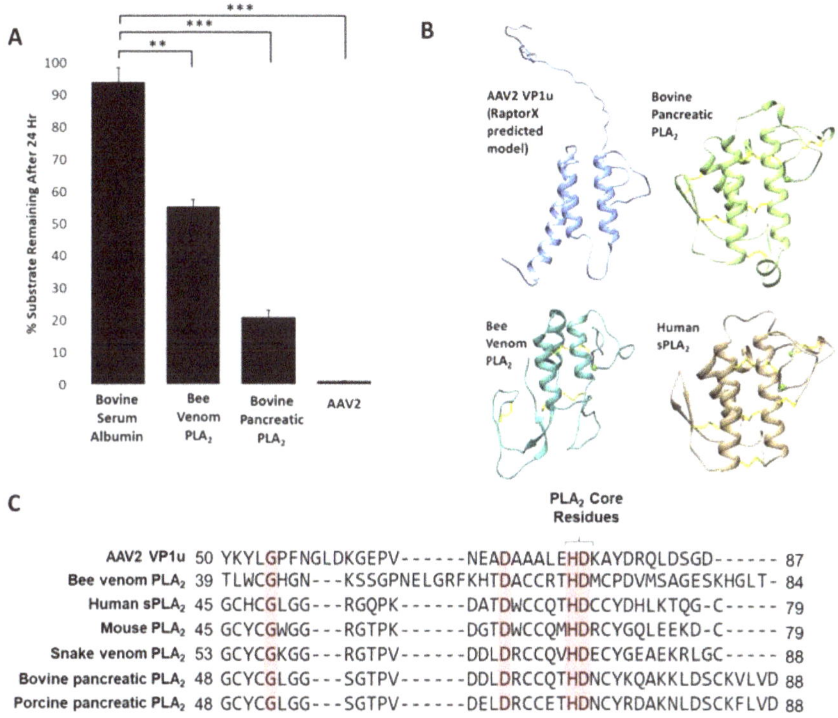

Figure 5. Protease activity is a general property of PLA_2 enzymes: (**A**) Quantification of casein substrate degraded by bee venom PLA_2, bovine pancreatic PLA_2 and AAV2. The y- and x-axes are as described in Figure 4. (**B**) Predicted structure of AAV2 VP1u compared to bee venom PLA_2 (PDB ID: 1POC), bovine pancreatic PLA_2 (PDB ID: 1UNE) and human $sPLA_2$ (PDB ID: 1KQU). (**C**) Partial amino acid sequence alignment of PLA_2 enzymes (conserved residues are highlighted in red). Statistical significance as indicated by asterisk annotations (*) are described in Material and Methods section.

Site directed mutagenesis was used to better characterize the determinants of AAV2 VP1u protease function based on conserved sequence and structural homology with other PLA_2 enzymes (Figure 5B,C and Figure 6A). In addition to the "HD" PLA_2 motif, a sequence alignment highlighted other identical residues, including a glycine residue located in the calcium-binding loop (residue 54) and an aspartic acid (residue D69) (Figure 5C), which was selected for mutagenesis. Previously, it had been shown for AAV2 that deletion of the VP1u calcium-binding loop containing the conserved glycine was detrimental to PLA_2 function [8] but a potential role for the conserved aspartic acid (D69, VP1 AAV2 numbering) has not been delineated. Another residue mutated was D97, conserved in parvovirus PLA_2 domains and previously shown to result in defective transduction when substituted [45]. Finally, the two remaining histidine residues in VP1u, H38 and H95, were modified because histidines are commonly associated with enzyme active sites [46] and often studied for their role in catalysis (Figure 6A).

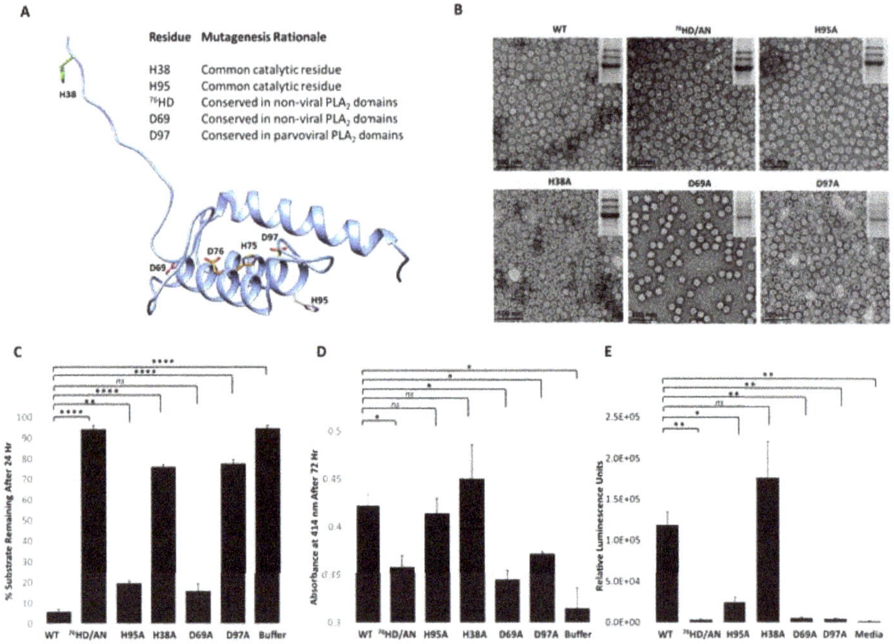

Figure 6. Functional phenotypes of AAV2 VP1u variants. (**A**) Location of amino acid substitutions in the AAV2 VP1u listed and shown in stick representation on a RaptorX model. Residues colored in orange represent those with PLA_2 and protease defects when substituted, pink for defect to PLA_2 only, green for defect to protease only and gray for no defect to either PLA_2 or protease function. (**B**) Negative-stain EMs of wt AAV2 and variant capsids, confirming the capsid assembly of the viruses. SDS-PAGE gel insert shows expression of VP1, VP2 and VP3; (**C**) Quantification of the proteolysis of a casein substrate by wt AAV2 and the variants listed (*x*-axis) after 24 h. The *y*-axis is as described in Figure 2. (**D**) PLA_2 activity of wt AAV2 and variants. The *y*-axis depicts the level of lipid modification after 72 h at pH 8.0 and *x*-axis lists the samples tested. (**E**) Luciferase reporter activity expression (RLU) for wt AAV2 and variants. The *y*-axis depicts the relative luminescence units and *x*-axis lists the samples tested. Statistical significance of asterisk annotations (*) are described in Material and Methods section.

The five VP1u variants made, H38A, D69A, ^{76}HD/AN, H95A and D97A, all express VP1, VP2 and VP3 in the expected ratio of VP1:VP2:VP3 and assemble capsids (Figure 6B). The variants displayed various phenotypes with respect to protease and PLA_2 activity and transduction efficiency. The H38A, ^{76}HD/AN and D97A variants were observed to have an 8–10-fold decrease in protease activity compared to wt AAV2, with the most attenuation associated with the ^{76}HD/AN variant (Figure 6C). While D69A is active for protease function, it along with the ^{76}HD/AN and D97A variants displayed reduced PLA_2 activity and cellular transduction (~50-fold reduction in RLU compared to wt AAV2) (Figure 6D,E). In contrast, the H38A variant, with a protease defect, has no PLA_2 and transduction defect (Figure 6E). Since H38 is not conserved amongst non-viral PLA_2 enzymes (Figure 5C) or with other AAV serotypes, the mode by which it impacts protease function is not readily apparent. Although the sequence region around H38 is predicted to be structurally disordered (Figure 6A), the effect of this residue on protease function suggests that it could be positioned closer to the folded, globular domain with the alpha helices. The D69 residue is conserved between AAV2 and non-viral PLA_2s, and its amino substitution did not affect protease activity but did result in reduced PLA_2 function and reduced cellular transduction compared to wt AAV2. This suggests that D69 is involved in PLA_2 function and may be more critical to regulating this enzymatic function than previously understood (Figure 6E). The aspartic acid in the "HD" motif is predicted to coordinate the calcium ion interacting with the putative calcium binding loop of VP1u (Figure 2C). Thus, the substitution of this key amino-acid could perturb the calcium binding ability of the VP1u, resulting in a more defective protease activity phenotype as is observed for the ^{76}HD/AN variant, possibly due to reduced stability of the protein fold in absence of metal binding. The H95A variant had no effect on protease or PLA_2 function compared to wt AAV2 but did result in a decrease in cellular transduction, indicating that this phenotype is mediated by other factors. Interestingly, H95 is conserved in AAV VP1s but has no structurally analogous equivalent in other non-viral PLA_2s.

The observations with the five variants tested indicate that while a protease function exists in VP1u, there is significant overlap between the residues involved and those enabling the PLA_2 function within this capsid region. However, these residues are not identical and the data show that the PLA_2 function is the most essential for cellular transduction. A His-Asp-Ser catalytic triad is common in a wide variety of proteases but numerous variations to this common motif have also been seen, such as His-His-Ser (cytomegalovirus protease) and Ser-Lys (bacterial type I signal peptidase) [47]. Yet, there are no conserved serine residues among the different PLA_2 enzymes. Thus, it is possible that the AAV2 protease function and those observed for the bee venom and bovine pancreatic PLA_2 utilizes an alternate residue with a polar group as a nucleophile. The confirmation of a mechanistic model for this enzyme in AAV2 is thus awaiting a 3D structure not yet available.

4. Conclusions

This study shows that the VP1u region of AAV2 and AAV5 are responsible for protease function (Figure 1) in addition to the previously reported PLA_2 function. For AAV2, metal chelation with EDTA or EGTA reduced the rate of protease activity but did not eliminate function, providing evidence that metal binding to the VP1u region of AAV2 is not the sole determinant for catalysis but likely plays an ancillary role by maintaining structural integrity of the domain (Figure 2). Reduction of activity by human A2M indicates that this protease function can be partially inhibited by a non-specific protein inhibitor but an effect on the viral life cycle remains to be elucidated, because pre-incubation of AAV2 with A2M increases cellular transduction in HEK293 cells (Figure 3). Observations with the susceptible substrates, for example, native casein, gelatin and heat denatured BSA, suggest that the target for the VP1u protease function are disordered proteins (Figure 4). These exist at different points in the parvovirus life cycle, including during nuclear entry. Interestingly, these studies also show that other PLA_2 enzymes have proteolytic activity against casein, supporting a suggestion that the protease active site in AAV2 VP1u overlaps, in part, with the PLA_2 domain (Figure 5). This suggestion is further supported by the reduction of protease function in the AAV2 PLA_2 catalytic site variant ^{76}HD/AN. However, the protease and PLA_2 sites are not identical because H38, a non-PLA_2 residue affects protease function (Figure 6). Moreover, while the AAV PLA_2 activity is necessary for virion escape during the acidic conditions of the late endosome, the protease function described here operates at neutral pH, suggesting that the PLA_2 and protease functions of the VP1u have different roles in the cellular context. The findings of this study highlight a convergent evolution of the PLA_2 enzyme domain in active site sequence and structure and the acquisition of multiple enzyme functions within a single protein domain.

Author Contributions: Contributions to individual tasks are listed: plasmid mutagenesis; J.J.K. and A.B.; sample production, J.J.K. and J.A.H.; sample purification, J.J.K., J.C.Y. and W.M.C.; substrate preparation, J.J.K. and R.L.; protease assays, J.J.K. and W.M.C.; PLA_2 assays, J.J.K.; cellular transduction assays, J.J.K.; TEM imaging, J.J.K.; statistical analysis, J.J.K.; manuscript preparation, J.J.K., R.L., J.A.H., A.B., R.M. and M.A.-M.; project conception and design, R.M. and M.A.-M.

Funding: This work was supported by the NIH (5R01GM109524-04) and J.J.K. was partially supported by an NIH T32 Basic Microbiology and Infectious Diseases Training Grant (5T32AI007110-34) managed by David Bloom at the University of Florida.

Acknowledgments: The authors thank the University of Florida (UF) Interdisciplinary Center for Biotechnology Research (ICBR) for access to transmission electron microscopes that were utilized for negative-stain data collection. The Tecnai Spirit TEM was provided by UF College of Medicine (COM) and Division of Sponsored Programs

(DSP). The authors also thank Nicholas Muzyczka (University of Florida) for helpful discussions on the protease activities of the AAVs.

Conflicts of Interest: M.A.M. is a SAB member for Voyager Therapeutics, Inc. and AGTC, has a sponsored research agreement with AGTC, Voyager Therapeutics and Intima Biosciences, Inc. and is a consultant for Intima Biosciences, Inc. M.A.M. is a co-founder of StrideBio, Inc. This is a biopharmaceutical company with interest in developing AAV vectors for gene delivery application.

References

1. Gao, G.; Vandenberghe, L.H.; Alvira, M.R.; Lu, Y.; Calcedo, R.; Zhou, X.; Wilson, J.M. Clades of Adeno-Associated Viruses Are Widely Disseminated in Human Tissues. *J. Virol.* **2004**, *78*, 6381–6388. [CrossRef] [PubMed]
2. Van Vliet, K.; Mohiuddin, Y.; McClung, S.; Blouin, V.; Rolling, F.; Moullier, P.; Agbandje-McKenna, M.; Snyder, R.O. Adeno-Associated Virus Capsid Serotype Identification: Analytical Methods Development and Application. *J. Virol. Methods* **2009**, *159*, 167–177. [CrossRef] [PubMed]
3. Ylä-Herttuala, S. Endgame: Glybera Finally Recommended for Approval as the First Gene Therapy Drug in the European Union. *Mol. Ther.* **2012**, *20*, 1831–1832. [CrossRef] [PubMed]
4. Smalley, E. First AAV Gene Therapy Poised for Landmark Approval. *Nat. Biotechnol.* **2017**, *35*, 998–999. [CrossRef]
5. Snijder, J.; van de Waterbeemd, M.; Damoc, E.; Denisov, E.; Grinfeld, D.; Bennett, A.; Agbandje-McKenna, M.; Makarov, A.; Heck, A.J.R. Defining the Stoichiometry and Cargo Load of Viral and Bacterial Nanoparticles by Orbitrap Mass Spectrometry. *J. Am. Chem. Soc.* **2014**, *136*, 7295–7299. [CrossRef] [PubMed]
6. Dennis, E.A.; Cao, J.; Hsu, Y.H.; Magrioti, V.; Kokotos, G. Phospholipase A2 Enzymes: Physical Structure, Biological Function, Disease Implication, Chemical Inhibition and Therapeutic Intervention. *Chem. Rev.* **2011**, *111*, 6130–6185. [CrossRef] [PubMed]
7. Zádori, Z.; Szelei, J.; Lacoste, M.-C.; Li, Y.; Gariépy, S.; Raymond, P.; Allaire, M.; Nabi, I.R.; Tijssen, P. A Viral Phospholipase A2 Is Required for Parvovirus Infectivity. *Dev. Cell* **2001**, *1*, 291–302. [CrossRef]
8. Girod, A.; Wobus, C.E.; Zádori, Z.; Ried, M.; Leike, K.; Tijssen, P.; Kleinschmidt, J.A.; Hallek, M. The VP1 Capsid Protein of Adeno-Associated Virus Type 2 Is Carrying a Phospholipase A2 Domain Required for Virus Infectivity. *J. Gen. Virol.* **2002**, *83*, 973–978. [CrossRef] [PubMed]
9. Salganik, M.; Venkatakrishnan, B.; Bennett, A.; Lins, B.; Yarbrough, J.; Muzyczka, N.; Agbandje-McKenna, M.; McKenna, R. Evidence for pH-Dependent Protease Activity in the Adeno-Associated Virus Capsid. *J. Virol.* **2012**, *86*, 11877–11885. [CrossRef]
10. Tong, L. Viral Proteases. *Chem. Rev.* **2002**, *102*, 4609–4626. [CrossRef]
11. Choi, H.-K.; Tong, L.; Minor, W.; Dumas, P.; Boege, U.; Rossmann, M.G.; Wengler, G. Structure of Sindbis Virus Core Protein Reveals a Chymotrypsin-like Serine Proteinase and the Organization of the Virion. *Nature* **1991**, *354*, 37–43. [CrossRef]
12. Rabinowitz, J.E.; Rolling, F.; Li, C.; Conrath, H.; Xiao, W.; Xiao, X.; Samulski, R.J. Cross-Packaging of a Single Adeno-Associated Virus (AAV) Type 2 Vector Genome into Multiple AAV Serotypes Enables Transduction with Broad Specificity. *J. Virol.* **2002**, *76*, 791–801. [CrossRef]
13. Bennett, A.; Patel, S.; Mietzsch, M.; Jose, A.; Lins-Austin, B.; Yu, J.C.; Bothner, B.; McKenna, R.; Agbandje-McKenna, M. Thermal Stability as a Determinant of AAV Serotype Identity. *Mol. Ther. Methods Clin. Dev.* **2017**, *6*, 171–182. [CrossRef]
14. DiMattia, M.; Govindasamy, L.; Levy, H.C.; Gurda-Whitaker, B.; Kalina, A.; Kohlbrenner, E.; Chiorini, J.A.; McKenna, R.; Muzyczka, N.; Zolotukhin, S.; et al. Production, Purification, Crystallization and Preliminary X-Ray Structural Studies of Adeno-Associated Virus Serotype 5. *Acta Crystallogr. Sect. F. Struct. Biol. Cryst. Commun.* **2005**, *61*, 917–921. [CrossRef]
15. Xiao, X.; Li, J.; Samulski, R.J. Production of High-Titer Recombinant Adeno-Associated Virus Vectors in the Absence of Helper Adenovirus. *J. Virol.* **1998**, *72*, 2224–2232.
16. Zolotukhin, S.; Potter, M.; Hauswirth, W.W.; Guy, J.; Muzyczka, N. A "Humanized" Green Fluorescent Protein CDNA Adapted for High-Level Expression in Mammalian Cells. *J. Virol.* **1996**, *70*, 4646–4654.
17. Matsushita, T.; Elliger, S.; Elliger, C.; Podsakoff, G.; Villarreal, L.; Kurtzman, G.; Iwaki, Y.; Colosi, P. Adeno-Associated Virus Vectors Can Be Efficiently Produced without Helper Virus. *Gene Ther.* **1998**, *5*, 938–945. [CrossRef]

18. Zolotukhin, S.; Byrne, B.J.; Mason, E.; Zolotukhin, I.; Potter, M.; Chesnut, K.; Summerford, C.; Samulski, R.J.; Muzyczka, N. Recombinant Adeno-Associated Virus Purification Using Novel Methods Improves Infectious Titer and Yield. *Gene Ther.* **1999**, *6*, 973–985. [CrossRef]
19. Brooke, D.; Movahed, N.; Bothner, B. Universal Buffers for Use in Biochemistry and Biophysical Experiments. *AIMS Biophys.* **2015**, *2*, 336–342. [CrossRef]
20. Mietzsch, M.; Grasse, S.; Zurawski, C.; Weger, S.; Bennett, A.; Agbandje-McKenna, M.; Muzyczka, N.; Zolotukhin, S.; Heilbronn, R. OneBac: Platform for Scalable and High-Titer Production of Adeno-Associated Virus Serotype 1–12 Vectors for Gene Therapy. *Hum. Gene Ther.* **2014**, *25*, 212–222. [CrossRef]
21. Källberg, M.; Wang, H.; Wang, S.; Peng, J.; Wang, Z.; Lu, H.; Xu, J. Template-Based Protein Structure Modeling Using the RaptorX Web Server. *Nat. Protoc.* **2012**, *7*, 1511–1522. [CrossRef]
22. Pettersen, E.F.; Goddard, T.D.; Huang, C.C.; Couch, G.S.; Greenblatt, D.M.; Meng, E.C.; Ferrin, T.E. UCSF Chimera–a Visualization System for Exploratory Research and Analysis. *J. Comput. Chem.* **2004**, *25*, 1605–1612. [CrossRef]
23. DeLano, W.L. Pymol: An open-source molecular graphics tool. *CCP4 Newsl. Protein Crystallogr.* **2002**, *40*, 82–92.
24. Sievers, F.; Wilm, A.; Dineen, D.; Gibson, T.J.; Karplus, K.; Li, W.; Lopez, R.; McWilliam, H.; Remmert, M.; Soding, J.; et al. Fast, Scalable Generation of High-Quality Protein Multiple Sequence Alignments Using Clustal Omega. *Mol. Syst. Biol.* **2014**, *7*, 539. [CrossRef]
25. Suikkanen, S.; Antila, M.; Jaatinen, A.; Vihinen-Ranta, M.; Vuento, M. Release of Canine Parvovirus from Endocytic Vesicles. *Virology* **2003**, *316*, 267–280. [CrossRef]
26. Vestling, M.M.; Murphy, C.M.; Fenselau, C. Recognition of Trypsin Autolysis Products by High-Performance Liquid Chromatography and Mass Spectrometry. *Anal. Chem.* **1990**, *62*, 2391–2394. [CrossRef]
27. Vajda, T.; Garai, A. Comparison of the Effect of Calcium(II) and Manganese(II) Ions on Trypsin Autolysis. *J. Inorg. Biochem.* **1981**, *15*, 307–315. [CrossRef]
28. Grieger, J.C.; Johnson, J.S.; Gurda-Whitaker, B.; Agbandje-McKenna, M.; Samulski, R.J. Surface-Exposed Adeno-Associated Virus Vp1-NLS Capsid Fusion Protein Rescues Infectivity of Noninfectious Wild-Type Vp2/Vp3 and Vp3-Only Capsids but Not That of Fivefold Pore Mutant Virions. *J. Virol.* **2007**, *81*, 7833–7843. [CrossRef]
29. Kronenberg, S.; Böttcher, B.; von der Lieth, C.W.; Bleker, S.; Kleinschmidt, J.A. A Conformational Change in the Adeno-Associated Virus Type 2 Capsid Leads to the Exposure of Hidden VP1 N Termini. *J. Virol.* **2005**, *79*, 5296–5303. [CrossRef]
30. Venkatakrishnan, B.; Yarbrough, J.; Domsic, J.; Bennett, A.; Bothner, B.; Kozyreva, O.G.; Samulski, R.J.; Muzyczka, N.; McKenna, R.; Agbandje-McKenna, M. Structure and Dynamics of Adeno-Associated Virus Serotype 1 VP1-Unique N-Terminal Domain and Its Role in Capsid Trafficking. *J. Virol.* **2013**, *87*, 4974–4984. [CrossRef]
31. Nam, H.-J.; Gurda, B.L.; McKenna, R.; Potter, M.; Byrne, B.; Salganik, M.; Muzyczka, N.; Agbandje-McKenna, M. Structural Studies of Adeno-Associated Virus Serotype 8 Capsid Transitions Associated with Endosomal Trafficking. *J. Virol.* **2011**, *85*, 11791–11799. [CrossRef]
32. Canaan, S.; Zádori, Z.; Ghomashchi, F.; Bollinger, J.; Sadilek, M.; Moreau, M.E.; Tijssen, P.; Gelb, M.H. Interfacial Enzymology of Parvovirus Phospholipases A2. *J. Biol. Chem.* **2004**, *279*, 14502–14508. [CrossRef]
33. Gettins, P.G.; Hahn, K.H.; Crews, B.C. Alpha 2-Macroglobulin Bait Region Variants. A Role for the Bait Region in Tetramer Formation. *J. Biol. Chem.* **1995**, *270*, 14160–14167. [CrossRef]
34. Dickson, R.B.; Willingham, M.C.; Pastan, I. Binding and Internalization of 125I-Alpha 2-Macroglobulin by Cultured Fibroblasts. *J. Biol. Chem.* **1981**, *256*, 3454–3459.
35. Ashcom, J.D.; Tiller, S.E.; Dickerson, K.; Cravens, J.L.; Argraves, W.S.; Strickland, D.K. The Human Alpha 2-Macroglobulin Receptor: Identification of a 420-KD Cell Surface Glycoprotein Specific for the Activated Conformation of Alpha 2-Macroglobulin. *J. Cell Biol.* **1990**, *110*, 1041–1048. [CrossRef]
36. van der Valk, J.; Brunner, D.; De Smet, K.; Fex Svenningsen, Å.; Honegger, P.; Knudsen, L.E.; Lindl, T.; Noraberg, J.; Price, A.; Scarino, M.L.; et al. Optimization of Chemically Defined Cell Culture Media – Replacing Fetal Bovine Serum in Mammalian in Vitro Methods. *Toxicol. In Vitro* **2010**, *24*, 1053–1063. [CrossRef]

37. Wang, M.; Sun, J.; Crosby, A.; Woodard, K.; Hirsch, M.L.; Samulski, R.J.; Li, C. Direct Interaction of Human Serum Proteins with AAV Virions to Enhance AAV Transduction: Immediate Impact on Clinical Applications. *Gene Ther.* **2017**, *24*, 49–59. [CrossRef]
38. Horne, D.S. Casein Structure, Self-Assembly and Gelation. *Curr. Opin. Colloid Interface Sci.* **2002**, *7*, 456–461. [CrossRef]
39. Badii, F.; Howell, N.K. Fish Gelatin: Structure, Gelling Properties and Interaction with Egg Albumen Proteins. *Food Hydrocoll.* **2006**, *20*, 630–640. [CrossRef]
40. Takeda, K.; Wada, A.; Yamamoto, K.; Moriyama, Y.; Aoki, K. Conformational Change of Bovine Serum Albumin by Heat Treatment. *J. Protein Chem.* **1989**, *8*, 653–659. [CrossRef]
41. Van der Lee, R.; Buljan, M.; Lang, B.; Weatheritt, R.J.; Daughdrill, G.W.; Dunker, A.K.; Fuxreiter, M.; Gough, J.; Gsponer, J.; Jones, D.T.; et al. Classification of Intrinsically Disordered Regions and Proteins. *Chem. Rev.* **2014**, *114*, 6589–6631. [CrossRef]
42. Denning, D.P.; Patel, S.S.; Uversky, V.; Fink, A.L.; Rexach, M. Disorder in the Nuclear Pore Complex: The FG Repeat Regions of Nucleoporins Are Natively Unfolded. *Proc. Natl. Acad. Sci. USA* **2003**, *100*, 2450–2455. [CrossRef]
43. Porwal, M.; Cohen, S.; Snoussi, K.; Popa-Wagner, R.; Anderson, F.; Dugot-Senant, N.; Wodrich, H.; Dinsart, C.; Kleinschmidt, J.A.; Panté, N.; et al. Parvoviruses Cause Nuclear Envelope Breakdown by Activating Key Enzymes of Mitosis. *PLoS Pathog.* **2013**, *9*, e1003671. [CrossRef]
44. Cavigiolio, G.; Jayaraman, S. Proteolysis of Apolipoprotein A-I by Secretory Phospholipase A_2: A New Link between Inflammation and Atherosclerosis. *J. Biol. Chem.* **2014**, *289*, 10011–10023. [CrossRef]
45. Wu, P.; Xiao, W.; Conlon, T.; Hughes, J.; Agbandje-McKenna, M.; Ferkol, T.; Flotte, T.; Muzyczka, N. Mutational Analysis of the Adeno-Associated Virus Type 2 (AAV2) Capsid Gene and Construction of AAV2 Vectors with Altered Tropism. *J. Virol.* **2000**, *74*, 8635–8647. [CrossRef]
46. Rebek, J. On the Structure of Histidine and Its Role in Enzyme Active Sites. *Struct. Chem.* **1990**, *1*, 129–131. [CrossRef]
47. Ekici, O.D.; Paetzel, M.; Dalbey, R.E. Unconventional Serine Proteases: Variations on the Catalytic Ser/His/Asp Triad Configuration. *Protein Sci.* **2008**, *17*, 2023–2037. [CrossRef]

viruses

MDPI

Article

An Ancient Lineage of Highly Divergent Parvoviruses Infects both Vertebrate and Invertebrate Hosts

Judit J. Pénzes [1,*], William Marciel de Souza [2], Mavis Agbandje-McKenna [1] and Robert J. Gifford [3,*]

1 McKnight Brain Institute and Department of Biochemistry and Molecular Biology, University of Florida, 1149 Newell Dr, Gainesville, FL 32610, USA; mckenna@ufl.edu
2 Virology Research Center, School of Medicine of Ribeirão Preto of the University of São Paulo, Ribeirão Preto, Brazil; wmarciel2@gmail.com
3 Medical Research Council-University of Glasgow Centre for Virus Research, 464 Bearsden Road, Glasgow G61 1QH, UK
* Correspondence: judit.penzes@ufl.edu (J.J.P.); robert.gifford@glasgow.ac.uk (R.J.G.)

Received: 17 April 2019; Accepted: 5 June 2019; Published: 6 June 2019

Abstract: Chapparvoviruses (ChPVs) comprise a divergent, recently identified group of parvoviruses (family *Parvoviridae*), associated with nephropathy in immunocompromised laboratory mice and with prevalence in deep sequencing results of livestock showing diarrhea. Here, we investigate the biological and evolutionary characteristics of ChPVs via comparative in silico analyses, incorporating sequences derived from endogenous parvoviral elements (EPVs) as well as exogenous parvoviruses. We show that ChPVs are an ancient lineage within the *Parvoviridae*, clustering separately from members of both currently established subfamilies. Consistent with this, they exhibit a number of characteristic features, including several putative auxiliary protein-encoding genes, and capsid proteins with no sequence-level homology to those of other parvoviruses. Homology modeling indicates the absence of a β-A strand, normally part of the luminal side of the parvoviral capsid protein core. Our findings demonstrate that the ChPV lineage infects an exceptionally broad range of host species, including both vertebrates and invertebrates. Furthermore, we observe that ChPVs found in fish are more closely related to those from invertebrates than they are to those of amniote vertebrates. This suggests that transmission between distantly related host species may have occurred in the past and that the *Parvoviridae* family can no longer be divided based on host affiliation.

Keywords: chapparvovirus; parvovirus evolution; endogenous viral elements; *Parvoviridae*; densovirus; homology modeling; new viruses

1. Introduction

Parvoviruses (family *Parvoviridae*) are small, non-enveloped viruses with T = 1 icosahedral symmetry and linear, single-stranded DNA (ssDNA) genomes ~4–6 kilobases (kb) in length. The family has historically been divided into two subfamilies, *Parvovirinae* and *Densovirinae*, containing viruses that infect vertebrate and invertebrate hosts, respectively [1]. Despite exhibiting great variation in expression and transcription strategies, they have a relatively conserved overall genome structure: a non-structural (NS) expression cassette is located at the left side of the genome, while the structural viral proteins (VPs) are encoded by the right, and complex, hairpin-like DNA secondary structures are present at both genomic termini [2]. Small satellite proteins and an assembly-activating protein have been discovered as products of open reading frames (ORFs) overlapping the right-hand expression cassette, whereas additional auxiliary protein-encoding ORFs may be positioned between the two major cassettes [3,4].

Numerous novel parvoviruses have been identified in recent years, primarily via approaches based on high throughput sequencing (HTS) [5–11]. In addition, progress in whole genome sequencing of eukaryotes has revealed that sequences derived from parvoviruses occur relatively frequently in animal genomes [12–17]. These endogenous parvoviral elements (EPVs) are derived from the genomes of ancient parvoviruses that were incorporated into the gene pool of ancestral host species. This can presumably occur when infection of a germline cell leads to parvovirus-derived DNA becoming integrated into host chromosomes, and the cell containing the integrated sequences then goes on to develop into a viable organism [18]. Many EPVs are millions of years old, and are genetically "fixed" in the genomes of host species (i.e., all members of the species have the integrated EPV in their genomes). Such ancient EPV sequences are in some ways analogous to "parvovirus fossils", since they preserve information about the ancient parvoviruses that infected ancestral animals.

Among the novel parvovirus groups identified via sequencing, one—provisionally labeled "chapparvovirus"—stands out as being particularly unusual. These viruses, which have been primarily reported via metagenomic sequencing of animal feces, derive their name from an acronym (CHAP), referring to the host groups in which they were first identified (Chiropteran–Avian–Porcine) [15,16,19,20]. Subsequently, several additional chapparvovirus (ChPV) sequences have been reported, including some that were identified in whole genome sequence (WGS) data derived from vertebrates, including reptiles, mammals, and birds [9]. These sequences were picked up by in silico screens designed to detect EPVs. However, since all the ChPV sequences identified in WGS data lack clear evidence of genomic integration, it is likely that they actually derive from infectious ChPV genomes that contaminated WGS samples, rather than from endogenous elements [9].

Until relatively recently, evidence that the ChPVs detected via sequencing actually infected vertebrate hosts has been lacking. However, a recent study has claimed to demonstrate that a ChPV called mouse kidney parvovirus (MKPV) circulates among laboratory mice populations, in which it causes a kidney disease known as inclusion body nephropathy [21]. These findings, as well as their frequent presence in the feces of livestock, imply that ChPVs might be pathogenic and represent a potential disease threat to wildlife and domestic species. In addition, they have raised interest in the use of these viruses as experimental tools. In this study, we perform a comparative analysis of ChPV genomes and ChPV-derived EPVs, revealing new insights into the biology and evolution of this poorly understood group.

2. Materials and Methods

2.1. Genome Screening and Sequence Analysis

All WGS data were obtained from the National Center for Biotechnology Information (NCBI) genomes resource. We obtained all available genomes for eumetazoan animals as of October 2018. These data were screened for ChPV sequences using the database-integrated genome screening (DIGS) tool [22]. ChPV sequences were characterized and annotated using Artemis Genome Browser [23]. The NCBI Basic Local Alignment Search Tool (BLAST) program and its local executables were used to compare sequences and investigate predicted viral ORFs. To determine potential homology and sequence similarity, even between previously undescribed ORFs, we constructed a local database, including all ORFs exceeding 100 amino acids (aa) in length, derived from all the exogenous and endogenous sequences incorporated in this study, and used the local BLAST P and X algorithms to conduct similarity searches in it. Two ORFs were accepted as homologous if they gave a significant hit, in the case of an expectation value threshold of 1.

Promoters were predicted using the neural network-based promoter prediction server of the Berkeley Drosophila Genome Project and further verified by the Promoter Prediction 2.0 server [24,25]. Splice sites were also detected using the neural network-based applications of the Berkeley Drosophila Genome project and SplicePort [25,26]. Polyadenylation signals were predicted by the SoftBerry application POLYAH [27]. To verify that these applications were be capable of detecting the above-mentioned chapparvoviral transcription elements we ran MKPV through the workflow pipeline.

2.2. Phylogenetic Reconstructions

The derived aa sequences of ORFs disclosing homology to parvoviral NS1 proteins were aligned with at least five representatives of each parvovirus genus, or with one representative of each species of a given genus in cases where the number of species did not exceed five. To ensure the correct identification of the tripartite helicase domain, structural data was also incorporated into alignment construction using T-coffee Expresso [28] and Muscle [29]. The full-length NS1 derived aa sequences of the ChPV clade were aligned by Muscle and the M-coffee algorithm of T-coffee [30]. Model selection was carried out by ProTest and the substitution models RtREV+I+G, in cases of helicase-based inferences, and LG+I+G, for the complete chapparvoviral NS1 tree, were predicted to be the most suitable, based on both Akaike and Bayes information criteria. The PhyML-3.1 program was used to infer a maximum likelihood phylogenetic tree, with 100 bootstrap iterations [31], based on a guide tree previously constructed by the ProtDist and Fitch programs of the Phylip 3.697 package [32].

2.3. Homology Modeling and DNA Structure Prediction

Structural homology was detected by applying the pGenTHREADER and pDomTHREADER algorithms of the PSIPRED Protein Sequence Analysis Workbench [33]. The same workbench was used to map disordered regions using DISOPRED3 and to predict the secondary structure of the complete chapparvoviral VP protein sequences via the PSIPRED algorithm. The selected PDB structures were applied as templates for homology modeling, carried out by the I-TASSER Standalone Package v.5.1 [34]. To guide the modeling, the predicted secondary structures were applied as a restriction. The Oligomer Generator feature of the Viper web database (http://viperdb.scripps.edu/) [35] was used to construct 60-mers of the acquired putative VP monomer structures. Surface images of the capsids were rendered using the PyMOL Molecular Graphics System [36]. Capsid surface maps and VP monomer superposition were carried out by UCSF Chimera [37]. To predict the presence of potential DNA secondary structural elements, the DNA Folding Form algorithm of the mFold web server was utilized [38].

3. Results

3.1. Comparative Analysis of Previously Reported ChPV Genomes

We performed a comparative analysis of nine previously sequenced ChPV genomes so that we could: (i) identify genome features that characterize these viruses, and (ii) make inferences about aspects of ChPV biology and evolution (Figure 1). ChPV genomes tend toward the shorter end of the parvovirus genome size range (~4 kb). They encode a relatively long *rep* gene, and a relatively short *cap* gene. The *rep* gene product (NS) is ~650 amino acids (aa) in length, with the longest example being the 668 aa protein encoded by *Desmodus rotondus* ChPV (DrChPV). ChPV NS proteins contain ATPase and helicase domains, but these are the only regions exhibiting clear homology to those found in other parvovirus groups (Figure 1). Overlapping the *rep*, a predicted minor ORF, ~220 aa in length, is located in a position equivalent to that of the nucleoprotein (NP) ORF found in certain *Parvovirinae* genera (i.e., *Ave-* and *Bocaparvovirus*). However, it should be noted that the protein encoded by this gene—which we tentatively refer to as NP—exhibits no significant similarity to any other parvovirus NP proteins. Secondary structure predictions indicate that the vast majority of the NP protein has a helical structure, with numerous potential phosphorylation sites as well as a potentially protein-binding disordered N-terminus (Figure S1). Together, these observations suggest a non-structural function. The NP ORF, although of similar length in all genomes, has no canonical start codon in the case of porcine parvovirus 7 (PPV7) and simian parvo-like virus 3 (SiPV3). This would imply that in these viruses, splicing of the *rep* RNA is required for expression of the NP protein.

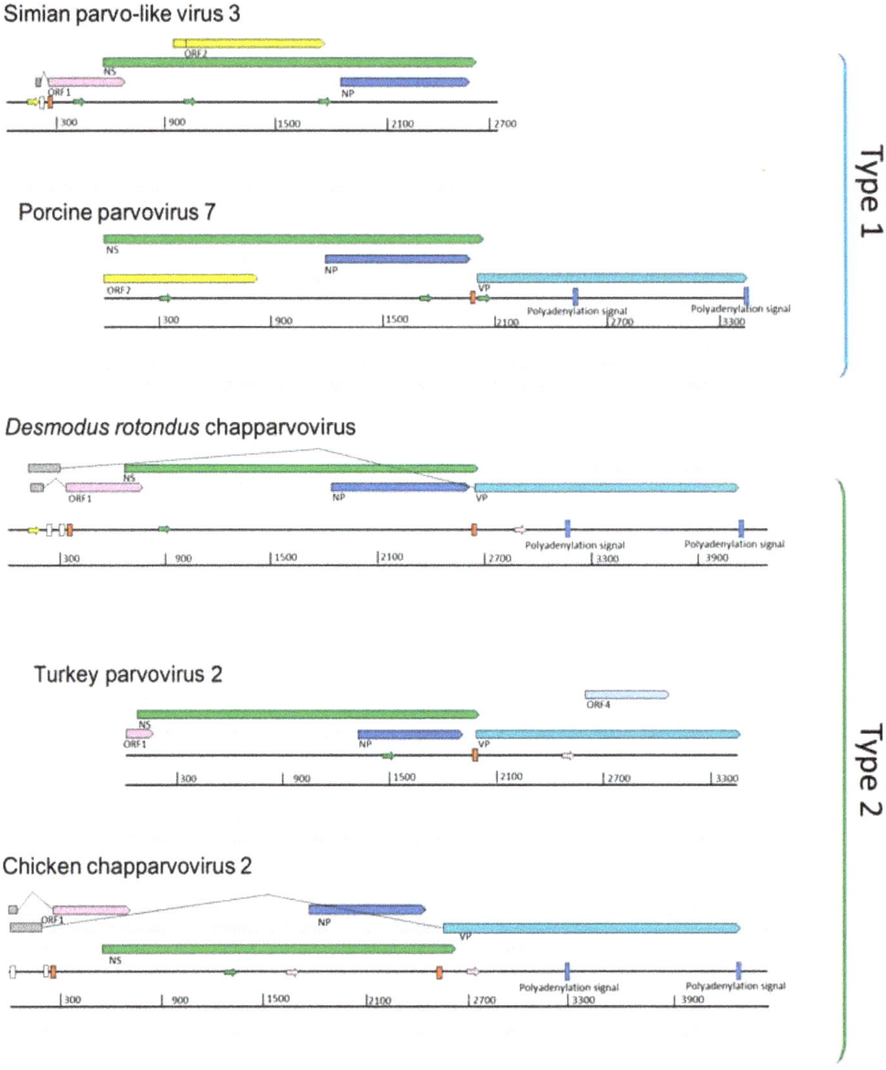

Figure 1. Representative complete coding sequence and partial genome organizations of the two distinct types of exogenous amniote chapparvoviruses (ChPVs). Open reading frames (ORFs) are represented by rectangular arrows, colored according to homology. Splice donor sites are marked by white-colored bars, acceptor sites by orange-colored bars. Blue-colored bars show predicted polyadenylation signals. Small arrows show predicted promoters and are colored according to prediction score (>0.95 = green; 0.9–0.95 = pink: <0.9 = yellow). Grey boxes indicate regions inferred to be transcribed but not translated. Note: ORF4 is unique to turkey parvovirus and is not found in other avian type 2 ChPVs, such as chicken ChPV2.

All ChPVs appear to be characterized by relatively short VP ORFs of 450–500 aa. VP proteins are typically ~650–820 aa in most other parvoviruses, the exception being the brevi- and penstyldensoviruses, which encode an even shorter VP. Notably, the VP proteins encoded by ChPVs share no significant sequence similarity with those of other parvoviruses. In all ChPVs, the first methionine of the VP ORF is preceded by a potential coding sequence, and in all published ChPV sequences, a canonical splice acceptor site is located immediately upstream. Possibly, the VP ORF encodes only the major capsid protein, and there may be other versions of this VP protein that are elongated at the N-terminus, and are incorporated into the capsid at a lower copy number, as found in the majority of parvoviruses [1]. However, the only splice donor sites we identified are located relatively far upstream. In MKPV, however, there are two large introns present, putting these upstream exons in frame with the VP encoding exon.

In addition to their fundamental NS–NP–VP genome organization, ChPVs encode various additional small ORFs. ORF1 is predicted to encode a small protein of approximately 15 kDa that contains a putative nuclear localization signal (NLS) in its C-terminal region. ORF1, which partially overlaps the N-terminal region of NS, is present in all genomes except PPV7. However, since the PPV7 genome also lacks the corresponding region of NS, this likely reflects a 5′ truncated genome sequence. The same is the case for turkey parvovirus (TPV2), although the C-terminal encoding region of the putative ORF1 protein could be revealed.

A second additional, putative ORF is present in only two of the ChPVs examined here: PPV7 and simian parvo-like virus 3. This ORF, referred to as ORF2, is located downstream from ORF1 in a position completely overlapping the NS ORF. The TPV2 genome also contains a unique, presumably genome-specific additional ORF (ORF4) that overlaps the C-term encoding region of VP, and may encode a predicted 17 kDa protein (Figure 1). Interestingly, this ORF was absent from the other, closely-related avian ChPVs.

Analysis in silico revealed at least three potential promoters in ChPV genomes. One of these is conserved throughout the clade, and is located upstream of all coding features, indicating that it likely drives early expression of virus genes. Moreover, its presence has been confirmed in MKPV by sequencing of cDNA derived from infected mouse tissue. None of the other potential promoters proved to be functional in the case of MKPV. The MKPV transcriptome includes three transcripts confirmed to undergo splicing. Of these, however, only the one with the shortest intron could be confidently predicted in all GenBank sequences with a complete or near complete coding region (Figure 1). Interestingly, DrChPV (similar to rodent-derived ChPVs) and chicken ChPV2 (similar to TPV2, but with a more complete 5′ end) were both predicted to possess the large intron of the putative VP transcript, and therefore appear to utilize a strikingly MKPV-like transcription mechanism, despite missing an acceptor site upstream of the NP start codon. In all ChPVs examined, with the exception of the 3′ truncated entries, we identified two potential polyadenylation signals in positions equivalent to those found in MKPV [21]. This implies that the polyadenylation strategy is a conserved feature of ChPV transcription.

3.2. Identification and Characterization of Novel ChPVs and ChPV-Derived EPVs

We systematically screened published WGS data and identified a total of 15 previously unreported ChPV-derived DNA sequences. Two were identified in vertebrates and 13 in invertebrates (Table 1). The majority of the novel ChPV sequences identified in our screen were derived from the non-structural protein gene (*rep*), but we identified complete sequences derived from both the *rep* and capsid (*cap*) genes in two species: the Gulf pipefish (*Syngnathus scovelli*) and the black widow spider (*Latrodectus hesperus*). Partial *cap* genes were identified in the scarab beetle (*Oryctes borbonicus*), taurus scarab (*Onthophagus taurus*), and Chinese golden scorpion (*Mesobuthus martensii*) elements (Figure 2).

We identified two chapparvoviral sequences in WGS assemblies of syngnathid fish (family Syngnathidae), including the tiger tail seahorse (*Hippocampus comes*) and the Gulf pipefish (*Syngnathus scovelli*). The pipefish sequence occurs in a relatively short scaffold (4002 nt) that is entirely comprised of viral sequence, displaying truncated, but nonetheless detectable, J-shaped terminal hairpin-like structures (Figure S2). This suggests it likely represents a virus contaminant, as suspected for other ChPV sequences recovered from vertebrate WGS data [9]. The virus from which this sequence was presumably derived was designated *Syngnathus scovelli* ChPV (ScChPV).

The seahorse and invertebrate sequences identified in our screen clearly represented EPVs (see below). However, the pipefish sequence lacked flanking genomic sequences and appeared to derive from an exogenous virus, encompassed by truncated hairpin-like secondary structure repeats (Figure S2). None of the ChPV-derived EPVs we identified shared homologous flanking sequences, indicating that each derives from a distinct germline incorporation event.

We identified a total of 13 EPV sequences that disclosed a relatively close phylogenetic relationship to ChPVs. These elements showed varying degrees of degradation. In many cases, only genome fragments were detected (Figure 2), and these usually included multiple nonsense mutations (Table 1). ChPV-derived elements were detected in three major arthropod clades that primarily occupy terrestrial habitats, namely arachnids of Chelicerata, chilopods of Myriapoda, as well as hexapod insects and entognaths.

We used maximum likelihood-based phylogenetic approaches and an alignment spanning the tripartite helicase domain of the NS protein to reconstruct the evolutionary relationships of ChPVs, ChPV-derived EPVs, and previously reported parvoviruses (Figure 3). Strikingly, reconstructions indicated that the family *Parvoviridae* consists of four major clades, rather than the two that have historically been recognized [1]. Of these four lineages, one corresponds to the subfamily *Parvovirinae* as in current taxonomic schemes. However, the subfamily *Densovirinae* is split into two clades; one encompassing all ambisense densoviruses along with viruses of the genus *Iteradensovirus* (which have monosense genomes) and the second, referred to here as HBP, containing the *Hepan-*, *Brevi-*, and *Penstyldensovirus* genera. Moreover, a fourth parvovirus lineage was evident, comprised of the ChPVs and ChPV-derived EPVs.

Table 1. Novel ChPV sequences identified in this study.

Host Common Name	Host Scientific Name	Virus/Element Name [a]	Gene Content	Nonsense Mutations [b]
		Vertebrates		
Gulf pipefish	*Syngnathus scovelli*	ScChPV	*rep+cap*	0; 0
Tiger tail seahorse	*Hippocampus comes*	ChPV.1-HipCom	*rep*	2; 2
		Invertebrates		
Black widow spider	*Latrodectus hesperus*	ChPV.2-LatHes	*rep+cap*	4; 1
		ChPV.3-LatHes	*rep+cap*	3; 1
		ChPV.4-LatHes	*rep* *	3; 3
		ChPV.5-LatHes	*rep*	4; 2
Chinese scorpion	*Mesobuthus martensii*	ChPV.6-MesMar	*rep+cap* *	2; 3
European centipede	*Strigamia maritima*	ChPV.7-StrMar	*rep*	2; 3
Northern forcepstail	*Catajapyx aquilonaris*	ChPV.8-CatAqu	*rep*	0; 0
Emerald ash borer	*Agrilus planipennis*	ChPV.9-AgrPla	*rep**	2; 0
Taurus scarab	*Onthophagus taurus*	ChPV.10-OntTau	*rep*	2; 3
		ChPV.11-OntTau	*rep*	0; 0
		ChPV.12-OntTau	*rep*	2; 1
Rhinocerous beetle	*Oryctes borbonicus*	ChPV.13-OryBor	*rep*	2; 0
		ChPV.14-OryBor	*rep*	0; 0

[a] For sequences that are presumed to derive from viruses, the proposed name of the virus is shown. For endogenous parvoviral elements (EPV) the locus name is given, following the standard nomenclature proposed for endogenous retrovirus (ERV) loci [39], except using the classifier "EPV" in the place of "ERV". The table shows a shortened version of the ID, used in the text of this manuscript, wherein the "EPV" classifier is omitted, and an abbreviated version of the species name is used within the taxonomic component of the ID (derived from the first three letters of each component of the Latin binomial scientific name of the host species). [b] Stop codons; frameshifts. * Asterisks indicate contigs that were truncated within the virus-derived portion of the sequence. Underlined names indicate the presence of the complete ORF.

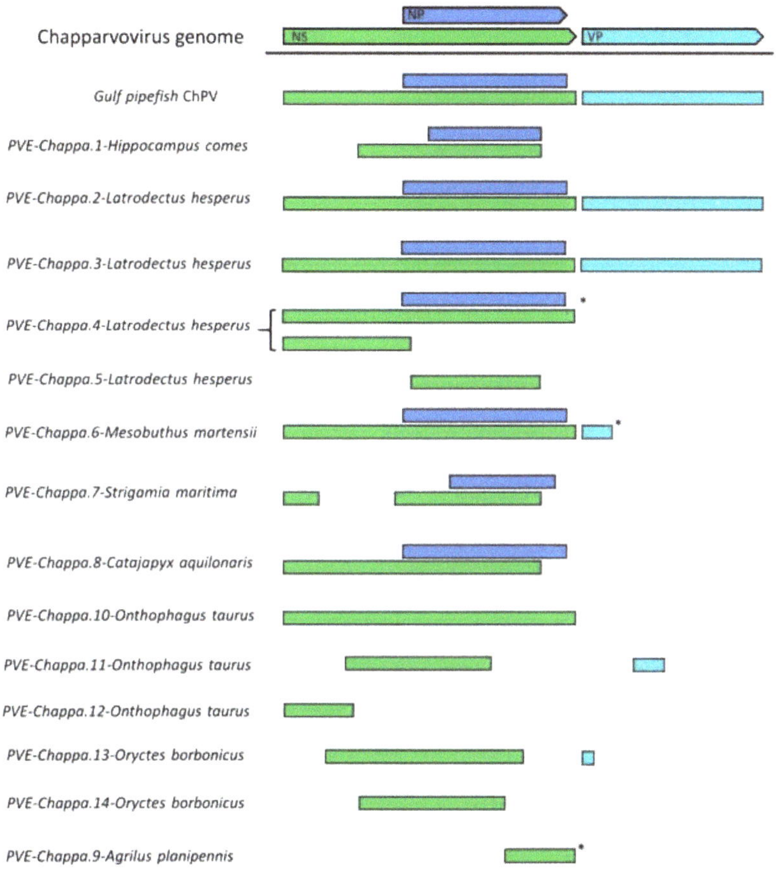

Figure 2. Basic gene content of newly identified chapparvoviruses (ChPVs) and ChPV-derived endogenous parvoviral element (EPV) sequences, shown in relation to a representative ChPV genome (mouse kidney parvovirus). Asterisks indicate contigs that were truncated within the virus-derived portion of the sequence. Abbreviations: non-structural protein (NS); capsid protein (VP); nucleoprotein (NP).

The branching relationships between ChPVs were not fully resolved by phylogenetic analysis of the helicase domain. The putative large non-structural proteins (NS1) of ChPVs displayed a high degree of amino acid variability, particularly toward their N- and C-term. However, a region ~500-aa-long could be aligned reliably throughout all complete and partial entries previously proven to cluster within the ChPV lineage in the case of the NS helicase-based inference. Phylogenies reconstructed from this alignment reveal the ChPV-related viruses to be comprised of three robustly supported monophyletic lineages (Figure 4). One of these includes ChPVs sampled from amniotes (reptiles, birds, and mammals), in which two robustly supported sublineages (labeled type 1 and 2) were observed, corroborating the helicase-based phylogeny. The amniote ChPVs form a sister clade to EPVs found in the arthropod subphyla Chelicerata (arachnids, camel spiders, scorpions, whip scorpions, harvestmen, horseshoe crabs, and kin) and Myriapoda (millipedes, centipedes, and kin) as well as syngnathe fish. A third lineage was also observed, containing sequences from the arthropod subphylum Hexapoda (insects, springtail, and forcepstail). Within this lineage, the beetle EPVs formed a well-supported monophyletic clade.

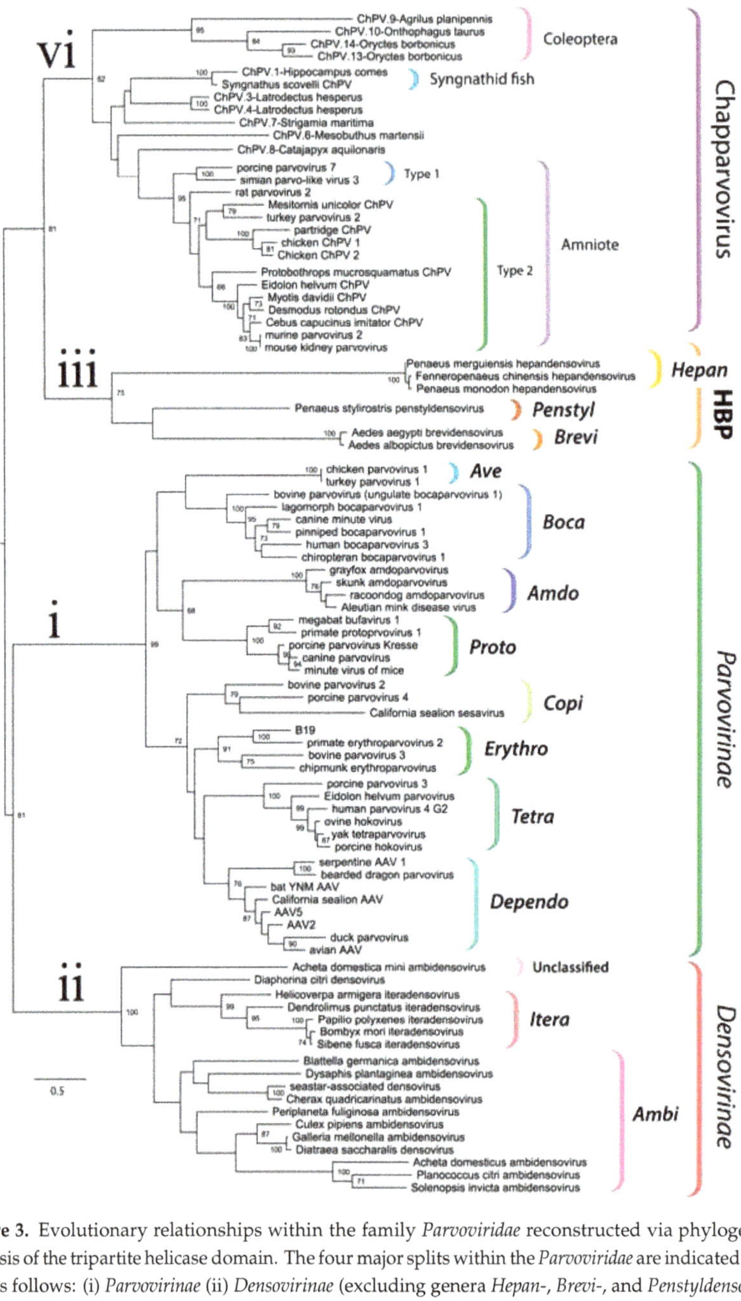

Figure 3. Evolutionary relationships within the family *Parvoviridae* reconstructed via phylogenetic analysis of the tripartite helicase domain. The four major splits within the *Parvoviridae* are indicated in the tree as follows: (i) *Parvovirinae* (ii) *Densovirinae* (excluding genera *Hepan-*, *Brevi-*, and *Penstyldensovirus*, abbreviated as HBP); (iii) HBP; (iv) Chapparvovirus (ChPV-related viruses and EPVs). Brackets to the right indicate taxonomic groups. The names of established genera are shown in bold italics in the abbreviated form (i.e., with the suffix "parvovirus" omitted). The scale bar shows evolutionary distance in substitutions per site. Numbers adjacent to tree nodes show bootstrap support (based on 100 bootstrap replicates) where >70%.

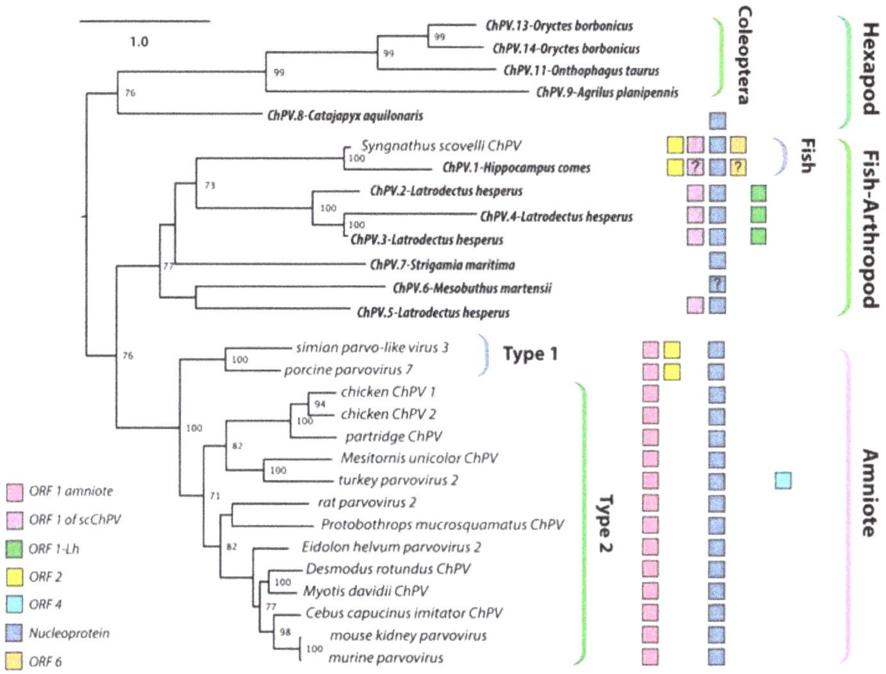

Figure 4. Maximum likelihood phylogenetic reconstructions of the ChPV clade based on the complete aligned amino acid sequences of the NS1. Colored boxes indicate the presence of auxiliary open reading frames (ORFs), as shown in the inset key. The "?" character indicates that the presence of an ORF is suspected but not confirmed. Taxa labels in bold italics indicate endogenous sequences, whereas italics indicate sequences known or believed to derive from viruses. Brackets to the right indicate taxonomic groups. The scale bar (top right) shows evolutionary distance in substitutions per site. Numbers adjacent to tree nodes show bootstrap support (based on 100 bootstrap replicates) where >70%.

3.3. *Characterization of Syngnathid ChPVs and EPVs*

The ScChPV genome encodes a long NS ORF (807 aa), a strikingly short VP (367 aa), and a ChPV-like NP (Figure 5). Furthermore, a homologue of the ORF2 protein found in the amniote parvoviruses PPV7 and SPV3 was present. A predicted ORF was present in a genomic position equivalent to that of ORF1, found in amniote ChPVs. However, the predicted protein sequence did not disclose any detectable similarity to its amniote counterpart. ORF6, identified in partial overlap with the VP C-term encoding region, encodes a small protein of 27.2 kDa (239 aa), exhibiting no detectable similarity to any other sequence in GenBank. Fold recognition, however, revealed a potential structural similarity to viral structural proteins, including the major envelope glycoprotein of the Epstein–Barr virus (PDB ID: 2H6O chain A, $p = 0.012$), the minor viral protein of the Sputnik virophage (PDB ID: 3J26, chain N, $p = 0.017$) and the surface region of *Galleria mellonella* ambidensovirus (PDB ID: 1DNV, $p = 0.021$). These findings imply ORF6 may encode an auxiliary structural protein.

The partial ChPV-like sequence identified in the genome of the tiger seahorse (*Hippocampus comes*) was flanked by extensive stretches of host genomic sequence, establishing that, unlike the ScChPV sequence identified in the Gulf pipefish genome assembly, it likely represents an EPV rather than a virus. Interestingly, however, phylogenies showed that both sequences obtained from syngnathe fish are relatively closely related, and cluster together with high bootstrap support (Figures 3 and 4).

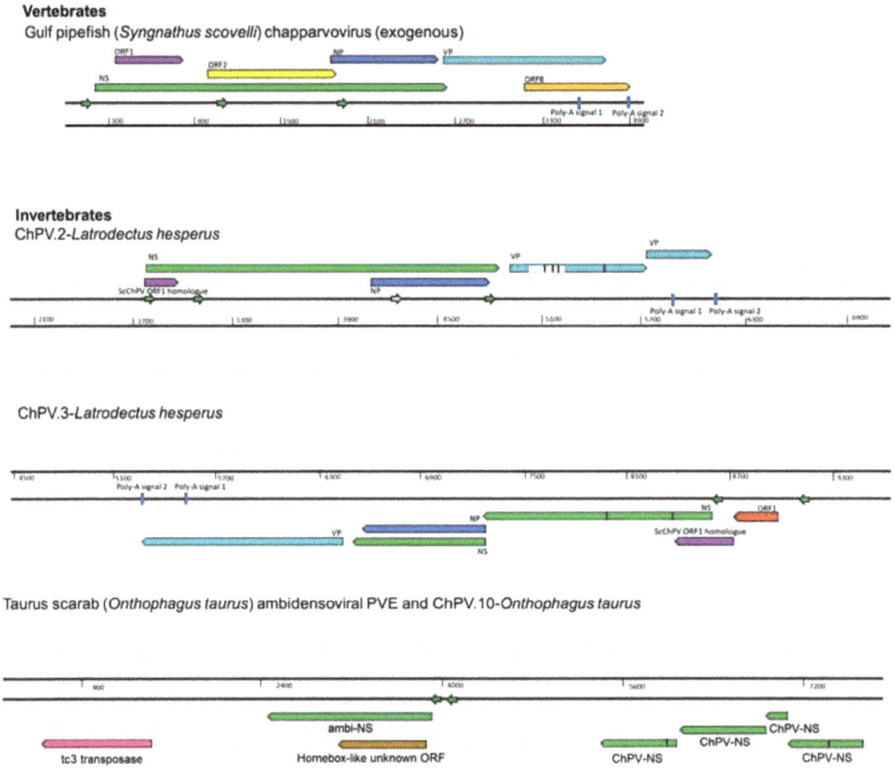

Figure 5. Genomic structures of newly identified chapparvoviruses (ChPVs) and ChPV-derived endogenous parvoviral element (EPV) sequences. The positions of putative open reading frames (ORFs) and predicted cis transcription elements of ChPVs are shown. ChPV.2-LatHes contains a previously unidentified repetitive element, present as multiple copies scattered in the *Latrodectus* genome, marked by the white box within the VP gene. The element ChPV.10-OntTau shares its integration site with another endogenous element, disclosing similarity to ambidensoviruses. ORFs are represented by rectangular arrows, colored according to homology. In-frame stop codons are shown as vertical lines. Splice donor sites are marked by white-colored bars, acceptor sites by orange-colored bars. Blue-colored bars show predicted polyadenylation signals. Small arrows show predicted promoters and are colored according to prediction score (>0.95 = green; 0.9–0.95 = pink: <0.9 = yellow). Grey boxes indicate regions inferred to be transcribed but not translated.

3.4. Characterization of ChPV-Derived EPVs in Invertebrate Genomes

Among the ChPV-derived EPVs we identified in invertebrates, the most complete were identified in the western black widow spider (*Latrodectus hesperus*) (Figure 5). Two of these elements spanned near complete genomes, including *rep*, *cap*, and NP genes, and a homologue of the ORF1 gene found in ScChPV. In addition, the ChPV.2-LatHes element encodes an apparently complete NS protein (690 aa), while ChPV.3-LatHes discloses an undisrupted ORF1 (113 aa) as well as an apparently intact *cap* gene encoding a 386-aa-long VP. The putative NS1 proteins encoded by these elements displayed only 62% identity at aa level. The disrupted *cap* gene of ChPV.2-LatHes was found to include an insertion of 74 aa, suspected to originate from a yet unknown repetitive element (revealed by sequence comparisons to be interspersed throughout the *L. hesperus* genome).

ChPV.3-LatHes, on the other hand, appeared to include an intact upstream region of the genome, revealing an additional small ORF of 81 aa length directly upstream of the ScChPV ORF1 homologue, designated ORF1-Lh. This ORF disclosed no detectable homology to any sequences to date. Upstream of this ORF, a potential promoter sequence could be identified with high confidence (0.98 of 1). Both elements included complete, NP-encoding ORFs of 233 aa, although a canonical ATG start codon could only be identified in one element (ChPV.3-LatHes).

We identified two further elements in the western black widow spider genome, although these only spanned disrupted *rep* genes. ChPV.4-LatHes encodes nearly complete NS and NP genes, as well as a complete homologue of the ScChPV ORF1 gene. The true extent of preservation could not be assessed for this EPV as it occurs on a short scaffold that terminated within the EPV *rep* sequence. The putative NS1 of ChPV.4-LatHes was 80% identical to its counterpart in ChPV.2-LatHes at aa level. Interestingly, this element contains additional, *rep*-encoding regions directly upstream of a larger, NS1- and ScChPV ORF1-encoding region. This second region encodes only the first 221 aa of the putative NS1 protein, together with the putative ScChPV ORF1 homologue and ORF1-Lh genes. The ORF1-Lh gene encoded by ChPV.4-LatHes lacks an ATG start codon. The upstream promoter was weakly predicted, with a score of 0.6. ChPV.5-LatHes displayed a highly divergent, partial *rep* of 216 aa, with only 42% identity to the ChPV.2-LatHes NS1 at aa level (Figure 5). This element clustered outside the monophyletic clade defined by the three other *Latrodectus* EPVs (Figure 4).

A single ChPV-derived EPV was identified in a second arachnid species—the Chinese golden scorpion (*Mesobuthus martensii*). This element was identified in a relatively short, unplaced scaffold, and comparison to the *Latrodectus* elements indicated that the contig was truncated within the EPV sequence, consequently the true extent of its preservation could not be assessed. Nevertheless, ORFs disclosing homology to the NS, NP, and VP proteins could be identified (Figure 2). While the first 100 or so codons of the NS ORF were absent, a complete NP ORF was detected, along with the first 46 codons of VP. All three ORFs were disrupted by frameshifts and stop codons. No homologues of any alternative ORFs identified in other ChPV genomes could be identified.

We identified a ChPV-derived EPV in the genome of a myriapod—the European centipede (*Strigamia maritima*). This element displayed partial homologues of the NS and NP encoding ORFs, both of which contained large deletions (Figure 2) as well as numerous nonsense mutations (Table 1). Moreover, the NS ORF was disrupted by an extensive stretch of an insertion of unknown origin. No homologues of any of the alternative ORFs found in other ChPVs could be identified in this endogenous sequence.

Seven ChPV-derived EPVs were identified in hexapod arthropods (subphylum Hexapoda). One occurs in the genome of a bristletail species—the Northern forcepstail (*Catajapyx aquillonaris*)—belonging to the entognath order Diplura. The other six were identified in three species belonging to the vast insect order Coleoptera: the emerald ash borer (*Agrilus planipennis*), the taurus scarab (*Onthophagus taurus*), and the scarab beetle (*Oryctes borbonicus*). The bristletail element contains a C-terminal truncated *rep* of at least 250 aa and a near full-length NP ORF. The partial *rep* was intact, but the NP ORF is disrupted and highly divergent, showing significant sequence similarity only in the conserved core region of the putative protein. The ash borer element ChPV.9-AgrPla occurs in a scaffold that is ~1 kb in length. One end of this scaffold contains a 592 nt region exhibiting homology to the NS ORF, which harboured an N-terminal deletion of at least 200 aa.

In ChPV.10-OntTau, a disrupted but almost complete NS ORF could be identified (Figure 5). Interestingly, a second EPV insertion was detected at the same locus. This element encodes an intact, potentially fully-expressible NS gene, homologous to the NS1 of ambidensoviruses (genus *Ambidensovirus*) and disclosing similarity to a recently reported ambidensovirus sequence that has been detected only at cDNA level in the transcriptome of two bumble bee species (*Bombus cryptarum* and *B. terrestris*) [40]. An additional intact, potentially expressible ORF was present in this ambidensoviral element, overlapping the putative NS1 gene, which harboured no significant similarity to any sequences deposited in GenBank to date. In its derived aa sequence, however, a homeobox domain could be revealed. The other two elements of the taurus scarab genome were located together in another assembly scaffold, only 2540 nts apart from each other. Both EPVs consisted of only a partial ORF, which disclosed similarity to chapparvoviral *reps*. None of these elements encompassed the tripartite helicase domain, hence they were not included in the phylogenetic inference.

Two EPVs were identified in the scarab beetle genome. One of these, designated ChPV.13-OryBor, harboured a near complete *rep* at 402 aa, as well as a short, partial *cap*, capable of encoding only the first 33 aa of the putative VP. The region of *rep* homology occurred within an ORF that was not disrupted by any frameshifts and could be extended without disruption upstream and downstream, suggesting that a longer gene product—potentially encoding a longer, divergent NS protein—may be present. However, these regions did not disclose sequence similarity to any proteins hitherto deposited to GenBank. The ChPV.14-OryBor element included only a heavily truncated NS of 254 aa.

3.5. Structural Characteristics of ChPV Capsids

We built 3D homology models to facilitate the comparison of ChPV capsid structures to those found in other parvoviruses. Interestingly, structural similarity with erythro-, proto-, and bocaparvoviruses can be detected for VP using fold recognition, even though the VP proteins of ChPVs share no significant sequence similarity with those of other parvoviruses (Figure 6a).

The derived polypeptide sequence of the complete VP ORF encoded by DrChPV was subjected to fold recognition, to identify suitable templates for homology modeling. This comparative analysis showed that the VP2 protein of parvovirus H1 (genus *Protoparvovirus*) (PDB ID: 4G0R) could potentially harbor the most structural similarity ($p = 9 \times 10^{-5}$), and this sequence was therefore used as the template for homology modeling. Due to the lack of sequence identity and the non-homologous nature of the ChPV VP genes to other parvoviral VPs, we used the final model obtained in this analysis as a template to construct homology models for four further ChPV VPs—rat parvovirus 2, PPV7, TPV2, and pit viper ChPV. This allowed us to overcome the stochastic aspect of model construction. Although the pitfalls of using models as templates have to be noted, this approach ensured that only those regions showed structural variability which would likely do so in the actual capsid structures.

We examined the VP sequences of two representatives of the second major ChPV clade (see Figure 4)—one derived from a presumably exogenous virus (ScChPV) and one from an EPV (ChPV.3-LatHes). For the VP protein encoded by ScChPV, fold recognition identified the following dependoparvovirus VP3 proteins as potential templates: adeno-associated virus 8, PDB ID: 2QA0, $p = 9 \times 10^{-4}$; Adeno-associated virus rh32.33, PDB ID: 4IOV, $p = 9 \times 10^{-4}$, while for the VP encoded by the black widow spider EPV the most reliable hit was the VP4 protein of an iteradensovirus (*Bombyx mori* densovirus 1, PDB ID: 3P0S, $p = 8 \times 10^{-4}$). When superimposing the obtained models with the VPs of AAV8 and BmDV1, however, structural similarity only covered the jelly roll core and the αA helix, and of the surface loops traditionally considered more variable, only the BC loop.

Modeling indicated that the ChPV VP monomer harbors an eight-stranded β-barrel "jelly roll" core and the αA helix at the two-fold symmetry axis, as found in all members of the family *Parvoviridae* to date [41] (Figure 6a). Equivalents of all short strands were present (β-C, H, E, F) as well, for four out of the five longer strands (β-B, D, I, G). However, no structural analogue to the outmost β-A could be identified (Figure 6). Examining the secondary structure prediction confirmed that a β-A analogue was not present, indicating β-B to be the closest to the N-term. The first strand of the *Syngnathus scovelli* ChPV VP appeared to fold outside of the jelly roll, leaving the longer sheet of the barrel without a β-B, comprised of only three strands—namely D, I, and G—despite a complete upper, CHEF sheet (Figure 6a). When modeling the complete $T = 1$ capsid polymer, this manifested as a hole, which is normally covered by β-B, even in the case of the smallest parvoviral capsids (Figure 6b). All VPs encoded by ChPVs and ChPV-derived EPVs displayed two canonical loops surrounding their five-fold axes, linking sheets D with E at the five-fold channel and sheets H with I on the floor surrounding the channel. In case of the amniote ChPVs, the pore displayed a tight opening. The sequence of the DE loop varied to some extent among these seven sequences, which also manifested in the models. The HI loop was, however, highly conserved throughout, containing only one variable position between the amniote ChPVs.

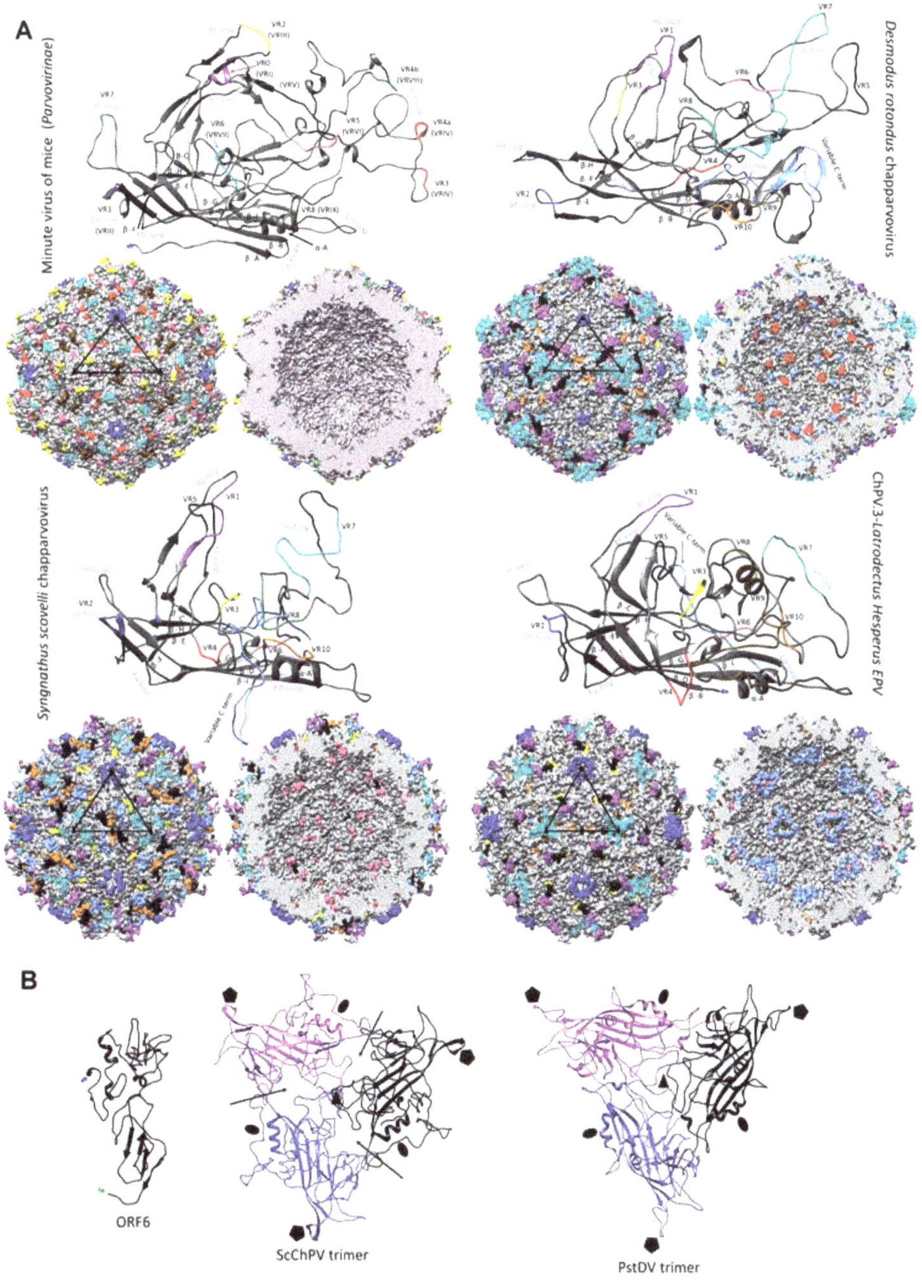

Figure 6. Structural variation and assembly interfaces of chapparvoviruses (ChPVs). (**A**) Comparison of VP monomer ribbon diagrams of the protoparvovirus minute virus of mice (PDB ID: 1Z14) from subfamily *Parvovirinae* to homology models of an amniote, a fish, and a ChPV-derived EPV from an arthropod genome (ChPV.3-LatHes). Variable regions (VRs) of the same number are marked by the

same color and mapped to the surface and luminal area of the $T = 1$ icosahedral capsid model constructed of 60 monomers. In the case of the minute virus of mice, the VRs are marked by both the traditional numbering established for dependoparvoviruses (Roman numerals) and by the special numbering applied for protoparvoviruses only (Arabic numerals). Blue signs indicate the names of the loops linking the beta strands of the conserved jelly roll core. Triangles mark the position of an asymmetric unit within the capsid, the five-fold symmetry axis is marked by a pentagon, the three-fold with the black filled triangles, and the two-fold with an ellipsoid. (**B**) Homology model of ORF6, the hypothetical structural protein of *Syngnathus scovelli* ChPV (ScChPV). The trimer of the ScChPV monomer model reveals a gap at each subunit interaction (arrows), unlike in the case of the trimer of even the hitherto smallest parvoviral capsid protein, *Penaeus stylirostris* densovirus. The gap might accommodate ORF6 in the assembled ScChPV capsid. Symmetry axes are marked by the same symbols as for panel A.

We mapped the chapparvoviral VRs identified by VP alignments (Figure S3) to both VP monomers and complete capsids, to examine how they manifest on the virion surface and make comparisons to parvoviruses of known structure, represented by the minute virus of mice (MVM), the prototypic member of subfamily *Parvovirinae* (PDB ID: 1Z14) (Figure 5). Out of ten chapparvoviral VRs identified (VR 1 to 10), shown in Figure S3a, only VR1, VR2, and VR9 proved to be similarly positioned and hence likely analogous to their counterparts in the MVM capsid. Some VRs (VR4 in all ChPVs examined, VR8 of the amniote ChPVs, and VR6 in ChPV.3-LatHes and ScChPV) appeared to be positioned at the luminal surface of the ChPV capsid, distinct from all parvoviruses studied to date. The only exception, however, is bovine parvovirus, a bocaparvovirus [42] in which VR8 is also located on the luminal surface of the capsid. Since the ChPV VRs appeared to be non-homologous to those established for either proto- or dependoparvoviruses, we re-defined them by numbering from N to C-term.

In addition to their distinctive VRs, ChPVs ubiquitously appeared to harbor a highly variable C-terminal region, with a length varying between 12 and 62 residues. The ChPV VP variable C-term appears to be buried in most cases, with the exception of ScChPV, where it is probably exposed. In the VP encoded by ChPV.3-LatHes it forms the luminal surface of the three-fold, whereas in the case of fish and amniote ChPVs it is located at the two-fold (Figure 6a).

The ScChPV and ChPV.3-LatHes VP lacked a VR6 homologous to that of the amniote ChPVs, albeit displayed variation in another position instead, still in the sixth-place counting from the N-term (Figure S3b). Moreover, both of them displayed truncated VRs 3, 5, and 7, compared to their amniote counterparts. VR9, furthermore, was absent from the ScChPV VP, whereas VR10 was missing from the VP of ChPV.2-LatHes (Figure S3b). As for the surface, the largest variable region for amniote ChPVs, namely DrChPV, is VR7, forming the entire three-fold protrusions, with VRs 1, and 9 forming small protrusions surrounding the aforementioned peaks.

The complete capsid models of non-amniote ChPVs were observed to harbor surface features that are strikingly distinct from those of the amniote ones, more closely resembling the capsids of the *Ambidensovirus-Iteradensovirus* clade of *Densovirinae* (see Figure 3), with a surface that is less spikey (Figure 7a). The homology model of ORF6 of ScCHPV, constructed based on the minor viral protein of the Sputnik virophage (PDB ID: 3J26) indicates that this potentially structural protein harbors multiple beta strands close to its C-term, out of which the outermost could potentially fill in the aforementioned gap caused by the lack of a β-B (Figure 6b).

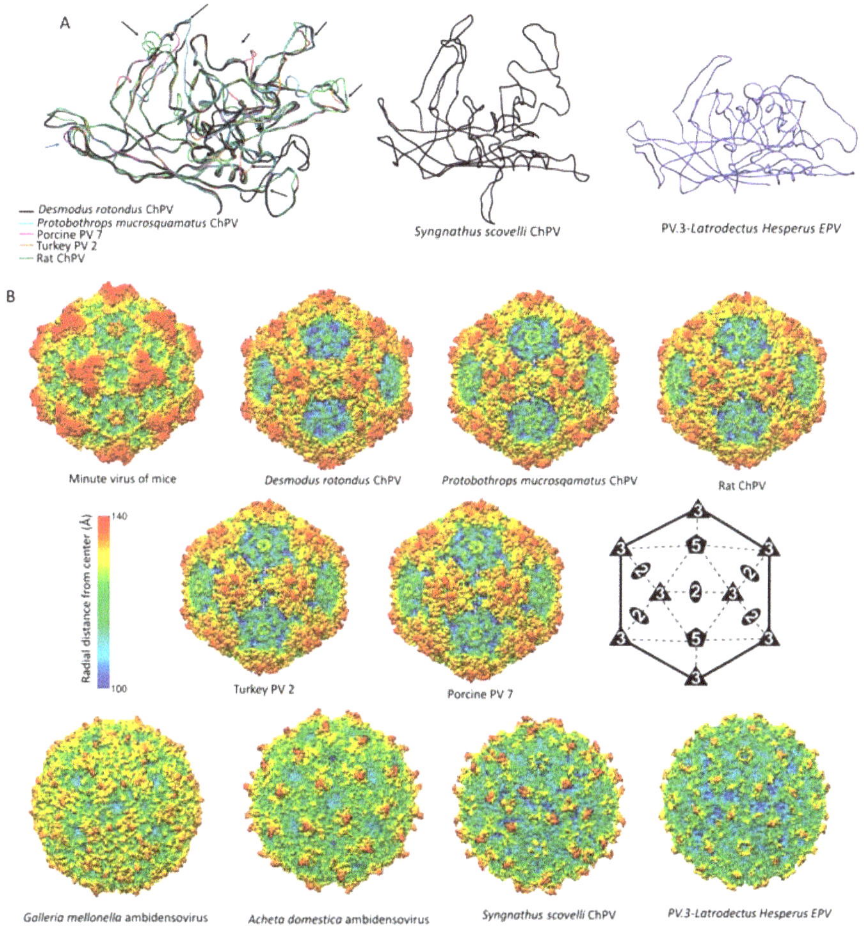

Figure 7. Comparison of chapparvoviruses (ChPV) capsid models of various host affiliations. (**A**) Homology models, shown as ribbon diagrams, representing the probable three different ChPV structural protein types. The first panel shows superposition of VP monomer homology models of amniote ChPV capsids, including reptilian, avian, rodent, chiropteran, and ungulate representatives. Black arrows show variable regions (VRs) previously identified by aligning the VP protein sequences. The next two panels show homology models of capsid monomers from a fish ChPV and an endogenous chapparvoviral element from an arthropod genome. (**B**) Capsid surface morphology of amniote ChPV homology models compared to that of the polymer structure of a prototypic parvovirus, the minute virus of mice (MVM) (PDB ID: 1Z14 at 3.25 Å resolution). Capsids are orientated by their two-fold symmetry axes, as shown in the line diagram, and are radially colored. Below, the comparison of homology models of complete viral capsid surface morphology of the newly identified fish ChPV and arachnid endogenous chapparvoviral element is shown, with that of the actual capsid structure of two densoviruses (subfamily *Densovirinae*, genus *Ambidensovirus*) (PDB ID: 4MGU at 3.5 Å resolution for *Acheta domestica* densovirus and 1DNV at 3.7 Å for *Galleria* densovirus).

4. Discussion

Historically, the family *Parvoviridae* has always been comprised of two subfamilies, with specificity for vertebrate or invertebrate hosts being the major demarcation criterion [2]. This division was initially supported by phylogenetic inference. However, as the number of densoviral genera increased, the heterogeneity of densoviruses, specifically their segregation into two clades, has not gone unnoticed [1]. Our study provides further evidence that the traditional division of parvoviruses into vertebrate-specific and invertebrate-specific subfamilies no longer holds, rather, it supports the division of the *Parvoviridae* into four major subgroups: the *Parvovirinae*, a split *Densovirinae*, and the ChPVs, as illustrated in Figure 3.

The data presented here show that ChPVs infect an exceptionally broad range of hosts, including both vertebrates and invertebrates. We show that ChPVs found in fish are more closely related to those that infected ancestral arachnoid arthropods than they are to those that infect amniote vertebrates (Figure 4), suggesting that ChPVs may have been transmitted between distantly related host species in the past. Furthermore, phylogenies indicate that all amniote ChPVs have a common origin (Figure 3), consistent with the overall conservation of their genome organization and some aspects of predicted transcriptional strategy (Figure 1).

While previous studies have suggested that ChPVs broadly co-diverged with host species [9], the present, expanded data set reveals that some transmission of ChPVs between vertebrate classes may have occurred (Figure 4). However, it should be kept in mind that almost all amniote ChPVs have been identified via metagenomic sequencing of environmental samples (mostly fecal viromes) and their true host affiliations remain uncertain.

The EPV sequences found in animal genomes overwhelmingly derive from a small proportion of parvovirus lineages [13,14,17,43,44]. For example, ambidensovirus-derived EPVs dominate invertebrate genomes [14], whereas vertebrate EPVs almost exclusively derive from the *Dependoparvovirus* and *Protoparvovirus* genera [12,13,43,44]. In this study, we found no trace of ChPV-derived EPVs in amniote genomes, despite recent evidence that ChPVs infect this host group [21,45]. By contrast, ChPV-derived EPVs are relatively common in arthropods, with some species harboring multiple, independently acquired elements, occasionally even in close proximity within the host genome (Table 1, Figure 4). The tendency of EPVs to derive from a subset of parvovirus genera likely has biological underpinnings. For example, in vertebrates it may reflect the ability of dependoparvoviruses to integrate into host DNA, and/or the requirement of protoparvoviruses to initiate DNA damage response (DDR) during replication [46,47]. Similar features of the viral life cycle could account for the biased distribution of ChPV-related sequences in animal genomes, i.e., arthropod and fish ChPVs might have adopted a replication strategy that favors germline integration, whereas that of amniote ChPVs precludes it. Notably, some arthropod species have integration sites containing multiple independently acquired EPVs of both ChPV and ambidensovirus origin, suggesting that hotspots of parvovirus integration and/or fixation might exist in their genomes.

Our discovery of ChPV-derived elements in fish and arthropod genomes establishes that ChPVs can infect these species in addition to amniotes [21,45]. Moreover, it provides evidence that the ChPVs are likely an ancient lineage of parvoviruses. Though we did not identify any orthologous ChPV insertions, the EPVs described here show extensive evidence of germline degradation. Through comparison to studies of EPVs in mammals (in which several orthologous EPVs have been described [13,48]), it appears likely that ChPVs have been present in animals for many millions of years. Moreover, as the hexapod EPVs appear to be monophyletic and mirror the evolution of their host species, the age of ChPVs could possibly correlate with the Insecta–Entognatha split, suggesting a minimum age of 400 million years [49].

Through comparative analysis of EPVs and ChPVs, we show that ChPV genomes exhibit a number of defining characteristics. Firstly, all possess a short, monosense genome, encoding a relatively large NS and a relatively short VP. The short VP proteins of ChPVs are clearly homologous to one another, but show no similarity to those found in other parvovirus lineages. Similar to those found in the penstyl-, hepan-, and brevidensoviruses, the VP proteins of ChPVs lack the phospholipase A2 (PLA2) domains that are required for infectivity in most other parvoviruses. Notably, these are also the genera to which ChPVs are most closely related in NS-based phylogenies (Figure 3).

Secondly, ChPVs typically encode multiple additional gene products besides the NS and VP. To begin with, almost all encode a nucleoprotein (NP) gene in an overlapping frame with *rep*. In this report, we show that putative NP ORFs are present in ChPV-derived EVEs, suggesting it is an ancestral, conserved feature of these viruses. However, its absence from the coleopteran lineage is intriguing, as it is still present in the EPV of the hexapod stem group Diplura of Entognatha. Phylogenetic reconstructions (and the extensive overlap with *rep*) imply it was acquired ancestrally and independently lost in the lineage derived from members of the hexapod crown group, Coleoptera (Figure 4).

A functional role for auxiliary ORF1 is supported by: (i) its conservation across the entire amniote ChPV clade; and (ii) limited experimental data indicating it is expressed in MKPV via a spliced transcript. Auxiliary ORF2 was only identified in a small subset of ChPV genomes, but a functional role for this ORF is suggested by the presence of homologues in distantly related ChPVs of amniotes and fish (see Figure 4). Interestingly, although all ChPVs appear to express ORF1 via splicing of a small intronic sequence (Figure 1), those harboring an ORF2 homologue are predicted to lack the peculiar large introns found in the expression of MKPV NP and VP transcripts [21]. ScChPV lacks an ORF1 homologue, but contains a predicted reading frame in the corresponding position. Homologues of this ScChPV ORF1 variant are present in all three arachnid EPVs, although not in the first, but in the second position. As only the three *Latrodectus* EPVs possess a homologue of ORF1-Lh, it is possible that this small ORF originated after the split from the syngnathe fish lineage, whereas the ScChPV ORF1 originates earlier. The distribution of homologous auxiliary genes across phylogenetic lineages of ChPVs implies that distinct lineages have acquired and/or lost these genes on multiple, independent occasions.

MKPV has been reported to possess only one promoter and two polyadenylation signals, as well as an extensive number of spliced transcripts. This transcription pattern, however, appears to be unique to only one of the two hitherto amniote ChPV lineages, comprising of rodent, chiropteran, New World primate, avian, and reptilian entries. As members of the "type 1" lineage, including PPV7, appear to display a genome organization specific for this clade and different from that of MKPV, they may utilize distinct transcription strategies as well.

Despite the potential pitfalls of homology modeling, and the use of distinct templates to reconstruct both the VP monomer and capsid structures, we obtained remarkably similar predicted structures for VP sequences found in closely related viruses/EPVs. Since the viral capsid plays an important role in mediating the interactions between parvoviruses and their hosts, comparisons of capsid structures can potentially reveal insights into parvovirus biology. Our analysis indicates that ChPV VPs would assemble into a complete, $T = 1$ icosahedral capsid, despite their relatively small size. Furthermore, their predicted structures are remarkably similar to those found in other parvoviruses, despite the lack of any detectable similarity in the sequences of their VP proteins. Structural similarities include the presence of a conserved jelly roll core and α-A helix, the existence of the D–E and H–I loops, and the presence of identifiable VRs. Interestingly, the amniote ChPV capsids appear to possess the same number of VRs as most of the vertebrate parvoviruses of subfamily *Parvovirinae*, even if only a few of them (namely VRs 1, 2, and 9) proved to be analogous features. In these virus capsids, variations were most prominent among the three-fold peaks and protrusions, as well as the two-fold depression, as observed in members of the *Parvovirinae* (Figure 7). The tendency of some VRs to manifest at the luminal surface of the capsid in models suggests these regions could play a role in intracellular host–virus interactions. For these regions to become accessible to intracellular signaling pathways would require either uncoating or conformational changes. Based on previous findings, however, the parvovirus capsid appears to traffic into the nucleus intact [50,51]. Considering this, these buried regions might play a role in processes linked to the nucleus. Interestingly, bovine parvovirus, the only other parvovirus in which buried VRs have previously been observed [52] is an enteric pathogen, and the association of amniote ChPVs with fecal viromes suggests these viruses might also be largely enteric.

In addition to the VRs, all ChPVs seem to harbor highly variable VP C-terms. A similar phenomenon has been observed in the case of iteradensoviruses, in which the last 40 C-terminal residues are disordered, hence the structure of this region cannot be resolved [53]. Although the location of the ChPV C-term appears to vary, its association with regions that are overtly involved in parvovirus–host interactions (e.g., the two- and three-fold peaks) is certainly intriguing.

MKPV is associated with the pathology of the urogenital system, whereas a related virus, murine ChPV, has been detected at a very high prevalence in murine liver tissue, suggesting it is a gastrointestinal agent [45]. The VPs of the two, however, only differ in six aa residues, located within VR3 and near VR2 on the surface and in the buried VR4, as well as in the similarly buried variable C-term (Figure S3a). Thus, these positions could constitute potential determinants of tissue tropism in murine ChPVs.

Parvovirus subfamilies *Parvovirinae* and *Densovirinae* utilize distinct strategies to stabilize their icosahedral capsids [54]. Vertebrate parvoviruses extend the longer side of the jellyroll fold with an additional, N-terminal strand by folding back β-A to interact with the two-fold axis of the very same monomer, hence creating an extended ABDIG sheet [55,56]. By contrast, the densovirus capsid preserves the symmetric arrangement of the jellyroll fold, and possesses a β-A which is a direct elongated N-terminal extension of the β-B instead, interacting with the β-B strand of the neighboring monomer toward the five-fold axis [57,58]. Strikingly, our data show that ChPV capsids lack β-A strands (and also the β-B strand, in the case of ScChPV). The functional implications of this are unclear—possibly ChPV capsids are stabilized in the absence of β-A via a yet unknown, additional VP. If ChPVs express additional structural proteins, they are presumably encoded by spliced transcripts (given the unusually small size of the *cap* gene). Alternatively, the ChPV capsid might assemble without the incorporation of an additional β strand, perhaps at the cost of losing the stability and resilience typical of parvoviruses in general. Potentially, this could account for the apparent presence of buried VRs. Interestingly, in studies of MKPV, viral proteins could be detected in the kidneys of infected mice, even though no assembled particles could be observed in inclusion body-affected tubular cells [21]. This, along with our structural predictions, suggests that the ChPV strategy for uncoating and cellular trafficking might be very different from that found in the *Parvovirinae* and *Densovirinae*.

Uniquely, the genome of ScChPV appears to include a putative additional structural protein (ORF6), in addition to the above-mentioned alternative ORFs. All parvoviruses to date—except those of genus *Penstyldensovirus*, with only one VP comprising the capsid [58]—have been reported to incorporate up to three additional minor VPs into the virion, which share a common C-terminal region. To encode a structural protein on an entirely separate ORF sharing, no mutual coding sequence with *cap* would be unique. Possibly, this unusual feature could be connected to the predicted lack of a β-B strand in the ScChPV VP monomer.

Taken together, the data presented here establish that the ChPVs belong to a parvovirus lineage that comprises a distinct lineage from all other parvoviruses, and infects an exceptionally broad range of host species, including both vertebrates and invertebrates. Consistent with this, their relatively complex genomes exhibit numerous unique features, implying that their life cycle might significantly differ from what has been established in the case of other members of the family. These findings underscore the need for further basic and comparative studies of ChPVs, to assess their potential impact on animal health, both wildlife and livestock. Furthermore, this is the first study to imply that vertebrate parvoviruses are not monophyletic, and that members of the family must have evolved to infect vertebrates on at least two separate occasions.

Supplementary Materials: The following are available online at http://www.mdpi.com/1999-4915/11/6/525/s1, Figure S1: Predictions of secondary structure, disordered regions and potential phosphorylation sites in case of an amniote exogenous and an endogenous invertebrate ChPV nucleoprotein (NP), Figure S2: Secondary structure predictions of the *Syngnathus scovelli* ChPV genome termini. Figure S3: Variable regions at the derived amino acid sequence level identified among ChPV capsid proteins.

Author Contributions: Conceptualization, R.J.G. and J.J.P.; Methodology, R.J.G. and J.J.P.; Software, R.J.G.; Validation, J.J.P., R.J.G and M.A.-M.; Resources, R.J.G. and M.A.-M.; Data Curation, J.J.P., R.J.G and W.M.d.S.; Writing—Original Draft Preparation, J.J.P and R.J.G.; Writing—Review & Editing, M.A.-M.; Funding Acquisition, R.J.G. and M.A.-M.

Funding: J.J.P. and M.A.-M. are funded by NIH R01 GM109524. R.J.G. was funded by the Medical Research Council of the United Kingdom (MC_UU_12014/12). W.M.d.S. is supported by the Fundação de Amparo à Pesquisa do Estado de São Paulo, Brazil (Scholarships No. 17/13981-0).

Conflicts of Interest: The authors declare no conflict of interest.

References

1. Cotmore, S.F.; Agbandje-McKenna, M.; Chiorini, J.A.; Mukha, D.V.; Pintel, D.J.; Qiu, J.; Soderlund-Venermo, M.; Tattersall, P.; Tijssen, P.; Gatherer, D.; et al. The family Parvoviridae. *Arch. Virol.* **2014**, *159*, 1239–1247. [CrossRef] [PubMed]
2. Tijssen, P.; Agbandje-McKenna, M.; Almendral, J.M.; Bergoin, M.; Flegel, T.W.; Hedman, K.; Kleinschmidt, J.; Li, Y.; Pintel, D.J.; Tattersall, P. Family Parvoviridae. In *Virus Taxonomy—Ninth Report of the International Committee on Taxonomy of Viruses*; King, A.M., Lefkowitz, E., Adams, M.J., Carstens, E.B., Eds.; Elsevier/Academic Press: London, UK, 2011; pp. 405–425.
3. Zádori, Z.; Szelei, J.; Tijssen, P. SAT: A late NS protein of porcine parvovirus. *J. Virol.* **2005**, *79*, 13129–13138. [CrossRef] [PubMed]
4. Sonntag, F.; Kother, K.; Schmidt, K.; Weghofer, M.; Raupp, C.; Nieto, K.; Kuck, A.; Gerlach, B.; Böttcher, B.; Müller, O.J.; et al. The assembly-activating protein promotes capsid assembly of different adeno-associated virus serotypes. *J. Virol.* **2011**, *85*, 12686–12697. [CrossRef] [PubMed]
5. Siqueira, J.D.; Ng, T.F.; Miller, M.; Li, L.; Deng, X.; Dodd, E.; Batac, F.; Delwart, E. Endemic infection of stranded southern sea otters (*Enhydra lutris* nereis). *J. Wildl. Dis.* **2017**, *53*, 532–542. [CrossRef] [PubMed]
6. Väisänen, E.; Fu, Y.; Hedman, K.; Söderlund-Venermo, M. Human protoparvoviruses. *Viruses* **2017**, *9*, 354. [CrossRef]
7. Geoghegan, J.L.; Pirotta, V.; Harvey, E.; Smith, A.; Buchmann, J.P.; Ostrowski, M.; Eden, J.-S.; Harcourt, R.; Holmes, E.C. Virological sampling of inaccessible wildlife with drones. *Viruses* **2018**, *10*, 300. [CrossRef]
8. De Souza, W.; Dennis, T.; Fumagalli, M.; Araujo, J.; Sabino-Santos, G.; Maia, F.; Acrani, G.; Carrasco, A.; Romeiro, M.; Modha, S.; et al. Novel parvoviruses from wild and domestic animals in Brazil provide new insights into parvovirus distribution and diversity. *Viruses* **2018**, *10*, 143. [CrossRef]
9. De Souza, W.M.; Romeiro, M.F.; Fumagalli, M.J.; Modha, S.; de Araujo, J.; Queiroz, L.H.; Durigon, E.L.; Figueiredo, L.T.M.; Murcia, P.R.; Gifford, R.J. Chapparvoviruses occur in at least three vertebrate classes and have a broad biogeographic distribution. *J. Gen. Virol.* **2017**, *98*, 225–229. [CrossRef]
10. Phan, T.G.; Gulland, F.; Simeone, C.; Deng, X.; Delwart, E. Sesavirus: Prototype of a new parvovirus genus in feces of a sea lion. *Virus Genes* **2015**, *50*, 134–146. [CrossRef]
11. Phan, T.G.; Dreno, B.; Da Costa, A.C.; Li, L.; Orlandi, P.; Deng, X.; Kapusinszky, B.; Siqueira, J.; Knol, A.-C.; Halary, F.; et al. A new protoparvovirus in human fecal samples and cutaneous T cell lymphomas (mycosis fungoides). *Virology* **2016**, *496*, 299–305. [CrossRef]
12. Belyi, V.A.; Levine, A.J.; Skalka, A.M. Sequences from ancestral single-stranded DNA viruses in vertebrate genomes: The parvoviridae and circoviridae are more than 40 to 50 million years old. *J. Virol.* **2010**, *84*, 12458–12462. [CrossRef] [PubMed]
13. Katzourakis, A.; Gifford, R.J. Endogenous viral elements in animal genomes. *PLoS Genet.* **2010**, *6*, e1001191. [CrossRef]
14. Liu, H.; Fu, Y.; Xie, J.; Cheng, J.; Ghabrial, S.A.; Li, G.; Peng, Y.; Yi, X.; Jiang, D. Widespread endogenization of densoviruses and parvoviruses in animal and human genomes. *J. Virol.* **2011**, *85*, 9863–9876. [CrossRef] [PubMed]
15. Reuter, G.; Boros, Á.; Delwart, E.; Pankovics, P. Novel circular single-stranded DNA virus from turkey faeces. *Arch. Virol.* **2014**, *159*, 2161–2164. [CrossRef] [PubMed]
16. Yang, S.; Liu, Z.; Wang, Y.; Li, W.; Fu, X.; Lin, Y.; Shen, Q.; Wang, X.; Wang, H.; Zhang, W. A novel rodent chapparvovirus in feces of wild rats. *Virol. J.* **2016**, *13*, 133. [CrossRef] [PubMed]
17. Kapoor, A.; Simmonds, P.; Lipkin, W.I. Discovery and characterization of mammalian endogenous parvoviruses. *J. Virol.* **2010**, *84*, 12628–12635. [CrossRef] [PubMed]

18. Holmes, E.C. The evolution of endogenous viral elements. *Cell Host Microbe* **2011**, *10*, 368–377. [CrossRef] [PubMed]
19. Baker, K.S.; Leggett, R.M.; Bexfield, N.H.; Alston, M.; Daly, G.; Todd, S.; Tachedjian, M.; Holmes, C.E.; Crameri, S.; Wang, L.-F.; et al. Metagenomic study of the viruses of African straw-coloured fruit bats: Detection of a chiropteran poxvirus and isolation of a novel adenovirus. *Virology* **2013**, *441*, 95–106. [CrossRef] [PubMed]
20. Palinski, R.M.; Mitra, N.; Hause, B.M. Discovery of a novel *Parvovirinae* virus, porcine parvovirus 7, by metagenomic sequencing of porcine rectal swabs. *Virus Genes* **2016**, *52*, 564–567. [CrossRef]
21. Roediger, B.; Lee, Q.; Tikoo, S.; Cobbin, J.C.; Henderson, J.M.; Jormakka, M.; O'Rourke, M.B.; Padula, M.P.; Pinello, N.; Henry, M.; et al. An atypical parvovirus drives chronic tubulointerstitial nephropathy and kidney fibrosis. *Cell* **2018**, *175*, 530–543. [CrossRef]
22. Zhu, H.; Dennis, T.; Hughes, J.; Gifford, R.J. Database-integrated genome screening (DIGS): Exploring genomes heuristically using sequence similarity search tools and a relational database. *bioRxiv* **2018**, 246835. [CrossRef]
23. Carver, T.; Harris, S.R.; Berriman, M.; Parkhill, J.; McQuillan, J.A. Artemis: An integrated platform for visualization and analysis of high-throughput sequence-based experimental data. *Bioinformatics* **2012**, *28*, 464–469. [CrossRef] [PubMed]
24. Knudsen, S. Promoter2.0: For the recognition of PolII promoter sequences. *Bioinformatics* **1999**, *15*, 356–361. [CrossRef] [PubMed]
25. Reese, M.G.; Eeckman, F.H.; Kulp, D.; Haussler, D. Improved splice site detection in genie. *J. Comput. Boil.* **1997**, *4*, 311–323. [CrossRef] [PubMed]
26. Dogan, R.I.; Getoor, L.; Wilbur, W.J.; Mount, S.M. SplicePort—An interactive splice-site analysis tool. *Nucl. Acids Res.* **2007**, *35* (Suppl. 2), W285–W291. [CrossRef]
27. Salamov, A.; Solovyev, V. Recognition of 3′ -processing sites of human mRNA precursors. *Bioinformatics* **1997**, *13*, 23–28. [CrossRef]
28. Armougom, F.; Moretti, S.; Poirot, O.; Audic, S.; Dumas, P.; Schaeli, B.; Keduas, V.; Notredame, C. Expresso: Automatic incorporation of structural information in multiple sequence alignments using 3D-Coffee. *Nucleic Acids Res.* **2006**, *34*, W604–W608. [CrossRef]
29. Edgar, R.C. MUSCLE: Multiple sequence alignment with high accuracy and high throughput. *Nucleic Acids Res.* **2004**, *32*, 1792–1797. [CrossRef]
30. Wallace, I.M.; O'Sullivan, O.; Higgins, D.G.; Notredame, C. M-Coffee: Combining multiple sequence alignment methods with T-Coffee. *Nucleic Acids Res.* **2006**, *34*, 1692–1699. [CrossRef]
31. Guindon, S.; Dufayard, J.F.; Lefort, V.; Anisimova, M.; Hordijk, W.; Gascuel, O. New algorithms and methods to estimate maximum-likelihood phylogenies: Assessing the performance of PhyML 3.0. *Syst. Boil.* **2010**, *59*, 307–321. [CrossRef]
32. Felsenstein, J. *PHYLIP (Phylogeny Inference Package), Version 3.6*; Department of Genome Sciences, University of Washington: Seattle, WA, USA, 2005.
33. Lobley, A.; Sadowski, M.I.; Jones, D.T. pGenTHREADER and pDomTHREADER: New methods for improved protein fold recognition and superfamily discrimination. *Bioinformatics* **2009**, *25*, 1761–1767. [CrossRef] [PubMed]
34. Yang, J.; Yan, R.; Roy, A.; Xu, D.; Poisson, J.; Zhang, Y. The I-TASSER suite: Protein structure and function prediction. *Nat. Methods* **2015**, *12*, 7–8. [CrossRef] [PubMed]
35. Carrillo-Tripp, M.; Shepherd, C.M.; A Borelli, I.; Venkataraman, S.; Lander, G.C.; Natarajan, P.; E Johnson, J.; Brooks, C.L.; Reddy, V.S. VIPERdb2: An enhanced and web API enabled relational database for structural virology. *Nucleic Acids Res.* **2009**, *37*, D436–D442. [CrossRef] [PubMed]
36. Schrödinger, L. *The PyMOL Molecular Graphics System, Version 2.0*; Wiley: Hoboken, NJ, USA, 2002.
37. Pettersen, E.F.; Goddard, T.D.; Huang, C.C.; Couch, G.S.; Greenblatt, D.M.; Meng, E.C.; Ferrin, T.E. UCSF Chimera? A visualization system for exploratory research and analysis. *J. Comput. Chem.* **2004**, *25*, 1605–1612. [CrossRef] [PubMed]
38. Zuker, M. Mfold web server for nucleic acid folding and hybridization prediction. *Nucleic Acids Res.* **2003**, *31*, 3406–3415. [CrossRef] [PubMed]
39. Gifford, R.J.; Blomberg, J.; Coffin, J.M.; Fan, H.; Heidmann, T.; Mayer, J.; Stoye, J.; Tristem, M.; Johnson, W.E. Nomenclature for endogenous retrovirus (ERV) loci. *Retrovirology* **2018**, *15*, 59. [CrossRef]

40. Schoonvaere, K.; Smagghe, G.; Francis, F.; De Graaf, D.C. Study of the metatranscriptome of eight social and solitary wild bee Species reveals novel viruses and bee parasites. *Front. Microbiol.* **2018**, *9*, 177. [CrossRef]
41. Chapman, M.S.; Agbandje-McKenna, M. Atomic structure of viral particles. In *Parvoviruses*; Kerr, J.R., Cotmore, F.C., Bloom, M.E., Linden, R.M., Parrish, C.R., Eds.; Hodder Arnold, Ltd.: London, UK, 2006; pp. 107–123.
42. Kailasan, S.; Agbandje-McKenna, M.; Parrish, C.R. Parvovirus family conundrum: What makes a killer? *Annu. Rev. Virol.* **2015**, *2*, 425–450. [CrossRef]
43. Pénzes, J.J.; Marsile-Medun, S.; Agbandje-McKenna, M.; Gifford, R.J. Endogenous amdoparvovirus-related elements reveal insights into the biology and evolution of vertebrate parvoviruses. *Virus Evol.* **2018**, *4*, vey026. [CrossRef]
44. Arriagada, G.; Gifford, R.J.; Beemon, K.L. Parvovirus-derived endogenous viral elements in two south American rodent genomes. *J. Virol.* **2014**, *88*, 12158–12162. [CrossRef]
45. Williams, S.H.; Che, X.; Garcia, J.A.; Klena, J.D.; Lee, B.; Muller, D.; Ulrich, W.; Corrigan, R.M.; Nichol, S.; Jain, K.; et al. Viral diversity of house mice in New York city. *mBio* **2018**, *9*, e01354-17. [CrossRef] [PubMed]
46. Deyle, D.R.; Russell, D.W. Adeno-associated virus vector integration. *Curr. Opin. Mol. Ther.* **2009**, *11*, 442–447. [PubMed]
47. Majumder, K.; Etingov, I.; Pintel, D.J. Protoparvovirus interactions with the cellular DNA damage response. *Viruses* **2017**, *9*, 323. [CrossRef] [PubMed]
48. Valencia-Herrera, I.; Cena-Ahumada, E.; Faunes, F.; Ibarra-Karmy, R.; Gifford, R.J.; Arriagada, G. Molecular properties and evolutionary origins of a parvovirus-derived myosin fusion gene in guinea pigs. *bioRxiv* **2019**, 572735. [CrossRef]
49. Willmann, R. Phylogenetic relationships and evolution of insects. In *Assembling the Tree of Life*; Cracraft, J., Donoghue, M.J., Eds.; Oxford University Press: Oxford, UK, 2004; pp. 330–344.
50. Cohen, S. Pushing the envelope: Microinjection of *Minute virus* of mice into *Xenopus* oocytes causes damage to the nuclear envelope. *J. Gen. Virol.* **2005**, *86*, 3243–3252. [CrossRef] [PubMed]
51. Sonntag, F.; Bleker, S.; Leuchs, B.; Fischer, R.; Kleinschmidt, J.A. Adeno-associated virus type 2 capsids with externalized VP1/VP2 trafficking domains are generated prior to passage through the cytoplasm and are maintained until Uncoating OCCURS in the nucleus. *J. Virol.* **2006**, *80*, 11040–11054. [CrossRef] [PubMed]
52. Kailasan, S.; Halder, S.; Gurda, B.; Bladek, H.; Chipman, P.R.; McKenna, R.; Brown, K.; Agbandje-McKenna, M. Structure of an enteric pathogen, bovine parvovirus. *J. Virol.* **2015**, *89*, 2603–2614. [CrossRef] [PubMed]
53. Kaufmann, B.; El-Far, M.; Plevka, P.; Bowman, V.D.; Li, Y.; Tijssen, P.; Rossmann, M.G. Structure of Bombyx mori Densovirus 1, a Silkworm Pathogen. *J. Virol.* **2011**, *85*, 4691–4697. [CrossRef] [PubMed]
54. Drouin, L.M.; Lins, B.; Janssen, M.; Bennett, A.; Chipman, P.; McKenna, R.; Chen, W.; Muzyczka, N.; Cardone, G.; Baker, T.S.; et al. Cryo-electron microscopy reconstruction and stability studies of the wild type and the R432A variant of adeno-associated virus type 2 reveal that capsid structural stability is a major factor in genome packaging. *J. Virol.* **2016**, *90*, 8542–8551. [CrossRef]
55. Simpson, A.A.; Hébert, B.; Sullivan, G.M.; Parrish, C.R.; Zádori, Z.; Tijssen, P.; Rossmann, M.G. The structure of porcine parvovirus: Comparison with related viruses. *J. Mol. Biol.* **2002**, *315*, 1189–1198. [CrossRef]
56. Xie, Q.; Bu, W.; Bhatia, S.; Hare, J.; Somasundaram, T.; Azzi, A.; Chapman, M.S. The atomic structure of adeno-associated virus (AAV-2), a vector for human gene therapy. *Proc. Natl. Acad. Sci. USA* **2002**, *99*, 10405–10410. [CrossRef] [PubMed]
57. Simpson, A.A.; Chipman, P.R.; Baker, T.S.; Tijssen, P.; Rossmann, M.G. The structure of an insect parvovirus (*Galleria mellonella* densovirus) at 3.7 å resolution. *Structure* **1998**, *6*, 1355–1367. [CrossRef]
58. Kaufmann, B.; Li, Y.; Szelei, J.; Tijssen, P.; Bowman, V.D.; Waddell, P.J.; Rossmann, M.G. Structure of Penaeus stylirostris densovirus, a shrimp pathogen. *J. Virol.* **2010**, *84*, 11289–11296. [CrossRef] [PubMed]

viruses

MDPI

Article

Chapparvovirus DNA Found in 4% of Dogs with Diarrhea

Elizabeth Fahsbender [1,2], Eda Altan [1,2], M. Alexis Seguin [3], Pauline Young [3], Marko Estrada [3], Christian Leutenegger [3] and Eric Delwart [1,2,*]

1 Vitalant Research Institute, San Francisco, CA 94118, USA; efahsbender@vitalant.org (E.F.); EAltan@vitalant.org (E.A.)
2 Dept. of Laboratory Medicine, University of California, San Francisco, CA 94118, USA
3 IDEXX Reference Laboratories, -Inc., West Sacramento, CA 95605, USA; alexis-seguin@idexx.com (M.A.S.); Pauline-Young@idexx.com (P.Y.); Marko-Estrada@idexx.com (M.E.); Christian-Leutenegger@idexx.com (C.L.)
* Correspondence: Eric.Delwart@ucsf.edu

Received: 22 March 2019; Accepted: 24 April 2019; Published: 27 April 2019

Abstract: Feces from dogs in an unexplained outbreak of diarrhea were analyzed by viral metagenomics revealing the genome of a novel parvovirus. The parvovirus was named cachavirus and was classified within the proposed *Chapparvovirus* genus. Using PCR, cachavirus DNA was detected in two of nine tested dogs from that outbreak. In order to begin to elucidate the clinical impact of this virus, 2,053 canine fecal samples were screened using real-time PCR. Stool samples from 203 healthy dogs were positive for cachavirus DNA at a rate of 1.47%, while 802 diarrhea samples collected in 2017 and 964 samples collected in 2018 were positive at rates of 4.0% and 4.66% frequencies, respectively (healthy versus 2017-2018 combined diarrhea *p*-value of 0.05). None of 83 bloody diarrhea samples tested positive. Viral loads were generally low with average real-time PCR Ct values of 36 in all three positive groups. The species tropism and pathogenicity of cachavirus, the first chapparvovirus reported in feces of a placental carnivore, remains to be fully determined.

Keywords: parvovirus; viral metagenomics; canine chapparvovirus

1. Introduction

Canine diarrhea is one of the most common illnesses treated by veterinarians with many possible causes of canine diarrhea, including bacteria, parasites, and viruses [1]. One of the most important dog enteric viruses is canine parvovirus 2 (CPV-2) in the *Carnivore protoparvovirus species 1* [2]. Parvoviruses are small, icosahedral, nonenveloped, single-stranded DNA viruses that are pathogenic to a variety of mammals [3–5]. The vertebrate-infecting parvoviruses are classified in the subfamily *Parvovirinae* in the *Parvoviridae* family (which also includes the insect infecting subfamily *Densovirinae*). The *Parvovirinae* subfamily is currently subdivided into eight officially recognized genera (*Dependoparvovirus*, *Copiparvovirus*, *Bocaparvovirus*, *Amdoparvovirus*, *Aveparvovirus*, *Protoparvovirus*, *Tetraparvovirus*, and *Erythroparvovirus* [6]). The recently proposed genus *Chapparvovirus* is currently comprised of a rat parvovirus 2 (KX272741) [7], *Eidolon helvum* fruit bat parvovirus 1 (MG693107.1) [8], and *E. helvum* bat parvovirus 2 (JX885610) [9], *Desmodus rotundus* bat parvovirus (NC032097.1) [10], simian parvo-like virus 3 (KT961660.1) [11], Turkey parvovirus TP1-2012/Hun (KF925531) [12], porcine parvovirus 7 (KU563733) [13], murine chapparvovirus (MF175078) [14], Tasmanian devil-associated chapparvovirus strains 1–6 (MK513528-MK53533) [15], red-crowned crane-associated parvovirus (KY312548, KY312549, KY312550, KY312551) [16], and chicken chapparvovirus 1 and 2 (MG846441 and MG846642) [17]. A close relative of murine chapparvovirus, initially reported in the feces of a wild *Mus musculus* from New York City [14], called murine kidney parvovirus (MH670588) was recently shown to cause nephropathy in immunocompromised laboratory mice [18]. A recent survey of eukaryotic genomes for chapparvovirus sequences has also shown the presence of a likely exogeneous chapparvovirus genome in a fish (Gulf pipefish or *Syngnathus scovelli*) and of mostly defective germline sequences in another fish (Tiger tail seahorse or *Hippocampus comes*) as well as in multiple invertebrates, indicating an ancient origin for chapparvoviruses [19]. A phylogenetic analysis of NS1 also indicated chapparvoviruses fall outside the traditional vertebrate-infecting *Parvovirinae* subfamily clade and closer to that of a subset of members of the subfamily *Densovirinae* [19].

Here an unexplained diarrhea outbreak among dogs was analyzed using viral metagenomics after diagnostic tests were negative for common canine enteric pathogens. The genome of a novel chapparvovirus was characterized and used to perform an epidemiological study to measure its prevalence and possible clinical significance.

2. Materials and Methods

2.1. Sample Collection and Pathogen Screening

Nine stool samples from dogs suffering from an infectious diarrhea outbreak in Colorado in October 2017 were submitted to IDEXX Reference Laboratories, Inc. (Sacramento, CA, USA) for pathogen testing. Fourteen dogs were involved in the initial outbreak which were identified by clinical signs that started with steatorrhea, progressed to hemorrhagic diarrhea with additional symptoms of lethargy, fever, and low lymphocyte counts pointing to a possible viral infection. At the time of feces collection, the nine sampled dogs were at various stages of the disease, with two of the dogs relapsing a month after initially experiencing parvo-like clinical signs. These stool samples were all negative for *Giardia* spp., *Cryptosporidium* spp., *Salmonella* spp., *Clostridium perfringens* enterotoxin gene (quantitative), *Clostridium perfringens* Alpha-toxin gene (quantitative), Canine enteric coronavirus (alphacoronavirus), Canine Parvovirus 2 and Canine Distemper virus using the IDEXX canine diarrhea profile real-time PCR tests.

2.2. Metagenomic Analysis

Stool samples were grouped into three pools of three and vortexed in phosphate buffer saline (PBS) with zirconia beads followed by microfuge centrifugation at 14,000 *rpm* for 10 min. The supernatants were passed through a 0.45 µm filter (Millipore, Burlington, MA, USA) and digested with a mixture of nuclease enzymes to enrich for viral particles [20,21]. RNA was extracted using the MagMAX kit (ThermoFisher, Waltham, MA, USA) which was transcribed into cDNA using a random RT-PCR step. The library was generated using the transposon-based Nextera™ XT Sample Preparation Kit (Illumina, San Diego, CA, USA) which was deep sequenced with the MiSeq platform (250 bases, paired-end reads) with dual barcoding. After demultiplexing the reads, they were trimmed and de novo assembled to produce contigs [22]. Both singlets and contigs were compared to all eukaryotic viral protein sequences in GenBank's non-redundant database using BLASTx [23].

2.3. Genome Assembly and Diagnostic PCR

Pairwise identity matrices using the amino acid sequence of the NS1 wasgenerated using Geneious R11 (Newark, NJ, USA). Amino acid sequences from the NS1 region of all available chapparvoviruses were aligned using MUSCLE and a Maximum likelihood tree was created using the Jones–Taylor–Thorton matrix-based model with 1,000 bootstrap replicates in MEGA6.0 [24–26].

A set of nested PCR primers were designed to screen for cachavirus in the nine stool samples from the diarrheal outbreak. DNA was extracted from each individual stool sample using the QIAamp MinElute Virus Spin kit (Qiagen, Hilden, Germany) and nested PCR assay primers were used to screen for cachavirus DNA. The first round of primers CPV_625F (5′-CAA CTA GCC GAA TGC AGG GA-3′) and CPV_948R (5′-CGA TAA CAT CCC CGG ACT GG-3′) were designed to target 323 nt of the NS1 region. The second round of primers CPV18_687FN (5′-AGC TCA GTT TGG CCC AGA TC-3′) and

CPV_911RN (5′-AGAGGGATCGCTGGATCTGT-3′) targeted a 224 nt region within the amplicon of the first round of primers. The PCR (containing a final concentration of 0.2 μm of each primer, 0.2 mM of dNTPs, 0.625 U of Amplitaq Gold® DNA polymerase (Applied Biosystems, Waltham, MA, USA), 1× PCR Gold buffer II, 1.5 mM of $MgCl_2$ and 1 μL of DNA template in a 25 μl reaction) proceeded as follows: 95 °C for 5 min, 40 cycles of (95 °C for 30 s, (52 °C for the first round and 54 °C for the second round of primers) for 30 s, and 72 °C for 30 s), followed by a final extension at 72 °C for 7 min. PCR products of the correct size were verified by gel electrophoresis and Sanger sequencing.

2.4. Prevalence

A proprietary real-time PCR assay with an amplification efficiency of 95% and an r^2 value of 0.99 was developed by IDEXX. One gram of feces was added to 3 mL of lysis buffer and 600 μL extracted into 200 μL nucleic acid eluate. Five μL of the eluate was tested in a PCR reaction with a limit of detection of 10 copies DNA for a sensitivity of 1,600 copies per gram of feces. A chi-square test comparing the proportion of healthy dogs that tested positive for cachavirus and those testing positive with diarrhea in 2017 and 2018 was performed in order to determine if the difference in frequency was statistically significant.

3. Results

Nine canine diarrheal samples from an unexplained outbreak of diarrhea were analyzed by viral metagenomics using three pools of three diarrhea samples each. Based on the BLASTx results, one of the three pools showed the presence of viral sequences most closely related to different chapparvoviruses reported from different vertebrates (0.05% of all reads). Other eukaryotic viral sequences observed were from Gyrovirus 4 (0.0003% of all reads), which has been reported in both chicken meat and human stool [27], indicating that it likely represents a dietary contaminant, and Torque teno canis virus (0.002% of reads), a common commensal canine blood virus [28].

Using de novo assembly and PCR paired with Sanger sequencing, a near complete genome of 4,123 bases containing the two main open reading frames of chapparvoviruses was generated (Figure 1, panel A). The available genome consisted of a 516 bases partial 5′UTR followed by an ORF encoding a 663 aa non-structural protein (NS) possessing the ATP binding Walker loop motif GPSNTGKS followed by a second ORF encoding a 505 aa viral capsid (VP) finishing with a 108 bases partial 3′UTR (Figure 1, panel A). When NS1 and VP1 proteins were compared to all available parvovirus sequences, the closest relative was from a Cameroonian fruit bat chapparvovirus (MG693107.1) [8] with an amino acid identity of 61 and 63% respectively (Table S1). A 210 amino acid ORF that is missing a start codon and is overlapping the NS1 ORF was also detected showing 57% identity to its homologue protein in mouse kidney parvovirus (AXX39021) [18] (Figure 1, panel A). This NP ORF is widely conserved among chapparvoviruses [19]. The 5′ UTR DNA sequence was 68% identical to that of the bat parvovirus sequence (MG693107.1)). The virus was named cachavirus (canine chapparvovirus) strain 1A (CachaV-1A).

Distance matrices of the NS1 showed that the cachavirus is sufficiently divergent based on ICTV criteria [6] (members of same species showing >85% NS1 identity) to qualify as a member of a tentative new species *Carnivore chapparvovirus species* 1 in the proposed *Chapparvovirus* genus (Table S1). A phylogenetic analysis of the NS1 ORF confirms its closest currently known relative is from a Cameroonian fruit bat (Figure 1, panel B).

Using a nested PCR, the other 8 samples were tested for the presence of this virus which was detected in a second diarrheic sample from that outbreak.

A.

B.

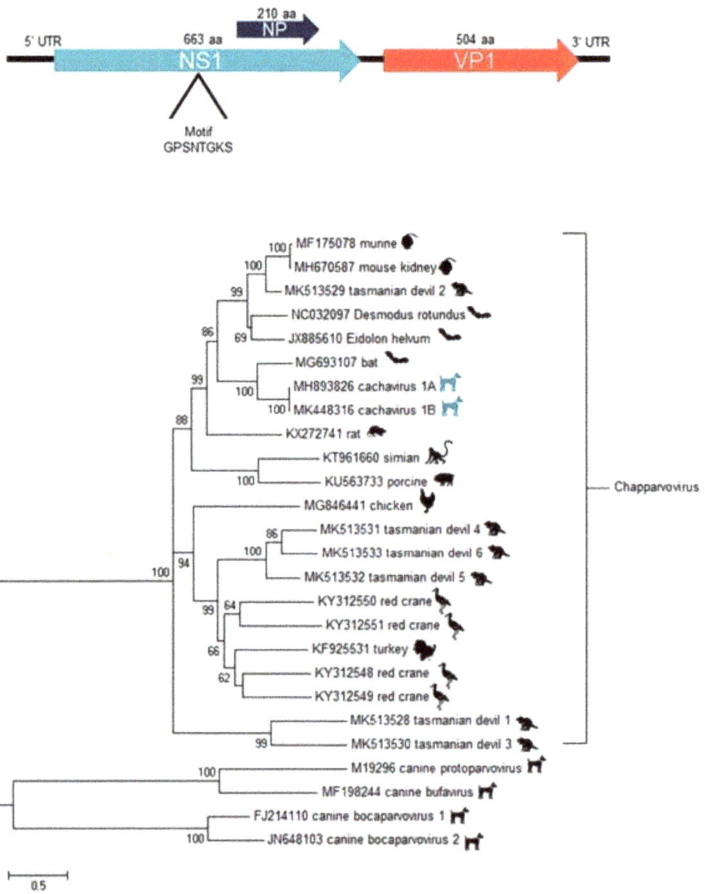

Figure 1. (**A**) ORF map and location of nucleotide-binding Walker loop motif. (B) Maximum likelihood tree of NS1 aa sequences of chapparvoviruses. Bar, 0.5 amino acid substitutions per site. Bootstrap values below 60 were removed.

A larger set of canine fecal samples were then tested using a real-time PCR assay. Of 2,053 fecal samples tested, a total of 80 were positive (Table 1). Fecal sample submissions from the same time frame as the outbreak (Sept-Oct 2017) were tested in order to determine the prevalence of CachaV-1 during that time. Healthy samples from fecal flotation samples submitted in 2018 for preventive care screening were available. A second set of diarrhea samples that were collected during the same time frame as the healthy samples was also analyzed to check for differences in prevalence across time, as was a set of 83 bloody diarrhea samples.

Three stool samples out of 203 healthy animals tested positive, 32 were positive out of 802 diarrhea submissions from September to October of 2017, and 45 were positive out of 965 diarrhea submissions from September to October of 2018. None of the 83 bloody diarrhea samples tested were positive (Table 1). When the fraction of PCR positive fecal samples was compared between the healthy animals (1.47% positive) and those with diarrhea, a statistically significant difference ($p < 0.05$) could be detected with the 965 diarrhea cases from 2018 (4.66% positive; $p = 0.037$), but not with the 803 diarrhea cases collected in 2017 (4.0% positive; $p = 0.08$). When 2017 and 2018 diarrhea samples were combined (4.35% positive) and compared to the healthy group (1.47% positive), we measured a *p*-value of 0.05.

Cachavirus viral load as reflected by the Ct value of the real-time PCR were low across all four cohorts, with Ct values ranging from 29 to 39 with an average value of 36 for all positive groups. The five dog samples with the lowest Ct values (highest viral load) were then analyzed by viral metagenomics. All five samples yielded cachavirus reads, but one yielded a near complete genome (cachavirus [1B]). This sample also yielded 0.001% reads that were related to anelloviruses. None of the other four animals showed the presence of other known mammalian viruses. The cachavirus-1B genome showed 98% overall nucleotide identity with the index IDEXX-1A strain. The NS1 and VP encoded protein showed 99 % identity.

Table 1. Real-time PCR results of cachavirus from four cohorts. A total of 2,053 samples were tested.

	Healthy Stool	Bloody Diarrhea	Diarrhea Submissions Sept-Oct 2017	Diarrhea Submissions Sept-Oct 2018	Total Diarrhea submissions (2017 + 2018)
number	203	83	802	965	1767
# Tested positive	3	0	32	45	77
Frequency	1.47%	0%	3.99%	4.66%	4.35%
Average Ct	36.49	-	36.48	36.38	36.15
p-value of frequency when compared to healthy cohort	-	-	0.08	0.037	0.05

4. Discussion

There are currently five other known canine parvovirus species belonging to two genera of the *Parvoviridae* family. Canine parvovirus 2 (CPV2) in the *Carnivore protoparvovirus 1* species is a highly pathogenic virus that is closely related to feline parvovirus (FPV), the cause of feline panleukopenia, and can infect other carnivores such as coyotes, wolfs, raccoons and pumas [29]. Canine bufavirus, a second protoparvovirus (in the species *Carnivore protoparvovirus 2*) was reported in 2018 in fecal and respiratory samples from both healthy and dogs with signs of respiratory illness [30]. That same protoparvovirus was recently reported as a frequent component of juvenile cats fecal and respiratory samples [31]. The canine minute virus (CnMV) in the *Carnivore bocaparvovirus 1* species is less pathogenic than CPV2 but can cause diarrhea in young pups and is frequently found in the context of co-infections [32]. Distantly related to CnMV, a second canine bocavirus in the *Carnivore bocaparvovirus 2* species was sequenced in dogs with respiratory diseases [33]. A third bocavirus was then characterized from the liver of a dog with severe hemorrhagic gastroenteritis [34].

Here, we describe the near complete genomes of two closely related cachaviruses, members of a new tentative species (*Carnivore chapparvovirus 1*) in a proposed genus *Chapparvovirus*, the third genera of viruses from the *Parvoviridae* family now reported in canine samples. The chapparvovirus was found in only two animals of the initial nine sampled. Many of the dogs in the outbreak analyzed were sampled more than 10 days after onset of clinical signs, increasing the possibility that they were no longer shedding viruses. Additionally, diarrhea is one of the top reasons for veterinary visits and some patients may have coincidentally presented with diarrhea from some other cause.

The two samples positive for CachaV-1 presented in the same week and were in the group of patients with the most severe clinical signs, requiring plasma transfusion and more aggressive supportive care. One of the two dogs, sampled at nine days after onset, died two days later. Because of the variable and often delayed feces sampling, it was therefore not possible to determine a clear disease association in this small group of diarrheic dogs (i.e., not all affected animals were shedding cachavirus).

A possible role for the cachavirus infection in canine diarrhea was further tested by comparing cachavirus DNA PCR detection in larger groups of healthy and diarrheic animals including a group of animals with bloody diarrhea. A statistically significant difference ($p = 0.037$) was seen when diarrhea samples from 2018 were compared to the feces from healthy animals collected the same year. When 2017 diarrheic samples were compared to e 2018 healthy samples, the p-value was 0.08. When 2017 and 2018 diarrhea samples were combined and compared to the healthy samples, the p-value was 0.05. The association of cachavirus with diarrhea is therefore borderline and the detection of viral DNA remains limited to ~4% of cases of diarrhea. The limited number of healthy samples available for PCR limited the statistical power of this analysis and a larger sample size will be required for further testing of disease association. The absence of detectable cachavirus DNA in 83 other cases of bloody diarrhea was unexpected given the similar signs that developed in the initial outbreak. Detection of viral DNA in feces may be related to timing of sample collection as shedding of the intestinal lining during hemorrhagic diarrhea may preclude viral replication and fecal shedding.

The detection of this virus in multiple fecal samples, the absence of prior cachavirus reports from tissues or fecal samples from other animals, and the confirmed vertebrate (murine) tropism of another chapparvovirus (mouse kidney parvovirus) [18], support the tentative conclusion that cachavirus infects dogs. Given its relatively low viral load and only borderline association with diarrhea, this virus' possible role in canine diarrhea or other diseases will require further epidemiological studies. Because viral nucleic acids in fecal samples may also originate from ingestion of contaminated food (rather than replication in gut tissues), the tropism of cachavirus for dogs will require further confirmation such as specific antibody detection, viral culture in canine cells, and/or evidence of replication in vivo such as RNA expression in enteric tissues of dogs shedding cachavirus DNA.

Supplementary Materials: The following are available online at http://www.mdpi.com/1999-4915/11/5/398/s1, Table S1: Percent identity between NS1 proteins of chapparvoviruses

Author Contributions: Conceptualization, E.F., M.A.S., P.Y., M.E. and C.L. and E.D.; Data curation, E.F., E.A., M.A.S., P.Y., M.E. and C.L.; Formal analysis, E.F., M.A.S., P.Y., and C.L.; Methodology, E.F.; Supervision, E.D.; Validation, M.E.; Writing—original draft, E.F.; Writing—review and editing, E.F. and E.D.

Acknowledgments: The authors would like to acknowledge IDEXX and the Vitalant Research Institute for funding.

Conflicts of Interest: At the time of this research, M.A.S., P.Y., C.L. and M.E. were employees of IDEXX Reference Laboratories, a division of IDEXX Laboratories, Inc., a company that provides veterinary diagnostics. IDEXX funded a portion of the work described in the article. The other authors declare no conflicts of interest.

References

1. Cave, N.J.; Marks, S.L.; Kass, P.H.; Melli, A.C.; Brophy, M.A. Evaluation of a routine diagnostic fecal panel for dogs with diarrhea. *J. Am. Vet. Med. Assoc.* **2002**, *221*, 52–59. [CrossRef]
2. Nandi, S.; Kumar, M. Canine parvovirus: Current perspective. *Indian J. Virol.* **2010**, *21*, 31–44. [CrossRef]
3. Conteville, L.C.; Zanella, L.; Marín, M.A.; Filippis, A.M.B.d.; Nogueira, R.M.R.; Vicente, A.C.P.; Mendonça, M.C.L.d. Parvovirus B19 1A complete genome from a fatal case in Brazil. *Mem. Inst. Oswaldo Cruz* **2015**, *110*, 820–821. [CrossRef]
4. Pérez, R.; Calleros, L.; Marandino, A.; Sarute, N.; Iraola, G.; Grecco, S.; Blanc, H.; Vignuzzi, M.; Isakov, O.; Shomron, N. Phylogenetic and genome-wide deep-sequencing analyses of canine parvovirus reveal co-infection with field variants and emergence of a recent recombinant strain. *PLOS ONE* **2014**, *9*, e111779. [CrossRef] [PubMed]
5. Miranda, C.; Parrish, C.R.; Thompson, G. Canine parvovirus 2c infection in a cat with severe clinical disease. *J. Vet. Diagn. Invest.* **2014**, *26*, 462–464. [CrossRef]
6. Cotmore, S.F.; Agbandje-McKenna, M.; Canuti, M.; Chiorini, J.A.; Eis-Hubinger, A.M.; Hughes, J.; Mietzsch, M.; Modha, S.; Ogliastro, M.; Penzes, J.J.; et al. ICTV Virus Taxonomy Profile: Parvoviridae. *J. Gen. Virol.* **2019**, *23*, 367–368. [CrossRef]
7. Yang, S.; Liu, Z.; Wang, Y.; Li, W.; Fu, X.; Lin, Y.; Shen, Q.; Wang, X.; Wang, H.; Zhang, W. A novel rodent Chapparvovirus in feces of wild rats. *Virol. J.* **2016**, *13*, 133. [CrossRef] [PubMed]
8. Yinda, C.K.; Ghogomu, S.M.; Conceicao-Neto, N.; Beller, L.; Deboutte, W.; Vanhulle, E.; Maes, P.; Van Ranst, M.; Matthijnssens, J. Cameroonian fruit bats harbor divergent viruses, including rotavirus H, bastroviruses, and picobirnaviruses using an alternative genetic code. *Virus Evol.* **2018**, *4*, vey008. [CrossRef] [PubMed]

9. Baker, K.S.; Leggett, R.M.; Bexfield, N.H.; Alston, M.; Daly, G.; Todd, S.; Tachedjian, M.; Holmes, C.E.; Crameri, S.; Wang, L.F.; et al. Metagenomic study of the viruses of African straw-coloured fruit bats: Detection of a chiropteran poxvirus and isolation of a novel adenovirus. *Virology* **2013**, *441*, 95–106. [CrossRef] [PubMed]
10. Souza, W.M.; Romeiro, M.F.; Fumagalli, M.J.; Modha, S.; de Araujo, J.; Queiroz, L.H.; Durigon, E.L.; Figueiredo, L.T.; Murcia, P.R.; Gifford, R.J. Chapparvoviruses occur in at least three vertebrate classes and have a broad biogeographic distribution. *J. Gen. Virol.* **2017**, *98*, 225–229. [CrossRef]
11. Kapusinszky, B.; Ardeshir, A.; Mulvaney, U.; Deng, X.; Delwart, E. Case-Control Comparison of Enteric Viromes in Captive Rhesus Macaques with Acute or Idiopathic Chronic Diarrhea. *J. Virol.* **2017**, *91*. [CrossRef] [PubMed]
12. Reuter, G.; Boros, A.; Delwart, E.; Pankovics, P. Novel circular single-stranded DNA virus from turkey faeces. *Arch. Virol.* **2014**, *159*, 2161–2164. [CrossRef] [PubMed]
13. Palinski, R.M.; Mitra, N.; Hause, B.M. Discovery of a novel Parvovirinae virus, porcine parvovirus 7, by metagenomic sequencing of porcine rectal swabs. *Virus Genes* **2016**, *52*, 564–567. [CrossRef]
14. Williams, S.H.; Che, X.; Garcia, J.A.; Klena, J.D.; Lee, B.; Muller, D.; Ulrich, W.; Corrigan, R.M.; Nichol, S.; Jain, K.; et al. Viral Diversity of House Mice in New York City. *MBio* **2018**, *9*, 01354–01317. [CrossRef] [PubMed]
15. Chong, R.; Shi, M.; Grueber, C.E.; Holmes, E.C.; Hogg, C.; Belov, K.; Barrs, V.R. Fecal viral diversity of captive and wild Tasmanian devils characterized using virion-enriched metagenomics and meta-transcriptomics. *J. Virol.* **2019**. [CrossRef] [PubMed]
16. Wang, Y.; Yang, S.; Liu, D.; Zhou, C.; Li, W.; Lin, Y.; Wang, X.; Shen, Q.; Wang, H.; Li, C.; et al. The fecal virome of red-crowned cranes. *Arch. Virol.* **2019**, *164*, 3–16. [CrossRef] [PubMed]
17. Lima, D.A.; Cibulski, S.P.; Tochetto, C.; Varela, A.P.M.; Finkler, F.; Teixeira, T.F.; Loiko, M.R.; Cerva, C.; Junqueira, D.M.; Mayer, F.Q.; et al. The intestinal virome of malabsorption syndrome-affected and unaffected broilers through shotgun metagenomics. *Virus Res.* **2019**, *261*, 9–20. [CrossRef]
18. Roediger, B.; Lee, Q.; Tikoo, S.; Cobbin, J.C.A.; Henderson, J.M.; Jormakka, M.; O'Rourke, M.B.; Padula, M.P.; Pinello, N.; Henry, M.; et al. An Atypical Parvovirus Drives Chronic Tubulointerstitial Nephropathy and Kidney Fibrosis. *Cell* **2018**, *175*, 530–543.e524. [CrossRef] [PubMed]
19. Pénzes, J.J.; de Souza, W.M.; Agbandje-McKenna, M.; Gifford, R.J. An ancient lineage of highly divergent parvoviruses infects both vertebrate and invertebrate hosts. *bioRxiv* **2019**. [CrossRef]
20. Allander, T.; Emerson, S.U.; Engle, R.E.; Purcell, R.H.; Bukh, J. A virus discovery method incorporating DNase treatment and its application to the identification of two bovine parvovirus species. *Proc. Nat. Acad. Sci. USA* **2001**, *98*, 11609–11614. [CrossRef] [PubMed]
21. Victoria, J.G.; Kapoor, A.; Li, L.; Blinkova, O.; Slikas, B.; Wang, C.; Naeem, A.; Zaidi, S.; Delwart, E. Metagenomic Analyses of Viruses in Stool Samples from Children with Acute Flaccid Paralysis. *J. Virol.* **2009**, *83*, 4642–4651. [CrossRef]
22. Deng, X.; Naccache, S.N.; Ng, T.; Federman, S.; Li, L.; Chiu, C.Y.; Delwart, E.L. An ensemble strategy that significantly improves de novo assembly of microbial genomes from metagenomic next-generation sequencing data. *Nucleic Acids Res.* **2015**, *43*. [CrossRef] [PubMed]
23. Zaretskaya, I.; Johnson, M.; McGinnis, S.; Raytselis, Y.; Merezhuk, Y.; Madden, T.L. NCBI BLAST: a better web interface. *Nucleic acids research* **2008**, *36*, W5–W9. [CrossRef]
24. Tamura, K.; Stecher, G.; Peterson, D.; Filipski, A.; Kumar, S. MEGA6: Molecular Evolutionary Genetics Analysis version 6.0. *Mol. Boil. Evol.* **2013**, *30*, 2725–2729. [CrossRef]
25. Edgar, R.C. MUSCLE: Multiple sequence alignment with high accuracy and high throughput. *Nucleic Acids Res.* **2004**, *32*, 1792–1797. [CrossRef]
26. Jones, D.T.; Taylor, W.R.; Thornton, J.M. The rapid generation of mutation data matrices from protein sequences. *Comput. Appl. Biosci.* **1992**, *8*, 275–282. [CrossRef]
27. Chu, D.K.; Poon, L.L.; Chiu, S.S.; Chan, K.H.; Ng, E.M.; Bauer, I.; Cheung, T.K.; Ng, I.H.; Guan, Y.; Wang, D.; et al. Characterization of a novel gyrovirus in human stool and chicken meat. *J. Clin. Virol.* **2012**, *55*, 209–213. [CrossRef] [PubMed]
28. Okamoto, H.; Takahashi, M.; Nishizawa, T.; Tawara, A.; Fukai, K.; Muramatsu, U.; Naito, Y.; Yoshikawa, A. Genomic characterization of TT viruses (TTVs) in pigs, cats and dogs and their relatedness with species-specific TTVs in primates and tupaias. *J. Gen. Virol.* **2002**, *83*, 1291–1297. [CrossRef] [PubMed]

29. Allison, A.B.; Kohler, D.J.; Fox, K.A.; Brown, J.D.; Gerhold, R.W.; Shearn-Bochsler, V.I.; Dubovi, E.J.; Parrish, C.R.; Holmes, E.C. Frequent cross-species transmission of parvoviruses among diverse carnivore hosts. *J. Virol.* **2013**, *87*, 2342–2347. [CrossRef]
30. Vito, M.; Gianvito, L.; Eszter, M.K.; Szilvia, M.; Renáta, V.-K.; Eszter, K.; Barbara Di, M.; Michele, C.; Nicola, D.; Canio, B.; et al. Novel Parvovirus Related to Primate Bufaviruses in Dogs. *Emerg. Infect. Dis. J.* **2018**, *24*, 1061. [CrossRef]
31. Diakoudi, G.; Lanave, G.; Capozza, P.; Di Profio, F.; Melegari, I.; Di Martino, B.; Pennisi, M.G.; Elia, G.; Cavalli, A.; Tempesta, M.; et al. Identification of a novel parvovirus in domestic cats. *Vet. Microbiol.* **2019**, *228*, 246–251. [CrossRef] [PubMed]
32. Carmichael, L.E.; Schlafer, D.H.; Hashimoto, A. Pathogenicity of minute virus of canines (MVC) for the canine fetus. *Cornell Vet.* **1991**, *81*, 151–171. [PubMed]
33. Kapoor, A.; Mehta, N.; Dubovi, E.J.; Simmonds, P.; Govindasamy, L.; Medina, J.L.; Street, C.; Shields, S.; Lipkin, W.I. Characterization of novel canine bocaviruses and their association with respiratory disease. *J. Gen. Virol.* **2012**, *93*, 341–346. [CrossRef] [PubMed]
34. Li, L.; Pesavento, P.A.; Leutenegger, C.M.; Estrada, M.; Coffey, L.L.; Naccache, S.N.; Samayoa, E.; Chiu, C.; Qiu, J.; Wang, C.; et al. A novel bocavirus in canine liver. *Virol. J.* **2013**, *10*, 10–54. [CrossRef] [PubMed]

viruses

MDPI

Article

Molecular Characterization and Evolutionary Analyses of *Carnivore Protoparvovirus 1 NS1* Gene

Francesco Mira [1,†], Marta Canuti [2,†], Giuseppa Purpari [1,†], Vincenza Cannella [1], Santina Di Bella [1,*], Leonardo Occhiogrosso [3], Giorgia Schirò [1], Gabriele Chiaramonte [1], Santino Barreca [1], Patrizia Pisano [1], Antonio Lastra [1], Nicola Decaro [3] and Annalisa Guercio [1]

1 Istituto Zooprofilattico Sperimentale della Sicilia "A.Mirri", Via Gino Marinuzzi n. 3, 90129 Palermo, Italy; dottoremira@gmail.com (F.M.); giuseppa.purpari@izssicilia.it (G.P.); vincenza.cannella@izssicilia.it (V.C.); giorgia.schiro@hotmail.it (G.S.); gabrielechiaramonte90@gmail.com (G.C.); santinobarreca@gmail.com (S.B.); pisano.patrizia@libero.it (P.P.); lastra.antonio77@gmail.com (A.L.); annalisa.guercio@izssicilia.it (A.G.)

2 Department of Biology, Memorial University of Newfoundland, 232 Elizabeth Ave., St. John's, NL A1B 3X9, Canada; marta.canuti@gmail.com

3 Department of Veterinary Medicine, University of Bari, Strada provinciale per Casamassima Km 3, 70010 Valenzano, Italy; leonardo.occhiogrosso@uniba.it (L.O.); nicola.decaro@uniba.it (N.D.)

* Correspondence: santinadibella78@gmail.com

† These authors contributed equally to this work.

Received: 25 February 2019; Accepted: 26 March 2019; Published: 29 March 2019

Abstract: *Carnivore protoparvovirus 1* is the etiological agent of a severe disease of terrestrial carnivores. This unique specie encompasses canine parvovirus type 2 (CPV-2) and feline panleukopenia virus (FPLV). Studies widely analyzed the main capsid protein (VP2), but limited information is available on the nonstructural genes (*NS1*/*NS2*). This paper analyzed the *NS1* gene sequence of FPLV and CPV strains collected in Italy in 2009–2017, along with worldwide related sequences. Differently from VP2, only one NS1 amino-acid residue (248) clearly and constantly distinguished FPLV from CPV-2, while five possible convergent amino-acid changes were observed that may affect the functional domains of the NS1. Some synonymous mutation in NS1 were non-synonymous in NS2 and vice versa. No evidence for recombination between the two lineages was found, and the predominance of negative selection pressure on NS1 proteins was observed, with low and no overlap between the two lineages in negatively and positively selected codons, respectively. More sites were under selection in the CPV-2 lineage. NS1 phylogenetic analysis showed divergent evolution between FPLV and CPV, and strains were clustered mostly by country and year of detection. We highlight the importance of obtaining the *NS1*/*NS2* coding sequence in molecular epidemiology investigations.

Keywords: *Carnivore protoparvovirus 1*; canine parvovirus; feline panleukopenia virus; NS1; NS2; sequence analysis; evolution

1. Introduction

Carnivore protoparvovirus 1 is a member of the *Protoparvovirus* genus (family *Parvoviridae*, subfamily *Parvovirinae*). As defined by the International Committee on Taxonomy of Viruses (ICTV) [1], both canine parvovirus type 2 (CPV-2) and feline panleukopenia virus (FPLV) are included in this unique specie, together with mink enteritis virus (MEV) and raccoon parvovirus (RaPV) [2,3]. In susceptible dogs and cats, *Carnivore protoparvovirus 1* commonly causes an acute and often lethal disease, inducing vomiting, enteritis, diarrhea, and acute lymphopenia [4].

FPLV is known since the beginning of the 20th century [5] and, during decades, it maintained a certain genetic stability [6]. Contrarily, CPV-2 emerged as a dog pathogen only in the late 1970s, most likely as a host variant of the feline virus or a related strain [7], and it displayed higher rates of nucleotide changes [8–11]. Indeed, soon after its emergence, the original CPV-2 type was replaced by two antigenic variants, CPV-2a and 2b [12,13], and in 2000 a third variant was detected, termed CPV-2c [14]. While dogs are susceptible only to the original CPV-2 and all its variants, cats are susceptible to both FPLV and CPV-2 variants [15–17], except the original CPV-2 type, despite the fact that FPLV remains the prevalent cause of parvovirus infection in domestic felines [18].

Carnivore protoparvovirus 1 includes small, non-enveloped, linear single-stranded DNA viruses. Their genome consists of an approximately 5200-nucleotide (nt) DNA molecule containing two large open reading frames (ORFs), encoding for two nonstructural (NS1 and NS2) and for two structural (VP1 and VP2) proteins, generated through alternative splicing of the same messenger RNAs (mRNAs) [4,19].

Among encoded structural proteins, VP2 is the major capsid protein, represents the main determinant of host range, and is subject to antibody-mediated selection [20,21]. On the other hand, the nonstructural proteins NS1 and NS2 are essential for viral replication, DNA packaging, cytotoxicity, and pathogenicity [22–24]. Due to the involvement of the VP2 capsid protein in host switch and due to its fast evolutionary rate, most studies on CPV and FPLV focused their attention on the *VP2* gene and on the structural analysis of the encoded protein. Contributions on the genetic analysis of the nonstructural genes [18,24] and on the structural analysis of the encoded proteins are limited, highlighting the limits of available sequence data [8,25–28]. The nonstructural protein 2 (NS2) of FPLV and CPV is produced by the conjunction of left-hand 260-nt and right-hand 238-nt genetic fragments of the NS1 open reading frame, but no studies were conducted on the NS2 amino-acid divergences within this viral species.

Only a few studies described the dynamics driving genetic changes of the CPV and FPLV *NS1* gene and the potential recombination events involving this gene [29,30], although recombination was hypothesized as a potential alternative source of genetic variations [18]. Moreover, the *NS1* gene molecular features, as a useful tool in outbreak tracing, were only recently reconsidered [31,32]. Despite the most recent sequence analyses on CPV also including this genomic ORF, there are still limited studies on the FPLV NS1 sequence [30,33–35].

The aim of this paper was to characterize NS1 sequences of FPLV and CPV strains, collected from cats and dogs in Italy, and to compare them to NS1 sequences available in public domain sequence databases. Sequence analyses, genetic diversity estimation, evaluation of potential recombination events, and phylogeny studies were performed to better elucidate the molecular features of NS1 and its role in the evolution of CPV-2 and FPLV. Moreover, the NS2 sequences were also characterized and the deduced amino-acid divergences were analyzed.

2. Materials and Methods

2.1. Sample Collection

The sequences analyzed in this study were obtained from samples collected from 18 cats and 29 dogs from 2009 to 2017. Samples or carcasses of animals with suspicion of parvovirus infection were submitted to the Istituto Zooprofilattico Sperimentale della Sicilia "A. Mirri" (Palermo, Italy) for necropsy for diagnostic purposes. Rectal swabs or organs (intestine, spleen, heart, brain) from domestic dogs and cats with different geographical origins and living conditions (client-owned or shelter animals) were collected and submitted for virological analyses. Details are summarized in Table 1.

Table 1. Origin and information on samples of cats and dogs. FPLV—feline panleukopenia virus; CPV—canine parvovirus.

Sample Id *	Date of Sampling	Origin	Sample	Type	Accession Number	Reference
72752/13	23 Oct 2013	Cat	Spleen	FPLV	MK413724 [a]	This study
4311/14	21 Jan 2014	Cat	Spleen	FPLV	MK413725 [a]	This study
149/15	05 Jan 2015	Cat	Intestine	FPLV	MK413726 [a]	This study
3201c1/15	24 Nov 2015	Cat	Intestine	FPLV	KX434461 [a]	This study
38056c2/15	26 Aug 2015	Cat	Intestine	FPLV	MK413727 [a]	This study
32369/15	14 Jul 2015	Cat	Intestine	FPLV	MK413728 [a]	This study
42807/15	24 Nov 2015	Cat	Rectal swab	FPLV	KX434462 [a]	This study
52333eva/15	18 Nov 2015	Cat	Heart	FPLV	MK413729 [a]	This study
55611/15	07 Dec 2015	Cat	Intestine	FPLV	MK413730 [a]	This study
58774/15	23 Dec 2015	Cat	Intestine	FPLV	MK413731 [a]	This study
PA285c2/16	12 Jan 2016	Cat	Intestine	FPLV	MK413732 [b]	This study
RG21/16	04 Jan 2016	Cat	Spleen	FPLV	MK413733 [b]	This study
PA12880Fe/16	11 Apr 2016	Cat	Intestine	FPLV	MK413734 [b]	This study
PA12880Re/16	11 Apr 2016	Cat	Spleen	FPLV	MK413735 [b]	This study
PA12880Mi/16	11 Apr 2016	Cat	Intestine	FPLV	MK413736 [b]	This study
PA11334/17	20 Apr 2017	Cat	Brain	FPLV	MK413737 [a]	This study
CT1375/17	20 Feb 2017	Cat	Spleen	FPLV	MK413738 [a]	This study
29451/09	10 Sep 2009	Dog	Intestine	CPV-2a	KX434454 [a]	This study
987/10	14 Jul 2010	Dog	Intestine	CPV-2a	KX434457 [a]	This study
PA40697/16	02 Nov 2016	Dog	Spleen	CPV-2a	MK413739 [b]	This study
PA43847/16	21 Nov 2016	Dog	Rectal swab	CPV-2a	MG434738 [a]	[32]
PA48686/16	21 Dec 2016	Dog	Intestine	CPV-2a	MG434739 [a]	[32]
PA3213/17	09 Feb 2017	Dog	Intestine	CPV-2a	MG434740 [a]	[32]
PA5610/17	03 Mar 2017	Dog	Rectal swab	CPV-2a	MG434741 [a]	[32]
PA10388/17	11 Apr 2017	Dog	Spleen	CPV-2a	MG434742 [a]	[32]
PA13577/17	15 May 2017	Dog	Spleen	CPV-2a	MG434743 [a]	[32]
PA13579id90/17	15 May 2017	Dog	Intestine	CPV-2a	MG434744 [a]	[32]
PA13579id93/17	15 May 2017	Dog	Spleen	CPV-2a	MG434745 [a]	[32]
PA30636/17	31 Oct 2017	Dog	Spleen	CPV-2a	MK413740 [a]	This study
PA31209/17	07 Nov 2017	Dog	Spleen	CPV-2a	MK413741 [a]	This study
PA13600/17	15 May 2017	Dog	Spleen	CPV-2b	MK413742 [a]	This study
23782/09	10 Sep 2009	Dog	Intestine	CPV-2c	KX434455 [a]	This study
25835/09	10 Sep 2009	Dog	Intestine	CPV-2c	KU508407 [a]	This study
45361/09	21 Oct 2009	Dog	Intestine	CPV-2c	KX434456 [a]	This study
2323/11	21 Jun 2011	Dog	Intestine	CPV-2c	KX434458 [a]	This study
27692c1/11	05 Jul 2011	Dog	Intestine	CPV-2c	KX434459 [a]	This study
52238/12	20 Oct 2012	Dog	Intestine	CPV-2c	KX434460 [a]	This study
PA15423/16	29 Apr 2016	Cat	Spleen	CPV-2c	MK413743 [a]	This study
PA36395/16	06 Oct 2016	Dog	Intestine	CPV-2c	MK413744 [a]	This study
PA39667/16	26 Oct 2016	Dog	Brain	CPV-2c	MK413745 [b]	This study
41113c1/16	03 Nov 2016	Dog	Rectal swab	CPV-2c	MF510158 [a]	[36]
PA41113c2/16	03 Nov 2016	Dog	Rectal swab	CPV-2c	MK413746 [a]	This study
PA45984/16	01 Dec 2016	Dog	Rectal swab	CPV-2c	MK413747 [a]	This study
2743/17	06 Feb 2017	Dog	Intestine	CPV-2c	MF510157 [a]	[36]
CT1839id0018/17	02 Mar 2017	Dog	Intestine	CPV-2c	MK413748 [a]	This study
CT1839id2213/17	02 Mar 2017	Dog	Intestine	CPV-2c	MK413749 [a]	This study
PA27184/17	29 Sep 2017	Dog	Rectal swab	CPV-2c	MK413750 [a]	This study

* Samples in bold correspond to strain isolated. [a] ORF1 and ORF2 sequences; [b] *NS1* gene sequence.

2.2. DNA Extraction and Parvovirus PCR

Viral DNA was extracted from 200 μL of swab/organ homogenate, obtained as previously described [37], using a DNeasy Blood and Tissue Kit (Qiagen S.p.A., Milan, Italy) according to the manufacturer's instructions. Presence of FPLV and CPV DNA was evaluated using a primer pair amplifying a 700-bp fragment of the *VP2* gene [38] following a previously described PCR protocol [32].

2.3. Viral Isolation

Samples that tested positive (in bold in Table 1) were processed as previously described [37] and supernatants were inoculated in 80% confluent cell (A-72, CrFK) monolayers, cultured in minimum essential medium (MEM) with 10% bovine fetal serum (EuroClone S.p.A., Pero, Italy), antibiotic and antifungal solution (100 U/mL penicillin G sodium salt, 0.1 mg/mL streptomycin sulfate, 0.25 ug/mL amphotericin B; PAA Laboratories GmbH, Austria), 1% sodium pyruvate (A-72 cells), and 0.1% lactalbumin (CrFK cells). Inoculated cells were daily monitored for a maximum of five days and viral growth was evaluated by detection of cytopathic effect (CPE) and PCR. A total of five passages were carried out before considering virus isolation as unsuccessful.

2.4. Sequence Analysis

CPV/FPLV DNA from positive samples and from cell cultures with CPE were submitted to sequencing. Analyses were conducted amplifying a long genomic sequence, encompassing both ORFs, NS and VP, using primers pairs described by Pérez et al. [28] and the commercial kit GoTaq® G2 DNA Polymerase (Promega Italia s.r.l., Milan, Italy). Reaction mixes were prepared as previously described [36], with minor modifications (thermal conditions: 2 min for the elongation steps). Positive amplicons were purified with Illustra™ GFX™ PCR DNA and Gel Band Purification Kit (GE Healthcare Life Sciences, Amersham, Buckinghamshire, UK) and submitted to BMR Genomics srl (Padua, Italy) for direct Sanger sequencing. Overlapping sequences were assembled using BioEdit ver. 7.2.5 software [39] and a nearly complete genomic sequence for each sample was obtained.

Ten positive cell culture supernatants were submitted to the Istituto Zooprofilattico Sperimentale della Lombardia e dell'Emilia Romagna "Bruno Ubertini" (Parma, Italy) for sequencing service using next-generation sequencing (NGS) methodologies. DNA was extracted using the One for All Vet Kit (Qiagen, Milan, Italy) and amplified using primers F194/NS-Rext and 2161F/R4848 described by Pérez et al. [28]. Sequencing libraries were prepared using the Nextera XT kit (Illumina Inc. San Diego, CA, USA) and sequenced using the Illumina MiSeq (Illumina Inc. San Diego, CA, USA) system. Read files generated by the sequencer were assembled and analyzed using the software SeqMan NGen 12.0.0 (DNASTAR, Madison, WI, USA).

The complete nucleotide *NS1* coding sequences (2007 nt) alignments were obtained using the ClustalW program included in the BioEdit software. Sequences were submitted to nBLAST [40] to search related sequences in public domain databases. In December 2017, 26 FPLV and 141 CPV complete *NS1* sequences were obtained from NCBI database, including two FPLV and 18 CPV sequences previously submitted to the same database from the Istituto Zooprofilattico Sperimentale della Sicilia "A. Mirri". Sequences originated from samples collected in years 1964–2016 (FPLV) and 1978–2017 (CPV), from domestic and wild animals in America (nine FPLVs and 34 CPVs from North America; 41 CPVs from South America), Europe (two FPLVs; three CPVs), Asia (14 FPLVs; 57 CPVs), and Oceania (one FPLV; four CPVs) (see Dataset S1, Supplementary Materials).

NS1 and *VP2* gene sequences were aligned with reference sequences obtained from the NCBI database, translated into amino-acid (aa) sequences (668 and 584 aa, respectively), and analyzed using the BioEdit software. The complete nucleotide *NS2* coding sequences (498 nt) were also obtained from the whole dataset of sequences using the ClustalW program and analyzed using the BioEdit software. Viral typing was based on the analysis of VP2 amino-acid (aa) residues discriminating the viral type (FPLV/CPV) and the CPV variants [41]. Sequence data were submitted to the DDBJ/EMBL/GenBank databases under accession numbers reported in Table 1.

2.5. Recombination and Selection Pressure Analyses

The NS1 alignment was tested for the presence of potentially recombinant sequences with all the different methods included in the RDP 4 software package [42], as described in Canuti et al. [43]. Detected recombination events were confirmed by constructing maximum-likelihood phylogenetic trees with MEGA7 software [44], inferred with the maximum-likelihood method based on the Hasegawa–Kishino–Yano and Kimura 2-parameter models [45,46], the best-fitting models after the model test analysis. A discrete Gamma distribution was used to model evolutionary rate differences among sites.

To estimate the presence of selection pressure, the overall average synonymous (dS) and non-synonymous (dN) substitutions for each alignment (whole dataset, CPV subset, and FPLV subset) were calculated with the Z-test of selection implemented in MEGA 7. The Nei–Gojobori method [47] was used to test hypotheses of deviation from strict neutrality (null hypothesis, dN = dS), test of neutrality (dN =/= dS), purifying selection pressure (dN < dS), and positive selection pressure (dN > dS). Variance was estimated with the bootstrap method and 1000 replicates.

Individual sites under positive and purifying selection were identified with FUBAR (Fast Unconstrained Bayesian Approximation for inferring selection) [48], while those under episodic diversifying selection were detected with MEME (Mixed-Effects Model of Evolution) [49]. Sites under selection were considered acceptable only when statistically significant ($p < 0.1$ for MEME and posterior probability >0.9 for FUBAR). Both methods are available on the Datamonkey Adaptive Evolution Server (https://www.datamonkey.org). FUBAR and MEME were performed on the FPLV and CPV branches separately, after excluding potentially recombinant sequences.

2.6. Phylogenetic Analysis

To elucidate the genetic relationships between the obtained CPV and FPLV strains and the reference sequences, a phylogenetic tree was constructed. Due to the high number of sequences in dataset 2, a subset of 86 sequences was generated by excluding highly identical or identical sequences derived from the same geographic area and the same year. The model selection was performed using the best-fit model of nt substitution with MEGA7 software [44]. A phylogenetic tree was constructed with the MEGA7 software using the maximum-likelihood (ML) method according to the Hasegawa–Kishino–Yano model [45] with discrete Gamma distribution (five rate categories) and bootstrap analyses with 1000 replicates. Viral type or CPV variants, based on the analysis of the VP2 aa residues as described above, were depicted in the phylogenetic tree for each NS1 sequence. Depicted clades and subclades in the phylogenetic tree were numbered with Roman numerals and are not meant as a classification of the type/variants, but rather to allow easier referencing in the text.

For comparison, a phylogenetic tree based on the *VP2* gene sequences of the same strains included in the NS1 tree was constructed with the MEGA7 software using the ML method according to the Tamura three-parameter model [45] with discrete Gamma distribution (five rate categories) and bootstrap analyses with 1000 replicates.

3. Results

3.1. Detection and Characterization of FPLV and CPV

All samples analyzed tested positive for *Carnivore protoparvovirus 1*. Positive samples were obtained from tissues commonly known as viral targets, such as intestine, spleen, and lymph nodes, as well as less tested tissues such as brain and cerebellum [50]. Based on the analysis of the VP2 amino-acid residues, 17 strains from the 18 cats were typed as FPLV and one was typed as CPV-2c. Among the samples collected from the 29 dogs, 13, one, and 15 strains were typed as CPV2a, CPV-2b, and CPV-2c variants, respectively. The CPV-2c strain collected from the cat (sample identifier PA15423/16) showed high identity with the other CPV-2c strains from this study collected from dogs (NS1: 100–99.75%; VP2: 99.94–99.71%) and the highest identity rates with the strain 41113c1/16, collected in the same year. Viral types/variants are listed in Table 1.

Interestingly, two unreported amino-acid changes were observed within the FPLV *VP2* gene sequences; the aa change A359G was also observed in two FPLV VP2 sequences (accession number KY083101–KY083104) from Singapore in 2015, and the aa change D311N, which was unique to the strains analyzed in this study, was never reported in other FPLV sequences. VP2 non-synonymous changes of analyzed FPLV and CPV strains are listed in Table S2 (Supplementary Materials).

3.2. Sequence Analysis of NS1 Gene

The *NS1* gene sequences of 2007 base pairs in length were obtained from each sample. Among FPLV *NS1* sequences, 17 nucleotide substitutions were observed, resulting in 12 synonymous and five non-synonymous (81V/I, 115I/V, 247H/Q, 595H/Q, 664Q/R) changes (Table 2).

Table 2. *NS1* non-synonymous changes of analyzed FPLV strains described in this study.

Strain	NS1 Amino Acids (Nucleotides) [a]						
	81 (241–243)	115 (343–345)	247 (739–741)	248 (742–744)	545 (1633–1635)	595 (1783–1785)	664 (1990–1992)
72752/13	V (GTT)	I (ATT)	H (CAT)	T (ACT)	E (GAA)	H (CAC)	Q (CAA)
4311/14	--	--	--	--	--	--	--
149/15	I (ATT)	V (GTT)	Q (CAA)	--	--	Q (CAA)	R (CGA)
3201c1/15	--	V (GTT)	Q (CAA)	--	--	Q (CAA)	R (CGA)
55611/15	--	V (GTT)	Q (CAA)	--	--	Q (CAA)	R (CGA)
RG21/16	--	V (GTT)	Q (CAA)	--	--	Q (CAA)	R (CGA)
38056c/15	--	--	--	--	--	--	--
32369/15	--	--	--	--	--	--	--
42807/15	--	--	--	--	--	--	--
52333eva/15	--	--	--	--	--	--	--
58774/15	--	--	--	--	--	--	--
PA285c2/16	--	--	--	--	--	--	--
PA12880Felix/16	--	--	--	--	--	--	--
PA12880Red/16	--	--	--	--	--	--	--
PA12880Miele/16	--	--	--	--	--	--	--
PA11334/17	--	--	--	--	--	--	--
CT1375/17	--	--	--	--	--	--	--

[a] Amino-acid and nucleotide (in brackets) positions refer to the prototype FPLV isolate FPV-4.us_64 (U.S.A.–1964; accession n.: EU659112). Sites where no variation was observed are marked by "--".

Among the CPV *NS1* sequences, 63 nucleotide substitutions were observed, resulting in 52 synonymous and 11 non-synonymous (60I/V, 239N/T, 350D/N, 397L/F, 544Y/F, 545E/V, 572K/E, 584T/A, 590P/S, 597L/P, 630L/P) changes (Table 4).

Table 3. *NS1* non-synonymous changes of analyzed CPV strains described in this study.

Strain	CPV Variant	NS1 Amino Acids (Nucleotides) [b]													
		60 (178–180)	239 (715–717)	247 (739–741)	248 (742–744)	350 (1048–1050)	397 (1189–1191)	544 (1630–1632)	545 (1633–1635)	572 (1714–1716)	584 (1750–1752)	590 (1768–1770)	595 (1783–1785)	597 (1789–1791)	630 (1888–1890)
29451/09	CPV-2a	I (ATT)	N (AAC)	Q (CAA)	I (ATT)	D (GAT)	L (CTT)	Y (TAT)	E (GAA)	K (AAA)	T (ACA)	P (CCT)	Q (CAA)	L (CTA)	L (CTT)
987/10	CPV-2a	–	–	–	–	N (AAT)	–	F (TTT)	–	E (GAA)	A (GCA)	–	–	–	–
PA40697/16	CPV-2a	–	–	–	–	N (AAT)	–	F (TTT)	–	E (GAA)	–	–	–	P (CCA)	–
PA43847/16	CPV-2a	–	T (ACC)	–	–	N (AAT)	–	F (TTT)	–	E (GAA)	–	–	–	P (CCA)	–
PA48686/16	CPV-2a	–	–	–	–	N (AAT)	–	F (TTT)	–	E (GAA)	–	–	–	P (CCA)	–
PA3213/17	CPV-2a	–	–	–	–	N (AAT)	F (TTT)	F (TTT)	–	E (GAA)	–	–	–	P (CCA)	–
PA5610/17	CPV-2a	–	–	–	–	N (AAT)	–	F (TTT)	–	E (GAA)	–	–	–	P (CCA)	–
PA10388/17	CPV-2a	–	–	–	–	N (AAT)	–	F (TTT)	–	E (GAA)	–	–	–	P (CCA)	–
PA13577/17	CPV-2a	–	–	–	–	N (AAT)	–	F (TTT)	–	E (GAA)	–	–	–	P (CCA)	–
PA13579id90/17	CPV-2a	–	–	–	–	N (AAT)	–	F (TTT)	–	E (GAA)	–	–	–	P (CCA)	–
PA13579id93/17	CPV-2a	–	–	–	–	N (AAT)	–	F (TTT)	–	E (GAA)	–	–	–	P (CCA)	–
PA30636/17	CPV-2a	–	–	–	–	N (AAT)	–	F (TTT)	–	E (GAA)	–	–	–	P (CCA)	–
PA31209/17	CPV-2a	–	–	–	–	N (AAT)	–	F (TTT)	–	E (GAA)	–	–	–	P (CCA)	–
PA13600/17	CPV-2b	–	–	–	–	– (AAC)	–	–	–	–	–	S (TCT)	–	P (CCA)	–
23782/09	CPV-2c	–	–	–	–	–	–	–	–	E (GAA)	– (ACG)	–	–	–	–
25835/09	CPV-2c	–	–	–	–	–	–	–	–	E (GAA)	– (ACG)	–	–	–	–
45361/09	CPV-2c	–	–	–	–	–	–	–	–	E (GAA)	– (ACG)	–	–	–	–
2323/11	CPV-2c	–	–	–	–	–	–	–	–	E (GAA)	– (ACG)	–	–	–	–
27692c1/11	CPV-2c	–	–	–	–	–	–	–	–	E (GAA)	– (ACG)	–	–	–	–
52238/12	CPV-2c	–	–	–	–	–	–	–	–	E (GAA)	– (ACG)	–	–	–	–
PA15423/16	CPV-2c	–	–	–	–	–	–	–	–	E (GAA)	– (ACG)	–	–	–	–

Table 4. *NS1* non-synonymous changes of analyzed CPV strains described in this study.

Strain	CPV Variant	NS1 Amino Acids (Nucleotides) [b]													
		60 (178–180)	239 (715–717)	247 (739–741)	248 (742–744)	350 (1048–1050)	397 (1189–1191)	544 (1630–1632)	545 (1633–1635)	572 (1714–1716)	584 (1750–1752)	590 (1768–1770)	595 (1783–1785)	597 (1789–1791)	630 (1888–1890)
PA36395/16	CPV-2c	--	--	--	--	--	--	--	--	E (GAA)	-- (ACG)	--	--	--	--
PA39667/16	CPV-2c	--	--	--	--	--	--	--	--	E (GAA)	-- (ACG)	--	--	--	--
41113c1/16	CPV-2c	--	--	--	--	--	--	--	--	E (GAA)	-- (ACG)	--	--	--	--
PA41113c2/16	CPV-2c	--	--	--	--	--	--	--	--	E (GAA)	-- (ACG)	--	--	--	--
PA45984/16	CPV-2c	--	--	--	--	--	--	--	--	E (GAA)	-- (ACG)	--	--	--	--
2743/17	CPV-2c	V (GTT)	--	--	--	--	--	F (TTT)	V (GTA)	E (GAA)	--	--	--	--	P (CCT)
CT1839id0018/17	CPV-2c	--	--	--	--	--	--	--	--	E (GAA)	-- (ACG)	--	--	--	--
CT1839id2213/17	CPV-2c	--	--	--	--	--	--	--	--	E (GAA)	-- (ACG)	--	--	--	--
PA27184/17	CPV-2c	--	--	--	--	--	--	--	--	E (GAA)	-- (ACG)	--	--	--	--

[b] Amino-acid and nucleotide (in brackets) positions refer to the prototype CPV strain CPV-N (U.S.A. – 1978; accession n.: M19296). Sites where no variation was observed are marked by "--".

Comparison of the analyzed sequences with those from the NCBI database evidenced only one aa change clearly distinguishing FPLV from CPV strains; at residue 248, FPLV showed T while CPV showed I, due to a nucleotide change in the second base of the codon (c743t).

Other differences among CPV and FPLV strains were found at aa residues 247, 545, and 595 (Tables 2 and 4; Dataset S1, Supplementary Materials). All CPV sequences showed a Q at residues 247 and 595 and an E at residue 545. The only exceptions were some strains of Asian origin, which showed V at residue 545. In contrast, FPLV sequences showed an H at residues 247 and 595, and a Q at residue 545. Unlike most of the FPLV sequences, nine analyzed FPLV sequences (Table 2; Dataset S1, Supplementary Materials) evidenced residues identical to CPV-2 at these sites (Q at residues 247 and 595, and E at residue 545). Change Q545E was evidenced in all FPLV strains collected in Italy.

In some FPLV sequences obtained from this study, two additional changes (V115I and R664Q) were evident (Table 2) that were previously observed only in three CPV sequences from China or Vietnam (Dataset S1, Supplementary Materials).

Only old FPLV strains from domestic/wild felids in the United States of America (USA) (M38246, EU659111, EU65913-15), Japan (AB000048-49, AB000057, AB000060, AB000062), and more recently from wild carnivores in Canada (MF069445-47) showed the specific changes N23D, V165I, and I443V (Dataset S1, Supplementary Materials).

Differences among CPVs were observed in strains collected in Italy in 2016–2017 (Table 4). Change D350N was also observed in older sequences (1983–2008), almost all collected in the USA. Changes Y544F and L597P were observed both in older sequences from the USA (1983–2010) and New Zealand (1994), as well as in more recent sequences from South America, Canada, and China.

Among sequences from CPV-2c strains, specific residues were observed in different geographic areas, such as Australia (11K, 25P, 72K, 73K, 74K), Uruguay and Brazil (351K), China and Vietnam, and in an Italian imported dog (MF510157) (60V, 630P).

3.3. Sequence Analysis of NS2 Gene

Nucleotide substitutions resulting in some non-synonymous changes in *NS1* also lie in the NS2-encoding sequence (V81I and H595Q, and I60V, T584A, P590S, L597P, and L630P of the FPLV and CPV NS1 sequences, respectively), while changes at codons 597 and 630 of *NS1* CPV-2 sequences did not result in any changes in the NS2 protein. Other changes generated the additional aa changes V81I and S105R, and 60I/V, D93G, and S99F in the NS2 of FPLV and CPV sequences, respectively (Dataset S3, Supplementary Materials).

Other amino-acid divergences in the CPV NS2-enconding sequences were observed among the analyzed strains: 94T/A, 109S/F, 110D/N, 151N/D, and 160E/Q. These changes were synonymous in the corresponding NS1 amino-acid residues. All these changes in the NS2 sequences are summarized in Dataset S3 (Supplementary Materials).

Divergences between FPLV and CPV were observed at aa residues 152 and 163. At residue 152, an M was observed in FPLV strains from the USA, Canada, Japan, and Australia, and a V was observed in the most recent FPLV strains from Europe (Italy and Belgium) and China. On the other hand, amino acid V was observed in almost all CPV strains, with the exception of old CPV-2 and CPV-2a strains from the USA, which showed M at the same residue. At residue 163, the FPLV strains, including the strains collected in Italy, showed the amino acid L, with the exception of some strains which showed F at the same residue. These changes in the *NS2* sequence resulted in silent mutations in the corresponding aa residues of the NS1 sequence of the same strains (aa 642 and 653).

3.4. Recombination and Selection Pressure Analyses

The analysis performed with RDP identified only one potential recombination event, involving three CPV sequences (recombinant: CPV-2a, KT382542; major parent: CPV-2b, KP749859; minor parent: CPV-2c, KP749873) (Recombination and Selection Pressures S4, Supplementary Materials), with one breakpoint (nt 1515), and this was confirmed by phylogenetic reconstructions (Recombination

S5, Supplementary Materials). Therefore, as positively selected sites may be overestimated when recombination is present [51], all selection pressure analyses were performed on the entire alignment after excluding the potentially recombinant sequence.

The *Z*-test allowed us to reject the null hypothesis of strict neutrality and detected an overall presence of purifying selection in all cases. FUBAR identified 124 and 42 sites to be under negative selection pressure in the CPV and FPLV clades, respectively (Table 5), and only nine and two of these sites were located within the helicase motives [23]. Only 13 sites were found to be under negative selection pressure in both clades (in bold in Table 5). Within the CPV clade, FUBAR identified five sites (19, 278, 545, 572, and 583) to be under pervasive positive selection and MEME identified two additional sites (597 and 647) under episodic positive selection. Interestingly, in correspondence of the positively selected site 545, a case of convergent mutation between the CPV and FPLV clades (mutation C to G in some FPLV strains) was identified. Finally, only one site (443) resulted as being subjected to pervasive positive selection in the FPLV clade. This site is located within the Walker motif B of the NS1 helicase domain (440 to 445, LIW(I/V)EE) and, whereas all analyzed CPV strains had the amino-acid I in this position, 13 out of 43 of the analyzed FPLV strains possessed a V. However, 443V was identified mainly in viruses from older cats (1967 to 1995 and only one in 2006) and in raccoons from a segregated environment [34].

Table 5. List of codons within *NS1* gene sequence identified as being under negative or positive selection pressure. FUBAR—Fast Unconstrained Bayesian Approximation for inferring selection; MEME—Mixed-Effects Model of Evolution.

	Sites Under Negative Selection Pressure *	Sites Under Positive Selection Pressure	
	FUBAR	**FUBAR**	**MEME**
CPV	7, 10, 14, 15, **31**, 32, 47, 53, 54, 56, 66, 68, 69, 83, 92, 99, **102**, 104, 105, 107, 114, 119, 123, 124, 132, 135, 137, 140, 154, 163, 164, 165, 170, 172, 179, 189, 200, 211, 219, 223, 240, 242, 250, 251, 279, 283, **284**, 297, **307**, 313, **323**, 324, 325, 333, 336, 337, 340, 341, 343, 349, 353, 360, 366, 371, 374, 378, 384, 388, 391, 393, 394, 395, **403**, 405, 408, 430, 432, **435**, 439, 444, 451, 459, 463, 467, 473, 474, 475, 476, 483, **488**, **489**, 494, 495, 497, 499, 503, 505, 506, 512, 514, **517**, 525, 527, 528, 529, 531, 536, 537, **541**, **543**, 554, **560**, 563, 564, 584, 591, 596, 633, 640, 641, 642, 657, 659, 662	19, 278, 545, 572, 583	278, 572, 583, 597, 647
FPLV	6, **31**, 39, 58, 60, 71, 97, **102**, 174, 177, 185, 201, 207, 270, **284**, **307**, **323**, 352, 357, **403**, 418, 422, 428, **435**, 462, 479, **488**, **489**, 493, 515, **517**, 520, 533, 540, **541**, **543**, 549, 551, **560**, 562, 653, 660	443	

* codons in bold correspond to those identified in both CPV and FPV lineages.

3.5. Phylogeny

Figure 1 shows the phylogenetic tree inferred from NS1 sequences. Unfortunately, likely because of high sequence identity, obtained bootstrap values were sometimes poor and only bootstrap-supported sub-clades are indicated in the Figure. For clarity, only viral type, origin and year of detection, and accession number of strains are reported, while the same tree with the full strain information is available in Figure S6 (Supplementary Materials). Although with a low support (bootstrap = 49), the sequences analyzed in this study clustered in separate clades according to the type of the virus (CPV/FPLV), but not the CPV variant. Indeed, CPV-2 strains (indicated in black in the figure) tended to segregate according to the country and the year of collection rather than according to the strain variant.

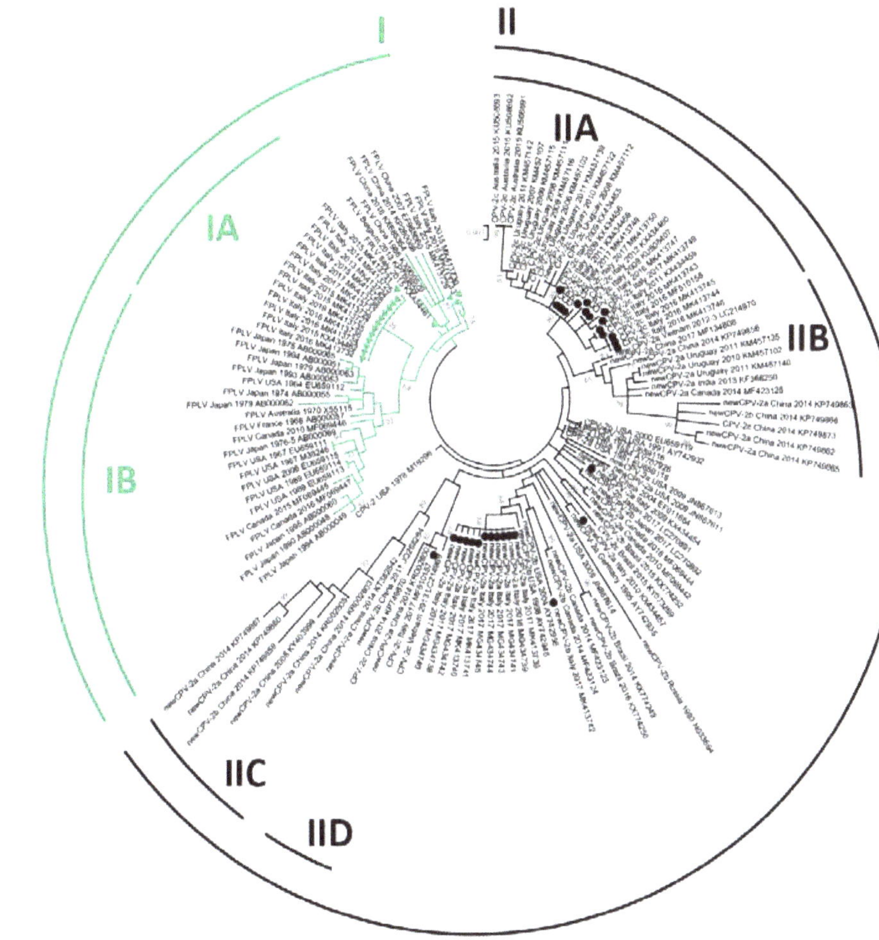

Figure 1. Maximum-likelihood tree based on 133 complete *NS1* gene sequences of feline panleukopenia virus (FPLV, in green) and canine parvovirus type 2 (CPV-2, in black) strains (bootstrap 1000 replicates; bootstrap values greater than 65 are shown). Green triangles and black dots indicate, respectively, FPLV and CPV strains analyzed in this study. Each sequence is indicated with virus type (FPLV/CPV) or variant (CPV-2, CPV-2a, CPV-2b, CPV-2c), country and year of collection, and accession number. The term "new" was used to distinguish the CPV-2a/2b strains with S297A main capsid protein (VP2) amino-acid changes from the early CPV-2a/2b variants. The same tree with more information about used strains (strain/isolate name) is available in Figure S6 (Supplementary Materials).

Most of the CPV-2c variants, with the exception of two strains (KP749873, KR002800), clustered in two distant subclades: the IIA subclade, in which strains collected in Italy, Uruguay, and Australia were included, and the IID subclade, which included strains with Asian origin. The CPV-2a/2b sequences collected from China were located together (subclade IIC) and were close to the CPV-2c strains of Asian origin (subclade IID), although the bootstrap support for this clade was low (bootstrap = 47). However, a common geographic origin was not maintained in the IIB subclade, which included CPV-2a/2b/2c viruses collected in Asia, Uruguay, and Canada.

Within clade I, including the FPLV strains, most of the recent Italian FPLV strains and the oldest FPLV strains clustered in statistically supported subclades (IA and IB, respectively), separately from those with convergent aa changes with CPV, which were located close to the CPV clade (between CPV and subclades IA/IB).

Figure S7 (Supplementary Materials) shows the phylogenetic tree inferred from the VP2 sequences of the same strains. Similar to the NS1 tree, the separation of the two main lineages was highly supported, whereby the FPLV sequences with convergent NS1 mutations were located closer to the CPV-2 clade, and geographic segregation of strains was partial. Finally, although without support, the CPV-2c sequences were separated from other strains.

4. Discussion

Almost all molecular studies on *Carnivore protoparvovirus 1* coding genes focused on the analysis of the *VP2* gene. The studies on the VP2 evolutionary dynamics helped clarify the spread of *Carnivore protoparvovirus 1* species, particularly after the first appearance of CPV-2. The VP2 protein determines the host range and antigenicity and, indeed, clear descriptions of the coding aa residues, which determine these features, were used to elucidate the host species jump from felids to canids [52–56]. Therefore, the separate evolution of FPLV and CPV was explained probably due to the different degree of the evolutive driving forces and to the different mutation rates among the viral types [8,57]. Moreover, studies based on the VP2 sequences evidenced the genetic stability of FPLV [11] and the continuous appearance of genetic mutants in CPV-2 [6,36,58]. In the current literature, there are only a few studies on the FPLV and CPV nonstructural genes [18], also due to the limited availability of updated *NS* genetic sequences for comparison [28], despite their essential role for viral replication, cytotoxicity, and pathogenicity [23,59,60]. To expand the current knowledge on the evolution of the *Carnivore protoparvovirus 1* members, this study provided a molecular characterization and evolutionary analysis of NS1 and NS2, comparing sequences of FPLV and CPV obtained from cats and dogs.

Early studies based on the comparison among only four FPLV and CPV NS1 sequences [61] evidenced a lesser degree of conservation of the NS1 aa sequence of CPV compared to FPLV, and 13 aa changes among the sequences of these viruses were described. Subsequent studies, based on few available sequences, detected only five or three aa differences in the NS1 protein between FPLV and CPV [25,26]. In the present study, all the distinctive aa residues between FPLV and CPV viral types in the *VP2* gene [41] were maintained; however, in the NS1-encoding sequence, only one amino-acid residue (248) clearly and constantly distinguished FPLV from CPV. Indeed, sequence analysis demonstrated that amino acids at specific residues (247, 545, and 595), previously potentially designated as discriminating the viral types, were present in nine FPLV strains collected in Italy, China, and Belgium, as well as in all the available CPV sequences. Previously, potential recombination events were hypothesized for some FPLV strains collected in China and Belgium [29,30,33,35] on the basis of the evidence of potential breakpoints located between the *NS1* and the *VP2* gene sequences, and of specific CPV-2 aa residues found in the NS1 sequence of FPLV strains. In this study, no evidence for recombination between FPLV and CPV was found within the NS1 sequence, although a larger sequence dataset in comparison to previous studies was evaluated. Moreover, specific amino acids supposed to be characteristic of CPV (247Q, 545E, and 595Q) were also observed among FPLV strains. Similarly, other substitutions (V115I and R664Q) emerged more recently both in FPLV and in CPV strains but in separate environments. These observations led us to conclude that these changes are more probably due to convergent substitutions that emerged independently in the two lineages (FPLV/CPV) rather than as a result of recombination events. According to these data, recombination does not seem to play an important role in shaping the evolution of the *NS1* gene of CPV and FPLV, as our dataset contained only one potentially recombinant sequence and no evidence for recombination between FPLV and CPV was found. However, due to the high sequence identity between these two viruses, it is possible that some recombination events went undetected and the importance of recombination may have been underestimated.

The circulation of CPV-2 variants in cats [15–17,62] arose questions about the epidemiological role of this species in parvovirus ecology [63] and suggested that cats may act as a potential source of new parvovirus variants [57]. Indeed, superinfection and co-infection with different species of parvovirus in the feline host led to a high genetic variability and the potential emergence of new viruses [57]. Unfortunately, no NS1 sequence is available for comparison with strains associated to superinfections or co-infections.

Moreover, our data do not confirm the detection of aa change L582S in the FPLV strains recovered from the central nervous system compared to strains collected in other tissues [35]. All samples from cerebral tissue of dogs and cats tested positive for *Carnivore protoparvovirus 1*, but no specific amino acid change was observed in any sample. This change occurred rather in CPV strains in the spleen tissues of coyotes in Canada in 2014 [34] and not in any other sequence of the analyzed dataset.

Several differences were found when studying selection pressure forces acting on the NS1 of CPV and FPLV. Firstly, considerably more amino acids were identified to be both positively and negatively selected in the CPV lineage compared to the FPLV lineage (7.0 and 3.4 times more, respectively). However, as only a limited number of FPLV sequences are currently available, it is possible that the wide FPLV diversity was not well represented in our dataset and, therefore, the number of positively and negatively selected site was underestimated. However, our results are consistent with those of previous studies that identified FPLV to be more stable and less subjected to positive selection [11,25].

Nevertheless, when we compared the sites that were subjected to selection pressure forces, surprisingly, there was only a minimal overlap between the two viruses. Only 13 negatively selected codons were identified in both viruses, while the vast majority of negatively selected codons were identified in either FPLV or CPV lineage (about 69% and 89.5%, respectively) and there was no overlap for positively selected codons. Our analyses evidenced a predominance of negative selection pressure on nonstructural proteins, slightly more marked among CPV strains. Interestingly, whereas two different amino acids could be observed among FPLV strains at residue 443 (V: 30%, I: 70%), within one of the functional domains (Walker B) of the viral helicase, only amino acid I was identified in all CPV strains. Although these two amino acids have very similar properties [64], keeping variation at this site might be important for the overall viral fitness. However, these findings need to be confirmed by specific mutagenesis studies.

Our results suggest that NS1 might be subjected to different evolutionary dynamics within the two lineages. Furthermore, the reduced viral diversity within the FPLV lineage (mean within-group distance: 0.6% for FPLV and 0.8% for CPV) could also reflect a different evolutionary behavior of these viruses. FPLV has been circulating within the feline population for a long time, whereas the CPV pandemic originated only recently and this virus was shown to evolve fast within the canine population [13]. This could partially explain our results. Furthermore, different evolutionary dynamics could be explained by the different infection dynamics and replication efficiency of the two viruses in the feline and the canine hosts. In fact, a more sustained transmission and, therefore, a shorter generation time favor a faster evolution [65]. These hypotheses highlight the need of acquiring the NS1 sequence of more strains in order to obtain a larger dataset, which is necessary to confirm our findings.

There are also limited studies on the NS1 protein, based only on evaluations of its functions [66–68] and on the potential location of its functional domains [10,22,23]. Changes in specific residues of NS1 CPV sequence [27] or affecting functional domains in others *Carnivore protoparvovirus 1* such as mink enteritis parvovirus [69] were hypothesized as potentially affecting the functions of this protein. According to a previous study [22], several described changes lay in the encoding sequence of ORI binding, helicase, and transactivation functional domains (Figure 2), despite only helicase domains being analyzed in great detail [23]. This region includes the convergent mutation between the CPV and FPLV clades (change Q to E in some FPLV strains) at the positively selected site 545 and the only residue subjected to positive selection pressure within the FPLV strains (site 443). Whereas residue 443 putatively lies in the β3-sheet of the Walker motif B of the helicase domain protein sequence, residues 350 and 544–545 are located between the α5- and α6-helices and just close to the α11-helix of the same domain, respectively, as illustrated in Canuti et al. [70] and Niskanen et al. [23]. The evidence of the convergent or divergent amino-acid changes between FPLV and CPV could contribute to further elucidate NS1 protein structure by clarifying any potential role of these residues. Moreover, the lack of studies on the *NS2* gene sequence [24] and its encoded protein highlights the need for additional investigations to advance any hypothesis on the effect of changes observed in the NS2 aa sequences.

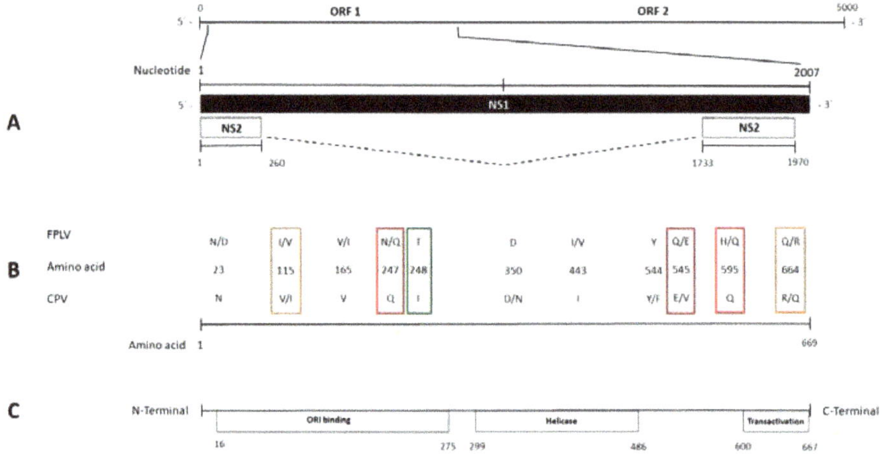

Figure 2. Schematic representation of the FPLV and CPV genome. The scheme, in the upper lines (**A**), represents the complete nucleotide (nt) length of the genome from the 5′ to the 3′ UTR and of the *NS1* and *NS2* genes. The relative positions of the described amino-acid changes in the *NS1* gene sequence are indicated in the middle lines (**B**). The lower line (**C**) represents the location of the potential functional domains within the *NS1* gene sequence, extended between the depicted amino-acid residues. Colored squares highlight the amino-acid changes distinguishing FPLV from CPV strains (green) and the convergent amino-acid changes between FPLV and CPV identified in the whole dataset (red) or only among the Italian FPLV strains (orange).

The analyzed sequences clustered mainly according to the viral lineage, suggesting divergent evolution between FPLV and CPV also for the *NS1* gene, but also according to the geographical area and the year of sample collection, especially for the CPV NS1 sequences. Separate clades in the phylogenetic tree included the FPLV and the CPV strains, and, although these differences are due to few aa changes, the molecular divergence could be considered as a useful tool in outbreak tracing [31,34]. Residues 23, 165, and 443 allow clustering old FPLV from domestic cats and wild carnivores from North America and Japan [34], suggesting a potential common origin. Similarly, common aa changes were also observed in the *NS2* encoding sequence of the FPLV strains from the USA and Canada. Although higher genetic stability compared to CPV was supposed, these few molecular markers contributed to distinguishing the FPLV strains and, therefore, we could consider changes at these residues as potential synapomorphies.

The lack of geographic segregation within the phylogenetic tree suggests the wide distribution of viruses, possibly by trading or transport of animals, as well as by contaminated equipment. As previously observed, infected animals represent a potential way of transport of CPV for long distances [36], as also evidenced for other canine viruses [71–73], and further analyses are necessary to evaluate both the spread and evolution within the canine population of variants that reach a new location.

The comparison with the phylogenetic tree inferred from VP2 sequences shows that, based on this dataset, the CPV sequences did not form clades corresponding to the CPV variant (2a/2b/2c) and showed different phylogenetic relationships, possibly because of the different evolutive forces acting on the different genes. As hypothesized by other authors, the CPV antigenic variants (CPV-2a/2b/2c) could be considered as variants of CPV-2a rather than distinct subtypes [74] and the classification system based on a single amino acid (VP2 426) to identify CPV variants does not reflect phylogenetic relationships of the strains; thus, it is not suitable to analyze CPV evolution [75]. Indeed, the molecular characterization of both ORFs allows possibly reconsidering the current typing of CPV (2a/2b/2c), which is not phylogenetically supported. The aa changes in the *VP2* gene considered for viral typing probably arose independently in different countries, also considering the global spread of CPV through animal movements, and they are not reliable in defining the viral evolution. Therefore, the molecular analysis based on long genome sequences encompassing both major ORFs could be helpful in the epidemiological surveillance of both CPV and FPLV, supporting the tracking of viral spread, and could contribute to further elucidate the evolution of *Carnivore protoparvovirus 1*.

In conclusion, a continuous molecular survey is necessary to better elucidate the ecology and distribution of the described strains and to evaluate their fit in the canine and feline populations. The reductionist evaluations based only on the *VP2* genomic sequence should be replaced by a holistic molecular approach, based on analysis of both ORFs, and the description of new CPV and FPLV mutants should include at least the major structural and nonstructural proteins.

Supplementary Materials: The following are available online at http://www.mdpi.com/1999-4915/11/4/308/s1: Dataset S1: Amino-acid sequence variations in the *NS1* gene sequence of CPV/FPLV and of the reference viruses from the NCBI database. Table S2: VP2 non-synonymous changes of analyzed FPLV/CPV strains described in this study. Dataset S3: Amino-acid sequence variations in the *NS2* gene sequence of CPV/FPLV collected in Italy. Recombination and Selection Pressure S4: Recombination and selection pressure file. Recombination S5: Phylogenetic reconstructions of the complete *NS1* gene of CPV-2 and FPLV strains based on different genomic regions located upstream and downstream the putative recombination breakpoint (nt 1515). Figure S6: Maximum-likelihood tree based on 133 complete *NS1* gene sequences of feline panleukopenia virus (FPLV, in green) and canine parvovirus type-2 (CPV-2, in black) strains (bootstrap 1000 replicates; bootstrap values shown greater than 65). Green triangles and black dots indicate, respectively, FPLV and CPV strains analyzed in this study. Each sequence is indicated with virus type (FPLV/CPV) or variant (CPV-2, CPV-2a, CPV-2b, CPV-2c), country and year of collection, strain/isolate name, and accession number. The term "new" was used to distinguish the CPV-2a/2b strains with S297A VP2 amino-acid change from the early CPV-2a/2b variants. Figure S7: Maximum-likelihood tree based on 132 complete *VP2* gene sequences of feline panleukopenia virus (FPLV, in green) and canine parvovirus type-2 (CPV-2, in black) strains (bootstrap 1000 replicates; bootstrap values greater than 65 are shown). Green triangles and black dots indicate, respectively, FPLV and CPV strains analyzed in this study. Each sequence is indicated with virus type (FPLV/CPV) or variant (CPV-2, CPV-2a, CPV-2b, CPV-2c), country and year of collection, strain/isolate name, and accession number. The term "new" was used to distinguish the CPV-2a/2b strains with S297A VP2 amino-acid change from the early CPV-2a/2b variants.

Author Contributions: Conceptualization, F.M., M.C., and G.P.; methodology, F.M., M.C., and G.P.; formal analysis, S.D.B., L.O., and G.S.; investigation, F.M., S.D.B., G.S., G.C., S.B., and P.P.; resources, G.P. and A.L.; data curation, F.M., G.P., and V.C.; writing—original draft preparation, F.M., M.C., and G.P.; writing—review and editing, F.M., M.C., G.P., N.D., and A.G.; visualization, S.D.B., G.S., and G.C.; supervision, G.P., N.D., and A.G.; project administration, G.P. and A.G.; funding acquisition, A.G.

Funding: The APC was funded by the Ministero della Salute (Italy), Ricerca Corrente IZS SI 03/18 RC "Studio del potenziale zoonosico e caratterizzazione genomica dei virus enterici del cane".

Conflicts of Interest: The authors declare no conflicts of interest. The funders had no role in the design of the study; in the collection, analyses, or interpretation of data; in the writing of the manuscript, or in the decision to publish the results.

References

1. Cotmore, S.F.; Agbandje-McKenna, M.; Canuti, M.; Chiorini, J.A.; Eis-Hubinger, A.-M.; Hughes, J.; Mietzsch, M.; Modha, S.; Ogliastro, M.; Pénzes, J.J.; et al. ICTV Virus Taxonomy Profile: Parvoviridae. *J. Gen. Virol.* **2019**, *100*, 367–368. [CrossRef] [PubMed]
2. Cotmore, S.F.; Agbandje-McKenna, M.; Chiorini, J.A.; Mukha, D.V.; Pintel, D.J.; Qiu, J.; Soderlund-Venermo, M.; Tattersall, P.; Tijssen, P.; Gatherer, D.; et al. The family Parvoviridae. *Arch. Virol.* **2014**, *159*, 1239–1247. [CrossRef]
3. Tijssen, P.; Agbandje-McKenna, M.; Almendral, J.M.; Bergoin, M.; Flegel, T.W.; Hedman, K.; Kleinschmidt, J.; Li, Y.; Pintel, D.J.; Tattersall, P. The family Parvoviridae. In *Virus Taxonomy—Ninth Report of the International Committee on Taxonomy of Viruses*; King, A.M.Q., Adams, M.J., Carstens, E.B., Lefkowitz, E.J., Eds.; Elsevier/Academic Press: London, UK, 2011; pp. 405–425.

4. Decaro, N.; Buonavoglia, C. Canine parvovirus—A review of epidemiological and diagnostic aspects, with emphasis on type 2c. *Vet. Microbiol.* **2012**, *155*, 1–12. [CrossRef] [PubMed]
5. Verge, J.; Christoforoni, N. La gastroenterite infectieuse des chats; est-elle due à un virus filtrable? *CR Seances Soc. Biol. Fil.* **1928**, *99*, 312.
6. Decaro, N.; Desario, C.; Miccolupo, A.; Campolo, M.; Parisi, A.; Martella, V.; Amorisco, F.; Lucente, M.S.; Lavazza, A.; Buonavoglia, C. Genetic analysis of feline panleukopenia viruses from cats with gastroenteritis. *J. Gen. Virol.* **2008**, *89*, 2290–2298. [CrossRef]
7. Truyen, U. Evolution of canine parvovirus—A need for new vaccines? *Vet. Microbiol.* **2006**, *117*, 9–13. [CrossRef]
8. Shackelton, L.A.; Parrish, C.R.; Truyen, U.; Holmes, E.C. High rate of viral evolution associated with the emergence of carnivore parvovirus. *Proc. Natl. Acad. Sci. USA* **2005**, *102*, 379–384. [CrossRef]
9. Pereira, C.A.D.; Leal, E.S.; Durigon, E.L. Selective regimen shift and demographic growth increase associated with the emergence of high-fitness variants of canine parvovirus. *Infect. Genet. Evol.* **2007**, *7*, 399–409. [CrossRef] [PubMed]
10. Hoelzer, K.; Shackelton, L.A.; Parrish, C.R.; Holmes, E.C. Phylogenetic analysis reveals the emergence, evolution and dispersal of carnivore parvoviruses. *J. Gen. Virol.* **2008**, *89*, 2280–2289. [CrossRef]
11. Decaro, N.; Desario, C.; Parisi, A.; Martella, V.; Lorusso, A.; Miccolupo, A.; Mari, V.; Colaianni, M.L.; Cavalli, A.; Di Trani, L.; et al. Genetic analysis of canine parvovirus type 2c. *Virology* **2009**, *385*, 5–10. [CrossRef]
12. Parrish, C.R.; O'Connell, P.H.; Evermann, J.F.; Carmichael, L.E. Natural variation of canine parvovirus. *Science* **1985**, *230*, 1046–1048. [CrossRef] [PubMed]
13. Parrish, C.R.; Aquadro, C.F.; Strassheim, M.L.; Evermann, J.F.; Sgro, J.Y.; Mohammed, H.O. Rapid antigenic-type replacement and DNA sequence evolution of canine parvovirus. *J. Virol.* **1991**, *65*, 6544–6552.
14. Buonavoglia, C.; Martella, V.; Pratelli, A.; Tempesta, M.; Cavalli, A.; Buonavoglia, D.; Bozzo, G.; Elia, G.; Decaro, N.; Carmichael, L. Evidence for evolution of canine parvovirus type 2 in Italy. *J. Gen. Virol.* **2001**, *82*, 3021–3025. [CrossRef] [PubMed]
15. Decaro, N.; Buonavoglia, D.; Desario, C.; Amorisco, F.; Colaianni, M.L.; Parisi, A.; Terio, V.; Elia, G.; Lucente, M.S.; Cavalli, A.; et al. Characterisation of canine parvovirus strains isolated from cats with feline panleukopenia. *Res. Vet. Sci.* **2010**, *89*, 275–278. [CrossRef] [PubMed]
16. Decaro, N.; Desario, C.; Amorisco, F.; Losurdo, M.; Colaianni, M.L.; Greco, M.F.; Buonavoglia, C. Canine parvovirus type 2c infection in a kitten associated with intracranial abscess and convulsions. *J. Feline Med. Surg.* **2011**, *13*, 231–236. [CrossRef]
17. Marenzoni, M.L.; Antognoni, M.T.; Baldelli, F.; Miglio, A.; Stefanetti, V.; Desario, C.; Di Summa, A.; Buonavoglia, C.; Decaro, N. Detection of parvovirus and herpesvirus DNA in the blood of feline and canine blood donors. *Vet. Microbiol.* **2018**, *224*, 66–69. [CrossRef] [PubMed]
18. Hoelzer, K.; Shackelton, L.A.; Holmes, E.C.; Parrish, C.R. Within-host genetic diversity of endemic and emerging parvoviruses of dogs and cats. *J. Virol.* **2008**, *82*, 11096–11105. [CrossRef] [PubMed]
19. Reed, A.P.; Jones, E.V.; Miller, T.J. Nucleotide sequence and genome organization of canine parvovirus. *J. Virol.* **1988**, *62*, 266–276.
20. Hueffer, K.; Parker, J.S.L.; Weichert, W.S.; Geisel, R.E.; Sgro, J.-Y.; Parrish, C.R. The natural host range shift and subsequent evolution of canine parvovirus resulted from virus-specific binding to the canine transferrin receptor. *J. Virol.* **2003**, *77*, 1718–1726. [CrossRef]
21. Nelson, C.D.S.; Palermo, L.M.; Hafenstein, S.L.; Parrish, C.R. Different mechanisms of antibody-mediated neutralization of parvoviruses revealed using the Fab fragments of monoclonal antibodies. *Virology* **2007**, *361*, 283–293. [CrossRef]
22. Niskanen, E.A.; Kalliolinna, O.; Ihalainen, T.O.; Häkkinen, M.; Vihinen-Ranta, M. Mutations in DNA binding and transactivation domains affect the dynamics of parvovirus NS1 protein. *J. Virol.* **2013**, *87*, 11762–11774. [CrossRef] [PubMed]
23. Niskanen, E.A.; Ihalainen, T.O.; Kalliolinna, O.; Häkkinen, M.M.; Vihinen-Ranta, M. Effect of ATP binding and hydrolysis on dynamics of canine parvovirus NS1. *J. Virol.* **2010**, *84*, 5391–5403. [CrossRef] [PubMed]
24. Wang, D.; Yuan, W.; Davis, I.; Parrish, C.R. Nonstructural protein-2 and the replication of canine parvovirus. *Virology* **1998**, *240*, 273–281. [CrossRef] [PubMed]

25. Horiuchi, M.; Yamaguchi, Y.; Gojobori, T.; Mochizuki, M.; Nagasawa, H.; Toyoda, Y.; Ishiguro, N.; Shinagawa, M. Differences in the evolutionary pattern of feline panleukopenia virus and canine parvovirus. *Virology* **1998**, *249*, 440–452. [CrossRef]
26. Parrish, C.R. Mapping specific functions in the capsid structure of canine parvovirus and feline panleukopenia virus using infectious plasmid clones. *Virology* **1991**, *183*, 195–205. [CrossRef]
27. Truyen, U.; Gruenberg, A.; Chang, S.F.; Obermaier, B.; Veijalainen, P.; Parrish, C.R. Evolution of the feline-subgroup parvoviruses and the control of canine host range in vivo. *J. Virol.* **1995**, *69*, 4702–4710.
28. Pérez, R.; Calleros, L.; Marandino, A.; Sarute, N.; Iraola, G.; Grecco, S.; Blanc, H.; Vignuzzi, M.; Isakov, O.; Shomron, N.; et al. Phylogenetic and genome-wide deep-sequencing analyses of canine parvovirus reveal co-infection with field variants and emergence of a recent recombinant strain. *PLoS ONE* **2014**, *9*, e111779. [CrossRef]
29. Ohshima, T.; Mochizuki, M. Evidence for recombination between feline panleukopenia virus and canine parvovirus type 2. *J. Vet. Med. Sci.* **2009**, *71*, 403–408. [CrossRef] [PubMed]
30. Liu, C.; Liu, Y.; Liu, D.; Qiu, Z.; Tian, J.; Guo, D.; Li, Z.; Liu, M.; Li, Y.; Qu, L. Complete Genome Sequence of Feline Panleukopenia Virus Strain HRB-CS1, Isolated from a Domestic Cat in Northeastern China. *Genome Announc.* **2015**, *3*, e01556-14. [CrossRef]
31. Ryt-Hansen, P.; Hagberg, E.E.; Chriél, M.; Struve, T.; Pedersen, A.G.; Larsen, L.E.; Hjulsager, C.K. Global phylogenetic analysis of contemporary aleutian mink disease viruses (AMDVs). *Virol. J.* **2017**, *14*, 231. [CrossRef]
32. Mira, F.; Dowgier, G.; Purpari, G.; Vicari, D.; Di Bella, S.; Macaluso, G.; Gucciardi, F.; Randazzo, V.; Decaro, N.; Guercio, A. Molecular typing of a novel canine parvovirus type 2a mutant circulating in Italy. *Infect. Genet. Evol.* **2018**, *61*, 67–73. [CrossRef] [PubMed]
33. Wang, X.; Li, T.; Liu, H.; Du, J.; Zhou, F.; Dong, Y.; He, X.; Li, Y.; Wang, C. Recombinant feline parvovirus infection of immunized tigers in central China. *Emerg. Microbes Infect.* **2017**, *6*, e42. [CrossRef] [PubMed]
34. Canuti, M.; Britton, A.P.; Graham, S.M.; Lang, A.S. Epidemiology and molecular characterization of protoparvoviruses infecting wild raccoons (*Procyon lotor*) in British Columbia, Canada. *Virus Res.* **2017**, *242*, 85–89. [CrossRef] [PubMed]
35. Garigliany, M.; Gilliaux, G.; Jolly, S.; Casanova, T.; Bayrou, C.; Gommeren, K.; Fett, T.; Mauroy, A.; Lévy, E.; Cassart, D.; et al. Feline panleukopenia virus in cerebral neurons of young and adult cats. *BMC Vet. Res.* **2016**, *12*, 28. [CrossRef] [PubMed]
36. Mira, F.; Purpari, G.; Lorusso, E.; Di Bella, S.; Gucciardi, F.; Desario, C.; Macaluso, G.; Decaro, N.; Guercio, A. Introduction of Asian canine parvovirus in Europe through dog importation. *Transbound. Emerg. Dis.* **2018**, *65*, 16–21. [CrossRef]
37. Purpari, G.; Mira, F.; Di Bella, S.; Di Pietro, S.; Giudice, E.; Guercio, A. Investigation on canine parvovirus circulation in dogs from Sicily (Italy) by biomolecular assay. *Acta Vet. (Beogr.)* **2018**, *68*, 80–94.
38. Touihri, L.; Bouzid, I.; Daoud, R.; Desario, C.; El Goulli, A.F.; Decaro, N.; Ghorbel, A.; Buonavoglia, C.; Bahloul, C. Molecular characterization of canine parvovirus-2 variants circulating in Tunisia. *Virus Genes* **2009**, *38*, 249–258. [CrossRef] [PubMed]
39. Hall, T.A. BioEdit: A user-friendly biological sequence alignment editor and analysis program for windows 95/98/NT. In *Nucleic Acids Symposium Series*; Information Retrieval Ltd.: London, UK, 1999; Volume 41, pp. 95–98.
40. Zhang, Z.; Schwartz, S.; Wagner, L.; Miller, W. A greedy algorithm for aligning DNA sequences. *J. Comput. Biol.* **2000**, *7*, 203–214. [CrossRef]
41. Martella, V.; Decaro, N.; Elia, G.; Buonavoglia, C. Surveillance activity for canine parvovirus in Italy. *J. Vet. Med. B Infect. Dis. Vet. Public Health* **2005**, *52*, 312–315. [CrossRef]
42. Martin, D.P.; Murrell, B.; Golden, M.; Khoosal, A.; Muhire, B. RDP4: Detection and analysis of recombination patterns in virus genomes. *Virus Evol.* **2015**, *1*, vev003. [CrossRef]
43. Canuti, M.; O'Leary, K.E.; Hunter, B.D.; Spearman, G.; Ojkic, D.; Whitney, H.G.; Lang, A.S. Driving forces behind the evolution of the Aleutian mink disease parvovirus in the context of intensive farming. *Virus Evol.* **2016**, *2*, vew004. [CrossRef]
44. Kumar, S.; Stecher, G.; Tamura, K. MEGA7: Molecular Evolutionary Genetics Analysis Version 7.0 for Bigger Datasets. *Mol. Biol. Evol.* **2016**, *33*, 1870–1874. [CrossRef]

45. Hasegawa, M.; Kishino, H.; Yano, T. Dating of the human-ape splitting by a molecular clock of mitochondrial DNA. *J. Mol. Evol.* **1985**, *22*, 160–174. [CrossRef]
46. Kimura, M. A simple method for estimating evolutionary rates of base substitutions through comparative studies of nucleotide sequences. *J. Mol. Evol.* **1980**, *16*, 111–120. [CrossRef] [PubMed]
47. Nei, M.; Gojobori, T. Simple methods for estimating the numbers of synonymous and nonsynonymous nucleotide substitutions. *Mol. Biol. Evol.* **1986**, *3*, 418–426. [PubMed]
48. Murrell, B.; Moola, S.; Mabona, A.; Weighill, T.; Sheward, D.; Kosakovsky Pond, S.L.; Scheffler, K. FUBAR: A fast, unconstrained bayesian approximation for inferring selection. *Mol. Biol. Evol.* **2013**, *30*, 1196–1205. [CrossRef]
49. Murrell, B.; Wertheim, J.O.; Moola, S.; Weighill, T.; Scheffler, K.; Kosakovsky Pond, S.L. Detecting individual sites subject to episodic diversifying selection. *PLoS Genet.* **2012**, *8*, e1002764. [CrossRef] [PubMed]
50. Decaro, N.; Martella, V.; Elia, G.; Desario, C.; Campolo, M.; Lorusso, E.; Colaianni, M.L.; Lorusso, A.; Buonavoglia, C. Tissue distribution of the antigenic variants of canine parvovirus type 2 in dogs. *Vet. Microbiol.* **2007**, *121*, 39–44. [CrossRef]
51. Shriner, D.; Nickle, D.C.; Jensen, M.A.; Mullins, J.I. Potential impact of recombination on sitewise approaches for detecting positive natural selection. *Genet. Res.* **2003**, *81*, 115–121. [CrossRef] [PubMed]
52. Palermo, L.M.; Hafenstein, S.L.; Parrish, C.R. Purified feline and canine transferrin receptors reveal complex interactions with the capsids of canine and feline parvoviruses that correspond to their host ranges. *J. Virol.* **2006**, *80*, 8482–8492. [CrossRef]
53. Truyen, U. Emergence and recent evolution of canine parvovirus. *Vet. Microbiol.* **1999**, *69*, 47–50. [CrossRef]
54. Parker, J.S.; Parrish, C.R. Canine parvovirus host range is determined by the specific conformation of an additional region of the capsid. *J. Virol.* **1997**, *71*, 9214–9222. [PubMed]
55. Truyen, U.; Evermann, J.F.; Vieler, E.; Parrish, C.R. Evolution of canine parvovirus involved loss and gain of feline host range. *Virology* **1996**, *215*, 186–189. [CrossRef] [PubMed]
56. Strassheim, M.L.; Gruenberg, A.; Veijalainen, P.; Sgro, J.Y.; Parrish, C.R. Two dominant neutralizing antigenic determinants of canine parvovirus are found on the threefold spike of the virus capsid. *Virology* **1994**, *198*, 175–184. [CrossRef] [PubMed]
57. Battilani, M.; Balboni, A.; Ustulin, M.; Giunti, M.; Scagliarini, A.; Prosperi, S. Genetic complexity and multiple infections with more Parvovirus species in naturally infected cats. *Vet. Res.* **2011**, *42*, 43. [CrossRef]
58. Zhou, P.; Zeng, W.; Zhang, X.; Li, S. The genetic evolution of canine parvovirus—A new perspective. *PLoS ONE* **2017**, *12*, e0175035. [CrossRef] [PubMed]
59. Nüesch, J.P.; Christensen, J.; Rommelaere, J. Initiation of minute virus of mice DNA replication is regulated at the level of origin unwinding by atypical protein kinase C phosphorylation of NS1. *J. Virol.* **2001**, *75*, 5730–5739. [CrossRef]
60. Ohshima, T.; Iwama, M.; Ueno, Y.; Sugiyama, F.; Nakajima, T.; Fukamizu, A.; Yagami, K. Induction of apoptosis in vitro and in vivo by H-1 parvovirus infection. *J. Gen. Virol.* **1998**, *79 (Pt 12)*, 3067–3071. [CrossRef]
61. Martyn, J.C.; Davidson, B.E.; Studdert, M.J. Nucleotide sequence of feline panleukopenia virus: Comparison with canine parvovirus identifies host-specific differences. *J. Gen. Virol.* **1990**, *71 (Pt 11)*, 2747–2753. [CrossRef]
62. Clegg, S.R.; Coyne, K.P.; Dawson, S.; Spibey, N.; Gaskell, R.M.; Radford, A.D. Canine parvovirus in asymptomatic feline carriers. *Vet. Microbiol.* **2012**, *157*, 78–85. [CrossRef]
63. Balboni, A.; Bassi, F.; De Arcangeli, S.; Zobba, R.; Dedola, C.; Alberti, A.; Battilani, M. Molecular analysis of carnivore Protoparvovirus detected in white blood cells of naturally infected cats. *BMC Vet. Res.* **2018**, *14*, 41. [CrossRef] [PubMed]
64. Pommié, C.; Levadoux, S.; Sabatier, R.; Lefranc, G.; Lefranc, M.-P. IMGT standardized criteria for statistical analysis of immunoglobulin V-REGION amino acid properties. *J. Mol. Recognit.* **2004**, *17*, 17–32. [CrossRef] [PubMed]
65. Duffy, S.; Shackelton, L.A.; Holmes, E.C. Rates of evolutionary change in viruses: Patterns and determinants. *Nat. Rev. Genet.* **2008**, *9*, 267–276. [CrossRef] [PubMed]
66. Ihalainen, T.O.; Niskanen, E.A.; Jylhävä, J.; Turpeinen, T.; Rinne, J.; Timonen, J.; Vihinen-Ranta, M. Dynamics and interactions of parvoviral NS1 protein in the nucleus. *Cell. Microbiol.* **2007**, *9*, 1946–1959. [CrossRef]

67. Ihalainen, T.O.; Willman, S.F.; Niskanen, E.A.; Paloheimo, O.; Smolander, H.; Laurila, J.P.; Kaikkonen, M.U.; Vihinen-Ranta, M. Distribution and dynamics of transcription-associated proteins during parvovirus infection. *J. Virol.* **2012**, *86*, 13779–13784. [CrossRef] [PubMed]
68. Mäntylä, E.; Salokas, K.; Oittinen, M.; Aho, V.; Mäntysaari, P.; Palmujoki, L.; Kalliolinna, O.; Ihalainen, T.O.; Niskanen, E.A.; Timonen, J.; et al. Promoter-Targeted Histone Acetylation of Chromatinized Parvoviral Genome Is Essential for the Progress of Infection. *J. Virol.* **2016**, *90*, 4059–4066. [CrossRef] [PubMed]
69. Zhang, X.; Wang, J.; Mao, Y.; Xi, J.; Yu, Y.; Liu, W. Induction and suppression of type I interferon responses by mink enteritis virus in CRFK cells. *Vet. Microbiol.* **2017**, *199*, 8–14. [CrossRef] [PubMed]
70. Canuti, M.; Williams, C.V.; Gadi, S.R.; Jebbink, M.F.; Oude Munnink, B.B.; Jazaeri Farsani, S.M.; Cullen, J.M.; van der Hoek, L. Persistent viremia by a novel parvovirus in a slow loris (Nycticebus coucang) with diffuse histiocytic sarcoma. *Front. Microbiol.* **2014**, *5*, 655. [CrossRef] [PubMed]
71. Martella, V.; Cirone, F.; Elia, G.; Lorusso, E.; Decaro, N.; Campolo, M.; Desario, C.; Lucente, M.S.; Bellacicco, A.L.; Blixenkrone-Møller, M.; et al. Heterogeneity within the hemagglutinin genes of canine distemper virus (CDV) strains detected in Italy. *Vet. Microbiol.* **2006**, *116*, 301–309. [CrossRef]
72. Decaro, N.; Campolo, M.; Elia, G.; Buonavoglia, D.; Colaianni, M.L.; Lorusso, A.; Mari, V.; Buonavoglia, C. Infectious canine hepatitis: An "old" disease reemerging in Italy. *Res. Vet. Sci.* **2007**, *83*, 269–273. [CrossRef]
73. Mira, F.; Purpari, G.; Di Bella, S.; Vicari, D.; Schirò, G.; Di Marco, P.; Macaluso, G.; Battilani, M.; Guercio, A. Update on canine distemper virus (CDV) strains of Arctic-like lineage detected in dogs in Italy. *Vet. Ital.* **2018**, *54*, 225–236. [PubMed]
74. Organtini, L.J.; Allison, A.B.; Lukk, T.; Parrish, C.R.; Hafenstein, S. Global displacement of canine parvovirus by a host-adapted variant: Structural comparison between pandemic viruses with distinct host ranges. *J. Virol.* **2015**, *89*, 1909–1912. [CrossRef] [PubMed]
75. Grecco, S.; Iraola, G.; Decaro, N.; Alfieri, A.; Alfieri, A.; Gallo Calderón, M.; da Silva, A.P.; Name, D.; Aldaz, J.; Calleros, L.; et al. Inter- and intracontinental migrations and local differentiation have shaped the contemporary epidemiological landscape of canine parvovirus in South America. *Virus Evol.* **2018**, *4*, vey011. [CrossRef]

viruses

MDPI

Communication

Metagenomic Next-Generation Sequencing Reveal Presence of a Novel Ungulate *Bocaparvovirus* in Alpacas

Deepak Kumar [1], Suman Chaudhary [1], Nanyan Lu [1], Michael Duff [1], Mathew Heffel [1], Caroline A. McKinney [2], Daniela Bedenice [2] and Douglas Marthaler [1,*]

[1] Kansas State Veterinary Diagnostic Laboratory, College of Veterinary Medicine, Kansas State University, Manhattan, KS 66506, USA

[2] Department of Clinical Sciences, Cummings School of Veterinary Medicine at Tufts University, 200 Westboro Road, North Grafton, MA 01536, USA

* Correspondence: marth027@umn.edu

Received: 24 May 2019; Accepted: 27 July 2019; Published: 31 July 2019

Abstract: Viruses belonging to the genus *Bocaparvovirus (BoV)* are a genetically diverse group of DNA viruses known to cause respiratory, enteric, and neurological diseases in animals, including humans. An intestinal sample from an alpaca (*Vicugna pacos*) herd with reoccurring diarrhea and respiratory disease was submitted for next-generation sequencing, revealing the presence of a BoV strain. The alpaca BoV strain (AlBoV) had a 58.58% whole genome nucleotide percent identity to a camel BoV from Dubai, belonging to a tentative ungulate BoV 8 species (UBoV8). Recombination events were lacking with other UBoV strains. The AlBoV genome was comprised of the NS1, NP1, and VP1 proteins. The NS1 protein had the highest amino acid percent identity range (57.89–67.85%) to the members of UBoV8, which was below the 85% cut-off set by the International Committee on Taxonomy of Viruses. The low NS1 amino acid identity suggests that AlBoV is a tentative new species. The whole genome, NS1, NP1, and VP1 phylogenetic trees illustrated distinct branching of AlBoV, sharing a common ancestor with UBoV8. Walker loop and Phospholipase A2 (PLA2) motifs that are vital for virus infectivity were identified in NS1 and VP1 proteins, respectively. Our study reports a novel BoV strain in an alpaca intestinal sample and highlights the need for additional BoV research.

Keywords: alpaca; virus; *Bocaparvovirus*; genome; next-generation sequencing; metagenomics

---

Bocaparvoviruses (BoVs) belong to the genus *Bocaparvovirus* and are emerging pathogens of the Parvoviridae family. BoVs are nonenveloped, single-stranded DNA viruses with an icosahedral symmetry and were originally named according to their first identified members, bovine parvovirus (BPV) and minute virus of canine (MVC) [1]. In the past few years, novel BoVs have been identified in a variety of animals, including bats [2], camels [3], gorillas [4], marmots [5], pigs [6], and rodents [7]. BoVs are comprised of 21 species, including carnivore BoV 1–6, chiropteran BoV 1–4, lagomorph BoV 1, pinniped BoV 1 and 2, primate BoV 1 and 2, and ungulate BoV (UBoV) 1–6. A few new UBoVs have been identified in dromedary camels (tentatively UBoV7 and UBoV8) [3] but have yet to be classified by the International Committee on Taxonomy of Viruses (ICTV).

Initially, the classification of parvoviruses required the isolation of the virus; however, reporting of the viral sequence containing all the non-structural and structural coding regions is now acceptable provided the genomic, serological, or biological data supports infectious etiology [8]. Most of the members of the *Bocaparvovirus* genus have been identified using molecular methods and lack isolation in cell culture [3,4,9]. Human BoVs cause severe respiratory and gastrointestinal infections in young children [10]. Bovine parvovirus (BPV) causes gastrointestinal and respiratory symptoms, reproductive failure, and conjunctivitis in cattle worldwide [11]. Another important member of the BoV genus, canine minute virus (MVC), causes sub-clinical disease and fetal infections often leading to neonatal respiratory disease or abortions [12]. However, Koch's postulates have yet to be fulfilled to link newly emerging BoVs with the clinical disease in animals [1,3,5].

Alpaca (*Vicugna pacos*) are domesticated members of the new world camelids closely related to llama (*Lama glama*), guanaco (*Lama guanicoe*), and vicuna (*Vicugna vicugna*) [13]. Over the past couple of decades, alpacas have gained significant popularity as pets, show animals, and fiber animals in the United States, with a total of 264,587 alpacas registered in the US as of May 2019 [14]. A variety of viruses have been identified in alpacas, including bovine viral diarrhea virus, coronavirus, adenovirus, equine viral arteritis virus, rotavirus, rabies, bluetongue virus, foot-and-mouth disease virus, bovine respiratory syncytial virus, influenza A virus, bovine papillomavirus, vesicular stomatitis virus, parainfluenza-3 virus, West Nile virus, and equine herpesvirus [12,15–20]. However, BoVs have yet to be reported in alpacas.

An alpaca farm in the mid-eastern United States reported recurrent diarrhea and respiratory failure in young alpacas, with a case fatality rate up to 100%. In 2017, an alpha coronavirus was identified as causing clinical disease in two animals, and vaccination was subsequently attempted. However, diarrhea and respiratory distress continued to occur in juvenile animals despite increased biosecurity measures and supportive herd management. In 2018, an intestinal sample from a deceased alpaca was submitted to Kansas State University Veterinary Diagnostic Laboratory for metagenomic next-generation sequencing (NGS) to further evaluate potential causes of disease. The intestinal sample was processed, extracted, and sequenced using previously described methods [21,22]. The raw data was analyzed using a custom bioinformatic pipeline [23]. Reads were trimmed, and the adapter/index sequences were removed using Trimmomatic [24], Sickle [25], and Scythe [26].

A total of 334,052 cleaned reads were classified as eukaryotes (41%), bacteria (28%), viral (7%), and other organisms (4%) by Kraken software, which applies a *k*-mer search strategy from a sequence database to taxonomically classify reads (Figure 1) [27]. Kraken revealed a majority of the viral reads (22,170) as BoV (77%); bacteriophages (14%); and miscellaneous viruses composed of retroviruses, bacteria viruses, and unclassified viruses (9%). Reads lacking classification (no hits, n = 67,604) and identified as viral reads (n = 22,170) were de novo assembled into contigs and BLAST (Basic Local Alignment Search Tool) against the National Center for Biotechnology Information (NCBI) database, identifying a contig with a 58.58% nucleotide percent identity to a camel BoV from Dubai (KY640435). A full-length genome (5155 nucleotides) of an alpaca BoV (AlBoV, GenBank number MK014742) had an average read coverage of 2440X. AlBoV was aligned with the 108 complete UBoV genomes from GenBank using Multiple Alignment using Fast Fourier Transform (MAFFT) [28] in Geneious Prime [29]. AlBoV shared a 57.77–58.58% whole genome nucleotide identity to the UBoV8 strains (Table 1). Recombination events were not detected in the UBoV alignment using RDP4 software [30], although single-stranded DNA viruses such as parvoviruses possess a mutation rate similar to single-stranded RNA viruses and a higher mutation rate than double-stranded DNA viruses [31].

AlBoV contained three open reading frames (ORFs), NS1, NP1, and VP1/VP2, which were 2154 bp (411 to 2564 bp), 507 bp (2701 to 3207 bp), and 1395bp (3194 to 4588 bp), respectively. ICTV indicates a new parvovirus species should have less than 85% amino acid identity of the NS1 protein with other parvovirus species. The AlBoV identified in the present study shared the highest NS1 amino acid percent identity (57.89–67.85%) with camel BoVs in UBoV8 (Table 1) and represents a tentative new BoV species, UBoV9. The ancillary protein NP1, which is a unique feature of BoVs, is known to influence RNA processing events by suppressing internal polyadenylation and splicing of an upstream intron [32]. Unlike some of the other BoV sequences, the coding region of NP1 of AlBoV did not overlap with the C-terminal region of NS1. Interestingly, VP1/VP2 gene of AlBoV was the shortest among the identified UBoVs in the GenBank (Figure 2). Frameshift mutation were lacking in the AlBoV VP1/VP2 sequence, and the nucleotide sequence after the VP1/VP2 stop codon varied among the 108 complete UBoV sequences in the GenBank.

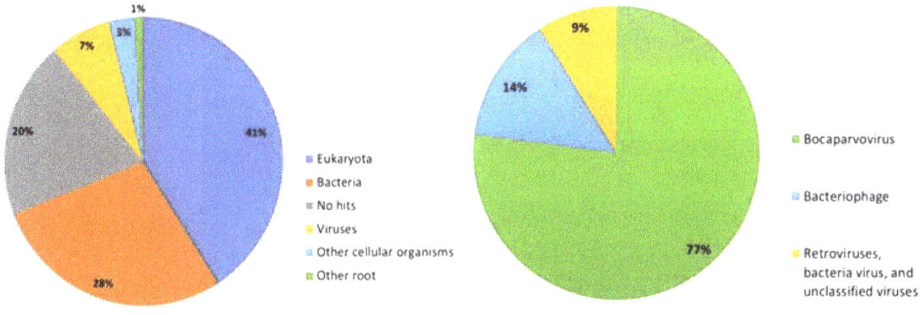

a b

Figure 1. Metagenomic (**a**) and virome (**b**) results from the alpaca intestinal sample.

Table 1. Nucleotide (nt) and amino acid (aa) percent identities of NS1, NP1, and VP1 genes of the alpaca bocaparvovirus (AlBoV) compared to the other ungulate BoV (UBoV) sequences (n = 108).

UBoV Virus	Species	Whole Genome (nt)	NS1		NP1		VP1	
			nt	aa	nt	aa	nt	aa
UBoV1 (n = 2)	Bovine	36.22–38.98	33.32–37.70	26.75–30.08	35.14–35.42	40.44–42.62	36.51–36.72	28.49–31.45
UBoV2 (n = 18)	Porcine	37.20–39.61	43.40–49.64	36.18–40.34	34.58–36.94	31.89–37.84	33.42–34.79	27.03–28.65
UBoV3 (n = 6)	Porcine	33.73–36.17	45.64–45.83	36.23–36.61	34.13–34.49	35.96	25.96–28.63	20.10–20.83
UBoV4 (n = 5)	Porcine	35.74–36.07	45.66–45.95	37.06–37.66	34.89–35.61	31.52–31.87	27.20–27.64	21.31–21.59
UBoV5 (n = 36)	Porcine	44.37–47.32	52.83–59.39	46.58–52.8	37.59–40.40	34.78–40.53	39.02–40.54	30.76–35.81
UBoV6 (n = 2)	Bovine	38.58–38.62	37.60–38.01	29.64	33.02	40.56–40.88	36.17–36.32	29.45–29.88
UBoV7 (n = 18)	Camel	36.49–36.76	39.01–39.64	33.08–33.98	36.91–38.93	32.24–33.88	26.05–27.11	21.08–21.84
UBoV8 (n = 21)	Camel	57.77–58.58	67.64–69.26	57.89–67.85	46.99–52.47	53.51–56.76	45.05–46.36	42.15–43.60

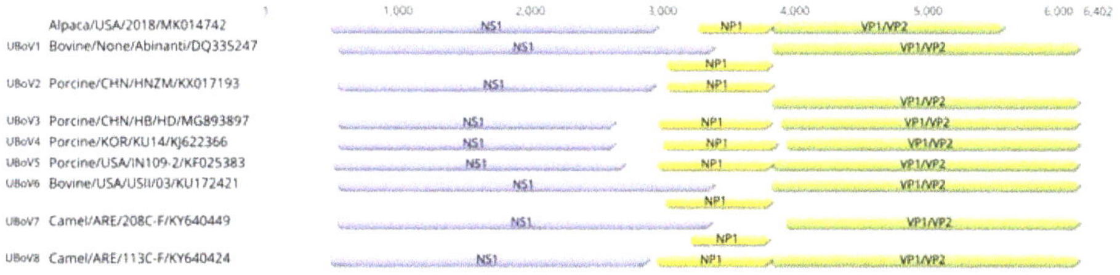

Figure 2. Genome organization of AlBoV compared to UBoV1–8. The purple, yellow, and green boxes indicate the NS1, NP1, and VP1/VP2 open reading frames (ORFs), respectively.

To study the phylogenetic relationship between AlBoV and other UBoVs, whole genome, NS1, NP1, and VP1 phylogenetic trees were created using a maximum likelihood method (phyML), using 500 bootstrap replicates in Geneious Prime. The trees were curated in FigTree (available from http://tree.bio.ed.ac.uk/software/figtree/) and Adobe Illustrator CS6 (Adobe Systems Inc, San Jose, CA, USA). Whole genome and NS1 phylogenetic trees illustrated that AlBoV shared a common ancestor with the UBoV8 species from camels (Figure 3). All eight species of UBoV (1–8) illustrated clear grouping in phylogenetic trees, which was observed in NP1 and VP1 phylogenetic trees as well.

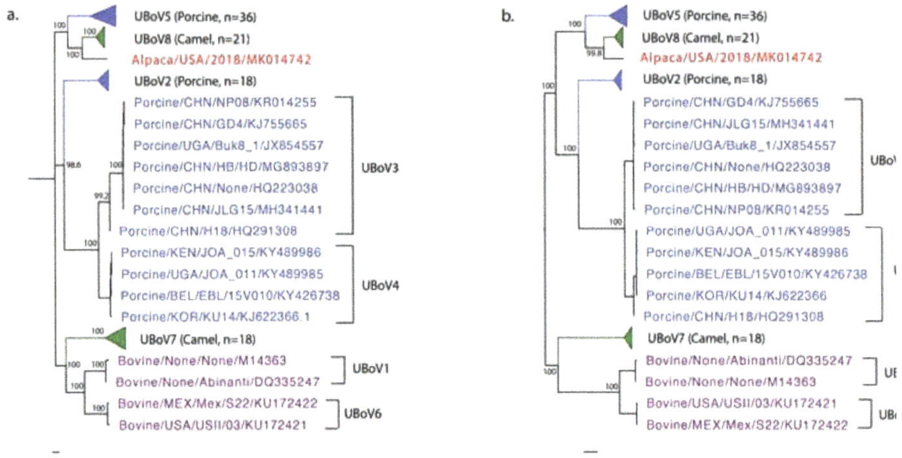

Figure 3. Mid-root Maximum Likelihood phylogenetic trees of AlBoV and other UBoV strains in the GenBank. (**a**) Whole genome phylogenetic tree. (**b**) Phylogenetic tree of NS1 amino acid sequences. Bootstrap values are indicated for major nodes. AlBoV is represented in red while the porcine, camel, and bovine UBoV strains are represented in blue, green, and purple, respectively.

To investigate and identify the presence of virulence attributes, AlBoV was screened for the ATP or GTP-binding Walker loop motif (GPASTGKT) and Phospholipase A2 (PLA2) motif with the calcium-binding loop and phospholipase catalytic residues; GPASTGKT and PLA2 were found in the NS1 and N-terminal of VP1 proteins, respectively (Figure 4). These protein motifs are conserved and are required for parvovirus infectivity. Phospholipase A2 activity, with the calcium-binding loop and phospholipase catalytic residues, is critical for efficient transfer of the viral genome from the late endosomes/lysosomes to the nucleus for the initiation of replication, and hence is considered essential for virus infectivity [33]. Mutations of critical amino acid residues in the VP1 protein of human parvovirus B19 induces a strong reduction in phospholipase A2 activity and virus infectivity [34]. Considering their vital role in parvovirus infectivity, PLA2 inhibitors are also targeted for antiviral drugs against parvovirus-associated diseases. The presence of the Walker loop and Phospholipase A2 motifs suggests that the newly identified alpaca BoV possesses the virulence determinants necessary to cause disease.

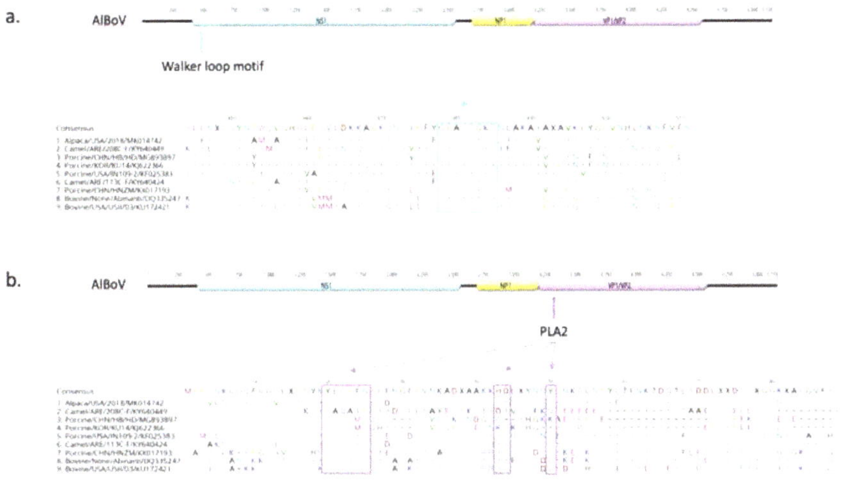

Figure 4. Detection of ATP and GTP-binding Walker-loop motif in NS1 protein (**a**) and Phospholipase A2 (PLA2) motif in N-terminal of VP1 protein (**b**). Dots indicate residues matching the consensus sequence and dashes represent gaps in the alignment.

A new species of UBoV was identified in an alpaca intestinal sample. Bocaparvoviruses cause respiratory and gastrointestinal infections in humans, bovines, and other animals. However, the causation of clinical disease in this alpaca farm is unclear. Establishing an association between the presence of BoV and clinical disease would require comprehensive PCR testing of the alpaca farms. Moreover, Koch's postulates is required to establish a virus–disease association. A causal association between the presence of BoV and clinical disease is often difficult due to prolonged viral shedding by the host after infection, high prevalence of BoV infection, and high rate of co-infections [35]. Nevertheless, the discovery of a new BoV will help in developing new PCR diagnostics to determine the prevalence of BoV in alpaca herds and also to develop vaccines to prevent clinical disease. Given the high mutation rate of BoVs and increasing domestication of alpacas, identification of a new BoV in alpaca presents a true risk of cross-species transmission to other mammals.

Author Contributions: Conceptualization: D.M.; Sample preparation and next generation sequencing: S.C.; next generation sequencing pipeline: N.L., M.H.; Formal analysis: D.K.; Phylogenetic trees: D.K., M.D.; Writing—original draft preparation: D.K.; writing—review and editing: D.M.; Case description and sample: D.B. and C.A.M.; Supervision: D.M.; Funding acquisition: D.M.

Funding: The study was partially supported by Marthaler's start up fund.

Acknowledgments: The authors would like to thank the Kansas State Veterinary Diagnostic Laboratory and Tufts University for supporting the project.

Conflicts of Interest: The authors declare no conflict of interest.

References

1. Wang, Y.; Zhao, J.; Zheng, M.; Liu, Z.; Yuan, J.; Zhao, J.; Shen, Q.; Fan, Z.; Jiang, L. Genome Sequence of a Porcine Bocavirus Detected in Feces of Domestic Minks in China. *Genome Announc.* **2017**, *5*, e01170-17. [CrossRef] [PubMed]
2. Lau, S.K.; Ahmed, S.S.; Yeung, H.C.; Li, K.S.; Fan, R.Y.; Cheng, T.Y.; Cai, J.P.; Wang, M.; Zheng, B.J.; Samson, S.Y.W.; et al. Identification and Interspecies Transmission of a Novel Bocaparvovirus among Different Bat Species in China. *J. Gen. Virol.* **2016**, *97*, 3345–3358. [CrossRef] [PubMed]

3. Woo, P.C.; Lau, S.K.; Tsoi, H.-W.; Patteril, N.G.; Yeung, H.C.; Joseph, S.; Wong, E.Y.M.; Muhammed, R.; Chow, F.W.N. Two novel dromedary camel bocaparvoviruses from dromedaries in the Middle East with unique genomic features. *J. Gen. Virol.* **2017**, *98*, 1349–1359.
4. Kapoor, A.; Mehta, N.; Esper, F.; Poljsak-Prijatelj, M.; Quan, P.L.; Qaisar, N.; Delwart, E.; Lipkin, W.L. Identification and characterization of a new Bocavirus species in Gorillas. *PLoS ONE* **2010**, *5*, e11948. [CrossRef] [PubMed]
5. Ao, Y.; Li, X.; Li, L.; Xie, X.; Jin, D.; Yu, J.; Lu, S.; Duan, Z. Two novel bocaparvovirus species identified in wild Himalayan marmots. *Sci. China Life Sci.* **2017**, *60*, 1348–1356. [CrossRef]
6. Gunn, L.; Collins, P.J.; Fanning, S.; McKillen, J.; Morgan, J.; Staines, A.; O'Shea, H. Detection and characterisation of novel bocavirus (genus Bocaparvovirus) and gastroenteritis viruses from asymptomatic pigs in Ireland. *Infect. Ecol. Epidemiol.* **2015**, *5*, 27270. [CrossRef] [PubMed]
7. Zhang, C.; Song, F.; Xiu, L.; Liu, Y.; Yang, J.; Yao, L.; Peng, J. Identification and characterization of a novel rodent bocavirus from different rodent species in China. *Emerg. Microbes Infect.* **2018**, *7*, 48. [CrossRef] [PubMed]
8. Cotmore, S.F.; Agbandje-McKenna, M.; Chiorini, J.A.; Mukha, D.V.; Pintel, D.J.; Qiu, J.; Soderlund-Venermo, M.; Tattersall, P.; Tijssen, P.; Gatherer, D.; et al. The family Parvoviridae. *Arch. Virol.* **2014**, *159*, 1239–1247. [CrossRef]
9. Cheng, W.-X.; Li, J.-S.; Huang, C.-P.; Yao, D.-P.; Liu, N.; Cui, S.-X.; Jin, Y.; Duan, Z.-J. Identification and nearly full-lengthg characterization of novel porcine Bocaviruses. *PLoS ONE* **2010**, *5*, e13583. [CrossRef]
10. Principi, N.; Piralla, A.; Zampiero, A.; Bianchini, S.; Umbrello, G.; Scala, A.; Bosis, S.; Fossali, E.; Baldanti, F. Bocavirus infection in otherwise healthy children with respiratory disease. *PLoS ONE* **2015**, *10*, e0135640. [CrossRef]
11. Kailasan, S.; Halder, S.; Gurda, B.; Bladek, H.; Chipman, P.R.; McKenna, R.; Brown, K.; Agbandje-McKenna, M. Structure of an enteric pathogen, bovine parvovirus. *J. Virol.* **2015**, *89*, 2603–2614. [CrossRef]
12. Binn, L.N.; Lazar, E.C.; Eddy, G.A.; Kajima, M. Recovery and characterization of a minute virus of canines. *Infect. Immun.* **1970**, *1*, 503–508.
13. McClenahan, S.D.; Scherba, G.; Borst, L.; Fredrickson, R.L.; Krause, P.R.; Uhlenhaut, C. Discovery of a Bovine Enterovirus in Alpaca. *PLoS ONE* **2013**, *8*, e68777. [CrossRef]
14. Alpaca Owners Association Inc Homepage. Available online: https://www.alpacainfo.com/about/statistics/alpacas-us (accessed on 22 May 2019).
15. Crossley, B.M.; Mock, R.E.; Callison, S.A.; Hietala, S.K. Identification and characterization of a novel alpaca respiratory coronavirus most closely related to the human coronavirus 229E. *Viruses* **2012**, *4*, 3689–3700. [CrossRef]
16. Brito, B.P.; Gardner, I.A.; Hietala, S.K.; Crossley, B.M. Variation in Bluetongue virus real-time reverse transcription polymerase chain reaction assay results in blood samples of sheep, cattle, and alpaca. *J. Vet. Diagn. Investig.* **2011**, *23*, 753–757. [CrossRef]
17. Kapil, S.; Yeary, T.; Evermann, J.F. Viral diseases of new world camelids. *Vet. Clin. N. Am. Food Anim. Pract.* **2009**, *25*, 323–337. [CrossRef]
18. Jin, L.; Cebra, C.K.; Baker, R.J.; Mattson, D.E.; Cohen, S.A.; Alvarado, D.E.; Rohrmann, G.F. Analysis of the genome sequence of an alpaca coronavirus. *Virology* **2007**, *365*, 198–203. [CrossRef]
19. Barrington, G.M.; Allen, A.J.; Parish, S.M.; Tibary, A. Biosecurity and biocontainment in alpaca operations. *Small Rum. Res.* **2006**, *61*, 217–225. [CrossRef]
20. Wernery, U.; Kaaden, O.R. Foot-and-mouth disease in camelids: A review. *Vet. J.* **2004**, *168*, 134–142. [CrossRef]
21. Hause, B.M.; Collin, E.A.; Anderson, J.; Hesse, R.A.; Anderson, G. Bovine rhinitis viruses are common in U.S. cattle with bovine respiratory disease. *PLoS ONE* **2015**, *10*, e0121998. [CrossRef]
22. Neill, J.D.; Bayles, D.O.; Ridpath, J.F. Simultaneous rapid sequencing of multiple RNA virus genomes. *J. Virol. Methods* **2014**, *201*, 68–72. [CrossRef]
23. Knutson, T.P.; Velayudhan, B.T.; Marthaler, D.G. A porcine enterovirus G associated with enteric disease contains a novel papain-like cysteine protease. *J. Gen. Virol.* **2017**, *98*, 1305–1310. [CrossRef]
24. Bolger, A.M.; Lohse, M.; Usadel, B. Trimmomatic: A flexible trimmer for Illumina sequence data. *Bioinformatics* **2014**. [CrossRef]

25. Joshi, N.; Fass, J. Sickle—A Windowed Adaptive Trimming Tool for FASTQ Files Using Quality. 2011. Available online: http://github.com/najoshi/sickle (accessed on 2 July 2019).
26. Buffalo, V. Scythe—A Bayesian Adapter Trimmer. 2011. Available online: http://github.com/vsbuffalo/scythe (accessed on 2 July 2019).
27. Wood, D.E.; Salzberg, S.L. Kraken: Ultrafast metagenomic sequence classification using exact alignments. *Genome Biol.* **2014**, *15*, R46. [CrossRef]
28. Katoh, K.; Standley, D.M. MAFFT Multiple Sequence Alignment Software Version 7: Improvements in Performance and Usability. *Mol. Biol. Evol.* **2013**, *30*, 772–780. [CrossRef]
29. Kearse, M.; Moir, R.; Wilson, A.; Stones-Havas, S.; Cheung, M.; Sturrock, S.; Buxton, S.; Cooper, A.; Markowitz, S. Geneious Basic: An integrated and extendable desktop software platform for the organization and analysis of sequence data. *Bioinformatics* **2012**, *28*, 1647–1649. [CrossRef]
30. Martin, D.P.; Murrell, B.; Golden, M.; Khoosal, A.; Muhire, B. RDP4: Detection and analysis of recombination patterns in virus genomes. *Virus Evol.* **2015**, *1*, vev003. [CrossRef]
31. Shackelton, L.A.; Parrish, C.R.; Truyen, U.; Holmes, E.C. High rate of viral evolution associated with the emergence of carnivore parvovirus. *Proc. Natl. Acad. Sci. USA* **2005**, *102*, 379–384. [CrossRef]
32. Fasina, O.O.; Dong, Y.; Pintel, D.J. NP1 protein of the bocaparvovirus minute virus of canines controls access to the viral capsid genes via its role in RNA processing. *J. Virol.* **2015**, *90*, 1718–1728. [CrossRef]
33. Zádori, Z.; Szelei, J.; Lacoste, M.-C.; Li, Y.; Gariépy, S.; Raymond, P.; Allaire, M.; Nabi, I.R.; Tijssen, P. A Viral Phospholipase A2 Is Required for Parvovirus Infectivity. *Dev. Cell* **2001**, *1*, 291–302. [CrossRef]
34. Deng, X.F.; Dong, Y.M.; Yi, Q.H.; Huang, Y.; Zhao, D.; Yang, Y.B.; Tijssen, P.; Qiu, J.M.; Liu, K.Y.; Li, Y. The determinants for the enzyme activity of human parvovirus b19 phospholipase a2 (pla2) and its influence on cultured cells. *PLoS ONE* **2013**, *8*, e61440. [CrossRef]
35. Castrignano, S.B.; Nagasse-Sugahara, T.K. The metagenomic approach and causality in virology. *Rev. Saúde Pública* **2015**, *49*, 21. [CrossRef]

viruses

MDPI

Article

Equine Parvovirus-Hepatitis Frequently Detectable in Commercial Equine Serum Pools

Toni Luise Meister [1,†], Birthe Tegtmeyer [2,†], Alexander Postel [3], Jessika-M.V. Cavalleri [4], Daniel Todt [1], Alexander Stang [1,‡] and Eike Steinmann [1,*,‡]

1 Department of Molecular and Medical Virology, Faculty of Medicine, Ruhr-University Bochum, 44801 Bochum, Germany; Toni.meister@rub.de (T.L.M.); Daniel.todt@rub.de (D.T.); Alexander.stang@rub.de (A.S.)

2 Institute for Experimental Virology, TWINCORE Centre for Experimental and Clinical Infection Research, a joint venture between the Medical School Hannover (MHH) and the Helmholtz Centre for Infection Research (HZI), 30625 Hannover, Germany; birthe.tegtmeyer@twincore.de

3 University of Veterinary Medicine Hannover, Institute of Virology, 30559 Hannover, Germany; alexander.postel@tiho-hannover.de

4 Department for Companion Animals and Horses, University of Veterinary Medicine, 1210 Vienna, Austria; Jessika.Cavalleri@vetmeduni.ac.at

* Correspondence: eike.steinmann@rub.de; Tel.: +49-234-32-23189

† Equally contributing first authors.

‡ Equally contributing last authors.

Received: 16 April 2019; Accepted: 17 May 2019; Published: 21 May 2019

Abstract: An equine parvovirus-hepatitis (EqPV-H) has been recently identified in association with equine serum hepatitis, also known as Theiler's disease. This disease was first described by Arnold Theiler in 1918 and is often observed after applications with blood products in equines. So far, the virus has only been described in the USA and China. In this study, we evaluated the presence of EqPV-H in several commercial serum samples to assess the potential risk of virus transmission by equine serum-based products for medical and research applications. In 11 out of 18 commercial serum samples, EqPV-H DNA was detectable with a viral load up to 10^5 copies/mL. The same serum batches as well as three additional samples were also positive for antibodies against the EqPV-H VP1 protein. The countries of origin with detectable viral genomes included the USA, Canada, New Zealand, Italy, and Germany, suggesting a worldwide distribution of EqPV-H. Phylogenetic analysis of the EqPV-H NS1 sequence in commercial serum samples revealed high similarities in viral sequences from different geographical areas. As horse sera are commonly used for the production of anti-sera, which are included in human and veterinary medical products, these results implicate the requirement for diagnostic tests to prevent EqPV-H transmission.

Keywords: equine parvovirus-hepatitis; horses; commercial horse serum; phylogeny

1. Introduction

Parvoviruses are small, non-enveloped viruses with a DNA genome typically encoding at least two major gene complexes with the non-structural protein (NS1, multidomain nuclear phosphoprotein) and capsid protein (VP1). In recent years, many viruses have been newly identified or reassigned to the family *Parvoviridae*, which is divided into two subfamilies, the *Densovirinae* and the *Parvovirinae*, according to whether they infect invertebrates or vertebrates, respectively [1,2]. Both subfamilies are further divided into various genera based on their genome organization.

The parvovirus subfamily *Parvovirinae* is a large family with a wide host range, divided into eight genera that can infect humans, domestic animals, and wild animals [1,3,4].

Recently, a novel equine parvovirus (equine parvovirus-hepatitis, EqPV-H) was discovered in the serum of a horse that died of Theiler's disease indicating that EqPV-H could be the causative agent of Theiler's disease and also of subclinical infections [5–7]. Theiler's disease is also known as equine serum hepatitis and was initially described by Sir Arnold Theiler in 1918 [8]. After experimental vaccination studies to prevent African horse sickness, Theiler observed hundreds of cases of a highly fatal form of hepatitis. Theiler's disease or serum hepatitis has since been reported worldwide after treatment with a variety of equine serum products, for instance tetanus antitoxin, botulinum antitoxin, antiserum against Streptococcus equi as well as pregnant mare's serum, and equine plasma [5,8–12]. The clinical disease among horses receiving these products has a high fatality rate, and the incidence of fulminant hepatitis in these outbreaks was in the range of 1.4%–18% [13]. Recent studies provided evidence for the association of EqPV-H and Theiler's disease. A prospective study on Theiler's disease cases described the detection of EqPV-H in 18 consecutive cases of Theiler's disease that occurred after administration of an equine-based biological product [13]. The same authors also reported EqPV-H infection in 9 out of 10 cases of Theiler's disease in the absence of an equine biological product administration and noted 54% virus positivity of tested in-contact horses [14].

Given the potential risk of EqPV-H contaminated equine serum products for medical as well as research applications, in this study we investigated the prevalence of EqPV-H among commercial equine serum pools from various countries worldwide. To this end, a total of 18 serum samples from different providers were analyzed for the presence of anti-EqPV-H-VP1-antibodies and EqPV-H DNA. The results indicate that EqPV-H is highly prevalent in commercial horse serum around the world and that blood-based products derived from equine donors should be tested for EqPV-H.

2. Materials and Methods

2.1. Serum Sample Collection

A total of 18 different horse serum samples were collected from a variety of providers. The samples were shipped and stored at −20 °C until further analysis. Thaw and freeze cycles were kept at a minimum.

2.2. Detection of EqPV-H DNA

Viral DNA was extracted with a viral DNA Kit from Qiagen (Cat. No. 1048147, Hilden, Germany) according to the manufacturer's recommendations. DNA samples were stored at −20 °C until further analysis. A probe-based quantitative real-time polymerase chain reaction (qRT-PCR) was used with primers and probe designed and provided by Dr. Amit Kapoor as described before [5]. A serial dilution of a plasmid containing the EqPV-H VP1 sequence was generated as standard row for the quantification of EqPV-H within the samples tested. Fluorescence was assessed with a LightCycler 480 (Roche, Mannheim, Germany).

2.3. Detection of Anti-EqPV-H Antibodies

Samples were analyzed regarding the presence of anti-EqPV-H-VP1 antibodies using the luciferase immunoprecipitation system (LIPS) as described by Burbelo et al. [15,16] and Pfaender et al. [17]. For the EqPV-H-LIPS, the antigen VP1 was produced as described by Divers et al. [5]. Relative light units (RLU) were measured in a plate luminometer (LB 960 XS3; Berthold, Bad Wildbad, Germany). For calculation of sensitivity, a cut-off limit, analogous to Burbelo et al. (2012) and Pfaender et al. (2015), was determined and defined as the mean RLU plus 3 standard deviations (SD) of a EqPV-H negative horse serum. A cross-reaction of the LIPS with other related parvoviruses cannot be excluded.

2.4. Sequencing and Phylogeny

For sequence analysis, two PCRs (I and II) were designed within the NS1 of EqPV-H (Table 1 and Figure 3A). PCR was performed using the Expand High Fidelity PCR System (Roche Diagnostics) in a total volume of 50 µL containing 5 µL of purified DNA, 5 µL of 10× buffer, 200 µM of each dNTP, 10 pmol of each primer, and 0.375 µL of Taq Polymerase.

The PCR profile was the following: 95 °C for 2 min, 45 cycles of 95 °C for 20 s, 60 °C for 30 s, and 72 °C for 1 min 30 s, followed by a final extension at 72 °C for 10 min. PCR products were visualized on a 2% agarose gel, excised, and purified using a Monarch® DNA Gel Extraction Kit (New England Biolabs). Purified products were then sent for Sanger sequencing using the applicable PCR primers.

Phylogenetic trees were constructed using the maximum likelihood method and general time reversible model [18,19] implemented in MEGA X version 10.0.5 [20]. The tree is drawn to scale, with branch lengths measured in the number of substitutions per site.

Table 1. Primer positions and sequences used for sequencing analysis.

PCR	Primer	Sequence
I	EPVf1	GGGTGGTAAATGCCTTCG
	EPVseqr01	TGGTTGGTGACGCCTGTC
II	EPVseqf01	GACAGGCGTCACCAACCA
	1104R[1]	GGGAATGTCATTGAACGGGAA

[1] Lu et al. [6].

2.5. Purification of Viral Particles

Particle associated nucleic acid (PAN) purification was performed in detail as originally described [21]: 11 mL of horse serum was clarified (3220 g, 30 min) and subsequently filtered through a 0.22 µm pore-size sterile filter to eliminate particles of higher density and mass such as bacteria, eukaryotic cells, or fragments of them. To concentrate virus particles and separate them from particles of lower density, 10 mL of sterile filtered serum was layered onto 2 mL of 30% (*wt/vol*) sucrose in PBS, followed by ultracentrifugation for 3 h in an SW41 rotor at 30,000 rpm. For preparation of DNA, the pellet was resuspended in 250 µL of PBS containing 20 mM $MgCl_2$. To degrade DNA that is not inside a particle, a DNase step was performed by the addition of 5 U of DNase I followed by incubation at 37 °C for 30 min, followed in turn by DNA extraction with a Blood-Mini-Kit (Qiagen).

3. Results and Discussion

3.1. EqPV-H DNA is Frequently Detectable in Commercial Horse Sera

To evaluate the potential presence of EqPV-H in commercial serum pools, eighteen different serum samples were obtained from different countries with a specific serum type and number of individual horses per pool (Table 2).

Table 2. General information about the serum samples regarding serum type, land of origin, and the number of individuals.

Serum ID	Serum Type	Origin	Number of Individuals
1	Horse Serum	New Zealand	donor herd
2	Fetal Horse Serum	Mexico	unknown
3	Donor Horse Serum	USA	pooled
4	Horse Serum	USA	donor herd

Table 2. *Cont.*

Serum ID	Serum Type	Origin	Number of Individuals
5	Horse Serum	USA	donor herd
6	Donor Horse Serum	Italy	pooled
7	Horse Serum	France	pooled
8	Donor Horse Serum	Canada	unknown
9	Donor Horse Serum	Chile	unknown
10	Donor Horse Serum	Germany	unknown
11	Donor Horse Serum	Italy	unknown
12	Fetal Horse Serum	Brazil	unknown
13	Donor Horse Serum (heat inactivated)	Chile	unknown
14	Horse Serum	Europe	pooled
15	Donor Horse Serum	Europe	pooled
16	Donor Horse Serum	USA	unknown
17	Horse Serum	New Zealand	unknown
18	Donor Horse Serum	Canada	unknown

Eleven out of 18 commercially available sera tested positive for EqPV-H DNA, illustrated using gel electrophoresis of the qPCR products (Figure 1A). As depicted in Figure 1B, quantification of the viral DNA revealed loads ranging from 10^2 to 10^5 DNA copies/mL (Figure 1B). Next, the commercial horse serum samples were tested for the presence of anti-VP1-antibodies via LIPS assay. All EqPV-H DNA positive samples also yielded positive results in the antibody assay, while three additional sera were exclusively anti-VP1-antibody positive (7, 9, and 13) (Figure 1C). However, the measured relative light units (RLU) of these three seropositive samples were lower compared to the eleven sera that had also been tested DNA positive (Figure 1C). Due to the pooling of sera from several horses for one commercial serum batch, a potential dilution has to be considered, and the detection limit of EqPV-H PCR was determined at 175 DNA copies/mL. In line with these results, tetanus-antitoxins as one of the most common medical products administered to horses tested positive for EqPV-H in several cases of Theiler's disease [13]. Importantly, an experimental infection study had previously confirmed transmission of EqPV-H from a PCR-positive biological product to seronegative horses [5]. To evaluate, if the detected parvovirus DNA was encapsidated or just plain unprotected DNA, we performed PAN DNA isolation [21] with serum 1 as one example. This method contains a DNAse treatment step, which degrades all unprotected DNA, thus selects highly specific for DNA protected by a capsid. After purification we performed quantitative PCR for both the DNA isolation with and without selection for PAN-DNA. We found that around 1% of total parvovirus DNA could be recovered using this method. A recovery rate of 1% corresponds to our own findings with various viruses (DNA, RNA, enveloped, and non-enveloped), spiked to PBS for evaluation of this method. The relatively high losses can be either explained by the high stringency of the method or simply by presence of non-protected nucleic acid naturally occurring for different viruses. Either way, for this horse serum it is highly likely that parvovirus DNA is encapsidated in viral particles and so viral particles are present. Due to the lack of an infection cell culture system, we could not determine if these particles are infectious.

Of note, serum samples 8 to 13 have also been tested previously by us for the presence of equine hepacivirus (EqHV), equine pegivirus (EPgV), and Theiler's disease associated virus (TDAV) [22]. All samples were shown to be EPgV and EqHV positive except serum sample 12, which tested negative for EqHV. Furthermore, TDAV was detected in samples 10, 11, and 13 [22]. In summary, these results demonstrate a frequent detection of EqPV-H in commercial serum pools with 61.10% PCR positivity and 77.70% sero-positivity.

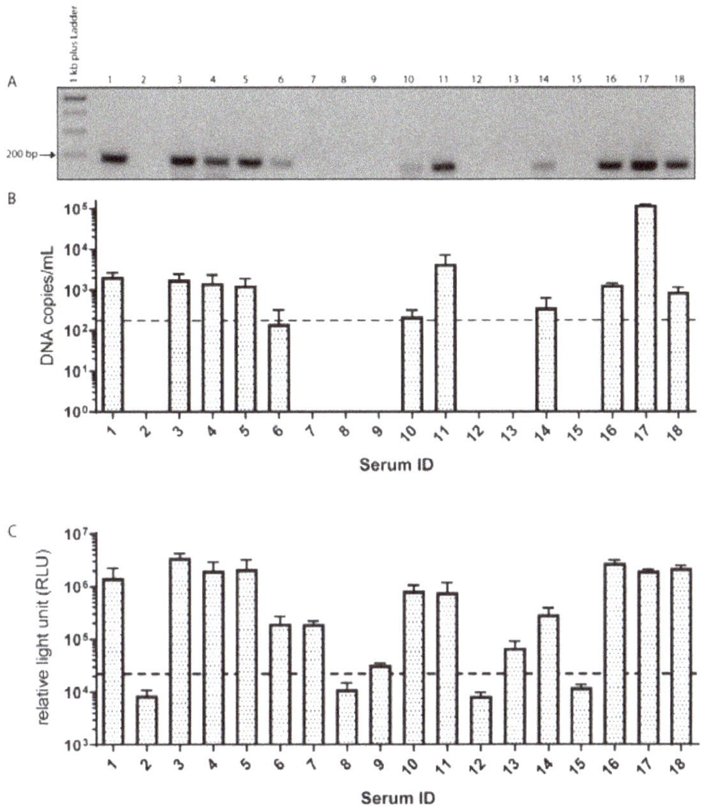

Figure 1. Occurrence of EqPV-H DNA and antibodies within commercial serum samples. (**A**) Agarose gel electrophoresis of quantitative PCR of commercial serum pools. (**B**) Viral loads of EqPV-H were determined using qPCR and are displayed in DNA copies/mL. The dotted line indicates the limit of detection. Every bar represents the mean of 5 technical replicates performed in 3 independent measurements. (**C**) Depicted are anti-EqPV-H antibodies as RLU measured in triplicates. The cut-off was determined by the mean value of the EqPV-H negative serum plus 3*SD and is indicated by a dashed line.

3.2. EqPV-H Can be Detected in Different Countries Worldwide

As the novel parvovirus has only been recently described [5], prevalence studies with EqPV-H have so far only been performed in the USA and China. Lu et al. showed that EqPV-H has a very low genetic diversity between farms in the same geographic region, similar to what has been observed in the USA [5,7]. When comparing the origin of the here-tested commercial sera regarding the presence of EqPV-H DNA and antibodies, all South American sera (green) tested negative for EqPV-H, while the majority of sera from North America (red), Europe (blue), and Oceania (orange) were positive for EqPV-H DNA and antibodies (Figure 2A). These included the countries New Zealand, the USA, Italy, Germany, and Canada indicating a worldwide circulation of EqPV-H. The two fetal horse sera that were included in the study tested EqPV-H PCR and antibody negative in contrast to the adult horse sera (Figure 2B,C). However, further investigations with more samples are needed to determine the importance of EqPV-H for vertical transmission and prevalence in young horses. However, PCR- and sero-negativity could also be a coincidence due to the origin of the fetal horse serum from Central and South America.

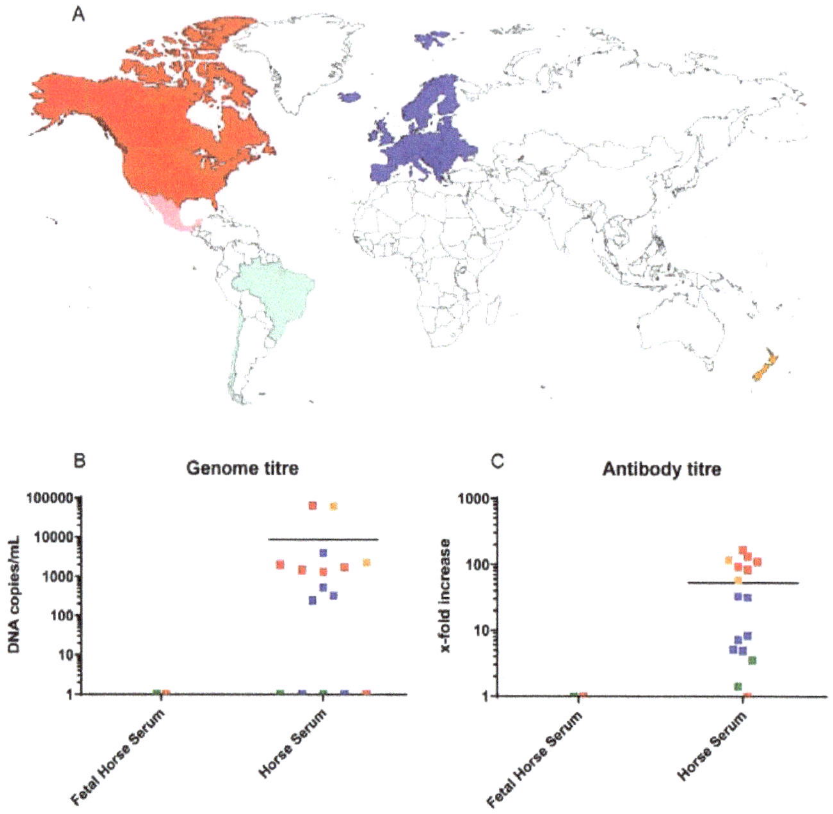

Figure 2. The origin of the serum pools is indicated on a world map (**A**). Reduced opacity indicates EqPV-H negative serum pools. Graphs (**B**) and (**C**) show the correlation of age (determined by the serum type) and origin on EqPV DNA and antibody prevalence, respectively. Every dot represents the mean of 5 technical replicates performed in two independent measurements. Negative samples were assigned the value 1. Red color corresponds to North America, while sera from South American countries are colored green. Blue indicates serum samples originating from Europe and orange belong to samples from Oceania (A–C).

3.3. Sequence and Phylogenetic Analysis of EqPV-H in Commercial Serum Pools

For a molecular characterization of the EqPV-H positive samples, primers (Table 1) in the NS1 gene were designed to obtain two PCR fragments (Figure 3A). Due to low viral loads being present for only some of the qPCR positive samples, sequencing of PCRI and II fragments was possible. We were able to recover 7/11 and 9/11 sequences for PCRI and II, respectively. These sequences were submitted to the GenBank database with the accession numbers indicated in Table 3. A maximum likelihood approach was used, and robustness of the trees tested with a bootstrap analysis was performed with a replicate rate of 1000. As depicted in Figure 3B,C, the obtained sequences were highly similar for all commercial serum pools around the world and clustered with the published American and Asian EqPV-H sequences (Figure 3B,C). This can be observed for two individually amplified regions in the NS1 gene. These results point to a high conservation between the world-wide circulating strains and low genetic variability of the EqPV-H strain.

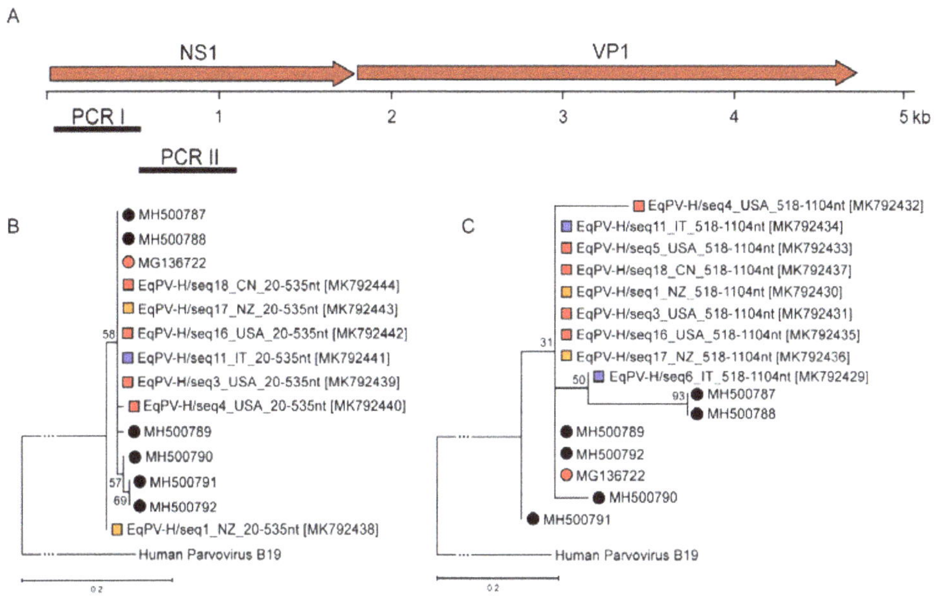

Figure 3. (**A**) Genomic organization of EqPV-H and primer positioning for PCR I-II. (**B**) Phylogenetic tree based on the fragments generated using PCR I. (**C**) Phylogenetic tree based on the fragments generated using PCR II. Evolutionary history was inferred by using the maximum likelihood method and general time reversible model. The trees with the highest log likelihood are shown. Red corresponds to North America, while blue indicates serum samples originating from Europe and orange matches samples from Oceania. Black corresponds to Asian strains. Circles indicate previously published EqPV-H sequences identified by various groups, whereas squares label newly found EqPV-H sequences within this study. Human parvovirus B19 was used as outgroup to root the tree.

Table 3. The newly identified specimens were submitted to NCBI and were assigned with respect to the serum ID and the land of origin.

Serum ID	EqPV Sequence Name	NCBI Accession Number
1	Equine Parvovirus H/seq1_NZ_518-1104nt	MK792430
3	Equine Parvovirus H/seq3_USA_518-1104nt	MK792431
4	Equine Parvovirus H/seq4_USA_518-1104nt	MK792432
5	Equine Parvovirus H/seq5_USA_518-1104nt	MK792433
6	Equine Parvovirus H/seq6_IT_518-1104nt	MK792429
11	Equine Parvovirus H/seq11_IT_518-1104nt	MK792434
16	Equine Parvovirus H/seq16_USA_518-1104nt	MK792435
17	Equine Parvovirus H/seq17_NZ_518-1104nt	MK792436
18	Equine Parvovirus H/seq18_CN_518-1104nt	MK792437
1	Equine Parvovirus H/seq1_NZ_20-535nt	MK792438
3	Equine Parvovirus H/seq3_USA_20-535nt	MK792439
4	Equine Parvovirus H/seq4_USA_20-535nt	MK792440
11	Equine Parvovirus H/seq11_IT_20-535nt	MK792441
16	Equine Parvovirus H/seq16_USA_20-535nt	MK792442
17	Equine Parvovirus H/seq17_NZ_20-535nt	MK792443
18	Equine Parvovirus H/seq18_CN_20-535nt	MK792444

4. Conclusions

In this study, we investigated the occurrence of EqPV-H DNA and antibodies within commercial horse sera. We showed that anti-EqPV-H DNA and EqPV-H antibodies are frequently detectable in commercially available horse sera from various origins indicating a worldwide circulation of EqPV-H infections. As horse sera are commonly used for production of anti-sera, which are licensed for various treatments in different animal species as well as humans (snake antivenom immunoglobulins and botulism antitoxin), these results should raise awareness for EqPV-H contaminations. Furthermore, other biologicals like live vaccines might harbor infectious EqPV-H, for instance when cell lines used for virus propagation were cultivated with horse serum. Sensitive diagnostic assays should be used for the detection of EqPV-H DNA and a careful risk assessment should be performed when using commercial horse sera in medical and research applications.

Author Contributions: Conceptualization, D.T., A.S., and E.S.; methodology, T.L.M., B.T., D.T., and A.S.; formal analysis, T.L.M.; investigation, T.L.M. and B.T.; resources, A.P. and J.V.M.C; data curation, T.L.M. and A.S.; writing—original draft preparation, T.L.M. and B.T.; writing—review and editing, T.L.M., B.T., A.P., J.V.M.C., D.T., A.S., and E.S.; visualization, T.L.M. and D.T.; supervision, E.S.; project administration, E.S.

Funding: This research received no external funding.

Acknowledgments: We are grateful to Amit Kapoor for providing us with the qPCR protocol and also thank Peter D. Burbelo (NIH, Maryland, USA) for providing the Renilla-luciferase-VP1 fusion plasmid. We would like to thank all members of the Department of Molecular and Medical Virology at the Ruhr-University Bochum and especially Rosemarie Bohr, Regina Bütermann, Monika Kopytkowski, Klaus Sure, and Ute Wiegmann-Misiek for technical support.

Conflicts of Interest: The authors declare no conflict of interest.

References

1. Cotmore, S.F.; Agbandje-McKenna, M.; Chiorini, J.A.; Mukha, D.V.; Pintel, D.J.; Qiu, J.; Soderlund-Venermo, M.; Tattersall, P.; Tijssen, P.; Gatherer, D.; et al. The family Parvoviridae. *Arch. Virol.* **2014**, *159*, 1239–1247. [CrossRef]
2. Kailasan, S.; Agbandje-McKenna, M.; Parrish, C.R. Parvovirus Family Conundrum, What Makes a Killer? *Annu. Rev. Virol.* **2015**, *2*, 425–450. [CrossRef]
3. Palinski, R.M.; Mitra, N.; Hause, B.M. Discovery of a novel Parvovirinae virus, porcine parvovirus 7, by metagenomic sequencing of porcine rectal swabs. *Virus Genes* **2016**, *52*, 564–567. [CrossRef]
4. Lau, S.K.P.; Woo, P.C.Y.; Yeung, H.C.; Teng, J.L.L.; Wu, Y.; Bai, R.; Fan, R.Y.Y.; Chan, K.-H.; Yuen, K.-Y. Identification and characterization of bocaviruses in cats and dogs reveals a novel feline bocavirus and a novel genetic group of canine bocavirus. *J. Gen. Virol.* **2012**, *93*, 1573–1582. [CrossRef]
5. Divers, T.J.; Tennant, B.C.; Kumar, A.; McDonough, S.; Cullen, J.; Bhuva, N.; Jain, K.; Chauhan, L.S.; Scheel, T.K.H.; Lipkin, W.I.; et al. New Parvovirus Associated with Serum Hepatitis in Horses after Inoculation of Common Biological Product. *Emerg. Infect. Dis.* **2018**, *24*, 303–310. [CrossRef]
6. Divers, T.J.; Tomlinson, J.E. Theiler's disease. *Equine Vet Educ.* **2019**, *19*, 120. [CrossRef]
7. Lu, G.; Sun, L.; Ou, J.; Xu, H.; Wu, L.; Li, S. Identification and genetic characterization of a novel parvovirus associated with serum hepatitis in horses in China. *Emerg. Microbes & Infect.* **2018**, *7*, 170.
8. Theiler, A. *Acute Liver-Atrophy and Parenchymatous Hepatitis in Horses*; Reports of the Director of Veterinary Research; CAB Direct: Glasgow, UK, 1918; pp. 7–164.
9. Aleman, M.; Nieto, J.E.; Carr, E.A.; Carlson, G.P. Serum Hepatitis Associated with Commercial Plasma Transfusion in Horses. *J. Vet. Intern. Med.* **2005**, *19*, 120–122. [CrossRef]
10. Thomsett, L.R. Acute Hepatic Failure in the Horse. *Equine Vet. J.* **1971**, *3*, 15–19. [CrossRef]
11. Chandriani, S.; Skewes-Cox, P.; Zhong, W.; Ganem, D.E.; Divers, T.J.; van Blaricum, A.J.; Tennant, B.C.; Kistler, A.L. Identification of a previously undescribed divergent virus from the Flaviviridae family in an outbreak of equine serum hepatitis. *Proc. Natl. Acad. Sci. USA* **2013**, *110*, E1407–E1415. [CrossRef]
12. Rose, J.A.; Immenschuh, R.D.; Rose, E.M. Serum hepatitis in the horse, Proceedings of the Twentieth Annual Conference of the American Association of Equine Practitioners. *Am. Assoc. Equine Pract.* **1974**, 175–185.

13. Tomlinson, J.E.; Kapoor, A.; Kumar, A.; Tennant, B.C.; Laverack, M.A.; Beard, L.; Delph, K.; Davis, E.; Schott Ii, H.; Lascola, K.; et al. Viral testing of 18 consecutive cases of equine serum hepatitis, A prospective study (2014–2018). *J. Vet. Intern. Med.* **2019**, *33*, 251–257. [CrossRef]
14. Tomlinson, J.E.; Tennant, B.C.; Struzyna, A.; Mrad, D.; Browne, N.; Whelchel, D.; Johnson, P.J.; Jamieson, C.; Löhr, C.V.; Bildfell, R.; et al. Viral testing of 10 cases of Theiler's disease and 37 in-contact horses in the absence of equine biologic product administration, A prospective study (2014–2018). *J. Vet. Intern. Med.* **2019**, *33*, 258–265. [CrossRef]
15. Burbelo, P.D.; Ching, K.H.; Klimavicz, C.M.; Iadarola, M.J. Antibody profiling by Luciferase Immunoprecipitation Systems (LIPS). *J. Vis. Exp.* **2009**, *32*, e1549. [CrossRef] [PubMed]
16. Burbelo, P.D.; Dubovi, E.J.; Simmonds, P.; Medina, J.L.; Henriquez, J.A.; Mishra, N.; Wagner, J.; Tokarz, R.; Cullen, J.M.; Iadarola, M.J.; et al. Serology-enabled discovery of genetically diverse hepaciviruses in a new host. *J. Virol.* **2012**, *86*, 6171–6178. [CrossRef] [PubMed]
17. Pfaender, S.; Cavalleri, J.M.V.; Walter, S.; Doerrbecker, J.; Campana, B.; Brown, R.J.P.; Burbelo, P.D.; Postel, A.; Hahn, K.; Anggakusuma, R.N.; et al. Clinical course of infection and viral tissue tropism of hepatitis C virus-like nonprimate hepaciviruses in horses. *Hepatology (Baltimore, Md.)* **2015**, *61*, 447–459. [CrossRef]
18. Waddell, P.J.; Steel, M.A. General time-reversible distances with unequal rates across sites, Mixing gamma and inverse Gaussian distributions with invariant sites. *Mol. Phylogenetics Evol.* **1997**, *8*, 398–414. [CrossRef]
19. Felsenstein, J. Evolutionary trees from DNA sequences, A maximum likelihood approach. *J. Mol. Evol.* **1981**, *17*, 368–376. [CrossRef]
20. Kumar, S.; Stecher, G.; Li, M.; Knyaz, C.; Tamura, K. MEGA X, Molecular Evolutionary Genetics Analysis across Computing Platforms. *Mol. Biol. Evol.* **2018**, *35*, 1547–1549. [CrossRef]
21. Stang, A.; Korn, K.; Wildner, O.; Uberla, K. Characterization of virus isolates by particle-associated nucleic acid PCR. *J. Clin. Microbiol.* **2005**, *43*, 716–720. [CrossRef]
22. Postel, A.; Cavalleri, J.-M.V.; Pfaender, S.; Walter, S.; Steinmann, E.; Fischer, N.; Feige, K.; Haas, L.; Becher, P. Frequent presence of hepaci and pegiviruses in commercial equine serum pools. *Vet. Microbiol.* **2016**, *182*, 8–14. [CrossRef] [PubMed]

viruses

MDPI

Communication

Methylation Status of the Adeno-Associated Virus Type 2 (AAV2)

Renáta Tóth [1,2], István Mészáros [1], Daniela Hüser [3], Barbara Forró [1], Szilvia Marton [1], Ferenc Olasz [1], Krisztián Bányai [1], Regine Heilbronn [3] and Zoltán Zádori [1,*]

1 Institute for Veterinary Medical Research, Centre for Agricultural Research, Hungarian Academy of Sciences, Hungária krt. 21, H-1143 Budapest, Hungary; toth.renata13@gmail.com (R.T.); meszaros.istvan@agrar.mta.hu (I.M.); barbara.forro@gmail.com (B.F.); marton.szilvia@agrar.mta.hu (S.M.); olasz.ferenc@agrar.mta.hu (F.O.); banyai.krisztian@agrar.mta.hu (K.B.)

2 Hungarian National Blood Transfusion Service, Laboratory of Transplantation Immunogenetics, Karolina út 19-21, H-1113 Budapest, Hungary

3 Institute of Virology, Campus Benjamin Franklin, Charité Medical School, Hindenburgdamm 27, 12203 Berlin, Germany; daniela.hueser@charite.de (D.H.); regine.heilbronn@charite.de (R.H.)

* Correspondence: zadori.zoltan@agrar.mta.hu

Received: 10 December 2018; Accepted: 4 January 2019; Published: 9 January 2019

Abstract: To analyze the methylation status of wild-type adeno-associated virus type 2 (AAV2), bisulfite PCR sequencing (BPS) of the packaged viral genome and its integrated form was performed and 262 of the total 266 CG dinucleotides (CpG) were mapped. In virion-packaged DNA, the ratio of the methylated cytosines ranged between 0–1.7%. In contrast, the chromosomally integrated AAV2 genome was hypermethylated with an average of 76% methylation per CpG site. The methylation level showed local minimums around the four known AAV2 promoters. To study the effect of methylation on viral rescue and replication, the replication initiation capability of CpG methylated and non-CpG methylated AAV DNA was compared. The in vitro hypermethylation of the viral genome does not inhibit its rescue and replication from a plasmid transfected into cells. This insensitivity of the viral replicative machinery to methylation may permit the rescue of the integrated heavily methylated AAV genome from the host's chromosomes.

Keywords: AAV2; adeno-associated virus; bisulfite PCR; CpG methylation; DNA virus; Parvoviridae

---

The *Parvoviridae* family consists of small, single-stranded DNA viruses with 4–6 kb linear genomes. It is a very diverse virus family with the capability to infect a wide range of hosts from insects to mammals [1]. Adeno-associated dependoparvoviruses (AAVs) are separated from other parvoviruses by their CpG island-like genome structure with high GC content (>50%) and high observed/expected CpG ratio (>70%) [2]. AAVs are also distinguished from other parvoviruses by their different reproductive strategy, because they require the presence of an unrelated helper DNA virus for successful reproduction. In the absence of a helper virus, they can establish a latent infection by preferentially integrating into the open chromatin structures of the host's genome or remaining latent as nuclear episomes [3,4].

AAVs are among the most frequently used gene therapy vectors, because they can infect many tissues in the human body without known adverse effects [5]. During the first months, recombinant AAV-mediated gene transfer results in a peak of transgene expression, but later this level decreases and reaches a reduced steady-state level [6,7]. Since CpG methylation can inhibit transcription [8], the methylation pattern of the promoter and vector in episomal adeno-associated dependoparvovirus A (AAV2)-based gene therapy constructs have been examined, but no significant CpG methylation has been found [9]. The methylation status of the replicative and the integrated form of the wild-type AAV2 remained unknown.

We previously determined that the genome of Ungulate protoparvovirus 1 (PPV) remains hypomethylated during the entire viral life cycle independent of its tissue of origin, and in vitro CpG methylation has no significant effect on viral replication [2]. The different reproductive strategy and the strikingly different genome composition of the AAV2 (AAV has 266 CpG sites, 54% GC content and 0.78 observed/expected CpG ratio (oCpGr) value compared to the 60 CpG sites, 38% GC content and 0.33 oCpGr of the PPV) suggested that CpG methylation may have a more significant role in the life cycle of the AAV2 than in the life cycle of the PPV. Therefore, we sought to investigate the methylation status of wild-type AAV2 genome during the different stages of the viral life cycle including the packaged viral DNA and the integrated and excisable form of the genome.

AAV2 virions were produced as previously described [10] by co-transfecting pTAV2-0 [11] and pDG [12] into HEK-293 cells. Freeze-thaw lysates were treated with benzonase (Merck, Darmstadt, Germany) to degrade non-encapsidated DNA, and AAV genomes were purified using proteinase K (Carl Roth, Karlsruhe, Germany) and phenol/chloroform extraction. The integrated viral genome was purified from latently infected Detroit 6 cells [13] using lysis buffer (1% N-lauroylsarcosine, 25 mM Tris-Cl pH 8.5, 10 mM EDTA pH 8.0) and proteinase K treatment followed by repeated phenol/chloroform extractions and ethanol precipitation.

To detect and separate the integrated form of the genome from spontaneously released AAV genomes, total Detroit 6 cell DNA was run on an agarose gel. Despite the typical low molecular weight AAV bands of 4.7 replicative form 1 (RF1) or 9.4 kb (RF2) were not being detected the high molecular weight chromosomal DNA was isolated by the Zymoclean Gel DNA Recovery Kit (Zymo Research, Irvine, CA, USA), as recommended by the manufacturer.

The methylation pattern of the AAV genomes derived from total Detroit 6 cell DNA, from the isolated high molecular weight DNA, and from the packaged viral DNA was determined by bisulfite PCR. The bisulfite treatment of the encapsidated, single-stranded DNA was performed with the EpiTect Bisulfite Kit (Qiagen, Venlo, The Netherlands) according to the manufacturer's instructions. Treatment of the genomic DNA was optimized by adding an extra denaturation step (95 °C, 5 min) followed by incubation at 60 °C for 2 h. The conversion efficiency of the unmethylated cytosines was verified by Sanger sequencing of several PCR fragments from the 27 CpG sites containing fragment AAV11 (Table 1). Sanger sequencing was performed with the BigDye Terminator v3.1 Cycle Sequencing Kit (Applied Biosystems, Foster City, CA, USA), according to the manufacturer's recommendations.

For the amplification of the modified CpG-containing DNA fragments, 22 PCR primer pairs were designed using the MethPrimer program [14] (Table 1). The 22 PCR fragments covered all CpGs of the AAV genome except the first and the last two sites (262 out of 266). DNA amplifications of most of the fragments were carried out by an initial denaturation for 5 min at 95 °C, followed by 35 cycles at 95 °C for 20 s, 52 °C for 20 s, and 72 °C for 20 s by using DreamTaq DNA Polymerase (Thermo Fisher Scientific, Waltham, MA, USA). For certain PCR fragments, the thermal conditions were altered. The temperature of the elongation step was changed to 58 °C at the 6th, 10th, 14th, 18th, 21st and 22nd fragments (Table 1), while the elongation occurred at 60 °C in the case of the 2nd and 20th fragments. The amplified fragments were purified from 1.2% agarose gel using the Zymoclean Gel DNA Recovery Kit. Finally, the PCR fragments were pooled in equal amounts and were sequenced with an Ion Torrent PGM sequencer. The CLC Genomics Workbench 7.0.4 was used for data analysis. The average read length was 213 nucleotides and 262 (of the total 266) CpG sites were mapped. The read depth of the 262 CpG sites of the virion-packaged DNA, the AAV genome from the total DNA and the AAV genome from the isolated chromosomal DNA were between 112 and 12603, 49 and 4335, and 71 and 4953, respectively.

Table 1. Primers used for bisulfite PCR.

Primer Name	Sequence	Product Size (bp)	CpGs in Product
AAV1F AAV1R	5′-TTGGTTATTTTTTTTTTGCGCGTT-3′ 5′-CCTCTAATACAAAACCTCCCTA-3′	205	19
AAV2F AAV2R	5′-GGGTTAGGGAGGTTTTGTATT-3′ 5′-ATTCAAATCCATATCAAAATCTAAC-3′	279	17
AAV3F AAV3R	5′-ATTTTGATATGGATTTGAATTTGATT-3′ 5′-AAAATATAACACTCATCCACCACCT-3′	343	23
AAV4F AAV4R	5′-AGGGAGAGAGTTATTTTTATATGTA-3′ 5′-TCTAATTCTCTTTATTCTACTCCTAC-3′	372	25
AAV5F AAV5R	5′-AAGGTGGTGGATGAGTGTTATATTT-3′ 5′-AACCTAATCCTCCTAAATCCACTACTT-3′	309	15
AAV6F AAV6R	5′-GGAGAAGTAGTGGATTTAGGAGGAT-3′ 5′-AATTACAAACCCAAACAACCAAATA-3′	298	14
AAV7F AAV7R	5′-GGAAAGATTATGAGTTTGATTAAAAT-3′ 5′-AAAAAATTCTCATTAATCCAATTTAC-3′	284	15
AAV8F AAV8R	5′-AATTGGATTAATGAGAATTTTTTTT-3′ 5′-AATAACCTTCCCAAAATCATAATCC-3′	315	21
AAV9F AAV9R	5′-TGATTTTGGGAAGGTTATTAAGTAG-3′ 5′-ACAAAAAAACAACATCAAATTCATAC-3′	274	17
AAV10F AAV10R	5′-TGATGTTGTTTTTTTGTAGATAATG-3′ 5′-TAAACCAAATTTAAACTTCCACCAC-3′	345	10
AAV11F AAV11R	5′-TGGTGGAAGTTTAAATTTGGTTTAT-3′ 5′-AAAAATTCAAAAACCCTCTTTTTC-3′	323	27
AAV12F AAV12R	5′-AAAAAGAGGGTTTTTGAATTTTTG-3′ 5′-TTCAATCTTTTTCTTACAAACTACTAACC-3′	152	6
AAV13F AAV13R	5′-TTTGGTTGAGGAATTTGTTAAGA-3′ 5′-TTATAAATAAACAAAACCCAAATTC-3′	369	18
AAV14F AAV14R	5′-GTTTTTTTTGGTTTGGGAATTAATA-3′ 5′-AAATCTATTAAAATCAAAATACCCCC-3′	282	12
AAV15F AAV15R	5′-TTGGGTTTTGTTTATTTATAATAATTATTT-3′ 5′-AATATTAAAAAACTTAAAATTAAATCTCTT-3′	217	4
AAV16F AAV16R	5′-AGATTTATTAATAATAATTGGGGATTT-3′ 5′-TACTCCAAACAATAAAATAAAAAAC-3′	299	18
AAV17F AAV17R	5′-AGTATGGATATTTTATTTTGAATAA-3′ 5′-AAAAACCAATTCCTAAACTAATCCC-3′	316	12
AAV18F AAV18R	5′-AGTTAAGGTTTTAGTTTTTTTAGGT-3′ 5′-AAATTAATTATCCTAATTTCCTCTTC-3′	340	12
AAV19F AAV19R	5′-AATGGTAGAGATTTTTTGGTGAATT-3′ 5′-AACCCCTAAAAATACACATCTCTATC-3′	317	9
AAV20F AAV20R	5′-AGGTATGGTTTGGTAGGATAGAGAT-3′ 5′-ATCCACAATAAAATCCACATTAACAA-3′	340	12
AAV21F AAV21R	5′-AGTGGGAGTTGTAGAAGGAAAATAGTA-3′ 5′-TAACCAACTCCATCACTAAAAATTC-3′	312	10
AAV22F AAV22R	5′-GTTTGTTAATGTGGATTTTATTGTGGAT-3′ 5′-TAACCACTCCCTCTCTACGCGCT-3′	360	22

In virion-packaged DNA, the ratio of the methylated cytosines was between 0–1.7% with an average of 0.6% methylation/CpG sites. In contrast, despite the CpG island-like genome structure, the integrated AAV2 genome was found to be hypermethylated, and the methylation ratio of the

CpG sites varied between 20.4% and 98.3% with an average of 76% methylation per site (Figure 1a). Sequencing of the isolated high molecular weight DNA yielded very similar results: the methylation of the CpG cytosines was between 21% and 98.8% with an average of 78.2% methylation per site (Figure 1b). Minimal differences (0.003–12.3%) were detected in the methylation status of CpGs determined from total cellular DNA or isolated chromosomal DNA, confirming that the overwhelming majority of the detected methylation pattern derived from integrated copies and not from episomal forms.

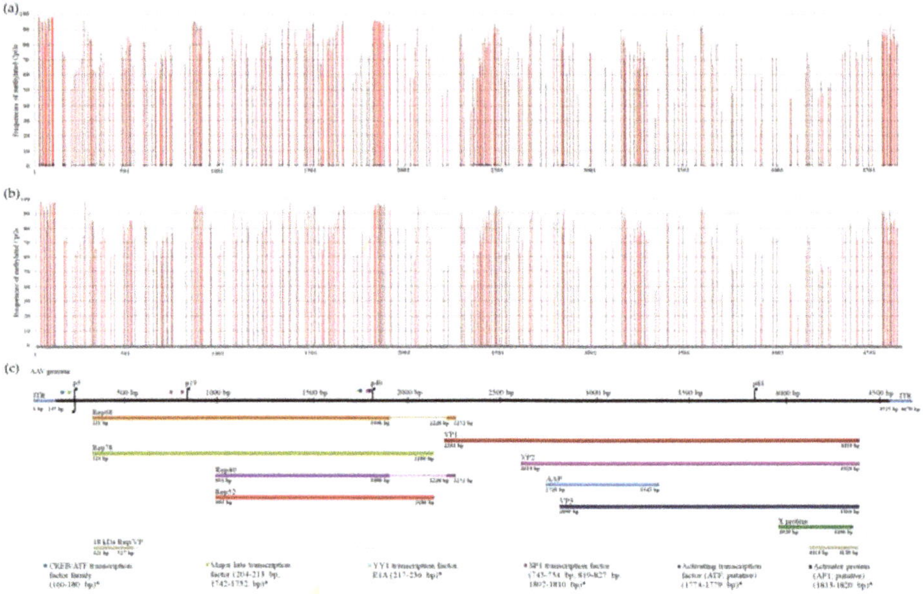

Figure 1. Deep sequencing of the bisulfite treated adeno-associated virus type 2 (AAV2) genomes. Vertical bars label the position of the CpGs in the AAV2 genomes in the diagrams: (**a**) Methylation values of the packaged AAV2 genome and the integrated AAV2 genome from total Detroit 6 DNA are represented by blue and red bars, respectively; (**b**) methylation values of the integrated AAV2 genome from purified chromosomal DNA; (**c**) the AAV2 genome and its transcription–translation map [15–17] is presented in scale showing the CpG-containing binding sites of transcription factors as well. The methylation-sensitive transcription factors are labelled by an asterisk.

The methylation level showed local minimums around the four promoters (p5, p19, p40 and p81) and the least methylated CpG sites were found in the X protein-coding ORF (Figure 1b,c). It is tempting to speculate that the lower level of methylation of these CpG sites might play a functional role in the reactivation of the promoters.

Our results indicate that the packaged and replicating AAV DNA is hypomethylated, as has been shown for other parvoviruses (PPV, B19) [2,18] and small- or medium-sized DNA viruses (e.g., papillomaviruses, adenoviruses) [19]. Hypomethylation is a characteristic feature of the replicating of small DNA viruses, despite the fact that unmethylated CpGs may provide an access of the host immune system to immunostimulatory, unmethylated CpGs during in vivo replication and cell lysis. It is likely that hypomethylation is the result of rapid replication, compartmentalization or active exclusion of the DNA methylases by the viral proteins from the replicating DNA [19].

Although the hypermethylation of the latently integrated AAV genome is not fully unexpected, it is somewhat surprising. Some of the earlier observations indeed implied methylation. Usually, newly integrated replication-incompetent viral fragments inserted into the host genome become rapidly methylated. Complete and replication-competent retrovirus sequences are also recognized by the host defense system (e.g., Daxx protein) and integrated proviruses are rapidly silenced by antiviral epigenetic responses including histone modification and DNA methylation [20].

On the other hand, the AAV2 genome was reported to integrate into transcriptionally active open chromatin regions and in CpG islands [4,21] and it can be released from latently infected Detroit 6 cells by helper virus infection [13]. Furthermore, the AAV genome has a CpG island-like genome composition that in the host genome most frequently remains unmethylated, and its methylation silences gene expression [22,23]. Thus, these data may suggest that the unique CpG island-like structure of the AAV genome evolved to avoid methylation and keep the open chromatin structure of the integrated genome to ensure easy access for transcription factors to viral promoters. However, our findings challenge this hypothesis.

For replication initiation, Rep proteins are needed to release the integrated AAV DNA from the host genome [24–28]. DNA hypermethylation is usually associated with transcriptional repression. Accordingly, the crucial question is how the RNAs of the viral Rep proteins are transcribed from the methylated integrated copies to supply the required proteins, especially because several methylation-sensitive transcription sites are localized in, or in close proximity of, the AAV promoters (Figure 1).

To further analyze how methylation influences viral rescue, we compared the replication initiation capability of CpG methylated and non-CpG methylated AAV DNA. The pTAV2-0 plasmid produced in bacteria supplied the non-CpG methylated genome (although it contained bacterial DAM and DCM methylation). For the production of CpG methylated AAV DNA, the pTAV2-0 plasmid was linearized by FastDigest *Eco*RV restriction enzyme (Thermo Fisher Scientific, Waltham, MA, USA) and in vitro methylated using the CpG methylase kit (Zymo Research, Irvine, CA, USA). The reaction mix included 2 μg DNA, 4 μL of 10× CpG Reaction Buffer, 6 μL of 20× SAM (12 mM), 2 μL of 4 U/μL CpG Methylase (M.SssI)) and distilled water to a final volume of 40 μL, and was incubated overnight at 30 °C.

The efficiency of hypermethylation was estimated to be more than 90% by the ImageJ program [29] after comparing the intensity of the linearized methylated undigested and the methylation-sensitive SsiI-enzyme digested (Thermo Fisher Scientific, Waltham, MA, USA), vector bands (Figure 2a, lanes 5 and 2 respectively).

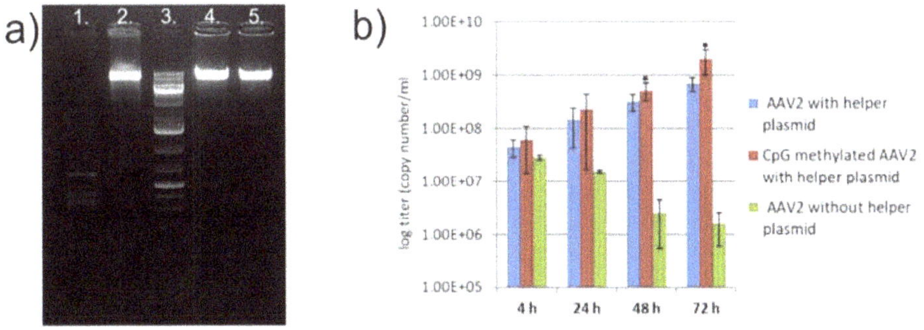

Figure 2. Replication initiated by differently methylated AAV DNAs: (**a**) digestion of the differently methylated pTAV2-0 DNAs. Lane 1, CpG unmethylated *Eco*RV linearized vector digested with SsiI (cutting at 57 sites); lane 2, CpG methylated *Eco*RV linearized vector digested with SsiI; lane 3, GeneRuler 1 kb Plus DNA Ladder; lane 4, CpG unmethylated *Eco*RV linearized vector; lane 5, CpG methylated *Eco*RV linearized vector; (**b**) copy numbers of the viral genome in the supernatant of cells transfected by differently methylated AAV2 plasmids. Vertical bars indicate twice the standard deviation in each case.

Linearized methylated and unmethylated plasmids were transfected together with pHelper plasmid [30] in equal amounts (0.5 μg each) into HEK-293 cells by TurboFect reagent (Thermo Fisher Scientific, Waltham, MA, USA) in triplicate according to the supplier's recommendations. Transfection of the unmethylated plasmid without pHelper was carried out as a negative control, also in triplicate. At 4, 24, 48 and 72 h post-transfection, the viral DNA was extracted from 200 μL tissue supernatant by the High Pure Viral Nucleic Acid Kit (Roche, Basel, Switzerland) according to the manufacturer's recommendations. The titer of progeny viruses was compared by qPCR from three independent transfection experiments. The PCR conditions were the following: initial denaturation for 5 min at 95 °C, followed by 30 cycles at 95 °C for 20 s, 64 °C for 20 s, and 72 °C for 20 s using DreamTaq DNA Polymerase, EvaGreen (Biotium, Fremont, CA, USA) DNA binding dye and a primer set (forward: 5′-TGC GTA AAC TGG ACC AAT GAG AAC-3′; reverse: 5′-TGT TGG TGT TGG AGG TGA CGA TCA-3′). The Mann–Whitney U test was applied for the statistical analysis of the data.

The result indicates that in vitro CpG hypermethylation of the viral genome does not inhibit its rescue from a plasmid. It also minimizes the possibility that helper rescue of integrated AAVs could be the result of the activation of incidentally existing un-methylated episomes [31,32] in these cells rather than the rescue of the integrated methylated genome. Hypermethylation has even a biologically minor but statistically significant positive effect (Figure 2b) on the output virus titers at 48 h and 72 h ($p = 0.00058$ and $p = 0.00018$).

Recently, it was found that AAV2 latency is mediated by rapid heterochromatin formation by the heterochromatin hallmark trimethylated histone 3 lysine 9 (H3K9me3) and the chromatin regulating KAP1 protein [33]. In addition to H3K9me3, the CpG hypermethylation of the DNA is one of the most characteristic features of the heterochromatin [34]. Accordingly, our data—that the integrated AAV2 is hypermethylated in Detroit 6 cells—give additional support to the heterochromatinization of the latent AAV2 genome.

Despite being hypermethylated, AAV2 is rescuable from Detroit 6 cells. We demonstrated that AAV indeed can be rescued even from in vitro hypermethylated plasmid DNA. Yet, the question can be raised of whether the results obtained from "naked plasmids" can be extrapolated to the chromatinized AAV genome [35]. However, transfected plasmid DNA, just like the nonintegrated wild-type AAV genome, is rapidly associated with histones and chromatinized [36], which makes it highly probable that similar mechanisms permit the rescue of the heavily methylated integrated AAV genome from transfected plasmids or from the host's chromosomes.

It is widely accepted that the binding of YY1 and MLTF to p5 is a key factor in the establishment and maintenance of latency [37,38]. However, the binding of these transcription factors to DNA is methylation-sensitive [39,40] and the effect of methylation to p5 binding was not considered in the original studies in the early 1990s. A recent publication of the epigenetic regulation of AAV latency [37] and our present data may warrant the reinvestigation of the role of these transcription factors in the maintenance of the latency of the methylated genome.

A voluminous literature demonstrates that the CpG methylation of the promoter regions is strongly associated with transcriptional repression, and DNA methylation is dominant over other epigenetic mechanisms for regulating gene expression. However, it is still unclear whether the changes in DNA methylation are the cause or the consequence of the altered gene expression [41,42]. Further studies of the methylated AAV genome release from latency can provide additional valuable data about the relationship between CpG methylation and the dynamics of the chromatin structure.

Funding: This research received no external funding.

Acknowledgments: This work was supported by NKFI K108607 and NKFI K119381.

Conflicts of Interest: The authors declare no conflict of interest.

References

1. Tattersall, P. The Evolution of Parvovirus Taxonomy. In *Parvoviruses*; Kerr, J.R., Cotmore, S.F., Bloom, M.E., Linden, R.M., Parrish, C.R., Eds.; Hodder Arnold: London, UK, 2006.
2. Tóth, R.; Mészáros, I.; Stefancsik, R.; Bartha, D.; Bálint, Á.; Zádori, Z. CpG distribution and methylation pattern in porcine parvovirus. *PLoS ONE* **2013**, *8*, e85986. [CrossRef]
3. Carter, B.J. Adeno-Associated Virus Helper Functions. In *Handbook of Parvoviruses*; Tijssen, P., Ed.; CRC-Press: Boca Raton, FL, USA, 1989.
4. Hüser, D.; Gogol-Döring, A.; Lutter, T.; Weger, S.; Winter, K.; Hammer, E.M.; Cathomen, T.; Reinert, K.; Heilbronn, R. Integration preferences of wildtype AAV-2 for consensus rep-binding sites at numerous loci in the human genome. *PLoS Pathog.* **2010**, *6*, e1000985. [CrossRef]
5. Rabinowitz, J.E.; Samulski, J. Adeno-associated virus expression systems for gene transfer. *Curr. Opin. Biotechnol.* **1998**, *9*, 470–475. [CrossRef]
6. Favre, D.; Blouin, V.; Provost, N.; Spisek, R.; Porrot, F.; Bohl, D.; Marme, F.; Cherel, Y.; Salvetti, A.; Hurtrel, B.; et al. Lack of an Immune Response against the Tetracycline-Dependent Transactivator Correlates with Long-Term Doxycycline-Regulated Transgene Expression in Nonhuman Primates after Intramuscular Injection of Recombinant Adeno-Associated Virus. *J. Virol.* **2002**, *76*, 11605–11611. [CrossRef]
7. Rivera, V.M.; Gao, G.P.; Grant, R.L.; Schnell, M.A.; Zoltick, P.W.; Rozamus, L.W.; Clackson, T.; Wilson, J.M. Long-term pharmacologically regulated expression of erythropoietin in primates following AAV-mediated gene transfer. *Blood* **2005**, *105*, 1424–1430. [CrossRef]
8. Attwood, J.T.; Yung, R.L.; Richardson, B.C. DNA methylation and the regulation of gene transcription. *Cell. Mol. Life Sci.* **2002**, *59*, 241–257. [CrossRef]
9. Léger, A.; Guiner, C.; Nickerson, M.L.; Im, K.; Ferry, N.; Moullier, P.; Snyder, R.O.; Penaud-Budloo, M. Adeno-associated viral vector-mediated transgene expression is independent of dna methylation in primate liver and skeletal muscle. *PLoS ONE* **2011**, *6*, e20881. [CrossRef]
10. Hüser, D.; Weger, S.; Heilbronn, R. Kinetics and frequency of adeno-associated virus site-specific integration into human chromosome 19 monitored by quantitative real-time PCR. *J. Virol.* **2002**, *76*, 7554–7559. [CrossRef]
11. Heilbronn, R.; Bürkle, A.; Stephan, S.; zur Hausen, H. The adeno-associated virus rep gene suppresses herpes simplex virus-induced DNA amplification. *J. Virol.* **1990**, *64*, 3012–3018.
12. Grimm, D.; Kern, A.; Rittner, K.; Kleinschmidt, J.A. Novel Tools for Production and Purification of Recombinant Adenoassociated Virus Vectors. *Hum. Gene Ther.* **1998**, *9*, 2745–2760. [CrossRef]
13. Berns, K.I.; Pinkerton, T.C.; Thomas, G.F.; Hoggan, M.D. Detection of adeno-associated virus (AAV)-specific nucleotide sequences in DNA isolated from latently infected Detroit 6 cells. *Virology* **1975**, *68*, 556–560. [CrossRef]
14. Li, L.C.; Dahiya, R. MethPrimer: Designing primers for methylation PCRs. *Bioinformatics* **2002**, *11*, 1427–1431. [CrossRef]
15. Ruffing, M.; Heid, H.; Kleinschmidt, J.A. Mutations in the carboxy terminus of adeno-associated virus 2 capsid proteins affect viral infectivity: Lack of an RGD integrin-binding motif. *J. Gen. Virol.* **1994**, *75*, 3385–3392. [CrossRef]
16. Cao, M.; You, H.; Hermonat, P.L. The X gene of Adeno-Associated Virus 2 (AAV2) is involved in viral DNA replication. *PLoS ONE* **2014**, *9*, e104596. [CrossRef]
17. Stutika, C.; Gogol-Döring, A.; Botschen, L.; Mietzsch, M.; Weger, S.; Feldkamp, M.; Chen, W.; Heilbronn, R. A Comprehensive RNA Sequencing Analysis of the Adeno-Associated Virus (AAV) Type 2 Transcriptome Reveals Novel AAV Transcripts, Splice Variants, and Derived Proteins. *J. Virol.* **2016**, *90*, 1278–1289. [CrossRef]
18. Bonvicini, F.; Manaresi, E.; Di Furio, F.; de Falco, L.; Gallinella, G. Parvovirus B19 DNA CpG dinucleotide methylation and epigenetic regulation of viral expression. *PLoS ONE* **2012**, *7*, e33316. [CrossRef]
19. Hoelzer, K.; Shackelton, L.A.; Parrish, C.R. Presence and role of cytosine methylation in DNA viruses of animals. *Nucleic Acids Res.* **2008**, *9*, 2825–2837. [CrossRef]
20. Shalginskikh, N.; Poleshko, A.; Skalka, A.M.; Katz, R.A. Retroviral DNA Methylation and Epigenetic Repression Are Mediated by the Antiviral Host Protein Daxx. *J. Virol.* **2013**, *87*, 2137–2150. [CrossRef]

21. Hüser, D.; Gogol-Doring, A.; Chen, W.; Heilbronn, R. Adeno-Associated Virus Type 2 Wild-Type and Vector-Mediated Genomic Integration Profiles of Human Diploid Fibroblasts Analyzed by Third-Generation PacBio DNA Sequencing. *J. Virol.* **2014**, *88*, 11253–11263. [CrossRef]
22. Deaton, A.M.; Bird, A. CpG islands and the regulation of transcription. *Genes Dev.* **2011**, *25*, 1010–1022. [CrossRef]
23. Jones, P.A. Functions of DNA methylation: Islands, start sites, gene bodies and beyond. *Nat. Rev. Genet.* **2012**, *13*, 484–492. [CrossRef]
24. Snyder, R.O.; Im, D.S.; Muzyczka, N. Evidence for covalent attachment of the adeno-associated virus (AAV) rep protein to the ends of the AAV genome. *J. Virol.* **1990**, *64*, 6204–6213.
25. Ward, P.; Urcelay, E.; Kotin, R.; Safer, B.; Berns, K.I. Adeno-associated virus DNA replication in vitro: Activation by a maltose binding protein/Rep 68 fusion protein. *J. Virol.* **1994**, *68*, 6029–6037.
26. Urcelay, E.; Ward, P.; Wiener, S.M.; Safer, B.; Kotin, R.M. Asymmetric replication in vitro from a human sequence element is dependent on adeno-associated virus Rep protein. *J. Virol.* **1995**, *69*, 2038–2046.
27. Linden, R.M.; Winocour, E.; Berns, K.I. The recombination signals for adeno-associated virus site-specific integration. *Proc. Natl. Acad. Sci. USA* **1996**, *93*, 7966–7972. [CrossRef]
28. Urabe, M.; Hasumi, Y.; Kume, A.; Surosky, R.T.; Kurtzman, G.J.; Tobita, K.; Ozawa, K. Charged-to-alanine scanning mutagenesis of the N-terminal half of adeno-associated virus type 2 Rep78 protein. *J. Virol.* **1999**, *73*, 2682–2693.
29. Schneider, C.A.; Rasband, W.S.; Eliceiri, K.W. NIH Image to ImageJ: 25 years of image analysis. *Nat. Methods* **2012**, *9*, 671–675. [CrossRef]
30. Xiao, X.; Li, J.; Samulski, R.J. Production of High-Titer Recombinant Adeno-Associated Virus Vectors in the Absence of Helper Adenovirus. *J. Virol.* **1998**, *72*, 2224–2232. [CrossRef]
31. Cheung, A.K.M.; Hoggan, M.D.; Hauswirth, W.W.; Berns, K.I. Integration of the Adeno-Associated Virus Genome into Cellular DNA in Latently Infected Human Detroit 6 Cells. *J. Virol.* **1980**, *33*, 739–748. [CrossRef]
32. Musatov, S.A.; Dudus, L.; Parrish, C.M.; Scully, T.A.; Fisher, K.J. Spontaneous mobilization of integrated recombinant adenoassociated virus in a cell culture model of virus latency. *Virology* **2002**, *294*, 151–169. [CrossRef]
33. Smith-Moore, S.; Neil, S.J.D.; Fraefel, C.; Linden, R.M.; Bollen, M.; Rowe, H.M.; Henckaerts, E. Adeno-associated virus Rep proteins antagonize phosphatase PP1 to counteract KAP1 repression of the latent viral genome. *Proc. Natl. Acad. Sci. USA* **2018**, *115*, E3529–E3538. [CrossRef]
34. Mazzio, E.A.; Soliman, K.F.A. Basic concepts of epigenetics impact of environmental signals on gene expression. *Epigenetics* **2012**, *7*, 119–130. [CrossRef]
35. Penaud-Budloo, M.; Le Guiner, C.; Nowrouzi, A.; Toromanoff, A.; Cherel, Y.; Chenuaud, P.; Schmidt, M.; von Kalle, C.; Rolling, F.; Moullier, P.; et al. Adeno-Associated Virus Vector Genomes Persist as Episomal Chromatin in Primate Muscle. *J. Virol.* **2008**, *16*, 7875–7885. [CrossRef]
36. Reeves, R.; Gorman, C.M.; Howard, B. Minichromosome assembly of non-integrated plasmid DNA transfected into mammalian cells. *Nucleic Acids Res.* **1985**, *13*, 3599–3615. [CrossRef]
37. Chang, L.-S.; Shi, Y.; Shenk, T. Adeno-Associated Virus P5 Promoter Contains an Adenovirus ElA-Inducible Element and a Binding Site for the Major Late Transcription Factor. *J. Virol.* **1989**, *63*, 3479–3488.
38. Shi, Y.; Seto, E.; Chang, L.S.; Shenk, T. Transcriptional repression by YY1, a human GLI-Krüppel-related protein, and relief of repression by adenovirus E1A protein. *Cell* **1991**, *67*, 377–388. [CrossRef]
39. Kim, J.; Kollhoff, A.; Bergmann, A.; Stubbs, L. Methylation-sensitive binding of transcription factor YY1 to an insulator sequence within the paternally expressed imprinted gene, Peg3. *Hum. Mol. Genet.* **2003**, *12*, 233–245. [CrossRef]
40. Molloy, P.L.; Watt, F. DNA methylation and specific protein-DNA interactions. *Philos. Trans. R. Soc. Lond. B Biol. Sci.* **1990**, *326*, 267–275. [CrossRef]

41. Bird, A. DNA methylation patterns and epigenetic memory. *Genes Dev.* **2002**, 6–21. [CrossRef]
42. Medvedeva, Y.A.; Khamis, A.M.; Kulakovskiy, I.V.; Ba-Alawi, W.; Bhuyan, M.S.I.; Kawaji, H.; Lassmann, T.; Harbers, M.; Forrest, A.R.R.; Bajic, V.B. Effects of cytosine methylation on transcription factor binding sites. *BMC Genom.* **2014**, *15*, 119. [CrossRef]

viruses

MDPI

Article

A Comprehensive RNA-seq Analysis of Human Bocavirus 1 Transcripts in Infected Human Airway Epithelium

Wei Zou [1], Min Xiong [2], Xuefeng Deng [1], John F. Engelhardt [3], Ziying Yan [3] and Jianming Qiu [1,*]

[1] Department of Microbiology, Molecular Genetics and Immunology, University of Kansas Medical Center, Kansas City, KS 66160, USA; zouw@umich.edu (W.Z.); Xuefeng.Deng@pennmedicine.upenn.edu (X.D.)
[2] The Children's Mercy Hospital, School of Medicine, University of Missouri Kansas City, Kansas City, MO 64108, USA; xiongminzw@icloud.com
[3] Department of Anatomy and Cell Biology, University of Iowa, Iowa City, IA 52242, USA; john-engelhardt@uiowa.edu (J.F.E.); ziying-yan@uiowa.edu (Z.Y.)
* Correspondence: jqiu@kumc.edu; Tel.: +1-913-588-4329

Received: 11 December 2018; Accepted: 2 January 2019; Published: 7 January 2019

Abstract: Human bocavirus 1 (HBoV1) infects well-differentiated (polarized) human airway epithelium (HAE) cultured at an air-liquid interface (ALI). In the present study, we applied next-generation RNA sequencing to investigate the genome-wide transcription profile of HBoV1, including viral mRNA and small RNA transcripts, in HBoV1-infected HAE cells. We identified novel transcription start and termination sites and confirmed the previously identified splicing events. Importantly, an additional proximal polyadenylation site (pA)p2 and a new distal polyadenylation site (pA)d$_{REH}$ lying on the right-hand hairpin (REH) of the HBoV1 genome were identified in processing viral pre-mRNA. Of note, all viral nonstructural proteins-encoding mRNA transcripts use both the proximal polyadenylation sites [(pA)p1 and (pA)p2] and distal polyadenylation sites [(pA)d1 and (pA)d$_{REH}$] for termination. However, capsid proteins-encoding transcripts only use the distal polyadenylation sites. While the (pA)p1 and (pA)p2 sites were utilized at roughly equal efficiency for proximal polyadenylation of HBoV1 mRNA transcripts, the (pA)d1 site was more preferred for distal polyadenylation. Additionally, small RNA-seq analysis confirmed there is only one viral noncoding RNA (BocaSR) transcribed from nt 5199–5340 of the HBoV1 genome. Thus, our study provides a systematic and unbiased transcription profile, including both mRNA and small RNA transcripts, of HBoV1 in HBoV1-infected HAE-ALI cultures.

Keywords: parvovirus; human bocavirus 1; RNA-seq; transcription profile; human airway epithelia

1. Introduction

Human bocavirus 1 (HBoV1) was identified from nasopharyngeal aspirates of pediatric patients with acute respiratory tract infections in 2005 [1,2]. HBoV1 genome has been frequently detected worldwide after respiratory syncytial virus, rhinovirus, and adenovirus infections in hospitalized young children under 2 or 5 years old with acute respiratory tract infections [3–8]. Severe and deadly cases, which are associated with high viral loads in respiratory specimens and with anti-HBoV1 IgM antibody detection, increased IgG antibody production, or viremia in serum samples, have been apparently linked to acute respiratory tract infections [9–14]. Using RNA-seq to detect the viral RNA genomes and also the viral mRNAs that are transcribed from both RNA and DNA viruses in respiratory secretions, a recent study has identified HBoV1 infections in a significantly greater proportion of patients with community-acquired pneumonia (18.6%) than in controls (2.2%), suggesting that mono-detection of HBoV1 infection is significantly associated with community-acquired pneumonia [15]. In vitro, HBoV1 infects polarized human bronchial airway epithelium (HAE) cultured at an air-liquid interface (ALI; HAE-ALI) and causes damage of the airway epithelium [16–20].

HBoV1 belongs to genus *Bocaparvovirus* of the *Parvoviridae* family. The two prototype members of this genus are minute virus of canines (MVC) and bovine parvovirus type 1 (BPV1) [21,22]. RNA transcription profiles of these three bocaparvoviruses have been well studied through the traditional RNA analysis methods: reverse transcription (RT)-PCR, RNase protection assay (RPA) and Northern blotting [16,21–26]. In HBoV1-infected HAE-ALI, through RT-PCR and RPA, we identified novel splicing donor and acceptor sites (D1′ and A1′) of viral pre-mRNA that are used to process HBoV1 mRNAs encoding novel viral nonstructural proteins NS2, NS3, and NS4 [24]. More importantly, we identified the first parvoviral long noncoding RNA (lncRNA), bocavirus-transcribed small RNA (BocaSR), during HBoV1 infection of HAE-ALI, which plays an important role in virus replication [26]. The identification of these novel HBoV1 RNA transcripts highlights the unique features of HBoV1 transcription among parvoviruses. In order to identify additional HBoV1 transcripts and avoid biases imparted by traditional RNA analysis methods, here, we utilized a systemic and unbiased approach to explore the transcription profile of HBoV1 during infection in human airway epithelia. RNA samples extracted from HBoV1-infected HAE-ALI cultures were analyzed with both mRNA-seq and small RNA-seq.

2. Materials and Methods

2.1. Human Airway Epithelium Cultured at an Air-Liquid Interface (HAE-ALI)

Primary human bronchial airway epithelial cells were isolated from the lungs of healthy donors at the Cell Culture Core of the Center for Gene Therapy, University of Iowa, under a protocol approved by the Institutional Review Board of the University of Iowa (IRB ID No. 9507432). Pseudostratified human airway epithelia as the polarized HAE-ALI cultures were differentiated from the isolated primary cells as previously described [17]. In brief, primary human airway epithelial cells were seeded on collagen-coated, permeable polyester membrane of Costar Transwell® inserts (Cat #3470, Corning, Tewksbury, MA, USA), and then were differentiated (polarized) at an air-liquid interface (ALI) for 3–4 weeks. Ultraser™-G (USG) serum substitute medium (Pall Corporation, Port Washington, NY, USA) was used for the polarization and maintenance of the HAE-ALI. HAE-ALI cultures with a transepithelial electrical resistance (TEER) of >2000 $\Omega\cdot cm^2$, as determined by Millicell ERS-2 Voltohmmeter (EMD Millipore, Burlington, MA, USA), were used for virus infection in this study.

2.2. Virus Infection and Quantification of Apically Released Virions

HBoV1 virions were produced in HEK293 cells transfected with pIHBoV1, a HBoV1 duplex form genome and purified as described previously [17]. HAE-ALI was infected the purified HBoV1 stock at a multiplicity of infection (MOI) of 1000 viral genome copy number (vgc)/cell, as described previously [17]. At 7 days post-infection, an aliquot of 100 µL of phosphate buffered saline (PBS), pH7.4, was added to the apical chamber of the HAE-ALI culture, and harvested as an apical wash. The presence of progeny virions in the apical washes was an indicator of the productive HBoV1 infection in HAE-ALI. All the apical washes were stored at 4 °C for quantification of vgc using a quantitative PCR (qPCR) with HBoV1-specific primers and probe, following the method described previously [17].

2.3. Immunofluorescence Analysis

We fixed a small piece of the insert membrane with 3.7% paraformaldehyde in PBS, and permeabilized with 0.2% Triton X-100 in PBS, followed by direct staining with an anti-HBoV1 NS1C antibody [23]. Immunofluorescence analysis was performed using a method described previously [17]. Confocal images were taken with an Eclipse C1 Plus confocal microscope (Nikon, Tokyo, Japan) controlled by Nikon EZ-C1 software. DAPI (4′,6-diamidino-2-phenylindole) was used to stain the nucleus.

2.4. RNA Extraction

At 7 days post-infection, mock- and HBoV1-infected cells were collected for total RNA isolation using miRNeasy Mini Kit (Qiagen, Valencia, CA, USA) following the manufacturer's instructions with DNase I treatment. HAE cells from two Transwell® inserts were used to prepare one RNA sample. A total of 6 RNA samples from HBoV1-infected HAE-ALI cultures (HBoV1 group) and 6 RNA samples from mock-infected HAE-ALI cultures (Mock group) were prepared. The quality of RNA samples was analyzed on an Agilent 2100 Bioanalyzer using an Agilent RNA 6000 Nano Kit for an RNA Integrity Number (RIN). Three RNA samples with RINs $\geq$ 8.0 were chosen randomly from each group and used for mRNA-seq and small RNA-seq.

2.5. mRNA-seq and Small RNA-seq

mRNA-seq was performed at Otogenetics Corporation (Atlanta, GA, USA). For mRNA-seq, the TruSeq Stranded Total RNA with Ribo-Zero HMR library Prep Kit (#RS-122-2201, Illumina, San Diego, CA, USA) was used to prepare the sequencing library from 1 μg of total RNA, and 2 × 106 bp paired-end sequencing in high output run mode was performed using Illumina HiSeq 2500 system. Small RNA-seq was performed at SeqMatic Company (Fremont, CA, USA). TailorMix miRNA V2 library preparation kit was used to prepare the small RNA library. 2 × 150 bp paired-end sequencing was performed using Illumina MiSeq system (San Diego, CA, USA).

2.6. mRNA-seq Read Mapping and Junction Analysis

The resulting base calling (bcl) files of mRNA-seq were converted to FASTQ files using Illumina's bcl2fastq v2.17.1.14 software (San Diego, CA, USA). TopHat 2.0.9 was used to map mRNA-seq reads against the HBoV1 full-length genome (GenBank accession no: JQ923422) using default parameters. Samtools were used to convert a BAM (.bam) file to a SAM (.sam) file. The HBoV1 mapping reads were extracted using an in-house-developed script. The alignment data were used to build the junction tracks by Integrative Genome View (IGV; http://software.broadinstitute.org/software/igv/home). The junctional events were identified only when a single read splits across two exons.

2.7. Detection of Polyadenylation Sites

We searched the paired-end mRNA-seq reads for polyadenine repeats of a length of 9 (i.e., AAAAAAAAA for R2, and TTTTTTTTT for R1), and then mapped those reads with the polyadenine repeats to the HBoV1 full-length genome by BWA (Burrows-Wheeler Aligner). It is noted that HBoV1 genome contains no polyadenine repeats longer than 8.

2.8. HBoV1 RNA Transcripts Assembling

Three samples FASTQ files were merged together. TopHat 2.0.9 was used to map RNA-seq reads against the HBoV1 full-length genome using default parameters. Based on the previous identified transcripts, splicing junctions and polyadenylation signals in the present study, we listed all possible HBoV1 mRNA transcripts as the reference viral transcript profile. Transcript assembly and abundance estimation were conducted with StringTie software and reported in Fragments Per Kilobase of exon per Million fragments mapped (FPKM).

2.9. Mapping of Small RNA-seq Reads and Transcript Abundance Estimation

The CAP-miRSeq v1.123 pipeline was employed for read pre-processing, alignment, mature/precursor/novel miRNA detection and quantification. In this pipeline, Cutadapt was used to trim reads adaptor at the 3′-end. After adaptor trimming, reads length less than 17 bp were discarded.

Then the reads were mapped to the full-length HBoV1 genome by mapper, identified as known and novel miRNA by miRDeep2, and quantified expression by quantifier. Meanwhile, we used Bowtie 2 to align small RNA-seq reads to HBoV1 genome for identification of all small RNA transcripts. The count of HBoV1 mapping reads was extracted using an in-house-developed script from an alignment file. The alignment data were used to build the coverage tracks by Integrated Genome Browser (IGB; http://igb.bioviz.org/).

3. Results

3.1. Virus Infection

To ensure a high infectivity, HAE-ALI cultures were infected with HBoV1 at an MOI of 1000 vgc/cell. At 7 days post-infection, immunofluorescence analysis revealed that majority HAE cells were infected (Figure 1), and qPCR for HBoV1 genome in the apical washes found that HBoV1 virions released from the apical side of the HAE-ALI culture reached a level of $>1.5 \times 10^{11}$ gc/mL, representing effective HBoV1 infections in HAE-ALI cultures [18]. Total RNA samples for next-generation RNA sequencing were extracted from these highly infected HAE-ALI cultures.

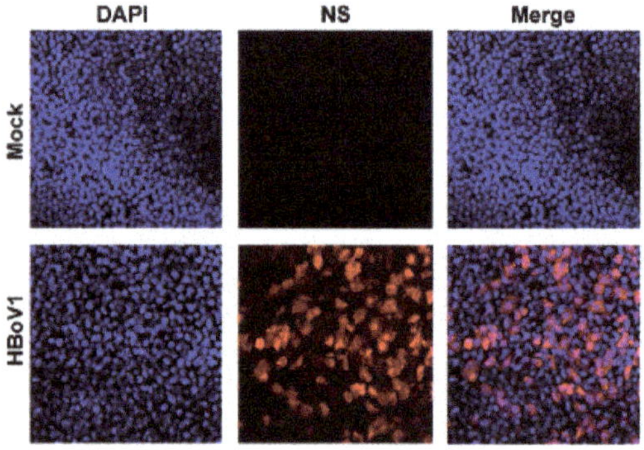

Figure 1. HBoV1 infection of HAE-ALI cells. HAE-ALI cultures were infected with HBoV1 at an MOI of 1000 vgc/cell, or mock-infected. At 7 days post-infection, the pieces of the inserts were fixed and subjected to direct immunofluorescence analysis. The membranes were stained with anti-HBoV1 NS1C antibody that detected all NS1-4 proteins. Images were taken using an Eclipse C1 Plus (Nikon) confocal microscope under 40×, which was controlled by Nikon EZ-C1 software. The nuclei were stained with DAPI (blue).

3.2. Illumina mRNA-seq Next-Generation Sequencing

We chose three total RNA samples isolated from HBoV1- or mock-infected HAE cells that had RIN values of ≥8 for Illumina mRNA-Seq. The complete raw and normalized mRNA-seq data have been deposited in the Gene Expression Omnibus of the National Center for Biotechnology Information (accession no. GSE102392). Reads between 71.8 and 92.3 million were obtained by Illumina RNA-Seq (Table 1). Approximate 75% of total reads were successfully mapped either to the human genome or to the HBoV1 genome. In three repeated RNA samples extracted from mock-infected HAE-ALI, all reads were mapped to the human genome except less than 20 reads that were mapped to the HBoV1 genome. In three repeated HBoV1 RNA samples, 0.21–0.47 million reads (0.23–0.55%) were mapped to the plus strand of the HBoV1 genome. Of note, there were also a few reads (9458–21,580) mapped to the minus strand of the viral genome, indicating the potential transcription capability of the minus strand. However, in this study, we only focused on these reads from the positive strand.

Table 1. Summary of mRNA-seq results.

Groups	Total Reads	No. (%) of Mapped Reads	No. (%) of Human Reads	No. (%) of HBoV1 reads		
				Plus Strand	Minus Strand	Ambiguous
Mock-8	92,255,534	69,845,826 (75.71)	69,845,805 (75.71)	19 (0.00)	2 (0.00)	0 (0.00)
Mock-9	83,459,160	63,548,966 (76.14)	63,548,950 (76.14)	15 (0.00)	1 (0.00)	0 (0.00)
Mock-10	95,389,110	72,602,804 (76.11)	72,602,787 (76.11)	17 (0.00)	0 (0.00)	0 (0.00)
HBoV1-11	86,814,188	64,362,968 (74.14)	63,865,552 (73.57)	474,990 (0.55)	21,580 (0.02)	846 (0.00)
HBoV1-20	90,567,600	68,650,250 (75.80)	68,429,393 (75.56)	208,998 (0.23)	9458 (0.01)	56 (0.00)
HBoV1-21	7,175,830	54,487,120 (75.93)	54,162,045 (75.48)	309,318 (0.43)	12,952 (0.02)	142 (0.00)

3.3. *mRNA-seq Reads Mapping on the HBoV1 Plus Strand*

We analyzed the reads mapped to the plus strand of HBoV1 genome. By sequence alignments, a coverage map of the HBoV1 genome was created, which displays the number of reads that are mapped to a specific position of the HBoV1 genome (Figure 2A). Although there were some variations between the three repeats in terms of total reads, we obtained a similar trend in the read coverages across the biologic replicates. Steep increases of mRNA-seq read counts are indicative of either transcription initiations or splicing events.

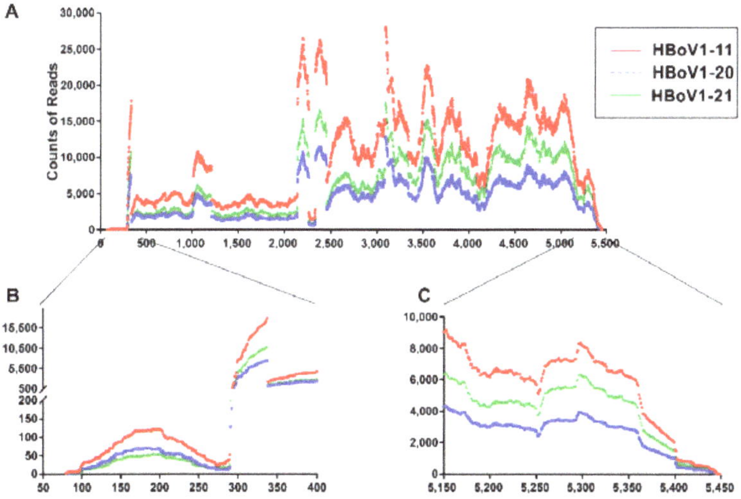

Figure 2. Coverage plots of viral mRNA-seq reads mapped to the HBoV1 genome. Red, blue and green lines represent three RNA samples of HBoV1-infected HAE-ALI cultures. (**A**) Reads mapped to HBoV1 full-length genome. The reads mapped to HBoV1 full-length genome are shown with the coverage across the entire HBoV1 genome (GenBank accession no: JQ923422). (**B** and **C**) Read coverages of the left- and right-hand ends. The read coverages of the left (nt 50–400) (**B**) and right (nt 5150–5450) (**C**) ends of the viral genome are enlarged for details.

From the mRNA-seq reads mapped to the HBoV1 full-length genome, it showed that viral mRNA transcripts initiated as early as nt 80, but at an abundance much lower than reads initiating at nt 291–296 (Figure 2B). These results confirmed transcriptional initiation from P5 promoter at nt 291–296, which was close to the previously determined initiation site at nt 282 [23], and suggest that the left-end hairpin (LEH) contains properties of promoter activity; this property is similar to what has been observed with the inverted terminal repeats (ITRs) of adeno-associated viruses (AAVs) [27,28]. On the right-hand hairpin (REH) end, all the three HBoV1 RNA samples contained viral mRNAs that ended as far as to nt 5499 (Figure 2C), suggesting an alternative distal polyadenylation signal. The results also confirmed the major mRNA transcripts ended at the previously identified polyadenylation site, (pA)d1, at nt 5171 immediately after capsid proteins (VP)-coding sequence [23].

3.4. Analyses of Alternative Splicing of the HBoV1 pre-mRNA

Previously, we and other groups had shown that there were six introns in the single HBoV1 pre-mRNA [16,23,24]. mRNA-seq reads confirmed all the six splice junctions including D1/A1′, D1′/A1, D1/A1, D1/A2, D2/A2, and D3/A3 (Figure 3 and Table 2). The junction reads revealed that the second intron splicing (D2/A2) had the highest frequency, which is consistent with a previous study showing that nearly 75% HBoV1 mRNAs splice out the second intron [23]. There was also a relatively high frequency of junction reads at the D3/A3 sites, splicing of which is required for production of VP-expressing mRNAs. However, the reads at the junctions for D1 to A1′ and D1′ to A1 splicing events were relatively low, indicating the virus only expresses few mRNAs that encode NS2, NS3, and NS4 [24]. Of note, two novel splicing events between sites of nt 337 and nt 1108 and sites of nt 337 and nt 2198 were identified in all three RNA samples of HBoV1 infection. The two novel acceptor sites nt 1108 and nt 2198 are close to the A1′ (nt 1017) and A1 (nt 2140) acceptor sites, respectively. There were also other novel splicing events that were detected in two or one of the samples (Table 2). Although all newly identified splicing events could produce novel HBoV1 transcripts, these spliced mRNAs have unchanged open reading frames (ORFs). Of note, we did not find any splicing events from D1 to A3 sites, which we previously predicted to produce VP-expressing mRNA R8 [23,25], indicating that R6 and R7 VP-expressing mRNAs are the only mRNA transcripts for production of capsid proteins.

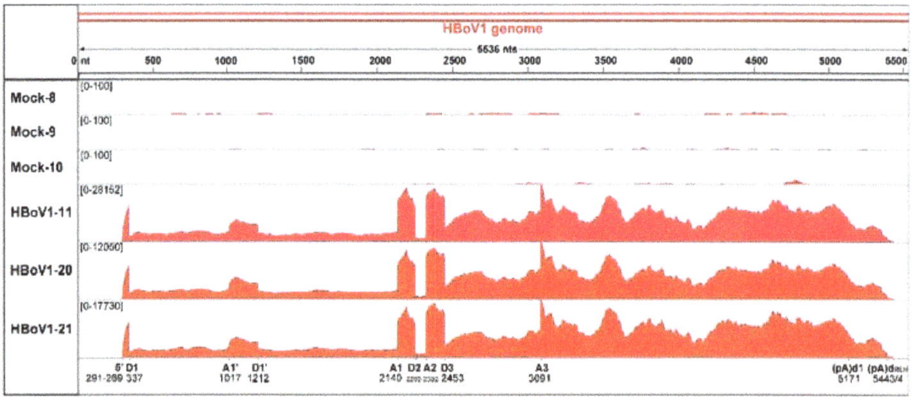

Figure 3. Analysis of alternative splicing of HBoV1 pre-mRNA. The mRNA-seq reads of three HBoV1-infected (HBoV1-11, 20, and 21) and three mock-infected (Mock-8, 9, and 10) RNA samples are mapped to HBoV1 genome. Histograms show the frequency of mRNA reads across the coverage of the HBoV1 genome. The junction events were identified only when at least a single read splits across two exons. The identified splicing junctions are labeled at the bottom with nucleotide numbers shown. The range of reads numbers are shown in each sample. The reads number of all identified splicing events including novel identified splicing and the donor and acceptor sites are shown in Table 2.

3.5. Analyses of Alternative Polyadenylation in the HBoV1 pre-mRNA

HBoV1 pre-mRNA is polyadenylated at (pA)p and distal (pA)d polyadenylation sites, although the mechanism controlling polyadenylation choice remains unclear [23]. There are five consensus polyA signals (CPSF160-binding site AAUAAA) [29] that can be used for polyadenylation at the proximal site, which are located at nt 3295–3300, nt 3329–3334, nt 3409–3414, nt 3440–3445, and nt 3485–3490 [25]. There is only one AAUAAA site located at the end of the genome (nt 5153–5158). By searching polyA sequences [>(A)9] in the mRNA-seq reads and mapping these reads containing a sequence of nine or more A residues to HBoV1 genome, we found that AAUAAA at nt 3329 and the previously identified AAUAAA at nt 3485 were most commonly used for proximal polyadenylations at the (pA)p2 and (pA)p1 sites, respectively (Table 3). While the previous reported distal polyadenylation site (pA)d1 at nt 5171 [23] was confirmed, our analyses also found a novel (pA)d_{REH} at the REH region where HBoV1 mRNA transcripts were cleaved and polyadenylated (Table 3). Of note, instead of adding polyA at a specific nucleotide, the polyadenylation at (pA)d_{REH} occurs in a wide range of 130 nts from nt 5369 to 5499 with hot sites at nt 5443 and 5444 (Figure 3).

Table 2. Detected splicing events in HBoV1 infected HAE cells.

Donor	Acceptor	Splicing Events	Strand	HBoV1-11	HBoV1-20	HBoV1-21	Ratio # (%)
337 §	1016	D1/A1′	+	2349	1081	1334	85.10
337	1060		+	35	0	0	
337	1108		+	327	144	160	14.90
337	1118		+	101	0	67	
337	2139	D1/A1	+	7962	2985	4698	97.82
337	2198		+	158	83	107	2.18
337	2331	D1/A2	+	4734	2084	3124	99.4
337	861		+	30	0	0	0.60
337	998		+	0	0	30	
1212	2139	D1′/A1	+	3818	1462	1814	95.12
1212	2198		+	0	89	111	4.88
1201	2187		+	0	52	112	
1212	2331	D1′/A2	+	95	71	46	14.73
1212	2372		+	414	0	0	
1630	2139		+	644	0	0	85.27
2250	2362		+	169	0	0	
2260	2331	D2/A2	+	14,175	6222	8782	98.86
2423	2576		+	228	107	0	1.14
2453	3090	D3/A3	+	12,973	5794	9006	99.44
3180	3865		+	0	0	156	0.56

§ Nucleotide numbers of the HBoV1 genome. # The ratio was only counted based on single splicing events.

Table 3. Assembled HBoV1 mRNA transcripts and expression level.

Transcripts (Splicing form)	mRNA Polyadenylation Sites			
	(pA)p1	(pA)p2	(pA)d1	(pA)d_{REH}
NS1 (D2A2)	15,342	16,071	10,029	9364
NS70	3686	3883	2440	2303
NS2 (D1′A1/D2A2)	11,700	12,500	6646	6243
NS2 (D1′A1)	5721	6105	3313	3098
NS3 (D1A1′/D2A2)	1938	2061	1155	1101
NS3 (D1A1′)	2102	2227	1268	1190
NS4 (D1A1′/D1′A1/D2A2)	4549	4998	2181	2007
NS4 (D1A1′/D1′A1)	4870	5350	2397	2213
NP1 (D1A1/D2A2)	11,434	12,782	5114	4667
NP1 (D1A2)	11,724	13,269	4971	4580
VP (D1A1/D2A2/D3A3)	NA	NA	26,107	4306
VP (D1A2/D3A3)	NA	NA	29,504	4378

Note: NA, not available.

3.6. Summarized HBoV1 mRNA Transcripts by RNA-seq

Due to the fact that different HBoV1 mRNA transcripts share the same exon sequences, but the alternative usage of the introns and alternative polyadenylation sites, it is hard to assemble de novo HBoV1 mRNA transcripts, based on the mRNA-seq reads. Thus, we used the newly identified (pA)p2 and (pA)d_{REH} and the previously identified mRNA transcripts as templates to assemble HBoV1 mRNA transcripts using the mRNA-seq data. The results showed that almost all NS- and NP1-coding mRNA transcripts used all four polyadenylation sites (pA)p1, (pA)p2, (pA)d1, and (pA)d$_{REH}$; whereas VP-expressing mRNAs only used (pA)d1 and (pA)d$_{REH}$ sites (Figure 4). All NS- and NP1-coding mRNAs showed the same expression levels at the (pA)p sites, (pA)p1 vs (pA)p2, as well as the (pA)d sites, (pA)d1 vs (pA)d$_{REH}$. Of note, they utilize the (pA)p site [(pA)p2 + (pA)p1] 1.5–2.5-fold more frequently than the (pA)d sites [(pA)d1 + (pA)d$_{REH}$] (Table 3 and Figure 4).

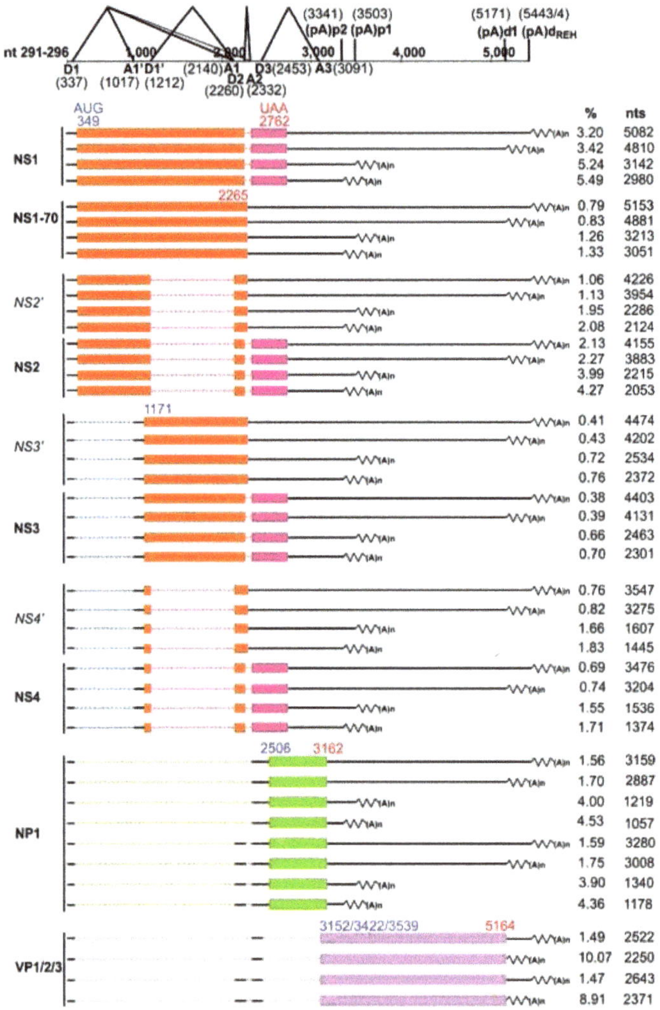

Figure 4. Analyses of all HBoV1 mRNA transcripts based on mRNA-seq data. HBoV1 genome is schematically diagramed with identified donor and acceptor sites, as well as the identified (pA)p1, (pA)p2, (pA)d1 and (pA)d$_{REH}$ polyadenylation sites, used during virus infection. Assembled transcripts of NS1, NS1-70, NS2, NS3, NS4, NP1, and VP using alternative splicing sites and alternative polyadenylation sites [(pA)p1, (pA)p2, (pA)d1 and (pA)d$_{REH}$] are diagramed. Percentage (%) of each transcript in total and the length of each transcript (nt), as determined from the initiation site at nt 291 to the cleavage site (minus the polyA tail), are shown to the right side. Boxes in color indicate ORFs of the exons. Nucleotide numbers of start (AUG; GUG at nt 3422 for VP2) and stop (e.g., UAA) are shown in the first appeared ORF. Introns in the mRNA transcript are diagrammed with dot lines.

NS1-coding transcripts spliced at D2/A2 sites were expressed at the highest level followed by NP1-, NS2- and NS4-coding transcripts in order, while NS1-70 and NS3 mRNAs were expressed at lower levels (Table 3). NS2 transcripts contain mRNA spliced at D1′/A1 and D2/A2 sites and mRNA spliced at D1′/A1 site, and the former mRNA showed an expression level twice more than the second one. NS3 transcripts contained two splicing forms, mRNA spliced at D1/A1′ and D2/A2 sites and mRNA spliced at D1/A1′ sites. NS4 transcripts contained mRNA spliced at D1/A1′, D1′/A1, and D2/A2 sites, and mRNA spliced at D1/A1′ and D1′/A1 sites. NP1 transcripts also had two splicing forms, mRNA spliced at D1/A1 and D2/A2 sites and mRNA spliced at D1/A2 site. The two splicing forms of NS3, NS4 and NP1 transcripts showed the similar expression level. All these NS- and NP1-coding mRNAs were polyadenylated at (pA)d1 and (pA)d$_{REH}$ sites at a similar ratio (Table 3 and Figure 4). VP-coding mRNA transcripts contain two spliced forms, mRNA spliced at D1/A1, D2/A2, and D3/A3 sites, and mRNA spliced at D1/A2 and D3/A3 sites. Importantly, the VP-coding mRNA transcripts polyadenylated at the (pA)d1 site was at a level of approximately 7-fold higher than those polyadenylated at (pA)d$_{REH}$ (Table 3 and Figure 4).

3.7. Small RNA-seq Analysis

The complete raw and identified viral small RNA read counts of small RNA-seq data have been deposited in the Gene Expression Omnibus of the National Center for Biotechnology Information (accession no. GSE GSE123253). Data of the small RNA-seq does not suggest that HBoV1 produce any classical miRNA, however, it revealed a small RNA hot spot located between nt 5199–5340 (Figure 5), which confirmed the expression of BocaSR encoded at nt 5199–5338 [26]. Of note, in addition to the full-length small RNA between 5199–5340, we also identified many smaller RNAs with different lengths located within this region (Table 4). However, we did not detect any of these smaller RNAs by Northern blotting using high percentage of polyacrylamide gels (data not shown), suggesting that these smaller RNAs detected by small RNA-seq might be artifacts of sequencing due to the secondary structure. Taken together, our results confirm that HBoV1 express small RNAs from the 3′ end of the genome at nt 5199–5340, but not from anywhere else of the viral genome.

Table 4. Top 20 identified small RNAs by small RNA-seq.

Start	End	Length	Strand	Sample 1 (Reads)	Sample 2 (Reads)	Sample 3 (Reads)	Total (Reads)
5199	5228	29	+	373	664	277	1314
5317	5340	23	+	316	532	421	1269
5221	5315	94	+	356	284	306	946
5221	5314	93	+	198	326	362	886
5199	5295	96	+	415	235	179	829
5199	5229	30	+	253	395	165	813
5199	5293	94	+	386	202	158	746
5199	5221	22	+	128	297	216	641
5200	5228	28	+	131	184	85	400
5317	5336	19	+	97	151	129	377
5317	5339	22	+	90	168	108	366
5199 #	5339	140	+	37	94	148	279
5221	5317	96	+	135	61	80	276
5199	5294	95	+	109	88	71	268
5317	5341	24	+	63	122	82	267
5199	5290	91	+	111	72	61	244
5199	5227	28	+	76	120	40	236
5221	5313	92	+	45	69	118	232
5199	5338	139	+	21	67	134	222
5199	5340	141	+	34	72	113	219

Numbers in red are indicative of coverages of the entire BocaSR.

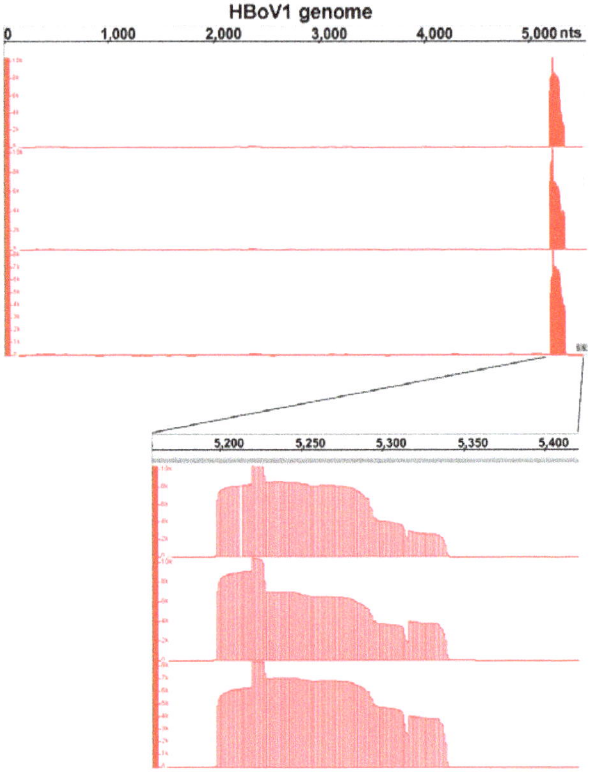

Figure 5. Coverage plots of viral small RNA-seq reads mapped to the HBoV1 genome. The small RNA-seq reads of three HBoV1-infected RNA samples are mapped to HBoV1 genome. Histograms show the frequency of small RNA reads that have the coverage across the HBoV1 genome. The reads coverage of the right ends (nt 5150–5400) of the HBoV1 genome are enlarged for detailed information, show as histograms at the bottom.

4. Discussion

Next generation RNA sequencing technology has been widely used in many aspects of biological research, including virology for the study of gene expression by both the host and virus. This technology is a powerful tool for the systematic and unbiased profiling of viral transcription/expression. Both mRNA-seq and small RNA-seq have been applied to profile gene expression of AAV2 in the presence or absence of coinfection of helper viruses, which identified novel AAV2 mRNA transcripts from both the positive and negative stands of the AAV2 genome, as well as viral miRNAs [30]. In the present study, we utilized mRNA-seq and small RNA-seq of RNA samples isolated from HBoV1-infected HAE-ALI cultures to study the transcription profile of HBoV1. Through this study, we have mapped HBoV1 transcriptional initiation sites, usage of different splicing donor and acceptor sites, and alternative polyadenylation sites. Importantly, the mRNA-seq also provided quantitative information on various HBoV1 mRNA transcripts, which will be useful for understanding HBoV1 transcription regulation from a single promoter.

Transcription start site. We previously identified the HBoV1 P5 promoter starts transcription at nt 282 from total RNA extracted from termini-less HBoV1 plasmid-transfected HEK293 cells [23], which was confirmed by this mRNA-seq. Additionally, our data also showed that a portion of HBoV1 mRNAs are transcribed as early as nt 80, which is located in the LEH region, suggesting the presence of cryptic promoter activity in the LEH. Interestingly, the LEH region of bocavirus BPV1 and the AAV ITRs also have promoter activities [22,27,28]. The reads covering nt 80–282 demonstrated a Poisson distribution (Figure 2). These extended 5′ untranslated regions (UTR) may also contain regulatory functions, though the abundance of these early mRNA transcripts is quite low.

Alternative RNA splicing sites. Pre-mRNA splicing is the key strategy that HBoV1 applies to generate different mRNA transcripts since all HBoV1 transcripts are generated from one pre-mRNA. There are nearly twenty matured mRNAs generated to encode nonstructural proteins (NS1/NS1-70, NS2/NS2′, NS3/NS3′, NS4/NS4′, and NP1) and structural proteins (VP1, VP2, and VP3) (Figure 4). The expression levels of NS2′, NS3′, and NS4′ were too low to be detected by Western-blotting [24]. Two novel donor sites (nt 1201 and nt 2423) and five acceptor sites (nt 1108, nt 1118, nt 2187, nt 2198 and nt 2576) were identified in at least two repeated RNA samples. The novel donor site at nt 1201 is closed to D1′ (nt 1212), and the one at nt 2423 is closed to D3 (nt 2453). Of note, both novel donor sites do not contain the canonical donor sequence of GU. All five novel acceptor sites contain classical AG sequence except the one at nt 2187 site. The acceptors at nt 1108 and nt 1118 are close to the A1′ site (nt 1017), and the ones at nt 2187 and nt 2198 are close to the A1 acceptor at nt 2140. Interestingly, the D1 donor site used three novel acceptor sites at nt 1108, nt 1118 and nt 2198. There are also mRNA transcripts spliced at D1′ donor and the acceptor at nt 2198. The donor at nt 1201 used the acceptor at nt 2187, and the donor at nt 2423 used the acceptor at nt 2576. Nevertheless, all these mRNA transcripts processed at these novel splice sites are predicated not to produce novel proteins as they do not have novel ORFs. We speculate that they may serve as backup mRNA transcripts that will be used in case the original donor or acceptor sites are mutated during virus replication. Therefore, these alternative donor and acceptor sites can still generate mRNA transcripts for production of viral proteins in the events that the viral genome has mutations.

Alternative polyadenylation. Both the NP1 of HBoV1 and MVC regulate proximal polyadenylation to facilitate production of VP-coding mRNAs, which ensures a productive infection [25,31–33]. We identified an additional (pA)p site [(pA)p2] used for proximal polyadenylation, in addition to the previously identified proximal polyadenylation site [called (pA)p1 here] [23], highlighting the complexity of internal polyadenylation regulation by the NP1 protein. The mRNA-seq data showed a ratio of 1.08 that the mRNAs are polyadenylated at the sites (pA)p2 vs (pA)p1, suggesting that HBoV1 mRNA is polyadenylated at the (pA)p2 site with a roughly equal efficiency at the (pA)p1 site, consistent with a previous report [34].

In addition to the previously identified (pA)d site at nt 5171 [(pA)d1], we identified a stretch of distal polyadenylation sites [(pA)d_{REH}] ranging from nt 5369 to nt 5499 with peak sites at nt 5443 and nt 5444, which was located in the REH. The (pA)d_{REH} might be a universal feature of bocaviral mRNA polyadenylation. In fact, bocaparvoviruses MVC and BPV1 utilize only the distal polyadenylation sites located at similar positions on the REH (close to the turn-round or the loop) [21,22]. However, there are no AAUAAA or degenerative polyA signals presented on or close to the HBoV1 REH. We hypothesize that the bocavirus REHs intrinsically contain strong upstream and downstream polyadenylation signals [35], and HBoV1 (pA)d_{REH} contains a non-canonical polyadenylation signal that helps addition of polyA resides at a long stretch of cleaved RNA ends that read through the (pA)d1. The feature that HBoV1 mRNAs utilize two polyadenylation sites at the distal end is unique among all parvoviruses, which warrants further characterization.

It has been reported that HBoV1 mRNAs, which were generated from transfection of a full-length HBoV1 clone in HEK293 cells, were polyadenylated dominantly at the (pA)d_{REH} site at nt 5445 [36]. However, analyses of the mRNA-seq on the RNA samples derived from HBoV1 infection in HAE-ALI suggests that the majority of HBoV1 mRNAs are distally polyadenylated at (pA)d1, with a ratio of the total RNA reads at (pA)d1 vs. (pA)d_{REH} of 2.09. We speculate that viral mRNA transcripts generated from a transfected plasmid are polyadenylated differently from those produced during virus infection.

HBoV1 mRNA transcripts. Identification of novel (pA)p2 and (pA)d_{REH} polyadenylation sites make the HBoV1 mRNA transcripts more diversified. Our previous study identified that NP1 plays an important role in regulating splicing at the A3 acceptor site and facilitates HBoV1 mRNAs to read through the (pA)p sites for production of VP-coding mRNAs [25]. We found that NP1 transcripts used (pA)p1 vs. (pA)p2 and (pA)d1 vs. (pA)d_{REH} equivalently. However, NS1-4 transcripts are preferred to use the proximal polyadenylation sites than the distal polyadenylation sites.

Although the mRNA-seq showed that NS1 transcripts are expressed at the highest level among these NS1-4-coding transcripts, the NS1 protein is expressed at a much lower level than NS2-4 in HBoV1-infected HAE cells [24]. The details of this regulatory mechanism warrant further investigation. It is hard to determine the protein expression levels of NS2 and NS3 in HBoV1- infected HAE cells because of their close molecular weight [24]. The fact that NS2 transcripts are expressed at a much higher level than NS3 transcripts may be associated with the observation that NS2 is indispensable to virus replication in HAE cells, whereas NS3 is dispensable [24].

HBoV1 small RNA transcripts. Recently, we identified a HBoV1 long noncoding RNA (BocaSR) located between nt 5199–5338 [26]. BocaSR regulates the expression of HBoV1-encoded non-structural proteins NS1, NS2, NS3, and NP1, but not NS4. BocaSR accumulates in the viral DNA replication centers within the nucleus and also plays a direct role in replication of the viral DNA [26]. The small RNA-seq further confirmed the expression of BocaSR. Interestingly, except for the BocaSR, we identified many smaller RNAs spanning this region; however, we did not find any canonical secondary structure in these detected smaller RNAs that might be suggestive of biologic function. Currently, we are unsure whether these detected small RNAs are degraded RNAs of BocaSR or artifacts of small RNA-seq.

In conclusion, we used both mRNA-seq and small RNA-seq data to profile RNA transcripts during HBoV1 infection of human airway epithelia. We identified novel polyadenylation sites not previously observed in other studies [34,36]. By using the previously established transcription map of HBoV1 [2], we were able to assemble a *de novo* HBoV1 transcription map. Small RNA seq data suggest that there is likely one viral small RNA transcribed during infection. Thus, our study provides an example to determine a comprehensive and unbiased parvoviral transcription profile using RNA-seq data.

Author Contributions: Conceptualization, Z.Y. and J.Q.; Formal analysis, W.Z. and M.X.; Funding acquisition, J.F.E., Z.Y. and J.Q.; Investigation, W.Z., M.X. and X.D.; Methodology, W.Z. and M.X.; Writing—original draft, W.Z. and J.Q.; Writing—review & editing, W.Z., X.D., J.F.E., Z.Y. and J.Q.

Funding: This study was funded by PHS grant R01 AI070723 (to J.Q.) and R21 R21AI139572 (to J.Q. and Y.Z.) from the National Institute of Allergy and Infectious Diseases and P30 DK054759 (to J.F.E.) from the National Institute of Diabetes and Digestive and Kidney Disease.

Acknowledgments: We would like to thank members in the Qiu lab for technical support and valuable discussions.

Conflicts of Interest: The authors declare no conflict of interest.

References

1. Allander, T.; Jartti, T.; Gupta, S.; Niesters, H.G.; Lehtinen, P.; Osterback, R.; Vuorinen, T.; Waris, M.; Bjerkner, A.; Tiveljung-Lindell, A.; et al. Human bocavirus and acute wheezing in children. *Clin. Infect. Dis.* **2007**, *44*, 904–910. [CrossRef]
2. Qiu, J.; Söderlund-Venermo, M.; Young, N.S. Human parvoviruses. *Clin. Microbiol. Rev.* **2017**, *30*, 43–113. [CrossRef] [PubMed]
3. Lin, F.; Zeng, A.; Yang, N.; Lin, H.; Yang, E.; Wang, S.; Pintel, D.; Qiu, J. Quantification of human bocavirus in lower respiratory tract infections in China. *Infect. Agent Cancer* **2007**, *2*, 3. [CrossRef] [PubMed]
4. Jartti, T.; Hedman, K.; Jartti, L.; Ruuskanen, O.; Allander, T.; Söderlund-Venermo, M. Human bocavirus-the first 5 years. *Rev. Med. Virol.* **2011**, *22*, 46–64. [CrossRef] [PubMed]
5. Don, M.; Söderlund-Venermo, M.; Valent, F.; Lahtinen, A.; Hedman, L.; Canciani, M.; Hedman, K.; Korppi, M. Serologically verified human bocavirus pneumonia in children. *Pediatr. Pulmonol.* **2010**, *45*, 120–126. [CrossRef]
6. Garcia-Garcia, M.L.; Calvo, C.; Falcon, A.; Pozo, F.; Perez-Brena, P.; De Cea, J.M.; Casas, I. Role of emerging respiratory viruses in children with severe acute wheezing. *Pediatr. Pulmonol.* **2010**, *45*, 585–591. [CrossRef]

7. Liu, W.K.; Liu, Q.; Chen, D.H.; Tan, W.P.; Cai, Y.; Qiu, S.Y.; Xu, D.; Li, C.; Li, X.; Lin, Z.S.; et al. Epidemiology of HBoV1 infection and relationship with meteorological conditions in hospitalized pediatric patients with acute respiratory illness: A 7-year study in a subtropical region. *BMC Infect. Dis.* **2018**, *18*, 329–3225. [CrossRef]
8. Praznik, A.; Vinsek, N.; Prodan, A.; Erculj, V.; Pokorn, M.; Mrvic, T.; Paro, D.; Krivec, U.; Strle, F.; Petrovec, M.; et al. Risk factors for bronchiolitis severity: A retrospective review of patients admitted to the university hospital from central region of Slovenia. *Influenza Other Respir Viruses* **2018**, *12*, 765–771. [CrossRef]
9. Ursic, T.; Steyer, A.; Kopriva, S.; Kalan, G.; Krivec, U.; Petrovec, M. Human bocavirus as the cause of a life-threatening infection. *J. Clin. Microbiol.* **2011**, *49*, 1179–1181. [CrossRef]
10. Korner, R.W.; Soderlund-Venermo, M.; van Koningsbruggen-Rietschel, S.; Kaiser, R.; Malecki, M.; Schildgen, O. Severe human bocavirus infection, Germany. *Emerg. Infect. Dis.* **2011**, *17*, 2303–2305. [CrossRef]
11. Edner, N.; Castillo-Rodas, P.; Falk, L.; Hedman, K.; Soderlund-Venermo, M.; Allander, T. Life-threatening respiratory tract disease with human bocavirus-1 infection in a four-year-old child. *J. Clin. Microbiol.* **2011**, *50*, 531–532. [CrossRef] [PubMed]
12. Jula, A.; Waris, M.; Kantola, K.; Peltola, V.; Söderlund-Venerm, M.; Hedman, K.; Ruuskanen, O. Primary and secondary human bocavirus 1 infections in a family, Finland. *Emerg. Infect. Dis.* **2013**, *19*, 1328–1331. [CrossRef] [PubMed]
13. Ursic, T.; Krivec, U.; Kalan, G.; Petrovec, M. Fatal human bocavirus infection in an 18-month-old child with chronic lung disease of prematurity. *Pediatr. Infect. Dis. J.* **2015**, *34*, 111–112. [CrossRef]
14. Eskola, V.; Xu, M.; Soderlund-Venermo, M. Severe Lower Respiratory Tract Infection Caused by Human Bocavirus 1 in an Infant. *Pediatr. Infect. Dis. J.* **2017**, *36*, 1107–1108. [CrossRef] [PubMed]
15. Schlaberg, R.; Queen, K.; Simmon, K.; Tardif, K.; Stockmann, C.; Flygare, S.; Kennedy, B.; Voelkerding, K.; Bramley, A.; Zhang, J.; et al. Viral Pathogen Detection by Metagenomics and Pan Viral Group PCR in Children with Pneumonia Lacking Identifiable Etiology. *J. Infect. Dis.* **2017**, *215*, 1407–1415. [CrossRef] [PubMed]
16. Dijkman, R.; Koekkoek, S.M.; Molenkamp, R.; Schildgen, O.; van der Hoek, L. Human bocavirus can be cultured in differentiated human airway epithelial cells. *J. Virol.* **2009**, *83*, 7739–7748. [CrossRef]
17. Huang, Q.; Deng, X.; Yan, Z.; Cheng, F.; Luo, Y.; Shen, W.; Lei-Butters, D.C.; Chen, A.Y.; Li, Y.; Tang, L.; et al. Establishment of a reverse genetics system for studying human bocavirus in human airway epithelia. *PLoS Pathog.* **2012**, *8*, e1002899. [CrossRef]
18. Deng, X.; Yan, Z.; Luo, Y.; Xu, J.; Cheng, Y.; Li, Y.; Engelhardt, J.; Qiu, J. In vitro modeling of human bocavirus 1 infection of polarized primary human airway epithelia. *J. Virol.* **2013**, *87*, 4097–4102. [CrossRef]
19. Deng, X.; Li, Y.; Qiu, J. Human bocavirus 1 infects commercially available primary human airway epithelium cultures productively. *J. Virol. Methods* **2014**, *195*, 112–119. [CrossRef]
20. Deng, X.; Yan, Z.; Cheng, F.; Engelhardt, J.F.; Qiu, J. Replication of an Autonomous Human Parvovirus in Non-dividing Human Airway Epithelium Is Facilitated through the DNA Damage and Repair Pathways. *PLoS Pathog.* **2016**, *12*, e1005399. [CrossRef]
21. Sun, Y.; Chen, A.Y.; Cheng, F.; Guan, W.; Johnson, F.B.; Qiu, J. Molecular characterization of infectious clones of the minute virus of canines reveals unique features of bocaviruses. *J. Virol.* **2009**, *83*, 3956–3967. [CrossRef] [PubMed]
22. Qiu, J.; Cheng, F.; Johnson, F.B.; Pintel, D. The transcription profile of the bocavirus bovine parvovirus is unlike those of previously characterized parvoviruses. *J. Virol.* **2007**, *81*, 12080–12085. [CrossRef] [PubMed]
23. Chen, A.Y.; Cheng, F.; Lou, S.; Luo, Y.; Liu, Z.; Delwart, E.; Pintel, D.; Qiu, J. Characterization of the gene expression profile of human bocavirus. *Virology* **2010**, *403*, 145–154. [CrossRef] [PubMed]
24. Shen, W.; Deng, X.; Zou, W.; Cheng, F.; Engelhardt, J.F.; Yan, Z.; Qiu, J. Identification and Functional Analysis of Novel Non-structural Proteins of Human Bocavirus 1. *J. Virol.* **2015**, *89*, 10097–10109. [CrossRef] [PubMed]
25. Zou, W.; Cheng, F.; Shen, W.; Engelhardt, J.F.; Yan, Z.; Qiu, J. Nonstructural Protein NP1 of Human Bocavirus 1 Plays a Critical Role in the Expression of Viral Capsid Proteins. *J. Virol.* **2016**, *90*, 4658–4669. [CrossRef] [PubMed]
26. Wang, Z.; Shen, W.; Cheng, F.; Deng, X.; Engelhardt, J.F.; Yan, Z.; Qiu, J. Parvovirus Expresses a Small Noncoding RNA That Plays an Essential Role in Virus Replication. *J. Virol.* **2017**, *91*, e02375-16. [CrossRef]

27. Flotte, T.R.; Afione, S.A.; Solow, R.; Drumm, M.L.; Markakis, D.; Guggino, W.B.; Zeitlin, P.L.; Carter, B.J. Expression of the cystic fibrosis transmembrane conductance regulator from a novel adeno-associated virus promoter. *J. Biol. Chem.* **1993**, *268*, 3781–3790.
28. Qiu, J.; Nayak, R.; Tullis, G.E.; Pintel, D.J. Characterization of the transcription profile of adeno-associated virus type 5 reveals a number of unique features compared to previously characterized adeno-associated viruses. *J. Virol.* **2002**, *76*, 12435–12447. [CrossRef]
29. Murthy, K.G.; Manley, J.L. The 160-kD subunit of human cleavage-polyadenylation specificity factor coordinates pre-mRNA 3′-end formation. *Genes Dev.* **1995**, *9*, 2672–2683. [CrossRef]
30. Stutika, C.; Mietzsch, M.; Gogol-Doring, A.; Weger, S.; Sohn, M.; Chen, W.; Heilbronn, R. Comprehensive Small RNA-Seq of Adeno-Associated Virus (AAV)-Infected Human Cells Detects Patterns of Novel, Non-Coding AAV RNAs in the Absence of Cellular miRNA Regulation. *PLoS ONE* **2016**, *11*, e0161454. [CrossRef]
31. Sukhu, L.; Fasina, O.; Burger, L.; Rai, A.; Qiu, J.; Pintel, D.J. Characterization of the nonstructural proteins of the bocavirus minute virus of canines. *J. Virol.* **2013**, *87*, 1098–1104. [CrossRef] [PubMed]
32. Fasina, O.O.; Dong, Y.; Pintel, D.J. NP1 Protein of the Bocaparvovirus Minute Virus of Canines Controls Access to the Viral Capsid Genes via Its Role in RNA Processing. *J. Virol.* **2015**, *90*, 1718–1728. [CrossRef] [PubMed]
33. Fasina, O.O.; Stupps, S.; Figueroa-Cuilan, W.; Pintel, D.J. The minute virus of canines (MVC) NP1 protein governs the expression of a subset of essential NS proteins via its role in RNA processing. *J. Virol.* **2017**, *91*, e00260-17. [CrossRef] [PubMed]
34. Dong, Y.; Fasina, O.O.; Pintel, D.J. The Human Bocavirus 1 NP1 Protein Is a Multifunctional Regulator of Viral RNA Processing. *J. Virol.* **2018**, *92*, e01187-18. [CrossRef]
35. Zhao, J.; Hyman, L.; Moore, C. Formation of mRNA 3′ ends in eukaryotes: Mechanism, regulation, and interrelationships with other steps in mRNA synthesis. *Microbiol. Mol. Biol. Rev.* **1999**, *63*, 405–445. [PubMed]
36. Hao, S.; Zhang, J.; Chen, Z.; Xu, H.; Wang, H.; Guan, W. Alternative Polyadenylation of Human Bocavirus at Its 3′ End Is Regulated by Multiple Elements and Affects Capsid Expression. *J. Virol.* **2017**, *91*, e02026-16. [CrossRef] [PubMed]

viruses

MDPI

Article

Parvovirus B19 Uncoating Occurs in the Cytoplasm without Capsid Disassembly and It Is Facilitated by Depletion of Capsid-Associated Divalent Cations

Oliver Caliaro [1], Andrea Marti [1], Nico Ruprecht [1,†], Remo Leisi [1], Suriyasri Subramanian [2], Susan Hafenstein [2,3] and Carlos Ros [1,*]

[1] Department of Chemistry and Biochemistry, University of Bern, Freiestrasse 3, 3012 Bern, Switzerland; oliver.caliaro@dcb.unibe.ch (O.C.); andrea.marti@students.unibe.ch (A.M.); nicoolivier.ruprecht@insel.ch (N.R.); remo.leisi@dcb.unibe.ch (R.L.)

[2] Department of Medicine, Pennsylvania State University College of Medicine, Hershey, PA 17033, USA; sxs1161@psu.edu (S.S.); suh21@psu.edu (S.H.)

[3] Department of Biochemistry and Molecular Biology, Pennsylvania State University, University Park, PA 16802, USA

* Correspondence: carlos.ros@dcb.unibe.ch; Tel.: +41-31-6314331

† Present address: Department of Diagnostic, Interventional and Pediatric Radiology, University Hospital, University of Bern, 3010 Bern, Switzerland.

Received: 17 April 2019; Accepted: 9 May 2019; Published: 10 May 2019

Abstract: Human parvovirus B19 (B19V) traffics to the cell nucleus where it delivers the genome for replication. The intracellular compartment where uncoating takes place, the required capsid structural rearrangements and the cellular factors involved remain unknown. We explored conditions that trigger uncoating in vitro and found that prolonged exposure of capsids to chelating agents or to buffers with chelating properties induced a structural rearrangement at 4 °C resulting in capsids with lower density. These lighter particles remained intact but were unstable and short exposure to 37 °C or to a freeze-thaw cycle was sufficient to trigger DNA externalization without capsid disassembly. The rearrangement was not observed in the absence of chelating activity or in the presence of $MgCl_2$ or $CaCl_2$, suggesting that depletion of capsid-associated divalent cations facilitates uncoating. The presence of assembled capsids with externalized DNA was also detected during B19V entry in UT7/Epo cells. Following endosomal escape and prior to nuclear entry, a significant proportion of the incoming capsids rearranged and externalized the viral genome without capsid disassembly. The incoming capsids with accessible genomes accumulated in the nuclear fraction, a process that was prevented when endosomal escape or dynein function was disrupted. In their uncoated conformation, capsids immunoprecipitated from cytoplasmic or from nuclear fractions supported in vitro complementary-strand synthesis at 37 °C. This study reveals an uncoating strategy of B19V based on a limited capsid rearrangement prior to nuclear entry, a process that can be mimicked in vitro by depletion of divalent cations.

Keywords: B19V; parvovirus; uncoating; divalent cations; capsid stability; genome externalization; trafficking; nuclear targeting

1. Introduction

Human parvovirus B19 (B19V) commonly causes a mild childhood disease known as *erythema infectiosum*, or fifth disease [1]. In adults, the virus can cause a range of clinical manifestations, and infection during pregnancy may result in *hydrops fetalis* and foetal death [2]. B19V is transmitted principally through the respiratory route and targets the bone marrow where it infects and kills erythroblast precursors. The single-stranded DNA genome of B19V is packaged into a small, nonenveloped, T = 1 icosahedral capsid consisting of 60 structural subunits, of which approximately 95% are VP2 (58 kDa) and 5% are VP1 (83 kDa). VP1 and VP2 are identical except for 227 additional amino acids at the VP1 N-terminal region, the so-called VP1 "unique region" (VP1u) [3].

Viral capsids assemble as highly stable structures to retain and protect the genome during their extracellular phase. However, they also have a built-in ability for disassembly when entering a new host cell. These apparently contradictory functions are possible because the robust protective capsids are metastable. They are conceived to rearrange upon specific cellular cues, adopting a sequence of structural configurations in a stepwise manner. Those configurations enable the intracellular transport of capsids and the release of the genome in the appropriate cell compartment for replication [4]. Viral capsids have evolved various strategies to balance their stability outside of the cell against their capacity to disassemble inside the cell. The switch between capsid stability and instability is mediated by specific cellular cues. Cellular receptors, attachment factors, proteases, kinases, ubiquitin or cellular motors among others facilitate virus uncoating by direct interaction with the capsid. A particular intracellular environment, such as the low endosomal pH, reducing conditions or low calcium concentrations may also provide cues for uncoating [5–7]. During cell entry, parvoviruses traffic through various cellular compartments before they reach the cell nucleus where the viral genome is delivered for replication [8]. The intracellular compartment where uncoating takes place, the required capsid structural rearrangements and the cellular cues involved in the process are poorly understood.

Similar to other parvoviruses, B19V enters the cell through clathrin-mediated endocytosis [9]. Although the endocytic elements involved and the sites of escape into the cytosol may vary among parvovirus species and cells [10,11], parvoviruses depend on the endosomal acidification, notably to trigger the exposure of VP1u and its constitutive phospholipase A_2 (PLA_2) activity, required to promote endosomal escape [12]. In contrast to other parvoviruses, B19V does not require endosomal acidification for VP1u exposure, which occurs already at the cell surface to promote virus uptake [13–16]. However, low pH is still required for efficient endosomal escape. Accordingly, bafilomycin A_1, which elevates the endosomal pH, but without compromising the integrity of endosomes, blocks the virus inside endocytic vesicles. In contrast, chloroquine, which induces endosomal vesicle enlargement and weakening, preventing their fusion to lysosomes [17], assists B19V infection by promoting endosomal escape [9]. The steps following the escape from endosomes are less well understood. Several studies have shown that cytoplasmic trafficking of parvovirus capsids is a microtubule-dependent process using cellular dynein as a motor protein [18,19]. However, other studies have shown that intracellular trafficking does not depend on dynein function or an intact microtubule network [20,21]. It has been proposed that parvoviruses enter the nucleus through the nuclear pore complex (NPC) via nuclear localization signals in the exposed VP1u [22–26]. A radically different mechanism has been suggested, which involves translocation of the capsids through discrete transient nuclear envelope (NE) breaks involving cell host caspases [27,28]. Through the NPC or through NE breaks, parvoviruses are small enough to enter the nucleus without capsid disassembly. However, it remains a matter of debate whether the infectious nuclear entry may still involve or not a disassembly process. Adeno-associated virus (AAV) infectivity can be blocked by injecting a neutralizing antibody against intact capsids into the nucleus [23]. However, other authors have shown that viruses enter the nucleus after partial or total disassembly in the cytosol or NPC [29].

A narrow channel at each five-fold vertex connecting with the interior of the particle is a common parvovirus structural feature and has been implicated in genome externalization and packaging [30–34]. In B19V capsids, the external end of the channel is closed, however, the presence of three consecutive glycine residues may provide the required flexibility to open the channel to allow the release of the viral DNA [35]. In agreement with this concept, in vitro studies have shown that parvovirus capsid disassembly is not required to externalize the viral genome [36–41]. Studies to understand the conditions required for DNA release at physiological conditions have shown that depletion of capsid-associated divalent cations in minute virus of mice (MVM) rendered the virions unstable and exposure to 37 °C was sufficient to trigger the externalization of the genome, which remained associated with the assembled capsid. The pressure of the encapsidated full-length viral DNA was important to promote the externalization at physiological temperatures [42]. A similar phenomenon was also observed in AAV, where the stability of virions containing full-length genomes required the presence of divalent cations in contrast to those containing subgenomic DNA [37,40].

Although the in vitro studies provide useful information, it remains uncertain whether the observed genome externalization without capsid disassembly can also occur in vivo during the process of virus entry. With the aim to gain insight into the mechanisms of B19V uncoating, conditions triggering viral DNA externalization at physiological temperatures were explored. To this end, virion density, capsid integrity and DNA accessibility were thoroughly examined in vitro upon exposure of virions to different conditions. Capsid rearrangements and uncoating were also followed in vivo during the process of cell entry. Viruses associated to cytoplasmic or to nuclear fractions were characterized at increasing times post-internalization by antibodies targeting capsid epitopes and phosphorylated amino acids. Additionally, the accessibility of the viral DNA was examined by immunoprecipitation and nuclease digestion and its suitability as a template for complementary-strand synthesis was evaluated by a primer hybridization and extension assay.

2. Materials and Methods

2.1. Cells and Viruses

The human megakaryoblastoid cell line UT7/Epo was cultured in Eagle's minimal essential medium (MEM), supplemented with 5% fetal calf serum (FCS), 2 U/mL recombinant human erythropoietin (Epo) and penicillin/streptomycin. A B19V-infected plasma sample with a high viral load (genotype 1) was obtained from CSL Behring (Bern, Switzerland). The virus was concentrated by ultracentrifugation through 20% sucrose cushion. The virus pellet was resuspended in MEM, 20 mM HEPES or PBS and immediately used or stored at 4 °C.

2.2. Antibodies and Chemicals

The monoclonal antibody 860-55D (referred as Caps) was obtained from Mikrogen (Neuried, Germany). The antibody recognizes a conformational epitope expanding three neighboring VP2 molecules related by a five-fold and by a three-fold axis [43], and does not recognize disassembled capsids. This antibody was obtained from an infected healthy adult and is neutralizing [44]. The polyclonal rabbit antibody against the PLA_2 region (referred as PLA2) was obtained as previously described [13]. The anti-phosphotyrosine mAb (clone 4G10), lambda phosphatase and the cytoplasmic dynein inhibitor ciliobrevin D (CbD) were purchased from EMD Millipore (Billerica, MA, USA). Anti-lamin A/C and anti-SERCA2 ATPase antibodies were obtained from Abcam (Cambridge, MA, USA). Bafilomycin A_1 ($BafA_1$) and chloroquine, were purchased from Sigma (St. Louis, MO, USA). CbD and $BafA_1$ were solved in DMSO and CQ was solved in water.

2.3. Quantitative PCR

Amplification of B19V DNA and real-time detection of PCR products were performed using a CFX96 Real Time Detection System (Bio-Rad, Hercules, CA, USA). Quantitative PCR (qPCR) was performed using the iTaq™ SYBR® Green Supermix kit (Bio-Rad) following the manufacturer's instructions. Primers used for B19V DNA amplification were as follows: B19V-forward, 5′-GGGCAGCCATTTTAAGTGTTT-3′; and B19V-reverse, 5′-GCACCACCAGTTATCGTTAGC-3′. Plasmids containing the complete genome of B19V were used at 10-fold dilutions as external standards.

2.4. Iodixanol Density Gradient Ultracentrifugation

The virus suspension was applied onto an iodixanol gradient containing 1.5 mL 55%, 2 mL 45%, 2 mL 40%, 2 mL 35% and 1.5 mL 15% iodixanol solution in 20 mM HEPES. The virus suspension was adjusted to 2 mL with the corresponding buffer and centrifuged at 35,000 rpm for 18 h at 18 °C in a swinging bucket rotor Beckman SW41Ti. After the centrifugation, 0.5 mL fractions were collected from the top. The refractive index was determined for each fraction and the presence of the virus was determined by dot-blot and qPCR.

2.5. Transmission Electron Microscopy

Purified B19V was resuspended in PBS alone or PBS supplemented with 1 mM $MgCl_2$ and stored at 4 °C for one month. Following a freeze/thaw cycle, 3 µL of each sample was applied to a freshly glow-discharged continuous carbon grid from Electron Microscopy Sciences (Hatfield, PA, USA), washed three times with dH_2O, and stained with 3 µL 1% (*w*/*v*) phosphotungstic acid. CCD images were acquired using a JEOL JEM 1200 EXII transmission electron microscope (Peabody, MA, USA) at 80 kV accelerating voltage, at 10,000× and 30,000× magnification.

2.6. Nuclease Assay

The presence of accessible DNA from the different virus samples was analysed by treatments with DNase I (Sigma). DNase I digestion was performed at 37 °C for 1 h in a buffer containing 40 mM Tris-HCl, pH7.9, 10 mM NaCl, 6 mM $MgCl_2$ and 1 mM $CaCl_2$. In order to test the DNase I activity, B19 viral particles were heated at 60 °C or 80 °C for 5 min. Native untreated virions served as controls. To stop the reaction, the viral DNA was extracted with the DNeasy blood and tissue kit (Qiagen, Venlo, Netherlands) and quantified as specified above.

2.7. Isolation of Cytoplasmic and Nuclear Fractions from Infected Cells

UT7/Epo cells (5×10^5) were incubated with B19V (2×10^4 virions per cell) for 1 h at 4 °C. The cells were subsequently washed four times at 4 °C with PBS, resuspended in MEM and further incubated at 37 °C to allow virus internalization. At increasing times post-internalization (pi), cytoplasmic or nuclear fractions were prepared. For cytoplasmic purification without nuclear contamination, cells were lysed in NP40 buffer (50 mM Tris-HCl, 150 mM NaCl, 1% NP-40) supplemented with a protease inhibitor cocktail (Complete Mini; Roche, Basel, Switzerland). After incubation on ice for 30 min, the cells were vortexed for 20 s and further incubated for 15 min on ice. Nuclei and cell debris were removed by centrifugation at 14,000× *g* for 10 min at 4 °C. The absence of nuclear contamination was determined by quantification of the human β-actin gene by qPCR.

For the isolation of nuclei, the cells were washed twice with ice-cold PBS and the pellets were resuspended in 100 µL EZ buffer (Sigma) and the volume completed to 1 mL with additional EZ buffer. The samples were vortexed and kept on ice for 5 min, then pelleted at 500× *g* for 5 min at 4 °C. This step was repeated once. Pellets were then resuspended in 500 µL EZ buffer containing 0.25 M sucrose and layered on top of 500 µL EZ buffer containing 0.5 M sucrose. The nuclei were collected by centrifugation at 500× *g* for 10 min at 4 °C, washed with 1 mL EZ buffer and resuspended in the desired buffer. The integrity of the isolated nuclei was assessed via light microscopy after trypan blue staining. The purity of the nuclei and the absence of cytoplasmic contamination were examined with antibodies against lamin A/C (marker for nuclear inner membrane), SERCA2 ATPase (marker for *endoplasmic reticulum*), and GAPDH (cytoplasmic marker). For immunoprecipitation, the nuclear pellets were resuspended in RIPA lysis buffer (50 mM Tris-HCl, 150 mM NaCl, 1% Triton X-100, 0.5% sodium deoxycholate, 0.1% SDS), supplemented with protease inhibitor cocktail (Complete Mini; Roche). The samples were incubated on ice for 20 min, vortexed for 20 s and further incubated for 15 min on ice. Nuclear debris was removed by centrifugation at 14,000× *g* for 10 min at 4 °C.

2.8. Immunoprecipitation

UT7/Epo cells were infected with B19V, as described above. At different times pi, viral particles were immunoprecipitated from cytoplasmic or from nuclear fractions with a B19V specific antibody against intact capsids (860-55D; Caps) or with an antibody against the PLA_2 region in VP1u (PLA2). For immunoprecipitation of phosphorylated capsids, an antibody against phosphorylated tyrosine was used (pTyr). After overnight incubation with 20 μL protein G agarose beads in LoBind tubes (Eppendorf, Hamburg, Germany) at 4 °C, the beads were washed four times (three times with PBSA-1% bovine serum albumin and once with PBS) and resuspended in protein loading buffer to analyse the immunoprecipitated capsids by Western blotting or in PBS to quantify the viral DNA by qPCR. Total DNA was extracted using the DNeasy blood and tissue kit (Qiagen) and quantified as specified above. The immunoprecipitated capsids were also used for complementary-strand synthesis, as specified below. The antibody 860-55D (Caps) was also used in immunoprecipitation experiments and dot-blot assays to test the integrity of the capsids.

2.9. Infectivity Assay

Virus infectivity was examined by quantification of NS1 mRNA. Cells were transferred 24 h pi to RNase-free tubes (Safe-Lock Tubes 1.5 mL, Eppendorf Biopur®) and pelleted. The pellet was washed twice with PBS and stored at −20 °C until use. Total poly-A-mRNA was isolated with a Dynabeads mRNA direct kit (Invitrogen). Following reverse transcription, cDNA was quantified by using iTaq™ Universal SYBR® Green One-Step reagent kit (Bio-Rad, Hercules, CA, USA). Primers were chosen to amplify a 133 nt-long NS1 cDNA fragment: NS1 forward (5′-GGGGCAGCATGTGTTAAAG-3′ (nucleotide 1017–1035) and NS1 reverse (5′-CCATGCCATATACTGGAACACT-3′ (nucleotide 1129–1150).

2.10. Complementary-Strand Synthesis

The presence of externalized DNA from the immunoprecipitated capsids and its suitability as a template for initiation of DNA synthesis was examined by a primer hybridization and extension reaction as previously described [38]. Briefly, primers consisting of a 3′ virus-specific and a 5′ virus-unrelated sequence were used. The hybridization reaction was performed in 40 μL volumes containing 20 μL of immunoprecipitated virus bound to protein G beads, 4 μL 5× hybridization buffer (40 mM Tris-HCl, pH 7.5, 20 mM $MgCl_2$ and 50 mM NaCl) and 2 μL primer (0.5 pmol), at 37 °C for 15 min. The hybridized primer was extended by adding 2 μL DTT (100 mM), 2 μL dNTPs (200 μM each) and 4 μL (3.25 U) of T7 DNA polymerase (Sequenase; USB, Cleveland, OH, USA) and incubated at 37 °C for 15 min or 0 min (negative control). The reaction was stopped, and DNA was purified by using the Wizard® SV Gel and PCR Clean-Up System (Promega, Madison, WI, USA). The primer-extended DNA was amplified by PCR as previously described [38] and the amplicons were separated by electrophoresis and visualized by staining with GelRed (Biotium, Hayward, CA, USA).

3. Results

3.1. Depletion of Capsid-Associated Divalent Cations Destabilizes the B19V Capsid

Iodixanol density gradient ultracentrifugation and qPCR were used to detect and to quantify changes in B19V capsid density. The density of native B19V from infected human plasma was compared to the virus pelleted through a 20% sucrose cushion and resuspended in PBS. Native capsids in human plasma and in PBS peaked at 1.22 g/mL, representing the density of intact native capsids (Figure 1A,B). A dot-blot confirmed the presence of capsids in the same fractions as the viral DNA (Figure 1C). Virus in PBS and exposed to 60 °C or 80 °C for 5 min resulted in a density shift to 1.09 g/mL, which corresponds to free viral DNA (Figure 1D,E).

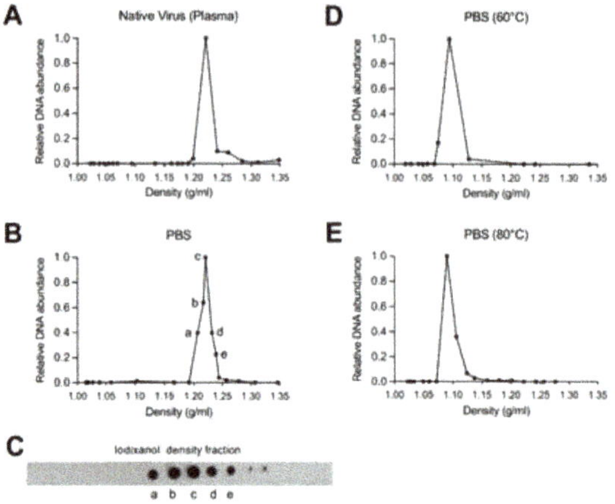

Figure 1. Buoyant density of native B19V from infected plasma or purified and resuspended in PBS. Fractions from iodixanol density gradient ultracentrifugation were collected and quantified by qPCR. (**A**) Density of B19V from infected human plasma. (**B**) Density of B19V purified from infected plasma by ultracentrifugation through 20% sucrose cushion and resuspended in PBS. (**C**) Detection of B19V capsids by dot-blot from density fractions of B19V in PBS. The corresponding fractions are indicated (a–e). (**D**) Density of B19V treated at 60 °C for 5 min. (**E**) Density of B19V treated at 80 °C for 5 min.

The density of B19V resuspended in MEM, HEPES and PBS and stored for a period of four weeks at 4 °C (prolonged exposure) was compared. While the virus density in MEM and HEPES did not change (1.22 g/mL), prolonged exposure to PBS induced a structural rearrangement resulting in capsids with lower density (1.20 g/mL) (Figure 2A). We next analysed the stability of B19V after prolonged exposure (four weeks at 4 °C) to the different buffers followed by a single freeze/thaw cycle. While the virus in MEM did not change, the virus in HEPES peaked at a similar density as the virus that was exposed to PBS for a prolonged time at 4 °C (1.19 g/mL). In contrast, a major density shift was observed after a freeze/thaw cycle in the virus exposed to PBS (1.11 g/mL). This shift was fully prevented when PBS was supplemented with 1 mM of $MgCl_2$ or 1 mM $CaCl_2$ (1.23 g/mL), suggesting that divalent cations have a stabilizing effect on the virion (Figure 2B). To further study the influence of divalent cations, the effect of the chelating agents EDTA and EGTA on the virus density was analysed. Prolonged exposure (four weeks at 4 °C) to HEPES supplemented with 1 mM EGTA or 1 mM EDTA provoked a density shift to 1.195 g/mL, similar to the shift observed in the virus exposed to PBS. However, these lighter particles were unstable and short exposure to 37 °C was sufficient to trigger a major density shift, similar to that of virus in PBS and exposed to a freeze/thaw cycle. The rearrangement at 37 °C was not observed in the absence of chelating agents (Figure 2C).

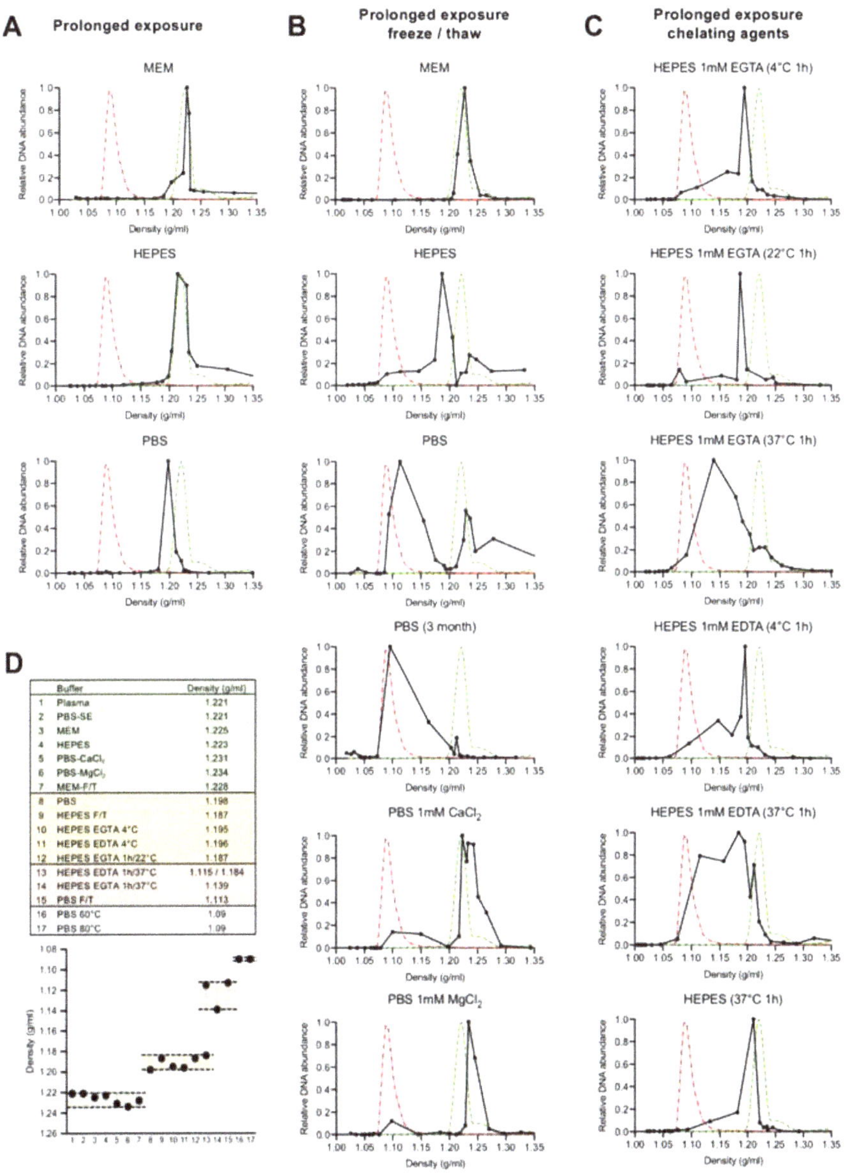

Figure 2. Influence of divalent cation depletion on the density of B19V. Virus from infected plasma was pelleted through 20% sucrose cushion, resuspended in different buffers and stored at 4 °C for one month. Fractions from iodixanol density gradient ultracentrifugation were quantified by qPCR. (**A**) Effect of prolonged (one month) incubation of B19V in MEM, HEPES and PBS at 4 °C. (**B**) Effect of a freeze/thaw cycle after prolonged incubation of B19V in MEM, HEPES, PBS and PBS supplemented with 1 mM $CaCl_2$ or 1 mM $MgCl_2$. (**C**) Effect of prolonged incubation of B19V in HEPES at 4 °C supplemented or not with 1 mM EGTA or 1 mM EDTA. Before separation by iodixanol density centrifugation, the virus suspensions were treated at 4 °C, 22 °C or 37 °C for 1 h. Green peak; density native virus. Red peak; density free viral DNA. (**D**) Upper panel; summary of the major density peaks (g/mL) of B19V in the different buffers and exposed to different conditions. Lower panel; graphic representation of the four distinct density groups. Similar densities appear grouped by colours.

In total, four density groups were identified (Figure 2D). Viruses in plasma or in buffers with divalent cations were stable and had a similar density around 1.22 g/mL. Viruses exposed to buffers with chelating activity peaked at a density of 1.19–1.20 g/mL. These particles shifted to 1.11–1.14 g/mL when exposed to 37 °C or to a freeze/thaw cycle. Free viral DNA generated by heat treatment of virions (60 °C or 80 °C for 5 min) peaked at 1.09 g/mL.

3.2. Depletion of Divalent Cations Facilitates B19V Uncoating without Capsid Disassembly

The capsid integrity of the different density populations was investigated by nuclease digestion and by immunoprecipitation with the antibody 860-55D against a conformational epitope (Caps), which recognizes only assembled capsids [44]. As shown in Figure 3A,B, capsids at densities ranging from 1.22–1.19 g/mL were mostly DNase I-resistant. Since the capsids were shortly exposed to 37 °C during the DNase I treatment, virions with densities around 1.19 g/mL showed a variable degree of nuclease sensitivity. However, capsids peaking at densities 1.11–1.14 g/mL were fully sensitive to nuclease digestion, similarly to control virus heated at 80 °C. The viral capsids could be immunoprecipitated under all tested conditions, except the control sample, which was exposed to 80 °C to provoke capsid disassembly (Figure 3C,D). This result indicates that the structural rearrangements resulting in DNA externalization do not compromise the integrity of the capsids, which remain assembled.

Negative stain transmission electron microscopy was used to visualize the effect on capsids and the packaged DNA in the absence of divalent cations. In PBS supplemented with 1 mM $MgCl_2$ (Figure 2B; density 1.23 g/mL), the capsids appear as stable, DNA-filled capsids. In contrast, in the absence of $MgCl_2$ and exposed to a freeze/thaw cycle (Figure 2B; major density peak at 1.11 and minor density peak at 1.22), a mixture of empty and DNA-filled capsids was observed. Some capsids showed an "eclipsing" effect, where the DNA appears condensed and rearranged, capturing an intermediate step during genome release (Figure 3E). The infectivity of the virus preparations used for TEM was evaluated by the quantification of the NS1 mRNA. While viruses supplemented with $MgCl_2$ were infectious, the infectivity dropped significantly in the absence of divalent cations (Figure 3F).

In summary, four density populations were characterized and are outlined in Figure 2D. Viruses in plasma or in buffers with divalent cations were stable, nuclease resistant and had a similar density around 1.22 g/mL. Viruses exposed for a prolonged time to buffers with chelating activity or to chelating agents at low temperatures remained assembled but their density shifted to 1.19–1.20 g/mL. These particles were unstable and exposure to 37 °C or to a freeze/thaw cycle was sufficient to trigger the externalization of the viral DNA without capsid disassembly and to provoke a major density shift to 1.11–1.14 g/mL. Finally, heating to 60 °C or 80 °C for 5 min caused the complete release of the viral DNA, which peaked at 1.09 g/mL. These results together suggest that capsid-associated divalent cations have a stabilizing role and their removal prepares the virus for uncoating at physiological temperatures without capsid disassembly.

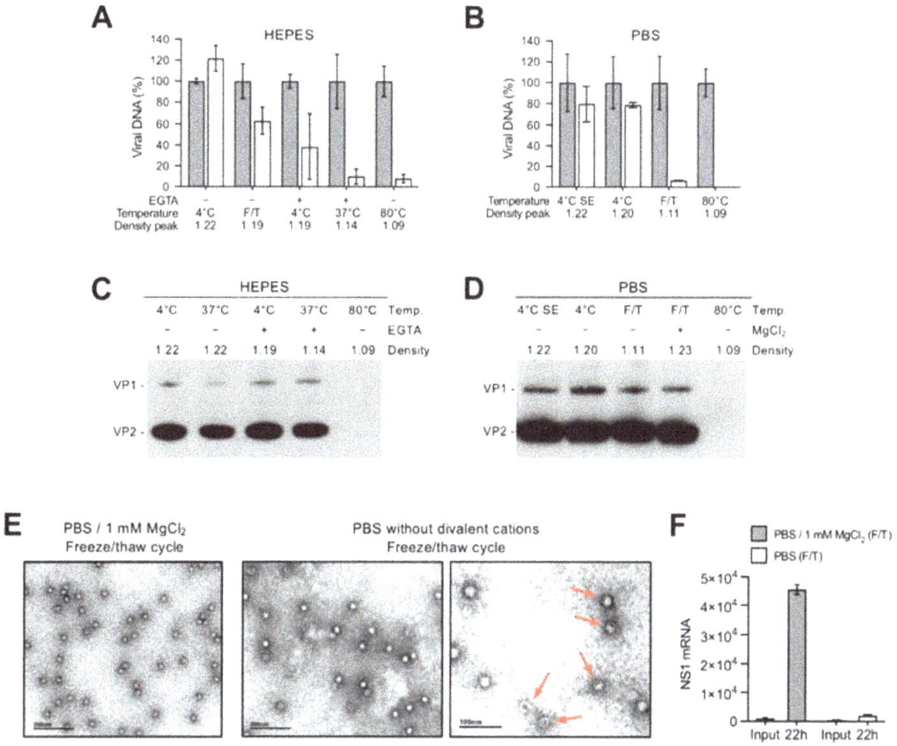

Figure 3. DNA accessibility and capsid integrity of the different B19V density populations. (**A**,**B**) Nuclease sensitivity of viruses in HEPES or in PBS displaying different densities. Virus samples from representative density populations were treated with DNase I at 37 °C for 1 h (white columns). Virus treated at 80 °C for 5 min was used as control. (**C**,**D**) Integrity of capsids in HEPES or in PBS displaying different densities. Virus samples from representative density populations were immunoprecipitated with the conformational antibody 860-55D against assembled capsids. Virus treated at 80 °C for 5 min was used as control. (**E**) Transmission electron microscopy (TEM) images of B19V in PBS alone and PBS supplemented with 1 mM $MgCl_2$ and exposed to a freeze/thaw cycle. Arrows indicate capsids with rearranged DNA. (**F**) Infectivity assay based on NS1 mRNA detection with the same B19V preparations used for TEM. SE; short exposure. F/T; freeze and thaw. Values correspond to genome equivalents per microliter (geq/μL).

3.3. *A Proportion of Incoming Capsids Uncoat in the Cytoplasm without Capsid Disassembly*

Cytoplasmic fractions were prepared from infected UT7/Epo cells. The lack of nuclear contamination was confirmed by quantitative detection of β-actin gene sequences (Figure 4A). The accessibility of the viral DNA from the incoming cytoplasmic virus was examined by nuclease digestion and qPCR. While at 5 min pi the viral DNA remained protected, approximately half of the incoming genomes became sensitive to nuclease digestion after 3 h pi (Figure 4B). The VP1u region is not accessible in native capsids but it becomes accessible upon interactions on the surface of susceptible cells [14,38]. As expected, cell-bound viruses were immunoprecipitated with the antibody targeting a conformational epitope in VP2 (Caps) and by the antibody targeting the PLA_2 region in VP1u (PLA2). During cell entry, the PLA_2 region remained accessible but the conformational epitope in VP2 became undetectable in an increasing proportion of incoming particles (Figure 4C). These results were further confirmed by immunoprecipitation and Western blot analysis of capsid proteins. Incoming viruses were immunoprecipitated with Caps and PLA2 antibodies at 3 h pi. The supernatant was used to immunoprecipitate remaining viruses with the heterologous antibody. While the PLA2 antibody detected all intracellular capsids, the Caps antibody did not recognize a significant proportion of incoming capsids (Figure 4D), suggesting that during entry some incoming virions rearrange and adopt a configuration that remained recognized by the PLA2 antibody but not by the VP2 conformational antibody.

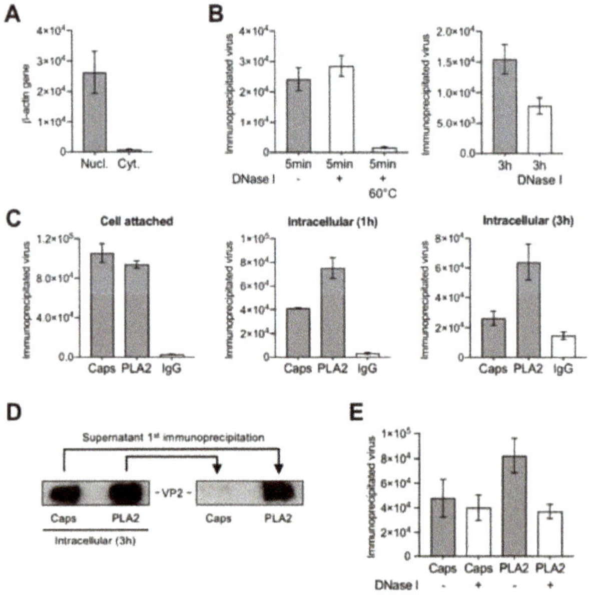

Figure 4. Capsid structural rearrangements and viral DNA externalization in the cytoplasm. (**A**) The purity of the cytoplasmic fraction and the absence of nuclear contamination were examined by quantitative detection of β-actin gene sequences. Values represent DNA copies per microliter. (**B**) Nuclease sensitivity of virions at 5 min and 3 h pi Virus treated at 60 °C for 5 min was used as control. (**C**) Accessibility of VP1u (PLA2 antibody) and VP2 conformational (Caps antibody) epitopes from membrane-bound or intracellular B19V. Virions were immunoprecipitated and quantified by qPCR. As control, an unrelated IgG was used. (**D**) Western blot of B19V immunoprecipitated at 3 h pi. The supernatants were used for a second immunoprecipitation with the indicated antibodies. (**E**) Nuclease sensitivity of B19V immunoprecipitated with the conformational antibody (Caps) or with the VP1u antibody (PLA2) at 1 h pi. All immunoprecipitation values represent geq/μL.

We next verified whether the observed capsid structural rearrangement rendered the viral DNA accessible. To explore this possibility, virions from cytoplasmic fractions were immunoprecipitated with the Caps or with the PLA2 antibody 3 h pi and the accessibility of the viral DNA from the immunoprecipitated capsids was examined by nuclease digestion and qPCR. The incoming capsids that remained detectable by the conformational antibody were resistant to nuclease digestion. In contrast, approximately half of the virions that were immunoprecipitated with the PLA2 antibody were sensitive to nuclease digestion (Figure 4E). This result suggests that a significant proportion of incoming capsids uncoat in the cytoplasm through a limited capsid rearrangement.

3.4. Uncoating Occurs after Endosomal Escape

In order to examine whether the detected capsid rearrangement and DNA externalization occur before or after endosomal escape, cells were treated with bafilomycin A_1 ($BafA_1$), which was previously shown to block endosomal escape of B19V [9]. The cells were fixed 30 min and 5 h pi and incoming viruses were detected with the conformational antibody (Caps). After 30 min, a similar signal with a characteristic endocytic distribution was observed in untreated or BafA1-treated cells. However, 5 h pi the number of capsids detectable with the conformational antibody decreased significantly in the untreated cells, but remained stable in the BafA$_1$-treated cells and displayed the same endocytic distribution, indicating that endosomal escape and the capsid rearrangement were inhibited (Figure 5A). The capsid rearrangement and the accessibility of the DNA were also examined by immunoprecipitation and nuclease digestion. As shown in Figure 5B, while in untreated cells a proportion of incoming capsids rearranged and became nuclease sensitive, in the presence of BafA$_1$ the capsids remained mostly unchanged.

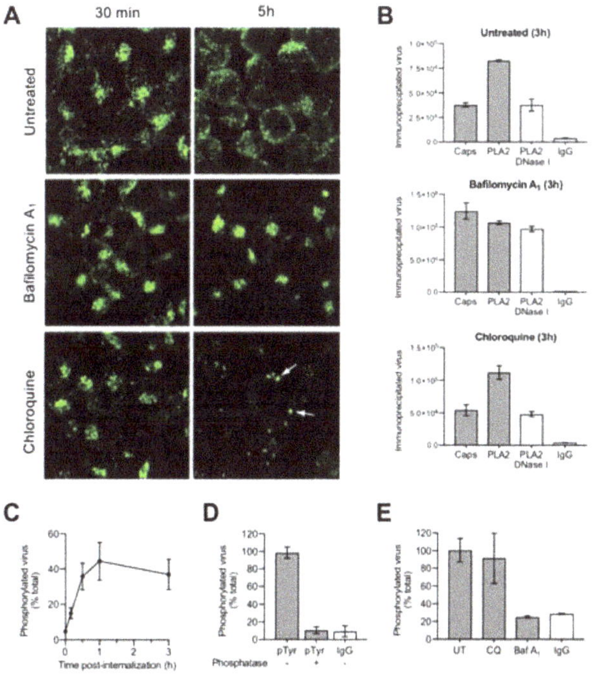

Figure 5. Conformational epitope rearrangement, DNA externalization and phosphorylation occur after endosomal escape. (**A**) Effect of BafA$_1$ and CQ on endosomal escape and conformational epitope integrity. Immunofluorescence images of infected cells treated or not with BafA$_1$ (20 nM) and CQ (25 µM). The integrity of the conformational epitope and the characteristic endocytic clustering of the virus was examined by staining with the conformational antibody (Caps) at 30 min and 3 h pi. Arrows indicate the presence of enlarged endosomes in cells treated with CQ. (**B**) Effect of BafA$_1$ and CQ on the conformational rearrangement and nuclease sensitivity of the incoming virions. The virions were immunoprecipitated from infected cells at 3 h pi and quantified by qPCR, values correspond to geq/µL. (**C**) Kinetics of B19V phosphorylation. At increasing times pi, virions were immunoprecipitated from cytoplasmic fractions with PLA2 (total virions) or with an antibody against phosphotyrosine and quantified by qPCR. (**D**) Phosphatase treatment abrogated the reactivity with the phosphospecific antibody. Before immunoprecipitation, the intracellular capsids were treated or not with lambda phosphatase (500 U) for 1 h at 30 °C. (**E**) Effect of BafA$_1$ (20 nM) or CQ (25 µM) on B19V phosphorylation. Virions from cytoplasmic fractions were immunoprecipitated with the phosphotyrosine antibody at 3h pi and quantified by qPCR. As control, an unrelated IgG was used.

These results are in line with our previous studies where we have shown that $BafA_1$ inhibits B19V infection by blocking endosomal escape. In the same studies, we observed that chloroquine (CQ), which also raises endosomal pH, did not hinder endosomal escape [9], an effect that was attributed to the vacuolization and damage of endocytic vesicles [17]. Accordingly, CQ was used to verify whether the inhibitory effect of BafA1 on the rearrangement and DNA accessibility is due to the raise in the endosomal pH or to the block of endosomal escape. As shown in Figure 5A,B, CQ induced the enlargement of endocytic vesicles and did not prevent the capsid rearrangement and viral DNA externalization, suggesting that these changes ensue only after endosomal escape and are not mediated by the low endocytic pH.

3.5. *Incoming Capsids Become Reactive to Phosphospecific Antibodies Following Endosomal Escape*

Cellular kinases have been shown to phosphorylate incoming parvovirus capsids following endosomal escape [45]. We investigated whether B19V is also phosphorylated after endosomal escape. To this end, cell-bound and internalized capsids were incubated with a phosphospecific antibody targeting tyrosine phosphorylation. Quantification of the immunoprecipitated capsids by qPCR revealed that by 1 h pi, approximately half of the internalized capsids became phosphorylated (Figure 5C). Capsid phosphorylation initiated as early as 10 min pi and was maximal between 30 min and 1 h pi. Incoming B19V were not reactive to phosphospecific antibodies following incubation with lambda phosphatase (Figure 5D). As expected, inhibition of endosomal escape by $BafA_1$ abrogated capsid phosphorylation. In contrast, phosphorylation was not prevented in the presence of CQ (Figure 5E), confirming our previous observations indicating that CQ does not hinder endosomal escape [9]. These results further demonstrate that the observed capsid rearrangement and DNA accessibility are not triggered by the endosomal low pH but following the delivery of incoming particles into the cytosol.

3.6. *Capsids Phosphorylated and with Accessible Genomes Accumulated Progressively in the Nuclear Fraction*

All the described capsid structural changes, i.e., conformational epitope rearrangement, phosphorylation and DNA externalization, were observed in virions isolated from the cytoplasmic fraction devoid of nucleus. We next analysed the presence of viral DNA and capsids in the nuclear fraction at increasing times pi. The integrity of the isolated nuclei was assessed by light microscopy after trypan blue staining and the purity of the nuclear fraction was verified by the absence of cytoplasmic contamination using antibodies against GAPDH (cytosolic marker), lamin A/C (nuclear inner membrane marker) and SERCA2 ATPase (endoplasmic reticulum marker) (Figure 6A). Nuclei isolated after 5 min or from cells treated with $BafA_1$ to prevent endosomal escape served as negative controls. Viral DNA was quantified from the purified nuclei by qPCR and the results were normalized by the quantification of the β-actin gene. An increasing amount of viral DNA accumulated in the nuclear fraction reaching a plateau by 2–3 h pi. In contrast, nuclear viral DNA did not increase significantly above the background level in cells treated with $BafA_1$ (Figure 6B).

The accessibility of the viral DNA accumulating in the nuclear fraction was examined by nuclease digestion. Purified nuclei were prepared at 5 min (negative control) and 3 h pi. While the DNA detected 5 min pi, representing the background, was resistant to nucleases, the viral DNA accumulated in the nuclear fraction at 3 h pi was mostly nuclease sensitive. Incubation of the nuclear fraction at 60 °C for 10 min was used to control the activity of DNase I (Figure 6C).

We next analysed whether the nuclear viral DNA signal originated from free or capsid-associated DNA. To this end, nuclear fractions were prepared at 5 min (negative control) and 3 h pi and used for immunoprecipitation with the Caps, PLA2 and phosphotyrosine antibody. The immunoprecipitated viruses were quantified by qPCR, as specified above. Additionally, the accessibility of the viral DNA was examined by treatments with DNase I. The results showed that only the capsids that underwent the structural modifications in the cytoplasm, i.e., conformational epitope rearrangement, phosphorylation and DNA externalization, were able to reach the nucleus (Figure 6D).

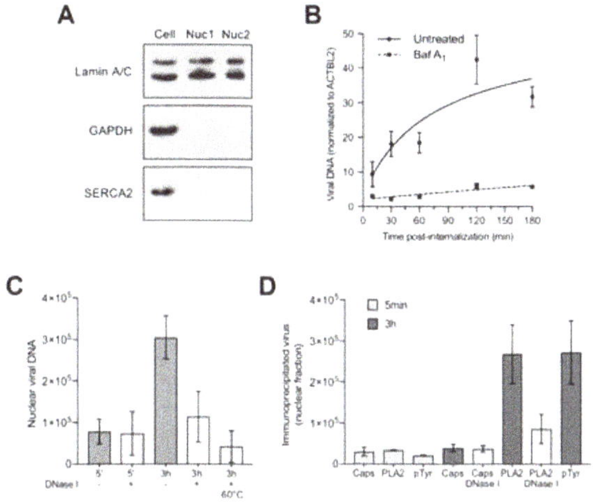

Figure 6. Characterization of incoming B19V associated to the nuclear fraction. (**A**) Isolation of intact nuclei without cytoplasmic contamination. The purity of the nuclear fraction and the absence of cytoplasmic contamination were examined by the detection of lamin A/C (nuclear marker) and SERCA2 ATPase (ER marker) and GAPDH (cytoplasmic marker) by Western blot. Nuc1 and Nuc2; two independent nuclear preparations. (**B**) Accumulation of B19V in the nuclear fraction at increasing times pi. Nuclei isolated after 5 min or from cells treated with $BafA_1$ served as negative controls. The results were normalized by the quantification of the β-actin-like gene 2 (ACTBL2). (**C**) Nuclease sensitivity of virions associated to the nuclear fraction. Nuclei isolated after 5 min served as background control. Nuclear fractions prepared 3 h pi were treated at 60 °C for 5 min to control the activity of DNase I. qPCR values represent geq/μL. (**D**) Immunoprecipitation of virions associated to the nuclear fraction. Nuclei isolated after 5 min served as background control. pTyr; phosphotyrosine antibody. qPCR values represent geq/μL.

3.7. Nuclear Targeting of B19V Is Mediated by the Microtubule-Dependent, Minus-End-Directed Motor Dynein

Cytoplasmic dynein mediates ATP-dependent retrograde movement of cargoes, including endocytic vesicles, along microtubules toward the centrosome near the nucleus [46]. Accordingly, endocytosed B19V can indirectly benefit from this transport. However, it remains unclear whether parvovirus particles can directly engage motor proteins when they are released in the cytosol for their own transport to the nuclear vicinity. In order to address this question, ciliobrevin D (CbD), which is a specific inhibitor of AAA+ ATPase motor cytoplasmic dynein, was used. CbD inhibits dynein function without altering microtubule structure and dynamics [47,48]. In order to not disturb dynein-mediated endocytic transport of B19V and release from endosomes, cells were treated with CbD 15 min after internalization, at a time when most of the intracellular viruses are in late endosomes [9]. Under these experimental conditions, the loss of the conformational epitope (Caps/PLA2 ratio), capsid phosphorylation and DNA externalization were not disturbed by CbD (Figure 7A,B). In contrast, the accumulation of viruses in the nuclear fraction was prevented. Release of the reversible CbD block resulted in an increased nuclear accumulation of viruses (Figure 7C). As expected, disruption of dynein function by CbD impaired B19V infection, but only when present early during virus entry and not at later times pi (Figure 7D).

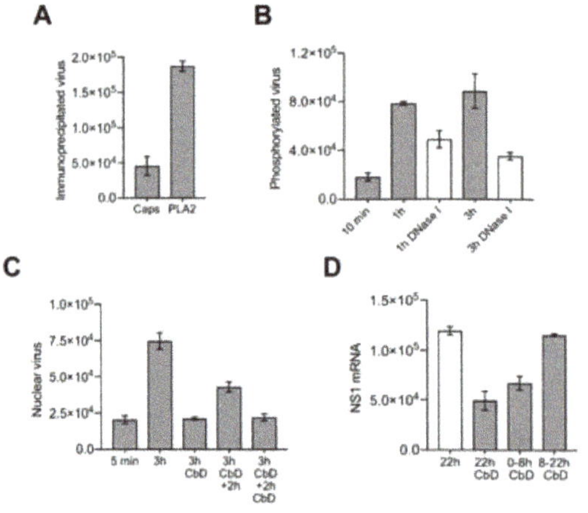

Figure 7. Inhibition of dynein-mediated nuclear targeting blocks the incoming viruses in the cytoplasm but does not prevent the capsid rearrangement, phosphorylation and uncoating (**A**) Effect of the dynein inhibitor ciliobrevin D (CbD; 100 μM) on conformational epitope integrity (Caps/PLA2 ratio). (**B**) Effect of CbD on phosphorylation and DNA externalization. (**C**) Effect of CbD on the nuclear accumulation of B19V DNA. After 5 min (background control) and 3 h pi, cells were washed and the amount of viral DNA was quantified by qPCR. Additionally, cells were incubated for two additional hours in the presence or absence of CbD. All values of qPCR correspond to geq/μL. (**D**) Effect of CbD on B19V infection. Cells were infected in the presence of CbD for the indicated times and the amount of NS1 mRNA was quantified by RT-qPCR at 22 h pi. Values represent NS1 mRNA copies/μL.

3.8. Capsids Immunoprecipitated from Cytoplasmic and from Nuclear Fractions Support Complementary-Strand DNA Synthesis

The strategy for complementary-strand synthesis is outlined in Figure 8A. Cytoplasmic and nuclear capsids were immunoprecipitated with the antibody against the PLA_2 region, which remains accessible during cell entry. The presence of externalized DNA in the immunoprecipitated capsids and its suitability as template for complementary-strand synthesis were examined by hybridization with primers targeting the 3′ or the 5′ region of the viral genome (outlined in Figure 8B). The oligonucleotides consisted of a 3′ virus-specific sequence (specific for a sequence stretch at the 3′ or 5′ regions) and a 5′ virus–unrelated sequence. Following the hybridization reaction at 37 °C, the extension was performed at 37 °C for 15 min. Negative controls consisted of viruses immunoprecipitated at 5 min pi or viruses immunoprecipitated at 3 h pi without the polymerase extension step. The reaction was stopped, and the primer-extended DNA was amplified by real-time PCR using a forward primer specific for the 5′ virus-unrelated sequences of the oligonucleotide and a virus-specific reverse primer. Only capsids immunoprecipitated from cytoplasmic fractions or from nuclear fractions at 3 h pi originated the expected PCR product, indicating the presence of accessible DNA templates from the immunoprecipitated capsids. Similar results were obtained by using primers targeting the 3′ or the 5′ region of the viral genome (Figure 8C). DNA accessibility was not detected from capsids immunoprecipitated after 5 min of internalization or in samples without polymerase extension. These results indicate that the viral DNA becomes accessible already in the cytoplasm prior to nuclear entry and supports complementary-strand synthesis while remaining associated to the assembled particle.

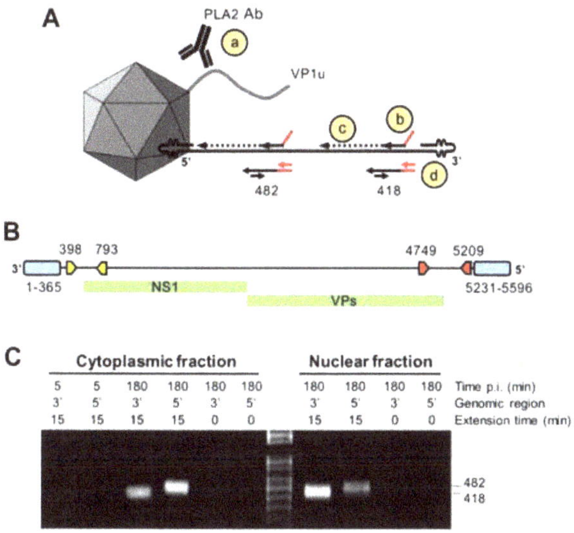

Figure 8. Complementary-strand DNA synthesis from cytoplasmic or nuclear capsids. (**A**) Depiction of the strategy for complementary-strand synthesis: (**a**) Immunoprecipitation of B19V capsids with the PLA2 antibody; (**b**) 5′ virus-unrelated sequence; (**c**) extension reaction by T7 polymerase at 37 °C; and (**d**) amplification of the primer-extended DNA by PCR. (**B**) Positions in the B19V genome of the 3′ (yellow) and 5′ (red) regions targeted by the hybridization and extension assay. (**C**) Viral particles were immunoprecipitated from cytoplasmic or from nuclear fractions with the antibody against the PLA_2 region (PLA2) and used for complementary-strand DNA synthesis. The primer-extended DNA was amplified by PCR and amplicons of the expected size were visualized by agarose gel electrophoresis. As controls, viruses were immunoprecipitated 5 min pi or incubated with the T7 polymerase for only a few seconds.

4. Discussion

Parvovirus infection critically depends on the processing of the incoming particles by cellular factors to promote their transport into the nucleus and the delivery of the viral genome for replication. How and where human parvovirus B19 (B19V) releases the viral DNA and which capsid rearrangement are required for the process is currently unknown. In this study, we combined in vitro and in vivo experiments to address the mechanism of uncoating of B19V.

A common parvovirus structural feature is the combination of antiparallel β-hairpins at the five-fold vertex enclosing a cylindrical structure that connects with the interior of the capsid [35,49–52]. Structural and in vitro studies suggest that these channels serve as portals for the externalization of N-terminal capsid protein sequences required during the process of virus entry and for the packaging and release of the viral genome [23,31–34,52–54]. Mutations that perturb the structure of the channel result in defective genome encapsidation, uncoating and VP1u externalization [30,31,39]. Those mutational studies have also confirmed that MVM cylinders can mediate progressive 3′-to-5′ genome release, suggesting that this is the strategy of uncoating, and that unknown cellular trigger(s) may initiate the DNA rearrangement during virus entry [39]. In B19V, the channel does not mediate the externalization of N-VP2 sequences, which are already exposed [55], and N-VP1 might also occupy a surface position not accessible to antibodies until the interaction of the virion with cellular receptors [14,15]. Accordingly, the main function of the channel in B19V would be the packaging and release of the viral genome. However, different to other parvoviruses, the channel in B19 VP2 capsids is constricted at its outside end, although three consecutive glycine residues at this site may provide enough flexibility to open the channel upon specific cellular cues [35].

Iodixanol density gradient ultracentrifugation followed by qPCR detection of the viral DNA proved to be a useful approach to detect and quantify structural rearrangements in the viral capsid. The method allowed to explore conditions triggering the uncoating reaction at physiological temperatures and to identify and characterize uncoating intermediates. Native capsids in human plasma or in MEM were stable and remained intact after exposure to 37 °C or to a freeze/thaw cycle. However, in the absence of divalent cations or in the presence of chelating activity at 4 °C, the viral capsids rearranged resulting in particles with a lower density and mostly resistant to nuclease digestion. These capsids however were rather unstable and incubation at 37 °C or a freeze/thaw cycle was sufficient to trigger viral DNA externalization without capsid disassembly. These rearrangements were prevented in the presence of 1 mM $MgCl_2$ or 1 mM $CaCl_2$, strongly suggesting that divalent cations have a stabilizing effect on the viral particle and their removal facilitates the uncoating reaction at physiological temperatures. The TEM images confirmed the presence of assembled particles with variable degree of DNA externalization (Figure 3E), explaining their broader iodixanol density profile (Figure 2). Similar results were obtained with minute virus of mice (MVM). Depletion of capsid-associated divalent cations in MVM rendered the virions unstable and exposure to 37 °C triggered the externalization of the genome, in a 3′-to-5′ direction, leaving the 5′ end of the DNA associated with the capsid. The process was not observed in the presence of divalent cations or in capsids with shorter genomes [42].

During packaging, the viral DNA is loaded at a high density into the small inner cavity of the pre-formed capsids in a 3′ to 5′ direction through the fivefold cylinder [31,33,56,57]. It is conceivable, that in order to condensate and stabilize the DNA-filled capsid, divalent cations may be incorporated into the B19 progeny particle during packaging to neutralize the negative charges of closely packed DNA phosphate backbones and eventually also negative charges in the particle lattice interior. The highly condensed DNA generates a considerable internal pressure and loss of capsid-associated divalent cations during entry may increase the internal tension and destabilize the whole structure, provoking the externalization of the viral genome through the fivefold channel without the need to disassemble the capsid. A direct correlation between the amount of encapsidated DNA and the sensitivity to chelating agents was demonstrated for a variety of of viruses [58,59], including different rAAV vectors and MVM [37,40,42]. Divalent cations may also bind the capsid to cement the structure, as it has been demonstrated for other viruses, and their removal was shown to destabilize the capsid and promote uncoating [60–64]. Prediction of metal ions binding sites by IonCom, which combines the ab initio model with multiple threading alignments [65], revealed a Mg^{2+} and Ca^{2+} binding site in close proximity on the surface of B19V capsid. While the Mg^{2+} binding domain was slightly buried, the Ca^{2+} binding site appeared on the surface surrounding the dimple-like depression at the icosahedral two-fold axis of symmetry (data not shown).

The similar response of MVM and B19V to divalent cation depletion may reflect a common uncoating strategy of parvoviruses based on a mechanism of DNA externalization without capsid disassembly. This strategy would allow the exceptionally stable parvoviral particles to deliver the genome inside the host cells, and since the particle and the viral DNA remain associated, the capsid can transport the externalized genome to the precise nuclear location to initiate replication and transcription. The destabilization and uncoating of B19 virions under divalent cation depletion in vitro suggests a mechanism for viral genome release in low-divalent-cation environments, such as those typically encountered within the cytosol of the cell, where the activities of ATP-driven Ca^{2+} pumps and Na^+/Ca^{2+} exchangers maintain the concentration of Ca^{2+} ions at a very low (10–100 nM) level [66]. Therefore, following endosomal escape, the virion is abruptly exposed to a divalent cation-depleted environment in the cytosol, which may destabilize the incoming particle. However, although the in vitro studies reveal important information on conditions allowing the uncoating reaction and allow the characterization of uncoating intermediates, these studies do not necessarily reflect the uncoating process in vivo, which may differ in its mechanism and be triggered by intracellular factor(s) other than divalent cation depletion. With the aim to get insights into the intracellular capsid processing required for B19V uncoating in vivo, we followed capsid modifications and changes in epitope and

DNA accessibility during B19V entry. These rearrangements were examined in UT7/Epo cells at various times pi from cytoplasmic and nuclear fractions and under different conditions restraining endosome and dynein functions.

The first detectable capsid rearrangement during B19V entry was the change in VP1u configuration occurring at the plasma membrane before virus internalization. For most parvoviruses, VP1u externalization occurs inside the endosomes triggered by the acidic environment [11,23,67–69]. However, we have previously shown that B19V operates differently. Upon interactions on the surface of susceptible cells, originally inaccessible VP1u sequences become exposed [13] and interact with as yet unknown highly restricted receptor required for virus uptake [14,15]. As expected, cell-bound virions were immunoprecipitated with the antibody against VP1u (PLA2) and the conformational antibody detecting exclusively intact capsids (Caps) (Figure 4C).

The second capsid rearrangement detected was more complex and occurred after endosomal escape in the cytoplasm. While the capsids remained detectable by the VP1u antibody, approximately half of them became undetectable by the conformational antibody against capsids (Figure 4C,D). The capsids that rearranged became sensitive to nuclease digestion in contrast to those that had not rearranged (Figure 4E). The conformational epitope expands three neighboring VP2 molecules related by a five-fold axis and by a three-fold axis [43], and its loss can be explained by a rearrangement occurring at this site. Alternatively, epitope masking by phosphorylation might prohibit antibody binding. In line with this assumption, approximately the same number of incoming capsids that rearranged became phosphorylated (Figure 5C), a process that can only occur after endosomal escape. As expected, endosomal alkalization by bafilomycin A1 ($BafA_1$) abrogated endosomal escape and all the capsid rearrangements, including the phosphorylation (Figure 5A,B,E). Similar to $BafA_1$, CQ also raises the endosomal pH but, in contrast to $BafA_1$, CQ promotes B19V endosomal escape by endosome swelling and rupture (Figure 5A) [9]. Accordingly, alkalization of endosomes by CQ had no effect on B19V capsid rearrangement and phosphorylation (Figure 5B,E).

Incoming B19V accumulated progressively in the nuclear fraction reaching a plateau by 2 h pi. As expected, blocking endosomal escape by $BafA_1$ prevented the nuclear accumulation of the capsids (Figure 6B). While the capsids present in the cytoplasmic fraction represented a mixture of intact and rearranged particles, the capsids associated to the nuclear fraction were mostly those that had rearranged, i.e., phosphorylated, undetectable by the conformational antibody and nuclease sensitive, suggesting the existence of a selective transport towards the nucleus for the capsids with accessible genomes. The accumulation of B19V capsids in the nuclear fraction was reversibly abrogated by ciliobrevin D (CbD), which is a specific inhibitor of the ATPase activity of cytoplasmic dynein [47]. CbD had no effect on the capsid rearrangements in the cytoplasm, including phosphorylation and genome externalization. The interference of dynein function had a significant inhibitory effect on the infection, but only when the reversible drug was present during the first hours of the infection (Figure 7), indicating that the accumulation of the incoming capsids with accessible genomes in the nuclear fraction is required for the infection. At present, it is uncertain how many of these particles are inside the nucleus and how many remain at the cytosolic side.

The primer hybridization and extension assay confirmed that incoming B19V particles expose the genome already in the cytoplasm prior to nuclear entry, and that the accessible DNA was an optimal template for complementary-strand synthesis (Figure 8). This observation suggests that initiation of DNA synthesis can proceed while the exposed genome remains associated to its capsid.

This study provides a better understanding of the conditions triggering B19V uncoating at physiological temperatures and allowed the identification of capsid structural transitions that precede genome release. Whether incoming viruses are destabilized by the low-cation environment of the cytosol, as suggested by the in vitro data or by another cellular cue, will have to be confirmed. However, our in vivo data reveal that during the process of entry, B19V employs a mechanism of DNA externalization following a limited capsid rearrangement in the cytoplasm to make the genome sufficiently accessible to the replication machinery of the cell.

Author Contributions: C.R. supervised project; C.R., O.C. and N.R. conceived and designed the experiments; O.C., N.R. and A.M. performed the experiments and analysed the data; S.S. and S.H. performed TEM; C.R. wrote the paper and O.C. and R.L. thoroughly revised it.

Funding: This research received no external funding.

Conflicts of Interest: The authors declare no conflict of interest.

References

1. Young, N.S.; Brown, K.E. Parvovirus B19. *N. Engl. J. Med.* **2004**, *350*, 586–597. [CrossRef] [PubMed]
2. Servey, J.T.; Reamy, B.V.; Hodge, J. Clinical presentations of parvovirus B19 infection. *Am. Fam. Physician* **2007**, *75*, 373–376. [PubMed]
3. Cotmore, S.F.; Mckie, V.C.; Anderson, L.J.; Astell, C.R.; Tattersall1, P.; Tattersall, P. Identification of the Major Structural and Nonstructural Proteins Encoded by Human Parvovirus B19 and Mapping of Their Genes by Procaryotic Expression of Isolated Genomic Fragments. *J. Virol.* **1986**, *60*, 548–557. [PubMed]
4. Kilcher, S.; Mercer, J. DNA virus uncoating. *Virology* **2015**, *479–480*, 578–590. [CrossRef] [PubMed]
5. Suomalainen, M.; Greber, U.F. Uncoating of non-enveloped viruses. *Curr. Opin. Virol.* **2013**, *3*, 27–33. [CrossRef] [PubMed]
6. Ravindran, M.S.; Tsai, B. Viruses Utilize Cellular Cues in Distinct Combination to Undergo Systematic Priming and Uncoating. *PLoS Pathog.* **2016**, *12*, e1005467. [CrossRef]
7. Yamauchi, Y.; Greber, U.F. Principles of Virus Uncoating: Cues and the Snooker Ball. *Traffic* **2016**, *17*, 569–592. [CrossRef]
8. Ros, C.; Bayat, N.; Wolfisberg, R.; Almendral, J.M. Protoparvovirus Cell Entry. *Viruses* **2017**, *9*, 313. [CrossRef]
9. Quattrocchi, S.; Ruprecht, N.; Bönsch, C.; Bieli, S.; Zürcher, C.; Boller, K.; Kempf, C.; Ros, C. Characterization of the early steps of human parvovirus B19 infection. *J. Virol.* **2012**, *86*, 9274–9284. [CrossRef]
10. Cotmore, S.F.; Tattersall, P. Parvoviral Host Range and Cell Entry Mechanisms. *Adv. Virus Res.* **2007**, *70*, 183–232.
11. Harbison, C.E.; Chiorini, J.A.; Parrish, C.R. The parvovirus capsid odyssey: From the cell surface to the nucleus. *Trends Microbiol.* **2008**, *16*, 208–214. [CrossRef]
12. Parrish, C.R. *Structures and Functions of Parvovirus Capsids and the Process of Cell Infection*; Springer: Berlin/Heidelberg, Germany, 2010; pp. 149–176.
13. Bönsch, C.; Kempf, C.; Ros, C. Interaction of parvovirus B19 with human erythrocytes alters virus structure and cell membrane integrity. *J. Virol.* **2008**, *82*, 11784–11791. [CrossRef]
14. Bönsch, C.; Zuercher, C.; Lieby, P.; Kempf, C.; Ros, C. The globoside receptor triggers structural changes in the B19 virus capsid that facilitate virus internalization. *J. Virol.* **2010**, *84*, 11737–11746. [CrossRef]
15. Leisi, R.; Ruprecht, N.; Kempf, C.; Ros, C. Parvovirus B19 uptake is a highly selective process controlled by VP1u, a novel determinant of viral tropism. *J. Virol.* **2013**, *87*, 13161–13167. [CrossRef]
16. Leisi, R.; Von Nordheim, M.; Ros, C.; Kempf, C. The VP1u Receptor Restricts Parvovirus B19 Uptake to Permissive Erythroid Cells. *Viruses* **2016**, *8*, 265. [CrossRef]
17. Zhang, W.; Tung, C.-H. Lysosome Enlargement Enhanced Photochemotherapy Using a Multifunctional Nanogel. *ACS Appl. Mater. Interfaces* **2018**, *10*, 4343–4348. [CrossRef]
18. Suikkanen, S.; Aaltonen, T.; Nevalainen, M.; Välilehto, O.; Lindholm, L.; Vuento, M.; Vihinen-Ranta, M. Exploitation of microtubule cytoskeleton and dynein during parvoviral traffic toward the nucleus. *J. Virol.* **2003**, *77*, 10270–10279. [CrossRef]
19. Kelkar, S.; De, B.P.; Gao, G.; Wilson, J.M.; Crystal, R.G.; Leopold, P.L. A common mechanism for cytoplasmic dynein-dependent microtubule binding shared among adeno-associated virus and adenovirus serotypes. *J. Virol.* **2006**, *80*, 7781–7785. [CrossRef]
20. Hirosue, S.; Senn, K.; Clément, N.; Nonnenmacher, M.; Gigout, L.; Linden, R.M.; Weber, T. Effect of inhibition of dynein function and microtubule-altering drugs on AAV2 transduction. *Virology* **2007**, *367*, 10–18. [CrossRef]
21. Lyi, S.M.; Tan, M.J.A.; Parrish, C.R. Parvovirus particles and movement in the cellular cytoplasm and effects of the cytoskeleton. *Virology* **2014**, *456–457*, 342–352. [CrossRef]
22. Vihinen-Ranta, M.; Kakkola, L.; Kalela, A.; Vilja, P.; Vuento, M. Characterization of a Nuclear Localization Signal of Canine Parvovirus Capsid Proteins. *Eur. J. Biochem.* **1997**, *250*, 389–394. [CrossRef]

23. Sonntag, F.; Bleker, S.; Leuchs, B.; Fischer, R.; Kleinschmidt, J.A. Adeno-Associated Virus Type 2 Capsids with Externalized VP1/VP2 Trafficking Domains Are Generated prior to Passage through the Cytoplasm and Are Maintained until Uncoating Occurs in the Nucleus. *J. Virol.* **2006**, *80*, 11040. [CrossRef]
24. Johnson, J.S.; Li, C.; DiPrimio, N.; Weinberg, M.S.; McCown, T.J.; Samulski, R.J. Mutagenesis of adeno-associated virus type 2 capsid protein VP1 uncovers new roles for basic amino acids in trafficking and cell-specific transduction. *J. Virol.* **2010**, *84*, 8888–8902. [CrossRef]
25. Popa-Wagner, R.; Porwal, M.; Kann, M.; Reuss, M.; Weimer, M.; Florin, L.; Kleinschmidt, J.A. Impact of VP1-Specific Protein Sequence Motifs on Adeno-Associated Virus Type 2 Intracellular Trafficking and Nuclear Entry. *J. Virol.* **2012**, *86*, 9163. [CrossRef]
26. Nicolson, S.C.; Samulski, R.J. Recombinant adeno-associated virus utilizes host cell nuclear import machinery to enter the nucleus. *J. Virol.* **2014**, *88*, 4132–4144. [CrossRef]
27. Cohen, S.; Marr, A.K.; Garcin, P.; Panté, N. Nuclear envelope disruption involving host caspases plays a role in the parvovirus replication cycle. *J. Virol.* **2011**, *85*, 4863–4874. [CrossRef]
28. Fay, N.; Panté, N. Old foes, new understandings: Nuclear entry of small non-enveloped DNA viruses. *Curr. Opin. Virol.* **2015**, *12*, 59–65. [CrossRef]
29. Lux, K.; Goerlitz, N.; Schlemminger, S.; Perabo, L.; Goldnau, D.; Endell, J.; Leike, K.; Kofler, D.M.; Finke, S.; Hallek, M.; et al. Green fluorescent protein-tagged adeno-associated virus particles allow the study of cytosolic and nuclear trafficking. *J. Virol.* **2005**, *79*, 11776–11787. [CrossRef]
30. Farr, G.A.; Tattersall, P. A conserved leucine that constricts the pore through the capsid fivefold cylinder plays a central role in parvoviral infection. *Virology* **2004**, *323*, 243–256. [CrossRef]
31. Bleker, S.; Sonntag, F.; Kleinschmidt, J.A. Mutational analysis of narrow pores at the fivefold symmetry axes of adeno-associated virus type 2 capsids reveals a dual role in genome packaging and activation of phospholipase A2 activity. *J. Virol.* **2005**, *79*, 2528–2540. [CrossRef]
32. Farr, G.A.; Cotmore, S.F.; Tattersall, P. VP2 cleavage and the leucine ring at the base of the fivefold cylinder control pH-dependent externalization of both the VP1 N terminus and the genome of minute virus of mice. *J. Virol.* **2006**, *80*, 161–171. [CrossRef]
33. Plevka, P.; Hafenstein, S.; Li, L.; D'Abrgamo, A.; Cotmore, S.F.; Rossmann, M.G.; Tattersall, P.; Tattersall, P. Structure of a packaging-defective mutant of minute virus of mice indicates that the genome is packaged via a pore at a 5-fold axis. *J. Virol.* **2011**, *85*, 4822–4827. [CrossRef]
34. Cotmore, S.F.; Tattersall, P. Parvoviruses: Small Does Not Mean Simple. *Annu. Rev. Virol.* **2014**, *1*, 517–537. [CrossRef]
35. Kaufmann, B.; Simpson, A.A.; Rossmann, M.G. The structure of human parvovirus B19. *Proc. Natl. Acad. Sci. USA* **2004**, *101*, 11628–11633. [CrossRef]
36. Cotmore, S.F.; D'Abramo, A.M.; Ticknor, C.M.; Tattersall, P. Controlled Conformational Transitions in the MVM Virion Expose the VP1 N-Terminus and Viral Genome without Particle Disassembly. *Virology* **1999**, *254*, 169–181. [CrossRef]
37. Turnbull, A.E.; Skulimowski, A.; Smythe, J.A.; Alexander, I.E. Adeno-Associated Virus Vectors Show Variable Dependence on Divalent Cations for Thermostability: Implications for Purification and Handling. *Hum. Gene Ther.* **2000**, *11*, 629–635. [CrossRef]
38. Ros, C.; Baltzer, C.; Mani, B.; Kempf, C. Parvovirus uncoating in vitro reveals a mechanism of DNA release without capsid disassembly and striking differences in encapsidated DNA stability. *Virology* **2006**, *345*, 137–147. [CrossRef]
39. Cotmore, S.F.; Tattersall, P. Mutations at the base of the icosahedral five-fold cylinders of minute virus of mice induce 3′-to-5′ genome uncoating and critically impair entry functions. *J. Virol.* **2012**, *86*, 69–80. [CrossRef]
40. Horowitz, E.D.; Rahman, K.S.; Bower, B.D.; Dismuke, D.J.; Falvo, M.R.; Griffith, J.D.; Harvey, S.C.; Asokan, A. Biophysical and ultrastructural characterization of adeno-associated virus capsid uncoating and genome release. *J. Virol.* **2013**, *87*, 2994–3002. [CrossRef]
41. Bernaud, J.; Rossi, A.; Fis, A.; Gardette, L.; Aillot, L.; Büning, H.; Castelnovo, M.; Salvetti, A.; Faivre-Moskalenko, C. Characterization of AAV vector particle stability at the single-capsid level. *J. Biol. Phys.* **2018**, *44*, 181–194. [CrossRef]
42. Cotmore, S.F.; Hafenstein, S.; Tattersall, P. Depletion of virion-associated divalent cations induces parvovirus minute virus of mice to eject its genome in a 3′-to-5′ direction from an otherwise intact viral particle. *J. Virol.* **2010**, *84*, 1945–1956. [CrossRef]

43. Sun, Y.; Klose, T.; Liu, Y.; Modrow, S.; Rossmann, M.G. Structure of parvovirus B19 decorated by Fabs from a human antibody. *J. Virol.* **2019**. [CrossRef]
44. Gigler, A.; Dorsch, S.; Hemauer, A.; Williams, C.; Kim, S.; Young, N.S.; Zolla-Pazner, S.; Wolf, H.; Gorny, M.K.; Modrow, S. Generation of neutralizing human monoclonal antibodies against parvovirus B19 proteins. *J. Virol.* **1999**, *73*, 1974–1979.
45. Zhong, L.; Li, B.; Jayandharan, G.; Mah, C.S.; Govindasamy, L.; Agbandje-McKenna, M.; Herzog, R.W.; Weigel-Van Aken, K.A.; Hobbs, J.A.; Zolotukhin, S.; et al. Tyrosine-phosphorylation of AAV2 vectors and its consequences on viral intracellular trafficking and transgene expression. *Virology* **2008**, *381*, 194–202. [CrossRef]
46. Roberts, A.J.; Kon, T.; Knight, P.J.; Sutoh, K.; Burgess, S.A. Functions and mechanics of dynein motor proteins. *Nat. Rev. Mol. Cell Biol.* **2013**, *14*, 713–726. [CrossRef]
47. Firestone, A.J.; Weinger, J.S.; Maldonado, M.; Barlan, K.; Langston, L.D.; O'Donnell, M.; Gelfand, V.I.; Kapoor, T.M.; Chen, J.K. Small-molecule inhibitors of the AAA+ ATPase motor cytoplasmic dynein. *Nature* **2012**, *484*, 125–129. [CrossRef]
48. Sainath, R.; Gallo, G. The Dynein Inhibitor Ciliobrevin D Inhibits the Bi-directional Transport of Organelles along Sensory Axons and Impairs NGF- Mediated Regulation of Growth Cones and Axon Branches. *Dev. Neurobiol.* **2015**, *75*, 757–777. [CrossRef]
49. Tsao, J.; Chapman, M.S.; Agbandje, M.; Keller, W.; Smith, K.; Wu, H.; Luo, M.; Smith, T.J.; Rossmann, M.G.; Compans, R.W.; et al. The three-dimensional structure of canine parvovirus and its functional implications. *Science* **1991**, *251*, 1456–1464. [CrossRef]
50. Chapman, M.S.; Rossmann, M.G. Structure, Sequence, and Function Correlations among Parvoviruses. *Virology* **1993**, *194*, 491–508. [CrossRef]
51. Llamas-Saiz, A.L.; Agbandje-McKenna, M.; Wikoff, W.R.; Bratton, J.; Tattersall, P.; Rossmann, M.G. IUCr Structure Determination of Minute Virus of Mice. *Acta Crystallogr. Sect. D Biol. Crystallogr.* **1997**, *53*, 93–102. [CrossRef]
52. Agbandje-McKenna, M.; Llamas-Saiz, A.L.; Wang, F.; Tattersall, P.; Rossmann, M.G. Functional implications of the structure of the murine parvovirus, minute virus of mice. *Structure* **1998**, *6*, 1369–1381. [CrossRef]
53. Kronenberg, S.; Böttcher, B.; von der Lieth, C.W.; Bleker, S.; Kleinschmidt, J.A. A conformational change in the adeno-associated virus type 2 capsid leads to the exposure of hidden VP1 N termini. *J. Virol.* **2005**, *79*, 5296–5303. [CrossRef]
54. Castellanos, M.; Pérez, R.; Rodríguez-Huete, A.; Grueso, E.; Almendral, J.M.; Mateu, M.G. A slender tract of glycine residues is required for translocation of the VP2 protein N-terminal domain through the parvovirus MVM capsid channel to initiate infection. *Biochem. J.* **2013**, *455*, 87–94. [CrossRef]
55. Kaufmann, B.; Chipman, P.R.; Kostyuchenko, V.A.; Modrow, S.; Rossmann, M.G. Visualization of the externalized VP2 N termini of infectious human parvovirus B19. *J. Virol.* **2008**, *82*, 7306–7312. [CrossRef]
56. Cotmore, S.F.; Tattersall, P. Genome packaging sense is controlled by the efficiency of the nick site in the right-end replication origin of parvoviruses minute virus of mice and LuIII. *J. Virol.* **2005**, *79*, 2287–2300. [CrossRef]
57. King, J.A.; Dubielzig, R.; Grimm, D.; Kleinschmidt, J.A. DNA helicase-mediated packaging of adeno-associated virus type 2 genomes into preformed capsids. *EMBO J.* **2001**, *20*, 3282–3291. [CrossRef]
58. Ivanovska, I.; Wuite, G.; Jönsson, B.; Evilevitch, A. Internal DNA pressure modifies stability of WT phage. *Proc. Natl. Acad. Sci. USA* **2007**, *104*, 9603–9608. [CrossRef]
59. Bauer, D.W.; Li, D.; Huffman, J.; Homa, F.L.; Wilson, K.; Leavitt, J.C.; Casjens, S.R.; Baines, J.; Evilevitch, A. Exploring the Balance between DNA Pressure and Capsid Stability in Herpesviruses and Phages. *J. Virol.* **2015**, *89*, 9288–9298. [CrossRef]
60. Shirley, J.A.; Beards, G.M.; Thouless, M.E.; Flewett, T.H. The influence of divalent cations on the stability of human rotavirus. *Arch. Virol.* **1981**, *67*, 1–9. [CrossRef]
61. Sherman, M.B.; Guenther, R.H.; Tama, F.; Sit, T.L.; Brooks, C.L.; Mikhailov, A.M.; Orlova, E.V.; Baker, T.S.; Lommel, S.A. Removal of divalent cations induces structural transitions in red clover necrotic mosaic virus, revealing a potential mechanism for RNA release. *J. Virol.* **2006**, *80*, 10395–10406. [CrossRef]
62. Plevka, P.; Kazaks, A.; Voronkova, T.; Kotelovica, S.; Dishlers, A.; Liljas, L.; Tars, K. The structure of bacteriophage phiCb5 reveals a role of the RNA genome and metal ions in particle stability and assembly. *J. Mol. Biol.* **2009**, *391*, 635–647. [CrossRef]

63. Llauró, A.; Coppari, E.; Imperatori, F.; Bizzarri, A.R.; Castón, J.R.; Santi, L.; Cannistraro, S.; de Pablo, P.J. Calcium ions modulate the mechanics of tomato bushy stunt virus. *Biophys. J.* **2015**, *109*, 390–397. [CrossRef]
64. Kawano, M.; Xing, L.; Tsukamoto, H.; Inoue, T.; Handa, H.; Cheng, R.H. Calcium Bridge Triggers Capsid Disassembly in the Cell Entry Process of Simian Virus 40. *J. Biol. Chem.* **2009**, *284*, 34703–34712. [CrossRef]
65. Hu, X.; Dong, Q.; Yang, J.; Zhang, Y. Recognizing metal and acid radical ion-binding sites by integrating ab initio modeling with template-based transferals. *Bioinformatics* **2016**, *32*, 3260–3269. [CrossRef]
66. Clapham, D.E. Calcium Signaling. *Cell* **2007**, *131*, 1047–1058. [CrossRef]
67. Vihinen-Ranta, M.; Wang, D.; Weichert, W.S.; Parrish, C.R. The VP1 N-terminal sequence of canine parvovirus affects nuclear transport of capsids and efficient cell infection. *J. Virol.* **2002**, *76*, 1884–1891. [CrossRef]
68. Ros, C.; Kempf, C. The ubiquitin–proteasome machinery is essential for nuclear translocation of incoming minute virus of mice. *Virology* **2004**, *324*, 350–360. [CrossRef]
69. Mani, B.; Baltzer, C.; Valle, N.; Almendral, J.M.; Kempf, C.; Ros, C. Low pH-dependent endosomal processing of the incoming parvovirus minute virus of mice virion leads to externalization of the VP1 N-terminal sequence (N-VP1), N-VP2 cleavage, and uncoating of the full-length genome. *J. Virol.* **2006**, *80*, 1015–1024. [CrossRef]

viruses

MDPI

Review

Advances in the Development of Antiviral Strategies against Parvovirus B19

Elisabetta Manaresi and Giorgio Gallinella *

Department of Pharmacy and Biotechnology, University of Bologna, I-40138 Bologna, Italy
* Correspondence: giorgio.gallinella@unibo.it; Tel.: +39-051-4290900

Received: 25 June 2019; Accepted: 17 July 2019; Published: 18 July 2019

Abstract: Parvovirus B19 (B19V) is a human pathogenic virus, responsible for an ample range of clinical manifestations. Infections are usually mild, self-limiting, and controlled by the development of a specific immune response, but in many cases clinical situations can be more complex and require therapy. Presently available treatments are only supportive, symptomatic, or unspecific, such as administration of intravenous immunoglobulins, and often of limited efficacy. The development of antiviral strategies against B19V should be considered of highest relevance for increasing the available options for more specific and effective therapeutic treatments. This field of research has been explored in recent years, registering some achievements as well as interesting future perspectives. In addition to immunoglobulins, some compounds have been shown to possess inhibitory activity against B19V. Hydroxyurea is an antiproliferative drug used in the treatment of sickle-cell disease that also possesses inhibitory activity against B19V. The nucleotide analogues Cidofovir and its lipid conjugate Brincidofovir are broad-range antivirals mostly active against dsDNA viruses, which showed an antiviral activity also against B19V. Newly synthesized coumarin derivatives offer possibilities for the development of molecules with antiviral activity. Identification of some flavonoid molecules, with direct inhibitory activity against the viral non-structural (NS) protein, indicates a possible line of development for direct antiviral agents. Continuing research in the field, leading to better knowledge of the viral lifecycle and a precise understanding of virus–cell interactions, will offer novel opportunities for developing more efficient, targeted antiviral agents, which can be translated into available therapeutic options.

Keywords: parvovirus B19; erythroid progenitor cells; antiviral compounds; intravenous immunoglobulin (IVIG); hydroxyurea; cidofovir; brincidofovir; coumarin derivatives; flavonoids

---

1. Introduction

Parvovirus B19 (B19V), a single-stranded DNA virus in the family *Parvoviridae* [1], is a human pathogenic virus, characterized by a selective but not exclusive tropism for erythroid progenitor cells. Globally diffuse, it is responsible for an ample range of clinical manifestations, whose characteristics and outcomes depend on the interplay between the viral properties as well as the physiological and immune status of the infected individuals. The clinical attitude towards B19V infection is normally conservative, in the idea that consequences of infections are mild, self-limiting, and controlled by the development of a specific immune response. However, clinical situations can be more complex, depending on the genetic or physiological background of the host, in the case of underlying diseases or inefficiency of the immune response, and in the evenience of maternal transmission to fetus. Thus, in many situations clinical care is needed, relying on the currently available treatments that are only supportive, symptomatic, or unspecific, and in many cases of limited efficacy. Research aimed at the development of antiviral strategies should therefore be considered of highest importance for increasing the available options for more specific and effective therapeutic treatments. This field of research has been explored in recent years, and a few published works already report some achievements as well as interesting future perspectives.

2. B19V Structure

B19V shares genetic and structural features common to the family (comprehensively reviewed in [2,3]). The genome, a linear ssDNA molecule of 5.6 kb, is organized in a unique internal region, containing all the coding sequences, flanked by inverted terminal regions that serve as origins of replication (ORF). In its internal region, the genome presents two major ORFs, in the left side for the non-structural protein (NS), and in the right side for the two colinear capsid proteins, VP1 and VP2. Minor ORFs can encode other non-structural proteins, including a 11 kDa protein and the less characterized 9.0 and 7.5 kDa proteins. The capsid forms an icosahedral structure in T = 1 arrangement, about 25 nm in diameter, composed of 5–10% VP1 and 90–95% VP2 proteins. It is resolved in its atomic structure for the capsid shell but not for the N-terminus of VP1 (VP1 unique region, VP1u) [4]. A schematic diagram of B19V genome organization is depicted in Figure 1.

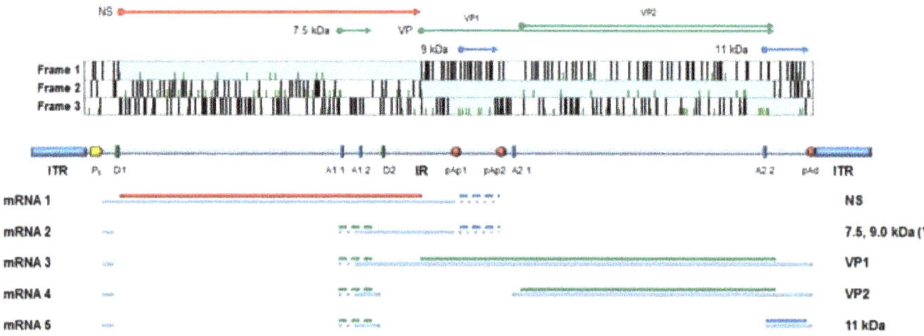

Figure 1. B19V genome organization. Top: major open reading frames identified in the positive strand of genome; arrows indicate the coding sequences for the viral proteins. NS, non-structural protein; VP, structural proteins, colinear VP1 and VP2, assembled in a T = 1 icosahedral capsid; and 7.5 kDa, 9.0 kDa, and 11 kDa: minor non-structural proteins. Center: a schematic diagram of B19V genome indicating the two inverted terminal regions (ITR), and the internal region (IR) with the distribution of cis-acting functional sites (P6, promoter; pAp1, pAp2, proximal cleavage-polyadenylation sites; pAd, distal cleavage-polyadenylation site; D1 and D2, splice donor sites; A1.1, A1.2, A2.1, and A2.2, splice acceptor sites). Bottom: simplified transcription map of B19V genome, indicating the five classes of mRNAs (mRNA 1–5) with respective alternative splicing/cleavage forms (dashed), and their coding potential. Adapted from Reference [5].

3. The Lifecycle

B19V shows a selective tropism for cells in the erythroid lineage in the bone marrow, cells that are susceptible to viral infection and permissive for a productive replicative cycle depending on their differentiation stage and proliferation rate. Such tropism, and a productive outcome of infection, can be considered the result of a double adaptation of virus to a specific cell population. The first involves the recognition and binding to specialized receptors that define as target cells a restricted cell population with a high proliferative potential, namely erythroid progenitor cells and in particular cells at the proerythroblast differentiation stage. The second involves a strict dependence of viral replication to the cellular response to convergent lineage-specific physiological stimuli, such as Erythropoietin (Epo) pathway activation and hypoxia. A schematic diagram of B19V lifecycle is depicted in Figure 2.

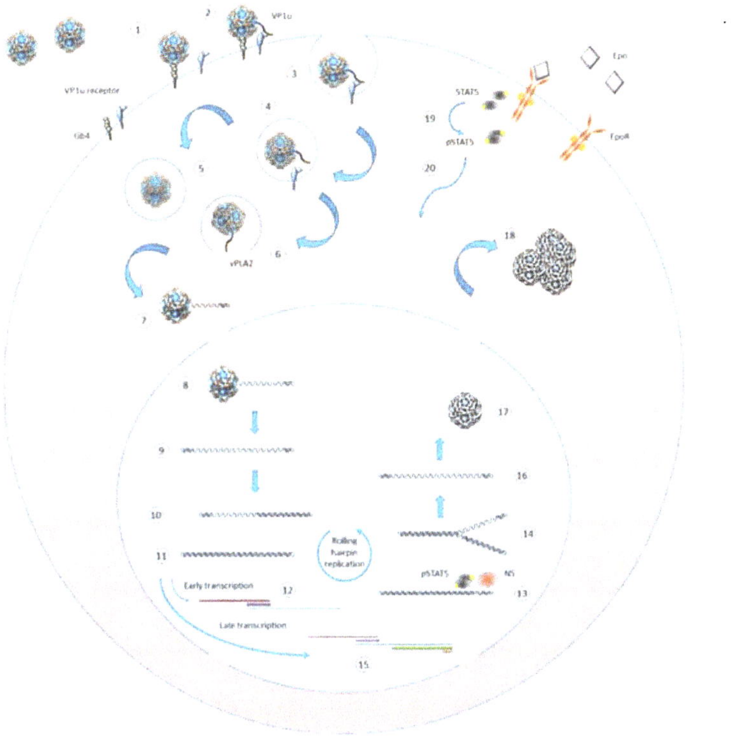

Figure 2. Outline of B19V replicative cycle in erythroid progenitor cells. 1: virion binding to globoside. 2: extrusion of VP1 unique (VP1u) region and binding to an erythroid specific receptor. 3: clathrin-mediated endocytosis. 4: virions in endosomal vesicles. 5: virion processing within endosomes. 6: VP1u-associated viral phospholipase (vPLA2) mediated virion escape from endosomes. 7: partial uncoating and externalization of viral ssDNA. 8: translocation in the nucleus and complete uncoating. 9: parental ssDNA and onset of macromolecular syntheses. 10: hairpin-primed second strand synthesis. 11: formation of dsDNA replicative intermediate. 12: early phase of transcription on the parental template, mainly of mRNAs for NS protein. 13: dsDNA nicked by NS and priming of replication in coordination with cellular proteins. 14: replication by a rolling hairpin mechanism, via self-primed single-strand displacement mechanisms. 15: late phase of transcription on the replicative intermediates, mainly of mRNAs for VP and 11kDa proteins. 16: progeny ssDNA released from the replicative intermediates. 17: incapsidation of progeny ssDNA molecules in newly formed virions. 18: accumulation of virions before their release via cell lysis or apoptosis. 19: Epo binding by Epo receptor (EpoR), EpoR activation, and STAT5 phosphorilation. 20: pSTAT translocation in the nucleus where it is essential for formation of a functional replicative complex.

Binding events involve domains on the viral capsid interacting with cellular receptors. An initial event is the interaction of the capsid shell with the membrane glycolipid globoside, which is present on erythroid progenitors, as well as on mature erythrocytes where it constitutes blood antigen P, but also on many other tissues mainly of mesodermic origin [6]. Since its first identification as a binding receptor [7], and the observation that its absence prevented infection in cells as well as individuals [8], subsequent reports presented contrasting evidence, either characterizing or questioning the binding of capsids to globoside as a necessary first step for cell infection [9–11]. However, even a transient binding of a capsid to globoside can trigger conformational modifications leading to exposure of the VP1u region [12], allowing interaction of its N-terminal region with a specific, but yet uncharacterized receptor whose distribution in cells of erythroid lineage matches the susceptibility of cells to productive infection [13–15]. Following binding, internalization via clathrin-mediated endocytosis can occur, the phospholipase activity associated to the VP1u region consents escape from the endosome, and by subsequent coordinated intracellular transport and uncoating events, a single-stranded genome is finally delivered in the nuclear environment [16,17].

In the nucleus, a series of macromolecular syntheses occurs leading to a productive replicative cycle [18,19]. On the single-stranded DNA template, cellular DNA repair synthesis generates a double-stranded DNA template that can serve for both transcription and replication of the viral genome. An early phase of transcription mainly produces mRNAs coding for the NS protein, which, acting together with cellular replicative machinery promote replication of the genome by a rolling hairpin mechanism. Replication is then followed by a late phase of transcription, mainly producing mRNAs coding for the structural VP and 11 kDa proteins. Accumulation of VP proteins eventually leads to the assembly of capsids, encapsidation of progeny single-stranded genomes, and release of virions from infected cells.

In the erythroid lineage, a productive viral replication and release of virus are restricted to differentiation stages ranging from colony forming unit-erythroid (CFU-E) to erythroblasts, indicating that both lineage- and differentiation-specific factors are necessarily involved in promoting viral macromolecular syntheses [20]. Viral replication is critically dependent on erythropoietin stimulation and is enhanced in hypoxic conditions [21,22], through a signaling cascade leading to formation of a functional replicative complex involving the viral NS in concert with cellular proteins, including the DNA replication polymerase δ and polymerase α [23]. A crucial role is exerted by phosphorylated STAT5 protein, which is a common terminal of Epo- and hypoxia-stimulated pathways [24]. A key event is the regulated switch from the early pattern of viral expression, characterized by transcription on the parental template mainly leading to NS protein production, to the late pattern of expression, with coordinated onset of DNA replication and enhanced transcription of the progeny templates leading to increased VP protein production [20]. In addition, the 11 kDa protein, expressed in the late phase, may also play a role in facilitating viral genome replication [25,26]. A deeper understanding of the mechanistic details of viral replication, including fine characterization of the molecular machinery and activation pathways involved, is in progress and will offer increasing opportunities to identify specific targets for the development of antiviral strategies.

In infected erythroid progenitors, the virus exerts a complex series of effects on the cellular environment, including induction of a DNA damage response, arrest of the cell cycle, and induction of apoptosis [27,28]. This cytotoxicity causes a temporary block in erythropoiesis and can lead to a transient or persistent erythroid aplasia. The interactions between the viral and cellular factors are still incompletely characterized, for example, in the possible activation of cellular sensors to viral infection, in the induction of cellular responses to restrict viral replication, or in priming of innate immunity. Therefore, in this subject area, a better understanding of the mechanistic details will probably offer opportunities to define novel antiviral strategies.

In addition to erythroid progenitors, the virus can also, although less efficiently, infect other cell types in diverse tissues. B Lymphocytes in tonsillar tissues have been shown to harbor the viral genome, and can be infected by an antibody-dependent uptake mechanism [29]. Endothelial cells constitute a diffuse cellular target susceptible to viral infection, also by an antibody-dependent mechanism [30]. The viral genome has progressively been detected in almost all solid tissues and organs, mostly in endothelial or stromal cells but occasionally also in parenchymal cells [31]. In non-erythroid tissues, infection is usually abortive, viral DNA can remain silent, and when transcription occurs this is normally at low levels. In these cases, transcription is mostly limited to early mRNAs—including those for the NS protein—and transcription of late mRNAs, including those for VP proteins, has been documented in tissues such as heart, liver, synovia, and skin. In these cells, a limited expression of viral proteins may contribute to pathological effects mainly by indirect mechanisms, such as modification of the cellular expression profile and the induction of inflammatory or autoimmune processes [31]. The frequent outcome is rather the persistence of the viral genome in tissues [32], probably in the episomal form although integration of the viral genome in the cellular genome of erythroid progenitor cells has been detected in an in vitro experimental system [33]. Reactivation, if it can happen, appears to be a sporadic event, not firmly documented in the literature. Notably, persistence of the viral genome in tissues appears to be lifelong and constitutes a repository of archived genomic sequences [34,35], also leading to exciting hints regarding the evolutionary history and genetic diversification within the species [36].

4. The Pathologies

B19V is a virus commonly diffuse in the population, and responsible for a wide spectrum of clinical manifestations (comprehensively reviewed in [2,3]). Following contact, normally through the respiratory route, the virus gains access to the circulation and reaches the bone marrow where it can infect erythroid progenitor cells. The pathogenic effects, typically in the form of pure red cell aplasia (PRCA), result from the capacity of the virus to induce cell-cycle arrest, block erythroid differentiation and proliferation, and eventually apoptosis of infected cells. The clinical impact on the host depends on the degree of inhibition of erythropoiesis, linked to the volume and turnover rate of the erythroid compartment, while the course of infection depends on the capacity of the immune system to mount an effective specific response [37].

In individuals with normal erythropoiesis and immune system response, bone marrow infection is limited in extent and temporal frame, is usually asymptomatic from hematological perspective, and is progressively cleared by the development of a neutralizing immune response. In the presence of an altered erythropoietic process and an expanded erythroid compartment, because of underlying genetic defects or stressed physiological conditions affecting the cellular turnover, infection can induce a more severe block in erythropoiesis, which usually manifests in the form of an acute episode of profound anemia. In the presence of defects of the immune system and a consequent inability to control, neutralize, and clear the virus, infection may become persistent and manifest with chronic anemia of different grades. Rarely, the infection has been linked to bone marrow necrosis [38], in addition to a wide variety of blood diseases and cytopenias of lineages other than the erythroid lineage [37], by mechanisms that still require investigation.

Productive replication in the bone marrow leads to a secondary viremic phase initially characterized by high viral load levels (up to 10^{12} virus/mL), followed by a systemic distribution of the virus and preluding to possible late clinical manifestations. In this later phase, both the virus and specific antibodies are present in the blood, so that immune-mediated inflammatory processes are mainly assumed to explain possible pathological processes. Different non-erythroid cell types, including endothelial, stromal, or synovial cells, can also be infected, and pathogenetic mechanisms directly related to the viral presence and activity can be hypothesized. However, only sporadically have some specific markers of viral activity been definitely localized within non-erythroid cells, and causally linked to pathological processes by viral-induced, usually proinflammatory, pathogenetic mechanisms [31].

Typically in this later phase, B19V infection is the cause of erythema infectiosum in children, and of arthropathies mainly in adult patients, with a tendency to chronicity. While B19V has been progressively detected and implicated in many clinical situations involving disparate tissues and organs, in particular it has been recognized as a relevant cardiotropic virus, responsible of acute myocarditis and possibly involved in the development of chronic cardiomyopathies (an intense debate recently summarized in [39]). B19V can be involved in the development of autoimmune disorders [40], and possible mechanisms involving epitope cross-reactivity [41] or the formation of apoptotic bodies induced by NS protein expression have been proposed [42,43].

B19V can cross the placenta and infect the fetus [44], where infection of erythroid progenitors can induce a block in fetal erythropoiesis whose effect will depend on the fetal developmental stage, the rate of expansion of the fetal erythroid compartment, and the maturity and efficacy of both maternal and fetal immune response. The virus can be detected in erythroid progenitor cells, located in liver and/or bone marrow depending on the gestational age, in erythroid cells circulating in the vessels of several tissues, in endothelial placental cells [45], and in the amniotic fluid [46]. Transplacental transmission can occur in about 30–50% of cases, and lead to fetal hydrops and/or fetal death in ~10% of cases (comprehensively reviewed in [47,48]).

5. Need for Treatment and Current Options

Although most infections are mild and self-limiting, there are situations where B19V infection can be severe and lead to the need of clinical care. These include hematological complications, from transient aplastic crisis to chronic pure red cell aplasia, to rarer clinical presentations involving bone marrow necrosis or autoimmune-mediated hematological disorders [37]. The role of B19V in acute or chronic myocarditis, although debated, is of relevance [39]. More classical manifestations such as arthropathies can chronicize and be invalidating to patients for extended time periods [40], and even dermatological manifestations can be atypical, severe, and lead to hospitalization [49]. Intrauterine transmission can severely affect the fetus, possibly leading to fetal death, development of fetal hydrops, and in rare cases congenital infection [44,47,48].

The diverse clinical presentations first of all call for an appropriate diagnostic approach [5]. B19V infections should be investigated not as a rare entity, but as a frequent possibility, especially in the context of peaks of incidence. Molecular and immunological diagnostic assays are now widely available and their rational use can lead to a prompt diagnosis and to appropriate clinical management. The clinical attitude towards B19V infection is normally conservative, in the idea that infection is self-limiting, and that the development of a specific immune response as measured by the production of specific and neutralizing antibodies will be effective in controlling the virus. However, this is not always the case. Acute infections can be clinically severe while an impaired immune response can lead to persistent infections. When required, supportive or symptomatic treatments can be used. Blood transfusions are required to overcome acute or chronic anemia, nonsteroidal anti-inflammatory drugs are generally used although with limited efficacy to relieve inflammatory symptoms in cases of arthritis and arthralgias, while scattered case reports suggest the utility of corticosteroids in cases of atypical inflammatory presentations. The management of intrauterine infections is also conservative, and when fetal Hb levels fall below a clinically defined threshold as measured by non-invasive Doppler ultrasonography determination of middle cerebral artery peak systolic velocity, it can rely with good success rates on intrauterine transfusions [50].

The gap in the development of antiviral strategies and in particular the availability of antiviral drugs directed against B19V as compared to other viruses is striking [51]. A vaccine against B19V is an attainable goal, technically feasible, composed of VLPs produced in heterologous expression systems, and following progressive development [52–54] now shows promising characteristics in terms of immunogenicity and absence of reactogenicity [55,56]. However, because of the lack of relevant animal models, it is still at the very beginning of clinical evaluation, and its implementation is not included among the WHO priorities. Administration of high doses of intravenous immunoglobulins (IVIG) is presently considered the only available option to neutralize infectious virus and mainly finds indication to control infections in cases of an impaired immune system response [57–59]. The beneficial effects of IVIG treatments are recognized, even if high-doses and repeated cycles may be required, and it is considered that IVIG are not sufficient to resolve infection unless a patient's own antiviral immune response develops and becomes effective.

Active research in the development and refinement of antiviral strategies directed against B19V should be considered of the highest relevance. In addition to the use of IVIG, the discovery of antiviral drugs with significant activity against B19V would offer important opportunities in the treatment and management of severe clinical manifestations. In particular, these would include the treatment of severe hematological complications in the acute phase of the infection, especially in subjects with stressed erythropoiesis, or the treatment of chronic infections in case of deficits of the immune system. Furthermore, antiviral compounds might be used in the implementation of prophylactic treatments, for example to reduce the risk of infection in immunosuppressed individuals as part of a general preventive or pre-emptive approach.

6. Passive Immunization

Administration of IVIG is currently the indicated treatment when patients are in need of controlling B19V infections, in the case of chronic infections or more rarely in acute infections with clinical severity, and inability of mounting an efficient immune response. Several accepted guidelines suggest cycles of 2 g/kg in 5-days courses, to be repeated if unsuccessful, but studies have not been carried out to determine an optimal therapeutic scheme. Efficacy of IVIG treatment has been assumed more on circumstantial and empirical evidence than on high-quality evidence-based assessments [60]. Available data obtained from small case series and literature reviews indicate that IVIG treatments are effective with good success rates [61], but IVIG treatments are likely to be underreported in the literature, and this more so in the case of failure.

The mechanism of action of IVIG is also not fully investigated. Possibilities include capacity of inhibiting the virus by direct binding of specific anti-B19 Ig, normally present in IVIG preparations, to functionally relevant epitopes on the viral capsid, thus preventing infectivity. However, in cellular models, binding and penetration steps may not be inhibited, while the successive phases of macromolecular synthesis can be severely impaired, both at transcriptional and replicative levels [62]. Possibly, binding to antibodies prevents the virions from correct intracellular trafficking, uncoating, and translocation of viral genome in the nucleus. In general, IVIGs may also exert their effect via immune modulatory mechanisms [63], and this might contribute to their efficacy, while the possibility exists that in peculiar situations the immune complex formation exacerbates inflammatory stimuli. A peculiar case came from the experience of treating the B19V-related chronic fatigue syndrome, with reports of successful treatments [64] as well as paradoxical response [65].

An alternative to IVIG would be the use of human/humanized monoclonal antibodies specifically targeted to B19V, as more and more are available for other infectious agents. This approach showed promising results in an early initial report [66], but would require further research to become an available option. In this case, a neat definition of relevant neutralizing epitopes is required. It is known from studies in the general population that antibodies recognize largely VP2 conformational antigens coupled to VP1u region linear antigens [67,68]. Neutralizing epitopes are distributed along most of the VP2 protein and in the N-terminal region of the VP1u [69–71]. A comprehensive epitope mapping on the capsid shell surface is still to be obtained, but recently a first structure of a parvovirus B19 capsid complexed to antigen-binding fragments (Fabs) from a human antibody has been obtained by cryo-electron microscopy (cryo-EM), showing binding to a quaternary structure epitope formed by residues from three neighboring VP2 capsid proteins [72]. The structure and location of VP1u is not determined, but it can be observed that the immunogenic region corresponds to the receptor-binding moiety essential for virus infectivity [73].

7. The Quest for Antiviral Agents

So far, some factors have been critically limiting in the search for compounds with antiviral activity against B19V. The virus requires demanding cell culture conditions and in vitro infections show a restrictive pattern with relatively low productivity, thus most experiments need to rely on the availability of the native virus obtained from viremic patients. Research in the field still offers an incomplete characterization of the viral lifecycle, of the viral proteome, and of the molecular machinery coopted to viral replication. The first problem limits the feasibility of a high-throughput screening against available chemical libraries, the second has until now hampered the rational design of specifically targeted drugs. To overcome these barriers, standardized model cell cultures and infectivity assays are required in the first instance. Then, these studies can also take advantage of the availability of cloned viral genomes that possess replicative competence and the ability to yield infectious viruses in standardized conditions.

Mainly, two cellular systems can be used to support viral replication in vitro and study the antiviral activity of tested compounds: primary erythroid progenitor cells (EPCs) and the cell line UT7/EpoS1. EPCs are primary cells that more closely resemble the natural target cells within the bone marrow environment [74]. EPCs obtained from peripheral blood can be cultured in conditions that promote proliferation and differentiation along the erythroid lineage [75], and progressively become permissive to viral replication, mostly at the proerythroblast stage [20]. However, in vitro culture conditions only approximate conditions in the bone marrow environment, and EPCs constitute a heterogeneous population with respect to the differentiation stage, proliferation rate, and metabolic activity. UT7/EpoS1 is a cell line of myeloblastoid origin, the most permissive and commonly used for B19V [76]. Although permissiveness is restricted to only a subset of cells [77], in these, the degree of replication of viral DNA is comparable to EPCs [78,79]. Both EPCs and UT7/EpoS1 cells require Epo stimulation to support viral replication. EPCs and UT7/EpoS1 cells thus provide manageable and appropriate models for investigating compounds with antiviral activity against B19V.

For infection, native virus obtained from viremic serum samples is normally used, with limitations implied due to both the limited availability and the unpredictable variation inherent in the use of individual clinical isolates within a heterogeneous biological matrix such as plasma or serum. The possibility of obtaining virus with complete biological activity starting from cloned DNA templates has been explored. Clone pM20 was established in 2004, has been shown to possess replicative activity, and it has been mainly used in transfection experiments [80]. More recently, functionally competent clones have been constructed starting from a synthetic consensus sequence (named EC01), possessing both replicative activity following transfection and the ability to yield infectious virus at high titers following serial amplification passages in EPCs [81]. In perspective, a crucial advantage of using virus obtained from cloned genomes is the possibility of conducing direct mutagenesis and sequence-function correlation studies to define targets relevant for antivirals.

In the experimental setup, the antiviral effects of tested compounds can be accurately evaluated by qPCR-based assays, to measure the variation in the abundance of viral DNA or mRNAs following a course of infection [78,79]. In situ hybridization (FISH) assays for viral nucleic acids or immunological (IIF) detection of viral proteins, can be used to measure variations in the frequency of productively infected cells [77]. Then, the extent of inhibition of viral replication exerted by the compounds can be determined by standard dose-response curve to yield the EC_{50} values. Concomitant effects of tested compounds on cell viability and cell proliferations rates need to be determined, usually by standard formazan-based, or equivalent assays, and by BrdU incorporation assays, to yield CC_{50} values. Selectivity indexes can then be calculated to assess the specificity of action of a tested compound.

Within this experimental frame, research can be aimed at the discovery of antiviral compounds targeted to crucial functions within the viral lifecycle. Antiviral compounds can be intended for conditioning the cellular environment as non-permissive, or specifically targeted to viral proteins as direct antiviral agents. Recent work in this field led to the first identification of compounds with antiviral activity against B19V. Alternative approaches to antiviral discovery have been followed until now: a strategy based on drug repositioning; a strategy based on investigation of known antiviral compounds for a possible activity against B19V; a serendipity approach in screening small chemical libraries of compounds with possible antiviral activity; and a search for direct antiviral compounds by targeted biochemical screening. The first approach yielded antiviral activity provided by the cell-proliferation inhibitor hydroxyurea (HU) [82], also used as a disease-modifying drug in the treatment of sickle cell disease. The second approach first yielded the acyclic nucleoside phosphonate cidofovir (CDV) [83,84], though with suboptimal activity, and then its lipid conjugate brincidofovir (BCV) [85], with substantially enhanced activity. By the third approach, a few coumarin derivatives showed promising characteristics [86]. In the search for direct antiviral agents, identification of a key function of viral NS protein allowed screening of a small molecule library by which a few compounds showed inhibitory activity, which were then assessed for inhibition of viral replication in a cell-based assay [87]. A summary of the results is reported in Table 1.

Table 1. Compounds with reported activity against B19V.

Compound/Cells	Max Inhibition	EC_{50} (μM [CI])	CC_{50} (μM [CI])	SI (CC_{50}/EC_{50})	References and Notes
HU					Ref [82]
UT7/EpoS1	100% at >1000 μM	96.2 [81.5–118.1]	581.9 [426.5–812.3]	6.0	moi in the range 10^1–10^4
EPCs	100% at >1000 μM	147.1 [121.4–190.4]	584.8 [478.5–722.3]	4.0	moi in the range 10^1–10^4
CDV					Ref [83,85]
UT7/EpoS1	100% at 500 μM	16.1 [12.9–20.2]	>500	ND	moi in the range 10^1–10^4
EPCs	ND	320.5 [173.9–590.7]	>500	ND	moi in the range 10^1–10^4
BCV					Ref [85]
UT7/EpoS1	100% at >10 μM	0.22 [0.19–0.25]	66.8 [62.0–72.9]	303.6	moi in the range 10^1–10^4
EPCs	100% at >100 μM	9.35 [8.84–9.89]	102.9 [87.6–120.8]	11.0	moi in the range 10^1–10^4
BCV (S)					Ref [85]
UT7/EpoS1	100% at >10 μM	0.63 [0.58–0.68]	59.9 [52.7–68.1]	95.1	moi 10^4
EPCs	100% at >100 μM	14.3 [11.8–17.3]	93.4 [68.9–126.6]	6.5	moi 10^4
BCV (R)					Ref [85]
UT7/EpoS1	100% at >100 μM	54.7 [42.7–69.9]	72.1 [62.5–83.1]	1.3	moi 10^4
EPCs	100% at >500 μM	93.0 [77.4–111.8]	146.2 [106.4–200]	1.6	moi 10^4
Coumarin derivatives					Ref [86]
UT7/EpoS1	82.1 at 12.5 μM	6.7	ND	4.0 at 12.5 μM	Compound #7; moi 10^4
EPCs	65.0 at 12.5 μM	ND	ND	2.7 at 12.5 μM	Compound #8; moi 10^4
Flavonoid compounds					Ref [87]
UT7/EpoS1					Following transfection (IIF)
Compound #7	NR	44.2 [25.6–62.8]	194.0 [171.0–216.3]	4.4	
Compound #135	NR	61.1 [60.8–61.4]	227.0 [206.0–248.0]	3.7	
Compound #201	NR	55.1 [47.2–63.0]	180.9 [160.4–201.4]	3.3	
EPCs					Following infection (IIF)
Compound #7	NR	37.6 [34.0–41.2]	55.9 [53.8–58.0]	1.5	
Compound #135	NR	53.9 [46.8–61.0]	89.8 [82.0–97.6]	1.7	
Compound #201	NR	33.5 [32.1–34.9]	60.0 [57.6–62.4]	1.8	

HU: hydroxyurea. CDV: cidofovir. BCV: brincidofovir. BCV (S), BCV (R): brincidofovir enantiomers S and R. SI: Selectivity Index. Moi: multiplicity of infection (genome copies/cell). ND: not determined. NR: not reported.

7.1. Hydroxyurea

Hydroxyurea (HU) is an inhibitor of DNA synthesis targeting cellular ribonucleotide reductase enzyme [88]. HU behaves as a 'virostatic' antiviral agent in combined therapy with deoxynucleoside analogs, with the assumption that HU depletes the intracellular deoxyribonucleotide pools required for viral replication, enhancing deoxynucleoside analogs incorporation [89–92]. Of relevance, the drug finds indication in the therapy for sickle cell disease (SCD) in adults [93], and increasingly in the pediatric SCD population [94], in which B19V infection is a major cause of severe complications.

Experimentally, HU demonstrated a measurable inhibitory effect on B19V replication in both EPCs and UT7/EpoS1 cells [82]. Complete inhibition of viral replication was obtained at >1 mM, and observed EC_{50} values were 96.2 μM and 147.1 μM in UT7/EpoS1 and EPCs, respectively. Cellular DNA replication was also affected with HU concentrations leading to a 50% reduction of DNA synthesis at 706.9 μM and 494.0 μM in UT7/EpoS1 and EPCs, respectively. A cytostatic effect was confirmed in both systems, with a 50% reduction of viability observed at 581.9 μM for UT7/EpoS1, and 584.8 μM for EPCs. The observed reduction in cell viability could be ascribed to the cytostatic effect of the drug rather to a cytotoxic effect related to loss of membrane integrity.

The effective concentrations of HU inhibiting B19V replication are comparable with those obtained for other human pathogenic viruses [89–92], and lower than those interfering with cell proliferation. In both cell systems, HU confirmed its cytostatic and 'virostatic' effects, in agreement with its inhibitory activity on cellular ribonucleotide reductase [88]. In EPCs, the variation in the distribution of cellular differentiation markers indicated an inhibitory effect on the differentiation of cell population and a reduction in the generation of more mature cells, exerted by both HU and virus with additive effects. HU prevented cells from leaving the G1/S phases with a related reduction of cells in G2/M, in both infected and uninfected cells. EPCs arrested with a 2N DNA content may be not competent to engage in B19V active replication, thus contributing to the antiviral effect of HU together with the lowering deoxyribonucleotide levels within cells.

As mentioned, HU is used as a disease-modifying drug in sickle cell disease, where it can exert a protective effect due to the inhibition of erythroid cell proliferation/differentiation [93,94]. SCD is a typical situation where infection with B19V can exert profound pathological effects, requiring hospitalization and intense supportive therapy, so a dual effect of the compound both on the course of the underlying disease and on the course of infection by its antiviral activity would be beneficial. In treated SCD patients, HU can reach peak plasma concentrations of ~250–400 mM [95], indicating that HU levels sufficient to reduce B19V replication in vitro are achievable in vivo. A survey of clinical records of SCD patients undergoing HU therapy showed indeed a protective effect of HU against B19V infection compared to non-treated patients, at least in terms of severity of disease and need for treatments [96]. As determination of peak viremic levels in the two group of patients were not presented, there are still two hypotheses to explain this observation, either that such protective effect is due to a lower viral replicative activity consequence of the antiviral activity of HU, and/or it can be indirectly linked to a prolonged lifespan of erythrocytes. Further clinical investigation would be helpful to explore the potential beneficial clinical effects of HU.

7.2. Nucleotide Analogues: Cidofovir (CDV) and Brincidofovir (BCV)

A different strategy involved the evaluation of broad-spectrum antiviral compounds for a possible activity against B19V. In particular, the acyclic nucleoside phosphonate cidofovir (CDV) has shown activity against all families of human, not retro-transcribing dsDNA viruses [51,97,98], including viruses not encoding their own DNA polymerase. B19V is a ssDNA virus, but depending for its replication on cellular DNA polymerase activity acting on a dsDNA replicative intermediate, so potentially inhibited by a nucleotide analogue incorporated in a nascent DNA molecule. Experimental results confirmed this working hypothesis [83,84].

In UT7/EpoS1 cells, CDV exerted a measurable inhibitory effect on B19V replication in the range 0–500 μM, achieving complete inhibition of viral replication at the higher concentration and EC_{50}

values in the range 7.45–41.27 μM (depending on the multiplicity of infection, in the range 10^1 to 10^4 geq/cell). Viral transcription was less affected by the presence of CDV, with a significant reduction only at the higher concentration tested, coupled with a block in the shift from an early to late pattern of transcription possibly correlated to the block in replicative activity. Concurrently, a progressive reduction in the number of FISH and IIF positive cells was observed with increasing the concentration of CDV. In these cells, CDV did not alter cell viability or proliferation to a statistically significant extent.

The inhibitory activity of CDV was much less relevant in EPCs. A statistically significant effect of CDV on viral DNA replication was evident only for the 500 μM concentration, and even at this highest concentration inhibition was not complete, but only in the range 68.2–92.8% depending on the multiplicity of infection. CDV added to cell cultures did not alter EPCs viability or proliferation to a statistically significant extent. These results suggest that the cellular environment is crucial to the activity of CDV, and different hypotheses to explain such dependency include a slower uptake of CDV within EPCs, a slower metabolic activity with reduced production of the active metabolite, CDV diphosphate (CDV-PP), or a difference in the replicative machinery involved in replication of viral genome with different sensitivity to CDV.

In EPCs, addition of CDV led to a decrease in the release of virus in the supernatant of cell cultures, and in a reduction of its infectivity in subsequent rounds of infection. At the highest multiplicity of infection tested, the overall reduction in virus yield and infectivity was >90%, a result arising as the additive effect of the inhibition of replication within EPCs, with a lower production of infectious virions (68–70% reduction), and a reduced replicative activity of viral DNA (75% reduction). It is possible to hypothesize that incorporation of CDV in progeny DNA strands is responsible for the reduced replicative activity observed.

The hypothesis that prolonged incubation with CDV could lead to a more profound inhibition in viral replication was tested by assessing at the highest multiplicity of infection and CDV concentration: (i) the effect of preincubation of cells with CDV prior to infection; (ii) the effect of an extended time course of infection in the presence of CDV; and (iii) the effect of serial passage of virus under antiviral pressure exerted by CDV. Reduction in viral replicative activity was observed in all of these situations. Preincubation with CDV reduced viral replication more than 90%, significantly higher than addition of CDV following infection. Extended incubation with CDV had modest effects on cell viability, although a reduction in cell proliferation up to 70% was observed, but inhibition of viral replication was observed at about 80%, coupled to a similar reduction in the amount of virus released in the cell culture supernatant. An overall reduction in viral replication higher than 96% was finally observed following three serial passages of virus in EPCs in the presence of CDV, suggesting that a constant pharmacological pressure exerted by CDV can alter the viral replication dynamics to a significant extent.

Overall, these results firstly indicated that inhibition of B19V replication could be achieved by effect of an antiviral agent, but the efficacy of CDV appeared critically dependent on the cellular environment. In primary EPCs, the inhibitory activity of CDV was significant only at the higher concentration tested and by extended exposure, which is impractical in clinical terms. Moreover, concerns of toxicity on CDV prevent its widespread use and would be a major obstacle in developing an effective treatment option for B19V, prompting for further research. Thus, in a development aimed at overcoming these limits, the antiviral activity of Brincidofovir (BCV) was further evaluated [85]. BCV (CMX001) is a modified form of CDV, where the acyclic nucleotide phosphonate has been conjugated to a lipid moiety, with the result of a more potent activity demonstrated against dsDNA viruses, better bioavailability and absence of toxicity [99–101].

Experimental investigation confirmed an enhanced antiviral activity of BCV compared to CDV in both cellular systems, and in particular in EPCs only BCV but not CDV yielded complete inhibition of viral replication [85]. For BCV, EC_{50} values were in the range 6.6–14.3 μM in EPCs and 0.22–0.63 μM in UT7/EpoS1 cells. In comparison, EC_{50} values for CDV were >300 μM in EPCs and 16.1 μM in UT7/EpoS1 cells. Accordingly, effects on cell viability were observed for BCV as opposed for CDV, with calculated CC_{50} values in the range 93.4–102.9 μM in EPCs and 59.9–66.8 μM in UT7/EpoS1. Specificity in the antiviral effect was confirmed by comparing the activity of the two enantiomeric forms of BCV, (S) and (R), where only BCV (S) and not BCV (R) is the active enantiomer. BCV (S) utilizes the lipid uptake pathway in cells, leading to an increase in the effective concentration of the active antiviral, CDV-PP, and therefore to enhanced antiviral potency [102]. In EPCs, the selectivity index values for BCV (S) and BCV (R), determined as the ratio CC_{50}/EC_{50}, were 6.5 and 1.6 respectively, yielding an S/R ratio of 4.0, and in UT7/EpoS1, SI values were 95.1 and 1.3, yielding an S/R ratio of 73.2. Such high S/R ratios indicate an active and specific antiviral role of CDV-PP, derived from BCV (S), as opposed to a nonspecific cytotoxic effect indirectly causing inhibition of viral replication.

As a common mechanism of action, the antiviral activity exerted by both BCV and CDV is due to CDV-diphosphate (CDV-PP) which is used as an alternate substrate for viral DNA synthesis [103]. Both BCV and CDV are broad-spectrum antivirals that possess activity against all dsDNA viruses, including those that do not encode their own polymerases [104–106], even though the mechanism of inhibition has not been fully explained in this case [107,108]. By also showing antiviral activity against B19V, the spectrum of activity of CDV-PP is thus expanded to include a ssDNA virus, even if it should be considered that the B19V genome replicative intermediates are actually dsDNA forms that utilize the host replication machinery and metabolic environment. The exact mechanism(s) of action of both CDV and BCV in the inhibition of B19V replication, and its dependence on the different cellular environments, warrants further investigation.

The identification of broad-spectrum antiviral compounds with in vitro demonstrated antiviral activity also including B19V might be considered of relevance as a rationale for evaluating the use of these drugs in the treatment of patients. Use of CDV is not recommended, but BCV proved effective in inhibiting B19V replication at concentrations that are attainable in vivo [109], has a known safety profile [110] and compares favorably with other antivirals in its activity against dsDNA viruses [111], thus opening the possibility of its use also to treat B19V infections, given a cautious approach required for clinical management.

7.3. Serendipity Approach: Coumarin Derivatives

As discussed, a high-throughput screen against available chemical libraries is hardly achievable, but a more targeted serendipity approach in the screening of small-scale chemical libraries is a practicable option. Small libraries might include compounds of different chemical nature, selected on the basis of known and potentially relevant biological activities, and can be investigated by using established biological and analytical protocols.

By this approach, an initial screening of a small chemical library was carried out indicating some coumarin derivatives as scaffold molecules with promising activity against B19V [86]. Coumarins are already in use as therapeutic agents in humans [112] and some products characterized by a coumarin nucleus are known to possess some antiviral activity in many model systems [113], although their precise mechanisms of action is unknown. Following the initial screening that led to identification of a compound with promising characteristics (3-(imidazo[2,1-b]thiazol-6-yl)-2H-chromen-2-one), serial chemical modifications of this molecular scaffold yielded a derived small chemical library that was further evaluated, leading to additional identification of differently substituted molecules with measurable specific antiviral activity. Overall, by testing these compounds at their highest attainable concentrations, inhibition of viral replication in both EPCs and UT7/EpoS1 was only partial, in the range 60–82% in the best case and mainly inUT7/Epos1 cells. Effects on cell viability were also relevant, with inhibition up to 30–40% in the worst case. However, for three of these compounds, prevalent antiviral compared to cytotoxic effects was observed, with SI > 2.4–4.0. Furthermore, in UT7/EpoS1 cells, the inhibition of viral replication followed a dose-response curve (calculated EC_{50} values ~6.4–6.7 μM) that was significantly different compared with a rather unspecific effect on cellular viability, suggesting that the mechanisms for the observed activity of these compounds could either involve inhibition of a viral target or of a cellular function specifically needed by the virus during its replicative cycle.

While such serendipity approach allows small-scale screening and can yield appreciable results, it is a laborious approach that can be hardly rewarding in terms of success. Even when screening molecules with promising characteristics, the hit rate is unpredictable, and in the presence of any antiviral activity the identification of the target, whether cellular or viral, is an endeavoring task. Nonetheless, by following this approach, characterization of both target and mechanisms of action would be required, not least due to the need to refine the design and synthesis of molecules better suited to exert their antiviral activity.

7.4. Direct Antiviral Agents

A different experimental approach can be followed in the search for direct antiviral agents. Detailed knowledge of the viral lifecycle and of mechanistic details of the molecular machinery involved, can allow the identification of critical targets, whose inhibition would prevent viral replication or at least viral cytotoxic effects. By this approach, functions crucial to the viral lifecycle should be attributed to specific genes, gene regions or even protein domains. In vitro assays, also using recombinant proteins, should be developed to measure correlate activities, so that any inhibition of these activities by tested compounds might be investigated firstly in screening experiments using biochemical assays, and then in cell-based assays. Such an approach has been reported in the literature, in the search for compounds that are able to inhibit the endonuclease activity associated with viral NS protein [87].

Within the B19V proteome, the NS protein is synthesized in the early phases and exerts crucial functions during the viral lifecycle [19]. The protein is involved in the terminal resolution reaction, which is essential for the rolling hairpin replication of viral DNA, and both an endonuclease and helicase activity are required, mapped to distinct domains of the protein. It has an activating role on the viral promoter as well as a heterologous trans-activating action on several cellular promoters, this activity is mapped to a different protein domain. The protein is responsible for interactions with cellular pathways, including the induction of a DNA damage response, dysregulation of cell cycle, and apoptosis. Since crystallographic studies related to the NS protein have not been produced, its molecular structure can be only predicted by analogy to other replicative molecules in the family, for example, rep proteins of Adeno-Associated Virus (AAV), but to an approximation that impairs the rational design of ligands and inhibitory molecules. The functional mapping of the NS protein indicates the presence of different domains and associated functions, localizes putative active sites, and allows the design of biochemical assays to measure functional activity.

The N-terminus (aa. 2–176) of NS1 possesses DNA binding and endonuclease activity, and an endonuclease motif resides between amino acids 137 and 145 [114]. The presence of a functional endonuclease domain is necessary for replication of the viral genome, by allowing terminal resolution and continuing rolling hairpin replication. This function can be monitored also by in vitro biochemical assays, by using a purified recombinant protein fragment obtained from a prokaryotic expression system and measuring activity by the amount of cleaved oligonucleotides of appropriate target sequence [115]. This biochemical assay, further improved using a fluorophore-based reporter system, proved suitable to evaluate a specific inhibitory activity of tested compound in a direct target-based assay [87]. The convenient assay format allowed screening of a selected chemical library and led to the identification of a subset of compounds with significant (>80%) in vitro endonuclease-inhibiting activity at concentrations <10 μM. Among these, three compounds of flavonoid-like structure were selected and further tested to determine their in vitro activity, in inhibiting the endonuclease nicking reaction, and in vivo to selectively inhibit B19V replication.

In vitro, dose-response curves showed IC_{50} values in the range 1.1–3.1 μM, making these compounds highly promising for subsequent evaluation in cell-based assays. In cell-based assays, involving both UT7/EpoS1 and EPCs, the selected compounds also showed a capacity to inhibit B19V replication as a dose- and time-dependent response, as determined by a cytometric assay to determine the fraction of productively infected cells. However, the inhibition of viral replication was only partial if not at the highest concentrations tested, at the expense of effects on cell viability. In UT7/EpoS1 cells, reported EC_{50} values were in the range 44.2–55.1 μM, compared to CC_{50} values in the range 180.9–227.0 μM, resulting in selectivity indexes of 3.3–4.4. In EPCs, EC_{50} values were in the range 33.5–53.9 μM, compared to CC_{50} values in the range 55.9–89.8 μM, resulting in selectivity indexes of 1.5–1.8. qPCR assay in EPCs following a 48 h infection course, the EC_{50} values were in the range 20.5–38.4, thus giving a selectively index in the range 2.4–2.7. Replication of the viral genome was already inhibited at an early time point post-infection, thus corroborating inhibition of the endonuclease function of the NS protein as a likely mechanism of antiviral activity.

Results of these studies, therefore, on one hand indicate that a target-oriented biochemical assay is feasible and useful, and that in principle it might be extended to investigate other viral functions crucial to the viral lifecycle. On the other hand, these results clearly indicate a major problem arising when considering the whole virus–cell system as a target, as opposed to isolated functions of protein domains. Issues of transport of compounds within cells, the metabolic fate of compounds, the accessibility of active sites in the context of a macromolecular assembly, and overall metabolic differences in cells, depending also on cell type, differentiation stage, proliferation rate, and metabolic activity, can all impact the efficacy of otherwise promising compounds in a crucial way.

7.5. Other Compounds

In the literature, a few other molecules have been reported, which possess measurable selective inhibitory activity on B19V or effects on B19V-infected cells. The assembly of a macromolecular machinery in the origin of replication of the viral genome requires not only a functional viral NS protein, but also cellular partners [23], including the phosphorylated form of STAT5, as a common terminus of the activation pathway triggered by Epo and enhanced by hypoxia [24]. The molecule pimozide is a known inhibitor of STAT5 phosphorylation, and accordingly it exerts an inhibitory effect on B19V replication, with only a minor effect on cell viability as determined by a colony formation inhibition assay. Pimozide is approved for use as an antipsychotic drug, so a dual use of the molecule might be conceivable but hardly proposed in the absence of aimed clinical studies.

The nucleotide analogue telbivudine, inhibitor of HBV reverse transcriptase, has been evaluated for its effects in B19V-infected endothelial progenitor cells, in the context of a pathogenetic mechanism proposed for B19V-induced endothelial disfunction and development of dilated inflammatory cardiomyopathy [116,117]. While telbivudine did not show any direct inhibitory effect on B19V replication or expression [116], it protected B19V infected endothelial progenitors by B19V-induced apoptosis [117], in a mechanism that possibly reverses B19V-induced dysregulation of BIRC3, thus intervening the apoptosis pathway and protecting susceptible cells from cell death.

Finally, the possible protective effects of IFN-beta have been evaluated in limited clinical trials for the treatment of dilated cardiomyopathies of supposed viral trigger, including B19V, considering its high prevalence in myocardial tissues, reporting promising results [118–120]. The interactions of B19V and the innate immune system are not yet well characterized, either in terms of sensor activation, induction of effector mechanism, and possible viral escape strategies. A better understanding of this aspect of virus–cell interaction will likely indicate novel antiviral strategies to pursue.

8. Conclusions and Perspectives

In conclusion, a few statements can be proposed. First, B19V infection should not be overlooked in clinical terms, and diagnostic uncertainties can be easily resolved when a correct diagnostic approach is followed. Thereafter, even if most infections do not require treatment, the management of more complicated cases would be advantageous with respect to the availability of dedicated treatments that incorporate both specific and unspecific antiviral agents, such as IVIG.

In the research on antivirals against B19V, some work has been done in recent years to close the gap with other viruses, first yielding compounds that are already in use and that could be retargeted to B19V. In the case of Hydroxyurea, available data already consent some clinical considerations, since continuous HU treatment is already used in SCD subjects that are at high risk of disease for

B19V infection, and retrospective clinical data show a measurable protective effect against severe hematological manifestations. In the case of nucleotide analogues, these have been used, or are being investigated, for viral infections other than B19V, so that their safety profiles are known. While CDV is not used because of its toxic side effects, BCV is qualified as a promising broad-range antiviral. Given its demonstrated in vitro activity, its possible use in off-label situations justified by severe and non-responsive B19V infection might offer a clue to its efficacy in in vivo situations. Furthermore, its possible use as a broad-range antiviral and prophylactic agent in immunosuppressed individuals would also offer the opportunity to evaluate its efficacy in preventing or controlling B19V infections in the follow-up of these subjects. Research on targeted direct antiviral agents, on the other hand, might offer better-suited molecules, but will need to face evaluation of clinical safety coupled to efficacy, a demanding task in many respects.

In this context, continuing research in the field, with an ever-increasing knowledge regarding the viral lifecycle, the molecular machinery involved, and a precise understanding of virus–cell interactions, will offer novel opportunities for developing more efficient, targeted antiviral agents, that can be translated to available therapeutic options in the near future.

Funding: This research received no external funding.

Acknowledgments: We gratefully acknowledged Vanessa D'Urbano (Department of Experimental, Diagnostic and Specialty Medicine, University of Bologna) for her graphical skills.

Conflicts of Interest: The authors declare no conflict of interest.

References

1. Cotmore, S.F.; Agbandje-McKenna, M.; Chiorini, J.A.; Mukha, D.V.; Pintel, D.J.; Qiu, J.; Soderlund-Venermo, M.; Tattersall, P.; Tijssen, P.; Gatherer, D.; et al. The family Parvoviridae. *Arch. Virol.* **2014**, *159*, 1239–1247. [CrossRef] [PubMed]
2. Gallinella, G. Parvovirus B19 Achievements and Challenges. *ISRN Virol.* **2013**. [CrossRef]
3. Qiu, J.; Soderlund-Venermo, M.; Young, N.S. Human Parvoviruses. *Clin. Microbiol. Rev.* **2017**, *30*, 43–113. [CrossRef] [PubMed]
4. Mietzsch, M.; Penzes, J.J.; Agbandje-McKenna, M. Twenty-Five Years of Structural Parvovirology. *Viruses* **2019**, *11*, 362. [CrossRef] [PubMed]
5. Gallinella, G. The clinical use of parvovirus B19 assays: Recent advances. *Expert Rev. Mol. Diagn.* **2018**, *18*, 821–832. [CrossRef] [PubMed]
6. Kaczmarek, R.; Buczkowska, A.; Mikolajewicz, K.; Krotkiewski, H.; Czerwinski, M. P1PK, GLOB, and FORS blood group systems and GLOB collection: Biochemical and clinical aspects. Do we understand it all yet? *Transfus. Med. Rev.* **2014**, *28*, 126–136. [CrossRef]
7. Brown, K.E.; Anderson, S.M.; Young, N.S. Erythrocyte P antigen: Cellular receptor for B19 parvovirus. *Science* **1993**, *262*, 114–117. [CrossRef]
8. Brown, K.E.; Hibbs, J.R.; Gallinella, G.; Anderson, S.M.; Lehman, E.D.; McCarthy, P.; Young, N.S. Resistance to parvovirus B19 infection due to lack of virus receptor (erythrocyte P antigen). *N. Engl. J. Med.* **1994**, *330*, 1192–1196. [CrossRef]
9. Chipman, P.R.; Agbandje-McKenna, M.; Kajigaya, S.; Brown, K.E.; Young, N.S.; Baker, T.S.; Rossmann, M.G. Cryo-electron microscopy studies of empty capsids of human parvovirus B19 complexed with its cellular receptor. *Proc. Natl. Acad. Sci. USA* **1996**, *93*, 7502–7506. [CrossRef]
10. Kaufmann, B.; Baxa, U.; Chipman, P.R.; Rossmann, M.G.; Modrow, S.; Seckler, R. Parvovirus B19 does not bind to membrane-associated globoside in vitro. *Virology* **2005**, *332*, 189–198. [CrossRef]
11. Nasir, W.; Nilsson, J.; Olofsson, S.; Bally, M.; Rydell, G.E. Parvovirus B19 VLP recognizes globoside in supported lipid bilayers. *Virology* **2014**, *456–457*, 364–369. [CrossRef] [PubMed]
12. Bonsch, C.; Zuercher, C.; Lieby, P.; Kempf, C.; Ros, C. The globoside receptor triggers structural changes in the B19 virus capsid that facilitate virus internalization. *J. Virol.* **2010**, *84*, 11737–11746. [CrossRef] [PubMed]
13. Leisi, R.; Ruprecht, N.; Kempf, C.; Ros, C. Parvovirus B19 uptake is a highly selective process controlled by VP1u, a novel determinant of viral tropism. *J. Virol.* **2013**, *87*, 13161–13167. [CrossRef] [PubMed]

14. Leisi, R.; Di Tommaso, C.; Kempf, C.; Ros, C. The Receptor-Binding Domain in the VP1u Region of Parvovirus B19. *Viruses* **2016**, *8*, 61. [CrossRef] [PubMed]
15. Leisi, R.; Von Nordheim, M.; Ros, C.; Kempf, C. The VP1u Receptor Restricts Parvovirus B19 Uptake to Permissive Erythroid Cells. *Viruses* **2016**, *8*, 265. [CrossRef] [PubMed]
16. Quattrocchi, S.; Ruprecht, N.; Bonsch, C.; Bieli, S.; Zurcher, C.; Boller, K.; Kempf, C.; Ros, C. Characterization of the early steps of human parvovirus B19 infection. *J. Virol.* **2012**, *86*, 9274–9284. [CrossRef] [PubMed]
17. Caliaro, O.; Marti, A.; Ruprecht, N.; Leisi, R.; Subramanian, S.; Hafenstein, S.; Ros, C. Parvovirus B19 Uncoating Occurs in the Cytoplasm without Capsid Disassembly and It Is Facilitated by Depletion of Capsid-Associated Divalent Cations. *Viruses* **2019**, *11*, 430. [CrossRef] [PubMed]
18. Luo, Y.; Qiu, J. Human parvovirus B19: A mechanistic overview of infection and DNA replication. *Future Virol.* **2015**, *10*, 155–167. [CrossRef]
19. Ganaie, S.S.; Qiu, J. Recent Advances in Replication and Infection of Human Parvovirus B19. *Front. Cell. Infect. Microbiol.* **2018**, *8*, 166. [CrossRef]
20. Bua, G.; Manaresi, E.; Bonvicini, F.; Gallinella, G. Parvovirus B19 Replication and Expression in Differentiating Erythroid Progenitor Cells. *PLoS ONE* **2016**, *11*, e0148547. [CrossRef]
21. Chen, A.Y.; Guan, W.; Lou, S.; Liu, Z.; Kleiboeker, S.; Qiu, J. Role of erythropoietin receptor signaling in parvovirus B19 replication in human erythroid progenitor cells. *J. Virol.* **2010**, *84*, 12385–12396. [CrossRef]
22. Chen, A.Y.; Kleiboeker, S.; Qiu, J. Productive parvovirus B19 infection of primary human erythroid progenitor cells at hypoxia is regulated by STAT5A and MEK signaling but not HIFalpha. *PLoS Pathog.* **2011**, *7*, e1002088. [CrossRef] [PubMed]
23. Zou, W.; Wang, Z.; Xiong, M.; Chen, A.Y.; Xu, P.; Ganaie, S.S.; Badawi, Y.; Kleiboeker, S.; Nishimune, H.; Ye, S.Q.; et al. Human Parvovirus B19 Utilizes Cellular DNA Replication Machinery for Viral DNA Replication. *J. Virol.* **2018**, *92*, e01881-17. [CrossRef]
24. Ganaie, S.S.; Zou, W.; Xu, P.; Deng, X.; Kleiboeker, S.; Qiu, J. Phosphorylated STAT5 directly facilitates parvovirus B19 DNA replication in human erythroid progenitors through interaction with the MCM complex. *PLoS Pathog.* **2017**, *13*, e1006370. [CrossRef]
25. Ganaie, S.S.; Chen, A.Y.; Huang, C.; Xu, P.; Kleiboeker, S.; Du, A.; Qiu, J. RNA Binding Protein RBM38 Regulates Expression of the 11-Kilodalton Protein of Parvovirus B19, Which Facilitates Viral DNA Replication. *J. Virol.* **2018**, *92*, e02050-17. [CrossRef]
26. Xu, P.; Chen, A.Y.; Ganaie, S.S.; Cheng, F.; Shen, W.; Wang, X.; Kleiboeker, S.; Li, Y.; Qiu, J. The 11-Kilodalton Nonstructural Protein of Human Parvovirus B19 Facilitates Viral DNA Replication by Interacting with Grb2 through Its Proline-Rich Motifs. *J. Virol.* **2019**, *93*, e01464-18. [CrossRef]
27. Chen, A.Y.; Qiu, J. Parvovirus infection-induced cell death and cell cycle arrest. *Future Virol.* **2010**, *5*, 731–743. [CrossRef] [PubMed]
28. Luo, Y.; Qiu, J. Parvovirus infection-induced DNA damage response. *Future Virol.* **2013**, *8*, 245–257. [CrossRef]
29. Pyoria, L.; Toppinen, M.; Mantyla, E.; Hedman, L.; Aaltonen, L.M.; Vihinen-Ranta, M.; Ilmarinen, T.; Soderlund-Venermo, M.; Hedman, K.; Perdomo, M.F. Extinct type of human parvovirus B19 persists in tonsillar B cells. *Nat. Commun.* **2017**, *8*, 14930. [CrossRef]
30. Von Kietzell, K.; Pozzuto, T.; Heilbronn, R.; Grossl, T.; Fechner, H.; Weger, S. Antibody-mediated enhancement of parvovirus B19 uptake into endothelial cells mediated by a receptor for complement factor C1q. *J. Virol.* **2014**, *88*, 8102–8115. [CrossRef] [PubMed]
31. Adamson-Small, L.A.; Ignatovich, I.V.; Laemmerhirt, M.G.; Hobbs, J.A. Persistent parvovirus B19 infection in non-erythroid tissues: Possible role in the inflammatory and disease process. *Virus Res.* **2014**, *190*, 8–16. [CrossRef] [PubMed]
32. Bua, G.; Gallinella, G. How does parvovirus B19 DNA achieve lifelong persistence in human cells? *Future Virol.* **2017**, *12*, 549–553. [CrossRef]
33. Janovitz, T.; Wong, S.; Young, N.S.; Oliveira, T.; Falck-Pedersen, E. Parvovirus B19 integration into human CD36+ erythroid progenitor cells. *Virology* **2017**, *511*, 40–48. [CrossRef] [PubMed]
34. Norja, P.; Hokynar, K.; Aaltonen, L.M.; Chen, R.; Ranki, A.; Partio, E.K.; Kiviluoto, O.; Davidkin, I.; Leivo, T.; Eis-Hubinger, A.M.; et al. Bioportfolio: Lifelong persistence of variant and prototypic erythrovirus DNA genomes in human tissue. *Proc. Natl. Acad. Sci. USA* **2006**, *103*, 7450–7453. [CrossRef] [PubMed]

35. Toppinen, M.; Perdomo, M.F.; Palo, J.U.; Simmonds, P.; Lycett, S.J.; Soderlund-Venermo, M.; Sajantila, A.; Hedman, K. Bones hold the key to DNA virus history and epidemiology. *Sci. Rep.* **2015**, *5*, 17226. [CrossRef] [PubMed]
36. Muhlemann, B.; Margaryan, A.; Damgaard, P.B.; Allentoft, M.E.; Vinner, L.; Hansen, A.J.; Weber, A.; Bazaliiskii, V.I.; Molak, M.; Arneborg, J.; et al. Ancient human parvovirus B19 in Eurasia reveals its long-term association with humans. *Proc. Natl. Acad. Sci. USA* **2018**, *115*, 7557–7562. [CrossRef] [PubMed]
37. Kerr, J.R. A review of blood diseases and cytopenias associated with human parvovirus B19 infection. *Rev. Med. Virol.* **2015**, *25*, 224–240. [CrossRef]
38. Tsitsikas, D.A.; Gallinella, G.; Patel, S.; Seligman, H.; Greaves, P.; Amos, R.J. Bone marrow necrosis and fat embolism syndrome in sickle cell disease: Increased susceptibility of patients with non-SS genotypes and a possible association with human parvovirus B19 infection. *Blood Rev.* **2014**, *28*, 23–30. [CrossRef]
39. Verdonschot, J.; Hazebroek, M.; Merken, J.; Debing, Y.; Dennert, R.; Brunner-La Rocca, H.P.; Heymans, S. Relevance of cardiac parvovirus B19 in myocarditis and dilated cardiomyopathy: Review of the literature. *Eur. J. Heart Fail.* **2016**, *18*, 1430–1441. [CrossRef]
40. Kerr, J.R. The role of parvovirus B19 in the pathogenesis of autoimmunity and autoimmune disease. *J. Clin. Pathol.* **2016**, *69*, 279–291. [CrossRef]
41. Lunardi, C.; Tinazzi, E.; Bason, C.; Dolcino, M.; Corrocher, R.; Puccetti, A. Human parvovirus B19 infection and autoimmunity. *Autoimmun. Rev.* **2008**, *8*, 116–120. [CrossRef]
42. Thammasri, K.; Rauhamaki, S.; Wang, L.; Filippou, A.; Kivovich, V.; Marjomaki, V.; Naides, S.J.; Gilbert, L. Human parvovirus B19 induced apoptotic bodies contain altered self-antigens that are phagocytosed by antigen presenting cells. *PLoS ONE* **2013**, *8*, e67179. [CrossRef]
43. Puttaraksa, K.; Pirttinen, H.; Karvonen, K.; Nykky, J.; Naides, S.J.; Gilbert, L. Parvovirus B19V Non-structural Protein NS1 Induces dsDNA Autoantibodies and End Organ Damage in Non-autoimmune Mice. *J. Infect. Dis.* **2018**, *219*, 1418–1429. [CrossRef]
44. Bonvicini, F.; Bua, G.; Gallinella, G. Parvovirus B19 infection in pregnancy-awareness and opportunities. *Curr. Opin. Virol.* **2017**, *27*, 8–14. [CrossRef]
45. Pasquinelli, G.; Bonvicini, F.; Foroni, L.; Salfi, N.; Gallinella, G. Placental endothelial cells can be productively infected by Parvovirus B19. *J. Clin. Virol.* **2009**, *44*, 33–38. [CrossRef]
46. Bonvicini, F.; Puccetti, C.; Salfi, N.C.; Guerra, B.; Gallinella, G.; Rizzo, N.; Zerbini, M. Gestational and fetal outcomes in B19 maternal infection: A problem of diagnosis. *J. Clin. Microbiol.* **2011**, *49*, 3514–3518. [CrossRef]
47. Bascietto, F.; Liberati, M.; Murgano, D.; Buca, D.; Iacovelli, A.; Flacco, M.E.; Manzoli, L.; Familiari, A.; Scambia, G.; D'Antonio, F. Outcome of fetuses with congenital parvovirus B19 infection: Systematic review and meta-analysis. *Ultrasound Obstet. Gynecol.* **2018**, *52*, 569–576. [CrossRef]
48. Xiong, Y.Q.; Tan, J.; Liu, Y.M.; He, Q.; Li, L.; Zou, K.; Sun, X. The risk of maternal parvovirus B19 infection during pregnancy on fetal loss and fetal hydrops: A systematic review and meta-analysis. *J. Clin. Virol.* **2019**, *114*, 12–20. [CrossRef]
49. Mage, V.; Lipsker, D.; Barbarot, S.; Bessis, D.; Chosidow, O.; Del Giudice, P.; Aractingi, S.; Avouac, J.; Bernier, C.; Descamps, V.; et al. Different patterns of skin manifestations associated with parvovirus B19 primary infection in adults. *J. Am. Acad. Dermatol.* **2014**, *71*, 62–69. [CrossRef]
50. Dijkmans, A.C.; de Jong, E.P.; Dijkmans, B.A.; Lopriore, E.; Vossen, A.; Walther, F.J.; Oepkes, D. Parvovirus B19 in pregnancy: Prenatal diagnosis and management of fetal complications. *Curr. Opin. Obstet. Gynecol.* **2012**, *24*, 95–101. [CrossRef]
51. De Clercq, E.; Li, G. Approved Antiviral Drugs over the Past 50 Years. *Clin. Microbiol. Rev.* **2016**, *29*, 695–747. [CrossRef]
52. Bansal, G.P.; Hatfield, J.A.; Dunn, F.E.; Kramer, A.A.; Brady, F.; Riggin, C.H.; Collett, M.S.; Yoshimoto, K.; Kajigaya, S.; Young, N.S. Candidate recombinant vaccine for human B19 parvovirus. *J. Infect. Dis.* **1993**, *167*, 1034–1044. [CrossRef]
53. Ballou, W.R.; Reed, J.L.; Noble, W.; Young, N.S.; Koenig, S. Safety and immunogenicity of a recombinant parvovirus B19 vaccine formulated with MF59C.1. *J. Infect. Dis.* **2003**, *187*, 675–678. [CrossRef]
54. Bernstein, D.I.; El Sahly, H.M.; Keitel, W.A.; Wolff, M.; Simone, G.; Segawa, C.; Wong, S.; Shelly, D.; Young, N.S.; Dempsey, W. Safety and immunogenicity of a candidate parvovirus B19 vaccine. *Vaccine* **2011**, *29*, 7357–7363. [CrossRef]

55. Chandramouli, S.; Medina-Selby, A.; Coit, D.; Schaefer, M.; Spencer, T.; Brito, L.A.; Zhang, P.; Otten, G.; Mandl, C.W.; Mason, P.W.; et al. Generation of a parvovirus B19 vaccine candidate. *Vaccine* **2013**, *31*, 3872–3878. [CrossRef]
56. Penkert, R.R.; Young, N.S.; Surman, S.L.; Sealy, R.E.; Rosch, J.; Dormitzer, P.R.; Settembre, E.C.; Chandramouli, S.; Wong, S.; Hankins, J.S.; et al. Saccharomyces cerevisiae-derived virus-like particle parvovirus B19 vaccine elicits binding and neutralizing antibodies in a mouse model for sickle cell disease. *Vaccine* **2017**, *35*, 3615–3620. [CrossRef]
57. Mouthon, L.; Lortholary, O. Intravenous immunoglobulins in infectious diseases: Where do we stand? *Clin. Microbiol. Infect.* **2003**, *9*, 333–338. [CrossRef]
58. Mouthon, L.; Guillevin, L.; Tellier, Z. Intravenous immunoglobulins in autoimmune- or parvovirus B19-mediated pure red-cell aplasia. *Autoimmun. Rev.* **2005**, *4*, 264–269. [CrossRef]
59. Mouthon, L.; Michel, M.; Gandre, C.; Montagnier-Petrissans, C.; Chevreul, K. Costs of intravenous immunoglobulin therapy in patients with unconfirmed parvovirus b19 pure red cell aplasia. *Clin. Infect. Dis.* **2015**, *60*, 488. [CrossRef]
60. Perez, E.E.; Orange, J.S.; Bonilla, F.; Chinen, J.; Chinn, I.K.; Dorsey, M.; El-Gamal, Y.; Harville, T.O.; Hossny, E.; Mazer, B.; et al. Update on the use of immunoglobulin in human disease: A review of evidence. *J. Allergy Clin. Immunol.* **2017**, *139*, S1–S46. [CrossRef]
61. Crabol, Y.; Terrier, B.; Rozenberg, F.; Pestre, V.; Legendre, C.; Hermine, O.; Montagnier-Petrissans, C.; Guillevin, L.; Mouthon, L.; Groupe d'experts de l'Assistance Publique-Hôpitaux de Paris. Intravenous immunoglobulin therapy for pure red cell aplasia related to human parvovirus b19 infection: A retrospective study of 10 patients and review of the literature. *Clin. Infect. Dis.* **2013**, *56*, 968–977. [CrossRef]
62. Modrof, J.; Berting, A.; Tille, B.; Klotz, A.; Forstner, C.; Rieger, S.; Aberham, C.; Gessner, M.; Kreil, T.R. Neutralization of human parvovirus B19 by plasma and intravenous immunoglobulins. *Transfusion* **2008**, *48*, 178–186. [CrossRef]
63. Chaigne, B.; Mouthon, L. Mechanisms of action of intravenous immunoglobulin. *Transfus. Apher. Sci.* **2017**, *56*, 45–49. [CrossRef]
64. Kerr, J.R.; Cunniffe, V.S.; Kelleher, P.; Bernstein, R.M.; Bruce, I.N. Successful intravenous immunoglobulin therapy in 3 cases of parvovirus B19-associated chronic fatigue syndrome. *Clin. Infect. Dis.* **2003**, *36*, e100–e106. [CrossRef]
65. Attard, L.; Bonvicini, F.; Gelsomino, F.; Manfredi, R.; Cascavilla, A.; Viale, P.; Varani, S.; Gallinella, G. Paradoxical response to intravenous immunoglobulin in a case of Parvovirus B19-associated chronic fatigue syndrome. *J. Clin. Virol.* **2015**, *62*, 54–57. [CrossRef]
66. Gigler, A.; Dorsch, S.; Hemauer, A.; Williams, C.; Kim, S.; Young, N.S.; Zolla-Pazner, S.; Wolf, H.; Gorny, M.K.; Modrow, S. Generation of neutralizing human monoclonal antibodies against parvovirus B19 proteins. *J. Virol.* **1999**, *73*, 1974–1979.
67. Manaresi, E.; Gallinella, G.; Zerbini, M.; Venturoli, S.; Gentilomi, G.; Musiani, M. IgG immune response to B19 parvovirus VP1 and VP2 linear epitopes by immunoblot assay. *J. Med. Virol.* **1999**, *57*, 174–178. [CrossRef]
68. Manaresi, E.; Zuffi, E.; Gallinella, G.; Gentilomi, G.; Zerbini, M.; Musiani, M. Differential IgM response to conformational and linear epitopes of parvovirus B19 VP1 and VP2 structural proteins. *J. Med. Virol.* **2001**, *64*, 67–73. [CrossRef]
69. Sato, H.; Hirata, J.; Furukawa, M.; Kuroda, N.; Shiraki, H.; Maeda, Y.; Okochi, K. Identification of the region including the epitope for a monoclonal antibody which can neutralize human parvovirus B19. *J. Virol.* **1991**, *65*, 1667–1672.
70. Sato, H.; Hirata, J.; Kuroda, N.; Shiraki, H.; Maeda, Y.; Okochi, K. Identification and mapping of neutralizing epitopes of human parvovirus B19 by using human antibodies. *J. Virol.* **1991**, *65*, 5485–5490.
71. Saikawa, T.; Anderson, S.; Momoeda, M.; Kajigaya, S.; Young, N.S. Neutralizing linear epitopes of B19 parvovirus cluster in the VP1 unique and VP1-VP2 junction regions. *J. Virol.* **1993**, *67*, 3004–3009.
72. Sun, Y.; Klose, T.; Liu, Y.; Modrow, S.; Rossmann, M.G. Structure of Parvovirus B19 Decorated by Fabs from a Human Antibody. *J. Virol.* **2019**, *93*, e01732-18. [CrossRef]
73. Zuffi, E.; Manaresi, E.; Gallinella, G.; Gentilomi, G.A.; Venturoli, S.; Zerbini, M.; Musiani, M. Identification of an immunodominant peptide in the parvovirus B19 VP1 unique region able to elicit a long-lasting immune response in humans. *Viral Immunol.* **2001**, *14*, 151–158. [CrossRef]

74. Hattangadi, S.M.; Wong, P.; Zhang, L.; Flygare, J.; Lodish, H.F. From stem cell to red cell: Regulation of erythropoiesis at multiple levels by multiple proteins, RNAs, and chromatin modifications. *Blood* **2011**, *118*, 6258–6268. [CrossRef]
75. Filippone, C.; Franssila, R.; Kumar, A.; Saikko, L.; Kovanen, P.E.; Soderlund-Venermo, M.; Hedman, K. Erythroid progenitor cells expanded from peripheral blood without mobilization or preselection: Molecular characteristics and functional competence. *PLoS ONE* **2010**, *5*, e9496. [CrossRef]
76. Wong, S.; Brown, K.E. Development of an improved method of detection of infectious parvovirus B19. *J. Clin. Virol.* **2006**, *35*, 407–413. [CrossRef]
77. Manaresi, E.; Bua, G.; Bonvicini, F.; Gallinella, G. A flow-FISH assay for the quantitative analysis of parvovirus B19 infected cells. *J. Virol. Methods* **2015**, *223*, 50–54. [CrossRef]
78. Bonvicini, F.; Filippone, C.; Delbarba, S.; Manaresi, E.; Zerbini, M.; Musiani, M.; Gallinella, G. Parvovirus B19 genome as a single, two-state replicative and transcriptional unit. *Virology* **2006**, *347*, 447–454. [CrossRef]
79. Bonvicini, F.; Filippone, C.; Manaresi, E.; Zerbini, M.; Musiani, M.; Gallinella, G. Functional analysis and quantitative determination of the expression profile of human parvovirus B19. *Virology* **2008**, *381*, 168–177. [CrossRef]
80. Zhi, N.; Zadori, Z.; Brown, K.E.; Tijssen, P. Construction and sequencing of an infectious clone of the human parvovirus B19. *Virology* **2004**, *318*, 142–152. [CrossRef]
81. Manaresi, E.; Conti, I.; Bua, G.; Bonvicini, F.; Gallinella, G. A Parvovirus B19 synthetic genome: Sequence features and functional competence. *Virology* **2017**, *508*, 54–62. [CrossRef]
82. Bonvicini, F.; Bua, G.; Conti, I.; Manaresi, E.; Gallinella, G. Hydroxyurea inhibits parvovirus B19 replication in erythroid progenitor cells. *Biochem. Pharmacol.* **2017**, *136*, 32–39. [CrossRef]
83. Bonvicini, F.; Bua, G.; Manaresi, E.; Gallinella, G. Antiviral effect of cidofovir on parvovirus B19 replication. *Antivir. Res.* **2015**, *113*, 11–18. [CrossRef]
84. Bonvicini, F.; Bua, G.; Manaresi, E.; Gallinella, G. Enhanced inhibition of parvovirus B19 replication by cidofovir in extendedly exposed erythroid progenitor cells. *Virus Res.* **2016**, *220*, 47–51. [CrossRef]
85. Bua, G.; Conti, I.; Manaresi, E.; Sethna, P.; Foster, S.; Bonvicini, F.; Gallinella, G. Antiviral activity of brincidofovir on parvovirus B19. *Antivir. Res.* **2019**, *162*, 22–29. [CrossRef]
86. Conti, I.; Morigi, R.; Locatelli, A.; Rambaldi, M.; Bua, G.; Gallinella, G.; Leoni, A. Synthesis of 3-(Imidazo[2,1-b]thiazol-6-yl)-2H-chromen-2-one Derivatives and Study of Their Antiviral Activity against Parvovirus B19. *Molecules* **2019**, *24*, 1037. [CrossRef]
87. Xu, P.; Ganaie, S.S.; Wang, X.; Wang, Z.; Kleiboeker, S.; Horton, N.C.; Heier, R.F.; Meyers, M.J.; Tavis, J.E.; Qiu, J. Endonuclease Activity Inhibition of the NS1 Protein of Parvovirus B19 as a Novel Target for Antiviral Drug Development. *Antimicrob. Agents Chemother.* **2019**, *63*, e01879-18. [CrossRef]
88. Gallicchio, V.S. Ribonucleotide reductase: Target therapy for human disease. *Expert Opin. Ther. Pat.* **2005**, *15*, 659–673. [CrossRef]
89. Neyts, J.; De Clercq, E. Hydroxyurea Potentiates the Antiherpesvirus Activities of Purine and Pyrimidine Nucleoside and Nucleoside Phosphonate Analogs. *Antimicrob. Agents Chemother.* **1999**, *43*, 2885–2892. [CrossRef]
90. Lori, F.; Foli, A.; Kelly, L.M.; Lisziewicz, J. Virostatics: A new class of anti-HIV drugs. *Curr. Med. Chem.* **2007**, *14*, 233–241. [CrossRef]
91. Bhave, S.; Elford, H.; McVoy, M.A. Ribonucleotide reductase inhibitors hydroxyurea, didox, and trimidox inhibit human cytomegalovirus replication in vitro and synergize with ganciclovir. *Antivir. Res.* **2013**, *100*, 151–158. [CrossRef]
92. Liu, X.; Xu, Z.; Hou, C.; Wang, M.; Chen, X.; Lin, Q.; Song, R.; Lou, M.; Zhu, L.; Qiu, Y.; et al. Inhibition of hepatitis B virus replication by targeting ribonucleotide reductase M2 protein. *Biochem. Pharm.* **2016**, *103*, 118–128. [CrossRef]
93. Platt, O.S. Hydroxyurea for the treatment of sickle cell anemia. *N. Engl. J. Med.* **2008**, *358*, 1362–1369. [CrossRef]
94. Green, N.S.; Barral, S. Emerging science of hydroxyurea therapy for pediatric sickle cell disease. *Pediatric Res.* **2013**, *75*, 196. [CrossRef]
95. McGann, P.T.; Ware, R.E. Hydroxyurea therapy for sickle cell anemia. *Expert Opin. Drug Saf.* **2015**, *14*, 1749–1758. [CrossRef]

96. Hankins, J.S.; Penkert, R.R.; Lavoie, P.; Tang, L.; Sun, Y.; Hurwitz, J.L. Parvovirus B19 infection in children with sickle cell disease in the hydroxyurea era. *Exp. Biol. Med.* **2016**, *241*, 749–754. [CrossRef]
97. De Clercq, E.; Holy, A. Acyclic nucleoside phosphonates: A key class of antiviral drugs. *Nat. Rev. Drug Discov.* **2005**, *4*, 928–940. [CrossRef]
98. De Clercq, E. Acyclic nucleoside phosphonates: Past, present and future. Bridging chemistry to HIV, HBV, HCV, HPV, adeno-, herpes-, and poxvirus infections: The phosphonate bridge. *Biochem. Pharm.* **2007**, *73*, 911–922. [CrossRef]
99. Aldern, K.A.; Ciesla, S.L.; Winegarden, K.L.; Hostetler, K.Y. Increased antiviral activity of 1-O-hexadecyloxypropyl-[2-(14)C]cidofovir in MRC-5 human lung fibroblasts is explained by unique cellular uptake and metabolism. *Mol. Pharmacol.* **2003**, *63*, 678–681. [CrossRef]
100. Williams-Aziz, S.L.; Hartline, C.B.; Harden, E.A.; Daily, S.L.; Prichard, M.N.; Kushner, N.L.; Beadle, J.R.; Wan, W.B.; Hostetler, K.Y.; Kern, E.R. Comparative activities of lipid esters of cidofovir and cyclic cidofovir against replication of herpesviruses in vitro. *Antimicrob. Agents Chemother.* **2005**, *49*, 3724–3733. [CrossRef]
101. Hostetler, K.Y. Alkoxyalkyl prodrugs of acyclic nucleoside phosphonates enhance oral antiviral activity and reduce toxicity: Current state of the art. *Antivir. Res.* **2009**, *82*, A84–A98. [CrossRef]
102. McMullan, L.K.; Flint, M.; Dyall, J.; Albarino, C.; Olinger, G.G.; Foster, S.; Sethna, P.; Hensley, L.E.; Nichol, S.T.; Lanier, E.R.; et al. The lipid moiety of brincidofovir is required for in vitro antiviral activity against Ebola virus. *Antivir. Res.* **2016**, *125*, 71–78. [CrossRef]
103. Magee, W.C.; Evans, D.H. The antiviral activity and mechanism of action of (S)-[3-hydroxy-2-(phosphonomethoxy)propyl] (HPMP) nucleosides. *Antivir. Res.* **2012**, *96*, 169–180. [CrossRef]
104. Johnson, J.A.; Gangemi, J.D. Selective inhibition of human papillomavirus-induced cell proliferation by (S)-1-[3-hydroxy-2-(phosphonylmethoxy)propyl]cytosine. *Antimicrob. Agents Chemother.* **1999**, *43*, 1198–1205. [CrossRef]
105. Randhawa, P.; Farasati, N.A.; Shapiro, R.; Hostetler, K.Y. Ether lipid ester derivatives of cidofovir inhibit polyomavirus BK replication in vitro. *Antimicrob. Agents Chemother.* **2006**, *50*, 1564–1566. [CrossRef]
106. Jiang, Z.G.; Cohen, J.; Marshall, L.J.; Major, E.O. Hexadecyloxypropyl-cidofovir (CMX001) suppresses JC virus replication in human fetal brain SVG cell cultures. *Antimicrob. Agents Chemother.* **2010**, *54*, 4723–4732. [CrossRef]
107. Andrei, G.; Topalis, D.; De Schutter, T.; Snoeck, R. Insights into the mechanism of action of cidofovir and other acyclic nucleoside phosphonates against polyoma- and papillomaviruses and non-viral induced neoplasia. *Antivir. Res.* **2015**, *114*, 21–46. [CrossRef]
108. Tsang, S.H.; Wang, R.; Nakamaru-Ogiso, E.; Knight, S.A.; Buck, C.B.; You, J. The Oncogenic Small Tumor Antigen of Merkel Cell Polyomavirus Is an Iron-Sulfur Cluster Protein That Enhances Viral DNA Replication. *J. Virol.* **2016**, *90*, 1544–1556. [CrossRef]
109. Painter, W.; Robertson, A.; Trost, L.C.; Godkin, S.; Lampert, B.; Painter, G. First pharmacokinetic and safety study in humans of the novel lipid antiviral conjugate CMX001, a broad-spectrum oral drug active against double-stranded DNA viruses. *Antimicrob. Agents Chemother.* **2012**, *56*, 2726–2734. [CrossRef]
110. Tippin, T.K.; Morrison, M.E.; Brundage, T.M.; Mommeja-Marin, H. Brincidofovir Is Not a Substrate for the Human Organic Anion Transporter 1: A Mechanistic Explanation for the Lack of Nephrotoxicity Observed in Clinical Studies. *Ther. Drug Monit.* **2016**, *38*, 777–786. [CrossRef]
111. Chemaly, R.F.; Hill, J.A.; Voigt, S.; Peggs, K.S. In vitro comparison of currently available and investigational antiviral agents against pathogenic human double-stranded DNA viruses: A systematic literature review. *Antivir. Res.* **2019**, *163*, 50–58. [CrossRef]
112. Penta, S. *Advances in Structure and Activity Relationship of Coumarin Derivatives*; Academic Press: Cambridge, MA, USA, 2015; pp. 1–182.
113. Hassan, M.Z.; Osman, H.; Ali, M.A.; Ahsan, M.J. Therapeutic potential of coumarins as antiviral agents. *Eur. J. Med. Chem.* **2016**, *123*, 236–255. [CrossRef]
114. Tewary, S.K.; Zhao, H.; Deng, X.; Qiu, J.; Tang, L. The human parvovirus B19 non-structural protein 1 N-terminal domain specifically binds to the origin of replication in the viral DNA. *Virology* **2014**, *449*, 297–303. [CrossRef]
115. Sanchez, J.L.; Romero, Z.; Quinones, A.; Torgeson, K.R.; Horton, N.C. DNA Binding and Cleavage by the Human Parvovirus B19 NS1 Nuclease Domain. *Biochemistry* **2016**, *55*, 6577–6593. [CrossRef]

116. Van Linthout, S.; Elsanhoury, A.; Klein, O.; Sosnowski, M.; Miteva, K.; Lassner, D.; Abou-El-Enein, M.; Pieske, B.; Kuhl, U.; Tschope, C. Telbivudine in chronic lymphocytic myocarditis and human parvovirus B19 transcriptional activity. *ESC Heart Fail* **2018**, *5*, 818–829. [CrossRef]
117. Zobel, T.; Bock, C.T.; Kuhl, U.; Rohde, M.; Lassner, D.; Schultheiss, H.P.; Schmidt-Lucke, C. Telbivudine Reduces Parvovirus B19-Induced Apoptosis in Circulating Angiogenic Cells. *Viruses* **2019**, *11*, 227. [CrossRef]
118. Zimmermann, O.; Rodewald, C.; Radermacher, M.; Vetter, M.; Wiehe, J.M.; Bienek-Ziolkowski, M.; Hombach, V.; Torzewski, J. Interferon beta-1b therapy in chronic viral dilated cardiomyopathy—Is there a role for specific therapy? *J. Card. Fail.* **2010**, *16*, 348–356. [CrossRef]
119. Schmidt-Lucke, C.; Spillmann, F.; Bock, T.; Kuhl, U.; Van Linthout, S.; Schultheiss, H.P.; Tschope, C. Interferon beta modulates endothelial damage in patients with cardiac persistence of human parvovirus b19 infection. *J. Infect. Dis.* **2010**, *201*, 936–945. [CrossRef]
120. Schultheiss, H.P.; Piper, C.; Sowade, O.; Waagstein, F.; Kapp, J.F.; Wegscheider, K.; Groetzbach, G.; Pauschinger, M.; Escher, F.; Arbustini, E.; et al. Betaferon in chronic viral cardiomyopathy (BICC) trial: Effects of interferon-beta treatment in patients with chronic viral cardiomyopathy. *Clin. Res. Cardiol.* **2016**, *105*, 763–773. [CrossRef]

viruses

MDPI

Communication

Telbivudine Reduces Parvovirus B19-Induced Apoptosis in Circulating Angiogenic Cells

Thomas Zobel [1], C.-Thomas Bock [2], Uwe Kühl [1], Maria Rohde [3], Dirk Lassner [3], Heinz-Peter Schultheiss [1,3] and Caroline Schmidt-Lucke [1,4,5,*]

1 Department of Cardiology and Pneumology, Charité-Universitätsmedizin Berlin, 10117 Berlin, Germany; Thomas.Zobel@Verwaltung.Uni-Muenchen.de (T.Z.); uwe.kuhl@charite.de (U.K.); heinz-peter.schultheiss@charite.de (H.-P.S.)
2 Department of Infectious Diseases, Robert-Koch-Institut, 13353 Berlin, Germany; bockc@rki.de
3 Institut für Kardiale Diagnostik und Therapie (IKDT), 12203 Berlin, Germany; maria.rohde@ikdt.de (M.R.); info@ikdt.de (D.L.)
4 MEDIACC GmbH, 10713 Berlin, Germany
5 Berlin-Brandenburg Centre for Regenerative Therapies, 13353 Berlin, Germany
* Correspondence: caroline.schmidt-lucke@mediacc.org; Tel.: +49-30-86439773; Fax: +49-30-86439774

Received: 26 January 2019; Accepted: 1 March 2019; Published: 6 March 2019

Abstract: Aims: Human parvovirus B19 (B19V) infection directly induces apoptosis and modulates CXCR4 expression of infected marrow-derived circulating angiogenic cells (CACs). This leads to dysfunctional endogenous vascular repair. Treatment for B19V-associated disease is restricted to symptomatic treatment. Telbivudine, a thymidine analogue, established in antiviral treatment for chronic hepatitis B, modulates pathways that might influence induction of apoptosis. Therefore, we tested the hypothesis of whether telbivudine influences B19V-induced apoptosis of CAC. **Methods and Results:** Pretreatment of two CAC-lines, early outgrowth endothelial progenitor cells (eo-EPC) and endothelial colony-forming cells (ECFC) with telbivudine before in vitro infection with B19V significantly reduced active caspase-3 protein expression (−39% and −40%, both $p < 0.005$). Expression of Baculoviral Inhibitor of apoptosis Repeat-Containing protein 3 (BIRC3) was significantly downregulated by in vitro B19V infection in ECFC measured by qRT-PCR. BIRC3 downregulation was abrogated with telbivudine pretreatment ($p < 0.001$). This was confirmed by single gene PCR ($p = 0.017$) and Western blot analysis. In contrast, the missing effect of B19V on angiogenic gene expression postulates a post-transcriptional modulation of CXCR4. **Conclusions:** We for the first time show a treatment approach to reduce B19V-induced apoptosis. Telbivudine reverses B19V-induced dysregulation of BIRC3, thus, intervening in the apoptosis pathway and protecting susceptible cells from cell death. This approach could lead to an effective B19V treatment to reduce B19V-related disease.

Keywords: telbivudine; B19V; circulating angiogenic cells; apoptosis; caspase-3; BIRC3 (cIAP-2)

1. Introduction

Human parvovirus B19 (B19V), belonging to the genus Erythrovirus of the Parvoviridae family, is a single-stranded DNA virus responsible for a wide range of clinical manifestations. Although the majority of clinical disorders are generally self-limiting and subclinical [1], in certain cases, the disease may turn chronic and clinically relevant. The latter may result from either direct virus-mediated injury, increased apoptosis [2], inadequacy of the specific anti-viral immune response [3] or dysregulated trafficking of cells involved in endothelial regeneration [4].

B19V replication and expression profiles highlight the very restricted cellular targets defined by a specific receptor status, erythroid lineage, and differentiation stage [2,5–8]. Recently, we have identified different cell types belonging to the heterogenous group of marrow-derived circulating angiogenic cells (CACs) with similarities to the erythroid and endothelial lineage, to be targets for B19 infection [2]. CAC play a key role in cardiovascular regeneration [9]. B19V directly induces apoptosis of CAC through the viral proteins NS1, VP1 [2], and the small 11kDa protein and impairs their trafficking [4]. Among CAC, the so-called early outgrowth endothelial progenitor cells (eo-EPC) have been shown to parallel disease progression in atherosclerosis [10]. Clonally distinct endothelial colony-forming cells (ECFC) with high proliferative potential expressing endothelial cell surface antigens form robust vascular structures in vivo and in vitro [11,12] and are associated with improved cardiac function [13].

Inhibitor of Apoptosis (IAP) gene products play an evolutionarily conserved role in regulating programmed cell death in diverse species [14]. The Baculoviral Inhibitor of apoptosis Repeat-Containing protein 3 (BIRC3; cellular inhibitor of apoptosis-2, cIAP-2) is a member of the Inhibitor of Apoptosis family [15,16] that inhibit apoptosis by interfering with the activation of caspases-3, -6, and -7 [14,17,18], including the effector caspase-9 [14] and caspase-8 [15,19]. We have previously shown the induction of apoptosis in CAC through activation of caspases-8 and -10 [2]. Expression of BIRC3 has been strongly linked to cell survival in virally-associated cancer and been classified as an oncogene [20]. Furthermore, BIRC3 was found to inhibit hepatitis B virus (HBV) protein synthesis, viral replication, and transcription [21,22] and ubiquitination of cellular factors essential for antiviral response [23].

The synthetic thymidine nucleoside analogue telbivudine, approved for the treatment of hepatitis B [24,25], inhibits DNA dependent second strand DNA synthesis [24,25]. Mechanistically, telbivudine-5′-triphosphate is incorporated into the nascent HBV DNA strand by the HBV DNA polymerase, competing with the natural substrate thymidine-5′-triphosphate, finally leading to chain termination. Furthermore, telbivudine modulates expression of the cytokines TNFα and Interferon-gamma (INFγ) [26–28] and influences NF-κB level [29] restoring cellular immune response. A direct effect of telbivudine on apoptosis has so far never been investigated.

Therefore, we tested the hypothesis of telbivudine influencing B19V-induced apoptosis of CAC We, therefore, analysed potential signalling pathway of apoptosis induction by B19V and the effect of telbivudine treatment in vitro.

2. Methods

2.1. Cell lines and Isolation of Primary Cells

Mononuclear cells (MNC) were isolated by density-gradient centrifugation with Biocoll (Biochrom) from peripheral blood of healthy donors. Cultivation of eo-EPC was performed as described previously [2], using the same seronegative male donors for corresponding experiments.

Human umbilical cord blood ECFC were purchased from Lonza and cultivated as recommended by the manufacturer. Experiments with ECFC were conducted at passage 5 to 7 since these yielded optimal results [2]. All in vitro experiments were conducted at least in triplicate. Cells were cultivated at 37 °C, 5% CO_2.

For the rationale to use different cell lines for the individual experiments, please see [2].

2.2. Telbivudine Treatment of Cell Cultures

Telbivudine (sc-222340, Santa Cruz Biotechnology) was dissolved in water and added at final concentrations of 10 ng/mL (41.3 nM) to the respective cell culture medium 2 h before infection.

2.3. Virus Stock and Infection

B19V belonging to genotype 1 was purified from the serum of a patient with B19V as described previously [2]. The concentration of virus particles was quantified by real-time PCR by means of B19V genome equivalents (GE). Uninfected, virus-free control plasma was purified using identical experimental conditions. Until otherwise indicated, cells were infected in the appropriate growth medium with 3000 GE/cell or treated with equal volumes of purified control plasma. As an internal control for successful B19V infection, detection of B19V DNA and RNA by nested PCR was performed as described previously with primers specific for the NS1 coding sequence [2] before performing the following experiments.

Consequently, 4 different experimental settings were compared: (a) plasma treatment, no telbivudine (plasma, no telbivudine); (b) plasma treatment, telbivudine (plasma, telbivudine); (c) B19V-infected plasma, no telbivudine (B19V, no telbivudine); (d) B19V-infected plasma, telbivudine (B19V, telbivudine).

2.4. *RNA Isolation and Reverse Transcriptase PCR*

Total RNA isolation with the RNeasy Kit (Qiagen, Hilden, Germany), DNase digestion of purified RNA with Turbo DNA-free DNase (Life Technologies, Waltham, Massachusetts, U.S.) and cDNA synthesis with M-MLV Reverse Transcriptase (RT) RNase H minus (Promega, Fitchburg, Wisconsin, USA) were performed according to the manufacturer's instructions. Turbo DNA-free digestion (Thermo Fisher Scientific, Waltham, Massachusetts, USA) was performed with 500 ng to 1.5 µg total RNA as recommended. At least 300 ng DNase-digested RNA was reverse transcribed with M-MLV RT as +RT reactions versus equal amounts of RNA under the same conditions without M-MLV RT as –RT reactions. cDNA synthesis was performed with oligo(dT) primers (Thermo Fisher Scientific).

2.5. *Fluorescence Associated Cell Sorting (FACS) Analysis for Active Caspase-3*

Active caspase-3 staining was performed with infected CAC as described previously [2]. CACs were harvested with Accutase (Thermo Fisher Scientific), fixed with 4% paraformaldehyde and washed. CACs were incubated for 15 min. at 4 °C with 2% human FcR-blocking reagent and washed once with phosphate buffered saline (PBS) (Sigma Aldrich, St. Louis, Missouri, USA). Afterwards, cells were permeabilized for intracellular caspase-3 staining with Cytofix/Cytoperm-solution (BD Cytofix/Cytoperm Permeabilization Kit, BD Biosciences) for 15 min. at 4 °C. Cells were resuspended in 100 µL BD Perm/Wash buffer and incubated with V450 rabbit anti-active caspase-3 antibody (1:33 diluted, BD Biosciences, Erembodegem, Belgium) for 20 min. at 4 °C in the dark. After the incubation, cells were washed once with BD Perm/Wash buffer and resuspended in PBS. FACS analyses were done on a BD FACSCanto II (BD Biosciences).

2.6. *PCR Array for Human Apoptosis and Angiogenesis*

A Human Apoptosis (PAHS-12Z) and Angiogenesis (PAHS-024Z) RT^2 Profiler PCR Array was performed with the RT^2 First Strand Kit and the RT^2 SYBR Green/ ROX Master Mix according to the manufacturer's instructions (Qiagen) using 500 ng input RNA. Data were analysed with the PCR Array Data Analysis Software (Qiagen). For this, only ECFC were used since this cell type can be cultivated in greater quantities independent of intersubject variability and expected confounders through the experimental manipulations.

2.7. *BIRC3 Single PCR Levels*

Quantitative PCR for BIRC 3 was performed using 50 ng cDNA with the Fast Blue qPCR MasterMix plus ROX (Eurogentec, Seraing, Belgium) and the BIRC3 TaqMan GeneExpression Assay (HS00985031_g1) according to the manufacturer's instructions. Standardization was performed with a primer/probe set against ribosomal Protein S29 (RPS29) using a primer and probe set designed by the Roche Universal Probe Library (UPL) Assay Design Center and using Universal Probe number 25 using the Fast Blue qPCR MasterMix plus ROX and 50 ng cDNA according to the manufacturer's instructions.

2.8. Statistical Analysis

All experiments except for the ones for the PCR-arrays (for apoptosis (n = 2) and for angiogenetic genes, n = 1) were performed as at least three independent experiments. Continuous variables were tested for normal distribution with the Kolmogorov–Smirnov test. Non-normally distributed continuous variables were compared by the Mann–Whitney-U test for two groups or by the Kruskal–Wallis test with more than two subgroups with post hoc analysis (Wilcoxon). Data are expressed as mean ± SD, unless otherwise stated. Comparison of categorical variables was generated by the Pearson $\chi 2$ test. Statistical significance was assumed if a null hypothesis could be rejected at $p \leq 0.05$. All statistical analysis was performed with SPSS 21.0 (SPSS, IBM, Armonk, New York, USA.).

3. Results

Telbivudine Inhibits Activation of B19V-Induced Apoptosis through Stabilisation of BIRC3 Levels

We have previously shown a strong induction of apoptosis in B19V-infected CAC [2]. Here, we assessed the magnitude of apoptosis in CAC after in vitro infection with B19V and the effect of pre-treatment with telbivudine, respectively. Pre-treatment with telbivudine significantly ($p < 0.001$) reduced B19V-induced apoptosis by 39%, as measured by activation of the effector caspase-3 in ECFC (B19V, no telbivudine 81.5 ± 11.7% vs. B19V, telbivudine 35.8 ± 19.3% active caspase-3 positive cells compared to plasma, no telbivudine 3.3 ± 2.4% vs. plasma, telbivudine 1.8 ± 1.3%; Figure 1A) and eo-EPC by 40%, ($p < 0.005$; B19V, no telbivudine 51.8 ± 2.3% vs. B19V, telbivudine 31.0 ± 5.6% active caspase-3 positive cells compared to plasma, no telbivudine 4.1 ± 1.7% vs. plasma, telbivudine 1.6 ± 0.4%; Figure 1B).

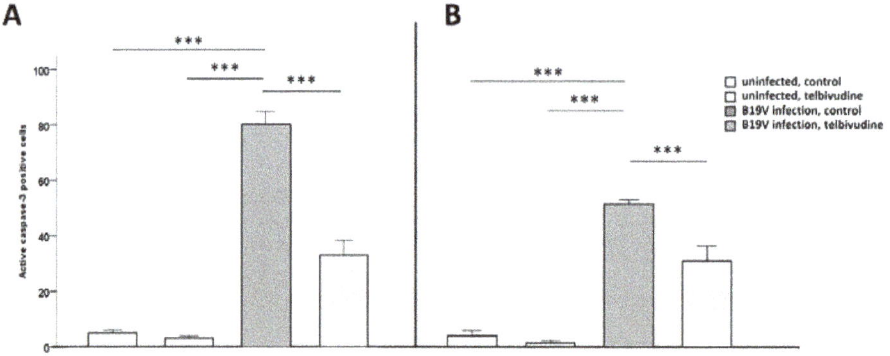

Figure 1. Reduced human parvovirus B19 (B19V)-induced apoptosis after telbivudine pre-treatment in B19V-infected early outgrowth endothelial progenitor cells (eo-EPC) and endothelial colony-forming cells (ECFC). Quantification of active caspase-3 positive in (**A**) ECFC and (**B**) eo-EPC. Data are means +SD, *** is $p < 0.001$.

To further dissect the underlying pathway, we analyzed multiple pathways through a PCR array for human apoptosis ($n = 1$) using ECFC. Infection with B19V led to strong downregulation of BIRC3 mRNA levels. Treatment of CAC with telbivudine before B19V infection reversed this effect (Figure 2A). This was confirmed by Single PCR ($n = 4$, Figure 2B), that showed BIRC3 levels to be less downregulated when ECFC were pretreated with elbivudine before B19V infection.

A

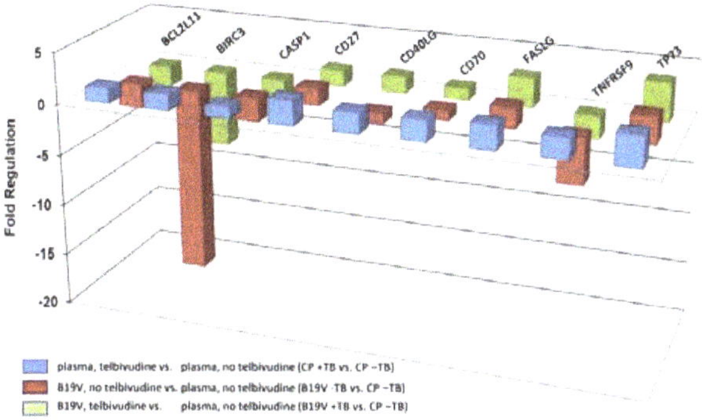

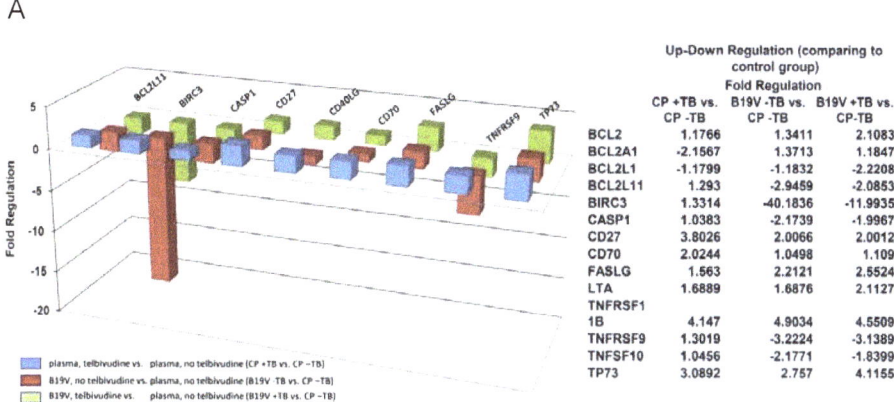

	Up-Down Regulation (comparing to control group) Fold Regulation		
	CP +TB vs. CP -TB	B19V -TB vs. CP -TB	B19V +TB vs. CP-TB
BCL2	1.1766	1.3411	2.1083
BCL2A1	-2.1567	1.3713	1.1847
BCL2L1	-1.1799	-1.1832	-2.2208
BCL2L11	1.293	-2.9459	-2.0853
BIRC3	1.3314	-40.1836	-11.9935
CASP1	1.0383	-2.1739	-1.9967
CD27	3.8026	2.0066	2.0012
CD70	2.0244	1.0498	1.109
FASLG	1.563	2.2121	2.5524
LTA	1.6889	1.6876	2.1127
TNFRSF11B	4.147	4.9034	4.5509
TNFRSF9	1.3019	-3.2224	-3.1389
TNFSF10	1.0456	-2.1771	-1.8399
TP73	3.0892	2.757	4.1155

B

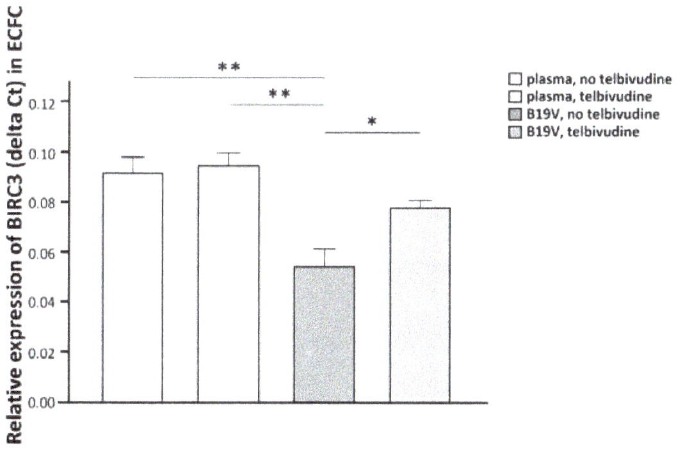

Figure 2. PCR Array for apoptosis and Baculoviral Inhibitor of apoptosis Repeat-Containing protein 3 (BIRC3) after telbivudine pre-treatment in B19V-infected ECFC. (**A**) Regulation of apoptotic genes in ECFC; plasma, telbivudine versus plasma, no telbivudine (blue bars), B19V, no telbivudine versus plasma, no telbivudine (red bars), and B19V, telbivudine versus plasma, no telbivudine (green bars). (**B**) Quantification of BIRC RNA in ECFC, * is $p < 0.05$, ** is $p < 0.01$.

Having shown that B19V infection affects trafficking of CAC [4], we subsequently analysed the effect of telbivudine on angiogenic genes with an RT2 Profiler PCR array analysis for angiogenic genes (n = 1). We saw very little changes in a few other genes, so that we postulate a post-transcriptional effect of B19V on CXCR4.

4. Discussion

The results of this study show for the first time an anti-apoptotic effect of the nucleoside analogue telbivudine through normalisation of BIRC3 levels in B19V-induced apoptosis in CACs, thus, providing a novel approach to protecting cells from B19V damage. These results extend the knowledge of activities of telbivudine against known human viruses. Thus, telbivudine may be an interesting candidate to unravel new insights into cellular mechanisms in B19V infection.

B19V infection is restricted to a small number of cell lines including erythroid progenitor cells, erythroblastoid cell line UT7/Epo-S1 [6,7] or CAC [2], the latter are important players in endogenous cardiovascular regeneration [30]. B19V infection in humans is associated with impaired endothelial regeneration through induction of apoptosis and dysregulated trafficking of infected CAC [2,4]. Therapy with interferon beta suppresses B19V replication (by 63%) and increases the viability of these erythroid progenitors [31]. However, an effective treatment option for B19V-associated disease is not available.

We, therefore, tested the effect of telbivudine, a thymidine analogon and therapeutic agent well established for treatment of chronic hepatitis B, in B19V infection of CAC focussing on apoptosis and trafficking. Reproducing previous results, B19V infection strongly induced apoptosis in CAC [2], and as demonstrated in this study, B19V-induced apoptosis is mediated through downregulation of the antiapoptotic inhibitors of apoptosis BIRC3 (cellular inhibitor of apoptosis-2 (cIAP2)), a potent suppressor of apoptotic cell death. With pretreatment of telbivudine, downregulation of the anti-apoptotic BIRC3 in CAC is reduced and apoptosis prevented. BIRC3 prevents the proteolytic processing of pro-caspases -3, -6 and -7 by blocking the cytochrome c-induced activation of pro-caspase-9 [14]. Whereas caspase-8 induced proteolytic activation of pro-caspase-3 is not inhibited by BIRC3 [14], the formation of a complex with the TNF-receptor associated factor 1 (TRAF1), TRAF2, and the TNFα receptor (TNFR), activating caspase-8, is hindered [15,19,32]. The direct anti-apoptotic effect of telbivudine in B19V-induced apoptosis could be shown on transcriptional levels of BIRC3. Further research on the precise pathway, on protein levels, up- and downstream signalling and to identify influencing player, i.e., RIP1, TRAF1, TRAF2, TRAIL, TNFR, caspase-8, caspase-6/7/9, is needed [33]. In erythroid progenitor cells, INFγ delays apoptosis, related to the expression of Bcl-x without the involvement of Fas [34]. The TNFα -inducible gene cIAP2 inhibits HBV protein synthesis, viral replication, and transcription [21]. Thus, since telbivudine alters the NF-κB level [29] and modulates expression of the cytokines TNFα and INFγ [26–28], the INFγ-mediated apoptosis pathways including NF-κB expression offer a further promising target [35–37].

Much to our surprise, no angiogenic gene modulations were detected, postulating a post-transcriptional effect of B19V on CXCR4 that needs to be further dissected.

The identification of compounds active against B19V-induced vascular damage might add therapeutic options to the treatment of B19 infection which, up to now, relies entirely on symptomatic treatment. It is tempting to speculate that the reduction of apoptosis of CAC by telbivudine could improve cell survival, thus, reducing the turn-over rate of CAC, which in turn could preserve the presumably finite pool of regenerative cells. This can be expected to preserve endothelial regenerative function. Whether our preliminary findings can be extended to a specific treatment in B19V-induced diseases in vivo, will have to be evaluated in detail in confirmatory in vitro and in vivo experimental and clinical studies. Furthermore, experiments to show the effect on apoptotic pathways apart from directly interfering with B19V replication are needed. Of interest, the results of these studies might have implications for angiogenesis related to tumour angiogenesis. The research on the role of B19V or its compounds might open new therapeutic approaches.

Author Contributions: T.Z., C.-T.B. and C.S.-L. conceived and designed the experiments; T.Z., M.R. and D.L. performed the experiments; T.Z. and C.S.-L. analyzed the data; M.R. and D.L. contributed reagents/materials/analysis tools; T.Z., H.-P.S. and C.S.-L. wrote the paper.

Funding: This study was supported by the Deutsche Forschungsgemeinschaft (SFB/TR 19 B6) and the Berlin-Brandenburg Centre for Regenerative Therapies (BCRT) to CSL and were supported by MEDIACC, Medico-academic Consultings, Berlin. The funders had no role in study design, data collection and analysis, decision to publish, or preparation of the manuscript.

Acknowledgments: We are grateful to Karen Boehme and Marzena Sosnowski for expert technical assistance. We thank Heinz Zeichhardt for his excellent support in virus purification and Stefan Weger for providing us with the virus lab facility.

Conflicts of Interest: None of the authors has any conflict of interest.

Abbreviations

B19V	human parvovirus B19
BIRC3	baculoviral inhibitor of apoptosis repeat-containing protein 3
CAC	circulating angiogenic cells
cIAP-2	cellular inhibitor of apoptosis-2
eo-EPC	early outgrowth endothelial progenitor cells
ECFC	endothelial colony forming cells
FACS	fluorescence associated cell sorting
GE	genome equivalents
HBV	hepatitis B virus
IAP	inhibitor of apoptosis
KDR	kinase insert domain receptor
MNC	mononuclear cells
PBS	phosphate buffered saline
RT	reverse transcriptase
RIP1	receptor interacting protein (RIP) kinases 1
TNF	tumor necrosis factor
TNFR	TNFα receptor
TRAF1	TNF receptor associated factor 1
TRAF2	TNF receptor associated factor 2
TRAIL	TNF-related apoptosis-inducing ligand

References

1. Cossart, Y.E.; Cant, B.; Field, A.M.; Widdows, D. Parvovirus-like particles in human sera. *Lancet* **1975**, *305*, 72–73. [CrossRef]
2. Schmidt-Lucke, C.; Zobel, T.; Schrepfer, S.; Kuhl, U.; Wang, D.; Klingel, K.; Becher, P.M.; Fechner, H.; Pozzuto, T.; Van Linthout, S.; et al. Impaired Endothelial Regeneration Through Human Parvovirus B19-Infected Circulating Angiogenic Cells in Patients with Cardiomyopathy. *J. Infect. Dis.* **2015**, *212*, 1070–1081. [CrossRef] [PubMed]
3. Brown, K.E.; Anderson, S.; Young, N.S. Erythrocyte P antigen: Cellular receptor for B19 parvovirus. *Science* **1993**, *262*, 114–117. [CrossRef] [PubMed]
4. Schmidt-Lucke, C.; Zobel, T.; Escher, F.; Tschope, C.; Lassner, D.; Kuhl, U.; Gubbe, K.; Volk, H.D.; Schultheiss, H.P. Human Parvovirus B19 (B19V) Up-regulates CXCR4 Surface Expression of Circulating Angiogenic Cells: Implications for Cardiac Ischemia in B19V Cardiomyopathy. *J. Infect. Dis.* **2018**, *217*, 456–465. [CrossRef] [PubMed]
5. Bua, G.; Manaresi, E.; Bonvicini, F.; Gallinella, G. Parvovirus B19 Replication and Expression in Differentiating Erythroid Progenitor Cells. *PLoS ONE* **2016**, *11*, e0148547. [CrossRef] [PubMed]
6. Wong, S.; Zhi, N.; Filippone, C.; Keyvanfar, K.; Kajigaya, S.; Brown, K.E.; Young, N.S. Ex Vivo-Generated CD36+ Erythroid Progenitors Are Highly Permissive to Human Parvovirus B19 Replication. *J. Virol.* **2008**, *82*, 2470–2476. [CrossRef] [PubMed]
7. Shimomura, S.; Komatsu, N.; Frickhofen, N.; Anderson, S.; Kajigaya, S.; Young, N. First continuous propagation of B19 parvovirus in a cell line. *Blood* **1992**, *79*, 18–24. [PubMed]
8. Kuhl, U.; Lassner, D.; Dorner, A.; Rohde, M.; Escher, F.; Seeberg, B.; Hertel, E.; Tschope, C.; Skurk, C.; Gross, U.M.; et al. A distinct subgroup of cardiomyopathy patients characterized by transcriptionally active cardiotropic erythrovirus and altered cardiac gene expression. *Basic Res. Cardiol.* **2013**, *108*, 372. [CrossRef] [PubMed]
9. Bearzi, C.; Leri, A.; Lo Monaco, F.; Rota, M.; Gonzalez, A.; Hosoda, T.; Pepe, M.; Qanud, K.; Ojaimi, C.; Bardelli, S.; et al. Identification of a coronary vascular progenitor cell in the human heart. *Proc. Natl. Acad. Sci. USA* **2009**, *106*, 15885–15890. [CrossRef] [PubMed]
10. Vasa, M.; Fichtlscherer, S.; Adler, K.; Aicher, A.; Martin, H.; Zeiher, A.; Dimmeler, S. Increase in circulating endothelial progenitor cells by statin therapy in patients with stable coronary artery disease. *Circulation* **2001**, *103*, 2885–2890. [CrossRef] [PubMed]

11. Ingram, D.A.; Mead, L.E.; Tanaka, H.; Meade, V.; Fenoglio, A.; Mortell, K.; Pollok, K.; Ferkowicz, M.J.; Gilley, D.; Yoder, M.C. Identification of a novel hierarchy of endothelial progenitor cells using human peripheral and umbilical cord blood. *Blood* **2004**, *104*, 2752–2760. [CrossRef] [PubMed]
12. Yoder, M.C.; Mead, L.E.; Prater, D.; Krier, T.R.; Mroueh, K.N.; Li, F.; Krasich, R.; Temm, C.J.; Prchal, J.T.; Ingram, D.A. Redefining endothelial progenitor cells via clonal analysis and hematopoietic stem/progenitor cell principals. *Blood* **2007**, *109*, 1801–1809. [CrossRef] [PubMed]
13. Meneveau, N.; Deschaseaux, F.; Séronde, M.-F.; Chopard, R.; Schiele, F.; Jehl, J.; Tiberghien, P.; Bassand, J.-P.; Kantelip, J.-P.; Davani, S. Presence of endothelial colony-forming cells is associated with reduced microvascular obstruction limiting infarct size and left ventricular remodelling in patients with acute myocardial infarction. *Basic Res. Cardiol.* **2011**, *106*, 1397–1410. [CrossRef] [PubMed]
14. Deveraux, Q.L.; Roy, N.; Stennicke, H.R.; Van Arsdale, T.; Zhou, Q.; Srinivasula, S.M.; Alnemri, E.S.; Salvesen, G.S.; Reed, J.C. IAPs block apoptotic events induced by caspase-8 and cytochrome c by direct inhibition of distinct caspases. *EMBO J.* **1998**, *17*, 2215–2223. [CrossRef] [PubMed]
15. Rothe, M.; Pan, M.G.; Henzel, W.J.; Ayres, T.M.; Goeddel, D.V. The TNFR2-TRAF signaling complex contains two novel proteins related to baculoviral inhibitor of apoptosis proteins. *Cell* **1995**, *83*, 1243–1252. [CrossRef]
16. Liston, P.; Roy, N.; Tamai, K.; Lefebvre, C.; Baird, S.; Cherton-Horvat, G.; Farahani, R.; McLean, M.; Ikeda, J.E.; MacKenzie, A.; et al. Suppression of apoptosis in mammalian cells by NAIP and a related family of IAP genes. *Nature* **1996**, *379*, 349–353. [CrossRef] [PubMed]
17. Roy, N.; Deveraux, Q.L.; Takahashi, R.; Salvesen, G.S.; Reed, J.C. The c-IAP-1 and c-IAP-2 proteins are direct inhibitors of specific caspases. *EMBO J.* **1997**, *16*, 6914–6925. [CrossRef] [PubMed]
18. Xu, Z.; Lu, G.; Wu, F. Simvastatin suppresses homocysteine-induced apoptosis in endothelial cells: Roles of caspase-3, cIAP-1 and cIAP-2. *Hypertens. Res.* **2009**, *32*, 375–380. [CrossRef] [PubMed]
19. Wang, L.; Du, F.; Wang, X. TNF-alpha induces two distinct caspase-8 activation pathways. *Cell* **2008**, *133*, 693–703. [CrossRef] [PubMed]
20. Dai, Z.; Zhu, W.G.; Morrison, C.D.; Brena, R.M.; Smiraglia, D.J.; Raval, A.; Wu, Y.Z.; Rush, L.J.; Ross, P.; Molina, J.R.; et al. A comprehensive search for DNA amplification in lung cancer identifies inhibitors of apoptosis cIAP1 and cIAP2 as candidate oncogenes. *Hum. Mol. Genet.* **2003**, *12*, 791–801. [CrossRef] [PubMed]
21. Liu, X.; Shao, J.; Xiong, W.; Yu, S.; Hu, Y.; Liu, J.; Wang, X.; Xiang, L.; Yuan, Z. Cellular cIAP2 gene expression associated with anti-HBV activity of TNF-alpha in hepatoblastoma cells. *J. Interf. Cytokine Res.* **2005**, *25*, 617–626. [CrossRef] [PubMed]
22. Wang, Z.; Ni, J.; Li, J.; Shi, B.; Xu, Y.; Yuan, Z. Inhibition of hepatitis B virus replication by cIAP2 involves accelerating the ubiquitin-proteasome-mediated destruction of polymerase. *J. Virol.* **2011**, *85*, 11457–11467. [CrossRef] [PubMed]
23. Mao, A.P.; Li, S.; Zhong, B.; Li, Y.; Yan, J.; Li, Q.; Teng, C.; Shu, H.B. Virus-triggered ubiquitination of TRAF3/6 by cIAP1/2 is essential for induction of interferon-beta (IFN-beta) and cellular antiviral response. *J. Biol. Chem.* **2010**, *285*, 9470–9476. [CrossRef] [PubMed]
24. Lai, C.L.; Gane, E.; Liaw, Y.F.; Hsu, C.W.; Thongsawat, S.; Wang, Y.; Chen, Y.; Heathcote, E.J.; Rasenack, J.; Bzowej, N.; et al. Telbivudine versus lamivudine in patients with chronic hepatitis B. *N. Engl. J. Med.* **2007**, *357*, 2576–2588. [CrossRef] [PubMed]
25. Tillmann, H.L.; McHutchison, J.G. Telbivudine versus lamivudine in patients with chronic hepatitis B. *N. Engl. J. Med.* **2008**, *358*, 1517–1518. [PubMed]
26. Chen, Y.; Li, X.; Ye, B.; Yang, X.; Wu, W.; Chen, B.; Pan, X.; Cao, H.; Li, L. Effect of telbivudine therapy on the cellular immune response in chronic hepatitis B. *Antivir. Res.* **2011**, *91*, 23–31. [CrossRef] [PubMed]
27. Ge, J.; Huang, Z.; Liu, H.; Chen, J.; Xie, Z.; Chen, Z.; Peng, J.; Sun, J.; Hou, J.; Zhang, X. Lower Expression of MicroRNA-155 Contributes to Dysfunction of Natural Killer Cells in Patients with Chronic Hepatitis B. *Front. Immunol.* **2017**, *8*, 1173. [CrossRef] [PubMed]
28. Wu, Z.G.; Yan, W.M.; Guo, W.; Chen, T.; Zou, Y.; Wang, H.W.; Wang, X.J.; Yang, X.J.; Lu, Y.L.; Luo, X.P.; et al. Telbivudine preserves T-helper 1 cytokine production and downregulates programmed death ligand 1 in a mouse model of viral hepatitis. *J. Viral Hepat.* **2010**, *17* (Suppl. 1), 24–33. [CrossRef] [PubMed]
29. Chen, J.; Li, D. Telbivudine attenuates UUO-induced renal fibrosis via TGF-beta/Smad and NF-kappaB signaling. *Int. Immunopharmacol.* **2018**, *55*, 1–8. [CrossRef] [PubMed]

30. Fadini, G.P.; Losordo, D.; Dimmeler, S. Critical Reevaluation of Endothelial Progenitor Cell Phenotypes for Therapeutic and Diagnostic Use. *Circ. Res.* **2012**, *110*, 624–637. [CrossRef] [PubMed]
31. Schmidt-Lucke, C.; Spillmann, F.; Bock, T.; Kuhl, U.; Van Linthout, S.; Schultheiss, H.P.; Tschope, C. Interferon beta modulates endothelial damage in patients with cardiac persistence of human parvovirus B19V infection. *J. Infect. Dis.* **2010**, *201*, 936–945. [CrossRef] [PubMed]
32. Chen, A.Y.; Zhang, E.Y.; Guan, W.; Cheng, F.; Kleiboeker, S.; Yankee, T.M.; Qiu, J. The small 11kDa nonstructural protein of human parvovirus B19 plays a key role in inducing apoptosis during B19 virus infection of primary erythroid progenitor cells. *Blood* **2010**, *115*, 1070–1080. [CrossRef] [PubMed]
33. Mahoney, D.J.; Cheung, H.H.; Mrad, R.L.; Plenchette, S.; Simard, C.; Enwere, E.; Arora, V.; Mak, T.W.; Lacasse, E.C.; Waring, J.; et al. Both cIAP1 and cIAP2 regulate TNFalpha-mediated NF-kappaB activation. *Proc. Natl. Acad. Sci. USA* **2008**, *105*, 11778–11783. [CrossRef] [PubMed]
34. Choi, I.; Muta, K.; Wickrema, A.; Krantz, S.B.; Nishimura, J.; Nawata, H. Interferon gamma delays apoptosis of mature erythroid progenitor cells in the absence of erythropoietin. *Blood* **2000**, *95*, 3742–3749. [PubMed]
35. Schoemaker, M.H.; Ros, J.E.; Homan, M.; Trautwein, C.; Liston, P.; Poelstra, K.; van Goor, H.; Jansen, P.L.; Moshage, H. Cytokine regulation of pro- and anti-apoptotic genes in rat hepatocytes: NF-kappaB-regulated inhibitor of apoptosis protein 2 (cIAP2) prevents apoptosis. *J. Hepatol.* **2002**, *36*, 742–750. [CrossRef]
36. Guo, S.; Messmer-Blust, A.F.; Wu, J.; Song, X.; Philbrick, M.J.; Shie, J.L.; Rana, J.S.; Li, J. Role of A20 in cIAP-2 protection against tumor necrosis factor alpha (TNF-alpha)-mediated apoptosis in endothelial cells. *Int. J. Mol. Sci.* **2014**, *15*, 3816–3833. [CrossRef] [PubMed]
37. Ebert, G.; Preston, S.; Allison, C.; Cooney, J.; Toe, J.G.; Stutz, M.D.; Ojaimi, S.; Scott, H.W.; Baschuk, N.; Nachbur, U.; et al. Cellular inhibitor of apoptosis proteins prevent clearance of hepatitis B virus. *Proc. Natl. Acad. Sci. USA* **2015**, *112*, 5797–5802. [CrossRef] [PubMed]

viruses

MDPI

Review

Systematic Review of PCR Proof of Parvovirus B19 Genomes in Endomyocardial Biopsies of Patients Presenting with Myocarditis or Dilated Cardiomyopathy

Angelos G. Rigopoulos [1,†], Bianca Klutt [2,†], Marios Matiakis [1], Athanasios Apostolou [3], Sophie Mavrogeni [4] and Michel Noutsias [1,*]

1 Mid-German Heart Center, Department of Internal Medicine III (KIM-III), Division of Cardiology, Angiology and Intensive Medical Care, University Hospital Halle-Wittenberg, Mid-German Heart Center, Martin-Luther-University Halle-Wittenberg, Ernst-Grube-Straße 40, D-06120 Halle (Saale), Germany; angelos.rigopoulos@uk-halle.de (A.G.R.); marios.matiakis@uk-halle.de (M.M.)

2 Department of Anesthesiology, Helios Hospital Herzberg/Osterode, Dr.-Frössel-Allee, D-37412 Herzberg am Harz, Germany; Bianca.Klutt@harz.de

3 School of Health Sciences, Faculty of Medicine, Department of Immunology & Histocompatibility, University of Thessaly, 41500 Larissa, Greece; thanosapostolou@gmail.com

4 Onassis Cardiac Surgery Center, Department of Cardiology, and National Kapodistrian University of Athens, Leoforou Andrea Siggrou 356, Kallithea, 17674 Athens, Greece; sophie.mavrogeni@gmail.com

* Correspondence: michel.noutsias@uk-halle.de; Tel.: +49-(151)-40236274; Fax: +49-(345)-5572072

† These authors contributed equally to this work.

Received: 27 May 2019; Accepted: 12 June 2019; Published: 18 June 2019

Abstract: Background: Diverse viral infections have been associated with myocarditis (MC) and dilated cardiomyopathy (DCM). In this meta-analysis, we summarize the published results on the association of parvovirus B19 (B19V) genomes with human MC/DCM versus controls. Methods: n = 197 publications referring to B19V and MC or DCM were retrieved using multiple PubMed search modes. Out of these, n = 29 publications met the inclusion criteria with data from prospective analyses on >10 unselected patients presenting with MC or DCM (dataset: MA01). Data retrieved simultaneously from both controls and MC/DCM patients were available from n = 8 from these publications (dataset: MA02). Results: In the dataset MA01 B19V genomes were detected in 42.6% of the endomyocardial biopsies (EMB) in this cohort by PCR. In the dataset MA02 comprising n = 638 subjects, there was no statistically significant different rate of B19V positivity in myocardial tissues comparing controls (mean: 38.8 + 24.1%) versus the MC/DCM-patients (45.5 + 24.3%; p = 0.58). There was also no statistical difference between the positivity rate of B19V genomes in myocardial tissues of MA01 (46.0 + 19.5%) and the two patient groups of MA02 (p > 0.05). Conclusions: This systematic review reveals that the mean rate of PCR detected B19V genomes in patients presenting with MC/DCM does not differ significantly from the findings in control myocardial tissues. These data imply pathogenetically insignificant latency of B19V genomes in a proportion of myocardial tissues, both in MC-/DCM-patients and in controls. More information (i.e., replicative status, viral protein expression) is pertinent to achieve a comprehensive workup of myocardial B19V infection.

Keywords: parvovirus B19; B19V; erythrovirus; diagnosis; dilated cardiomyopathy; inflammatory cardiomyopathy; myocarditis; prognosis

1. Introduction

Acute myocarditis (AMC) and dilated cardiomyopathy (DCM), more specifically inflammatory cardiomyopathy (DCMi), are etiopathogenically linked entities. The highly diverse courses and long-term outcomes after AMC are substantially influenced by complex virus–host interactions at the post-acute/subacute phase after AMC [1,2].

In ca. 60% of endomyocardial biopsies (EMB) of the patients presenting with AMC or DCM, chronic intramyocardial inflammation, as detected by immunohistological quantification [3], and/or genomes of diverse viruses can be detected, consistent with the diagnosis of DCMi [4,5]. The immunohistological proof of DCMi is associated with adverse prognosis (mortality and indication for heart transplantation) [6].

Cardiac magnetic resonance (CMR) is helpful for the non-invasive detection of intramyocardial inflammation in the setting of MC and DCM [7,8]. However, CMR fails to specifically detect myocardial viral infection, including B19V [9]. Serology for anti-B19V IgG and IgM antibodies provides indications for a past or recent primary infection with B19V, however, it shows no statistically significant association with the detectability of B19V nucleic acids in myocardial tissues [10]. Thus, proof of viral genomes by polymerase chain reaction (PCR), including B19V, remains the mainstay for virological analyses in the context of MC/DCM/DCMi [1,11].

Various viruses have been associated with MC and DCM, with parvovirus B19 (B19V) having by far the highest prevalence (ca. 40%) [4,12,13]. The proof of viral genomes in EMB has been attributed as a new entity in the MOGE(S) classification (etiology: V—viral infection) [14]. This classification entity may also have implications for rational treatment strategies. Whereas disease specificity of enterovirus (EV) (i.e., Coxsackievirus) in this setting has been confirmed by meta-analysis for MC/DCM/DCMi patients [15], this relationship has not been established for B19V genomes yet. For B19V, a high prevalence, increasing with age, is well documented for many tested healthy tissues, and is referred to as the "bioportfolio" phenomenon [16]. Regarding B19V, no prognostic relevance has been elucidated for the polymerase chain reaction (PCR) proof of viral genomes in EMB [6]. In contrast to MC/DCM/DCMi patients with EV (i.e., Coxsackievirus) persistence [17], no beneficial effects have been achieved by antiviral interferon treatment for B19V positive DCMi patients [18]. These discrepancies might be due to a possible lack of disease specificity and of prognostic relevance of the mere PCR proof of B19V genomes in EMB from patients presenting with MC or DCM.

2. Materials and Methods

Electronic literature searches were carried out using Medline (via PubMed), Web of Science, the Cochrane Library, and Embase following the PRISMA (Preferred Reporting Items for Systematic Reviews and Meta-Analyses) statement [19]. The databases were searched by two independent reviewers on April 29th, 2014 by BK and MN. We combined the following keywords/ MeSH terms to identify the publications in several queries: "Parvovirus B19 OR B19V OR PVB19" AND "dilated cardiomyopathy"; AND "myocarditis"; AND "inflammatory cardiomyopathy"; AND "cardiomyopathy". The literature search was conducted using EndNote Version X7.4 (Thomson Reuters, Eagan, MN, USA). We applied the following inclusion criteria: studies investigating >10 patients with clinically suspected myocarditis, DCM or DCMi, in whom EMB were obtained and processed for B19 genomes by PCR with defined protocols. We excluded publications referring to only animal experiments or in vitro experiments, human studies on <10 patients, case reports, congress reports, review articles, editorial letters, and publications written in languages other than English or German. Furthermore, we excluded publications reporting data from non-serially included patient groups, e.g., studies comparing pre-selected patient groups. The searches were reviewed by AGR. There were no discrepancies among the reviewers of the literature. We computed demographic data and the investigational results in a Microsoft Excel data table, which were then transferred to JMP statistical software (version 7.1; SAS Institute, Nancy, NC, USA).

Statistical Analysis

Statistical analyses were performed using the software packages JMP and R (The R Project for Statistical Computing; version 3.2.0) with the packages "meta" and "metaphor" were employed for calculation of heterogeneity between the studies, forest plots, and funnel plots [20]. A probability value of $p < 0.05$ was considered statistically significant.

3. Results

After exclusion of duplicates, $n = 197$ publications were found in the literature search. According to the inclusion criteria $n = 29$ publications with data from prospective analyses on 3424 subjects (dataset: MA01) were finally included in the synthesis. The study selection process is illustrated in the flow chart in Figure 1. The included publications without controls were $n = 21$, encompassing 2786 patients with clinically suspected MC or DCM. Data referring to controls ($n = 134$) and MC/DCM patients ($n = 504$) were available from $n = 8$ publications (dataset: MA02) (Table 1).

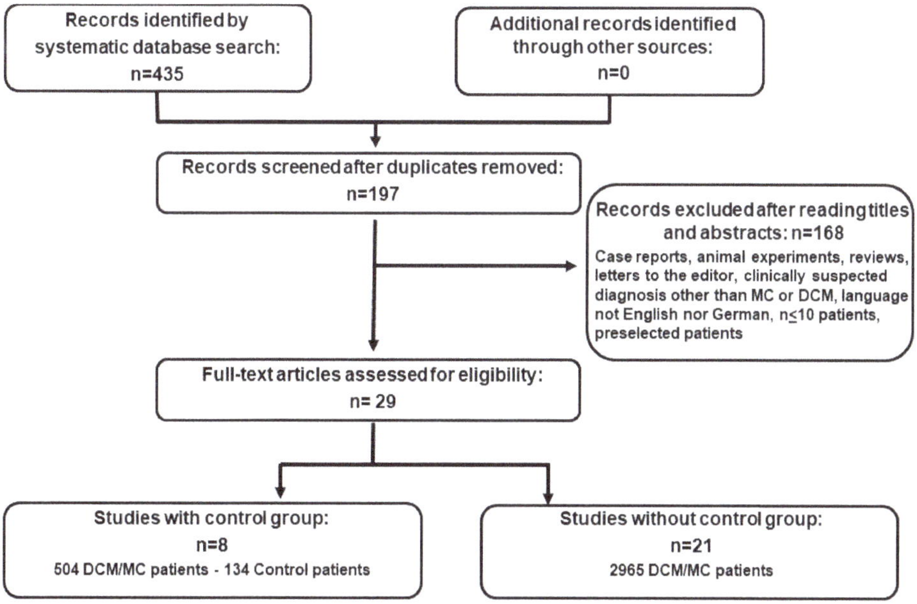

Figure 1. Flow chart for the selection of studies. The flow diagram shows the number of studies reviewed and included in the analysis as well as the number of the patients in the different study groups.

Table 1. Studies included in the meta-analysis.

Study Code	First Author	Year	Journal; Citation	Total Number of Study Subjects (n)	Number of Patients in the MC-/DCM-Group (n)	Number of Patients in the Control Group (n)
01	Kuhl	2003	Circulation; [21]	24	24	
02	Pankuweit	2003	Hum Pathol; [12]	138	110	28
03	Lotze	2004	Med Microbiol Immunol; [22]	62	52	10
04	Mahrholdt	2004	Circulation; [7]	32	32	
05	Vallbracht	2004	Circulation; [23]	124	124	
06	Kuhl	2005	Circulation; [13]	245	245	
07	Kuhl	2005	Circulation; [5]	172	172	
08	Kyto	2005	Clin Infect Dis; [24]	52	40	12
09	Tschöpe	2005	Circulation; [25]	70	70	
10	Mahrholdt	2006	Circulation; [26]	128	128	
11	Kuethe	2007	Am Heart J; [27]	197	197	
12	Escher	2008	Med Sci Monit; [28]	30	30	
13	Escher	2008	Med Sci Monit; [29]	62	62	
14	Kuhl	2008	J Med Virol; [30]	317	317	
15	Schenk	2008	J Clin Microbiol; [31]	69	69	
16	Yilmaz	2008	Heart; [32]	85	85	
17	Zimmermann	2009	Basic Res Cardiol; [33]	66	66	
18	Moulik	2010	J Am Coll Cardiol; [34]	94	94	
19	Zimmermann	2010	J Card Fail; [18]	110	110	
20	Lotze	2010	J Med Virol; [35]	34	24	10
21	Mahfoud	2011	Eur Heart J; [10]	124	124	
22	Ruppert	2011	J Med Virol; [36]	139	139	
23	Stewart	2011	Circ Heart Fail; [37]	100	100	
24	Dennert	2012	Clin Vaccine Immunol; [38]	179	159	20
25	Koepsell	2012	Cardiovasc Pathol; [39]	45	26	19
26	Kubanek	2012	Eur J Heart Fail; [40]	56	41	15
27	Moimas	2012	Heart Lung Circ; [41]	72	52	20
28	Kuhl	2013	Basic Res Cardiol; [42]	537	537	
29	Miranda	2014	Cardiol Young; [43]	61	61	

The included studies are listed in chronological order according to publication year and demonstrated with the study code for the meta-analysis and the name of the first author. The number of MC/DCM patients equals the total number of study subjects in the studies without a control group. DCM: dilated cardiomyopathy; MC: myocarditis.

The demographic data of the n = 3,424 patients of the dataset MA01 were as follows: mean age: 49.7 ± 14.9 years; n = 2,301 men (67.2%). Echocardiographic data showed a mean left ventricular ejection fraction (LVEF) of 42.4 ± 13.2% and a mean left ventricular end-diastolic diameter (LVEDD) of 59.0 ± 8.1 mm. B19V genomes were detected by PCR in 42.6% of the EMB in this cohort. The mean reported B19V-IgG positivity was 51.1%.

A demonstration of the characteristics of patients belonging to the study group in studies without a control group (S1) as well as in studies with a control group (S2) is shown in Table 2. In the 21 studies without a control group there were 2786 patients with a mean age of 50.6 ± 14.7 years, and 63.9% were male. The echocardiographic parameters showed a mean LVEF of 45.2 ± 11.6% and mean LVEDD of 60.0 ± 9.0 mm. The detection of the B19V with PCR was seen in 46.0% of those cases.

Table 2. Characteristics of the subgroups of the study group.

	S1	S2
Number of patients (DCM/MC) (n=)	2786	504
Male [%]	63.92	63.76
Age, mean ± SD [years]	50.62 ± 14.65	46.37 ± 12.2
LVEF, mean ± SD [%]	45.17 ± 11.64	34.18 ± 8.96
LVEDD, mean ± SD [mm]	59.95 ± 8.98	63.83 ± 7.56
PCR positive for B19V [%]	49.6	47.2

DCM: dilated cardiomyopathy, LVEDD: left ventricular end-diastolic diameter, LVEF: left ventricular ejection fraction, MC: myocarditis, PCR: polymerase chain reaction, S1: studies without control group, S2: studies with control group.

In the eight studies with an incorporated control group (S2), 504 patients were in the study group. The mean age was 46.4 ± 12.2 years, 63.8% of patients were male, mean LVEF was 34.2 ± 9.0%, and the mean LVEDD was 63.8 ± 7.6 mm. The PCR positivity for B19V DNA was 45.5%. Those studies comprised 134 control patients (healthy myocardial tissue from donor hearts, patients with known coronary artery disease or arterial hypertension). These control patients were 61.9% male, with a mean age of 61.8 ± 8.6 years, mean echocardiographic LVEF 62.8 ± 8.8%, and mean LVEDD of 36.0 ± 2.0 mm. The PCR detected positivity for B19V was 37.5%.

3.1. *Comparison of the Cardiac Parameters between Study and Control Groups*

In comparison to the low LVEF of the DCM/MC patients (38.6 ± 10.0%), the LVEF of the healthy control patients, with 62.8 ± 8.8%, is significantly higher ($p = 0.016$) (Figure 2). The study patients also had a very high LVEDD (62.8 ± 7.5 mm) in comparison to the normal LVEDD (36 ± 2.0 mm) of the control patients ($p = 0.007$) (Figure 2).

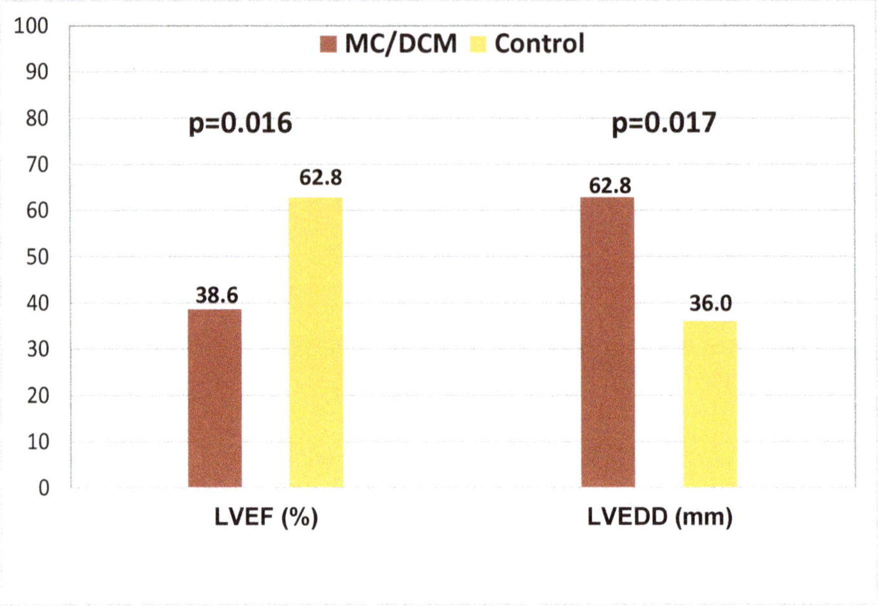

Figure 2. Comparing LVEF and LVEDD in the MC/DCM and in the control patients. The numbers on the bars represent the mean value. DCM: dilated cardiomyopathy; LVEF: left ventricular ejection fraction; LVEDD: left ventricular end-diastolic diameter; MC: myocarditis; DCM: dilated cardiomyopathy.

3.2. Virus Detection Methods

In the studies included in the meta-analysis, three different methods were used to prove the presence of B19V: polymerase chain reaction (PCR), serology, and immunohistochemistry (IHC). The detection of B19V with PCR was used in 29 (100%) of the included studies.

Endomyocardial biopsies (EMB) were obtained from patients via a femoral venous (right ventricular) or arterial (left ventricular) access and snap frozen in liquid nitrogen. The detection of virus DNA was performed with the use of PCR ($n = 19$) or of nested PCR (nPCR; $n = 15$) employing special primers for the VP1-/VP2-/NS1-coding regions. The virus load was assessed by quantitative PCR, and was reported in a minor portion of the publications, which made meaningful statistical analyses impossible. In the 29 studies, B19V could be detected in 1688 (49.3%) patients with a mean PCR positivity rate of 45.9% ± 20.4% in the study group versus 38.7% ± 24.1% in the control group, respectively ($p = 0.41$).

Serology was performed in 10 studies comprising 844 patients and the presence of antibodies (anti-B19 V immunoglobulins) was demonstrated. A positive finding for B19V specific antibodies was reported in 401 (47.5%) of the patients, with 46.1% ± 36.4% in the study group and 35.8% ± 37.8% in the control group ($p = 0.73$). The detection of IgM antibodies was reported in 18 (4.5%) of the patients, and of IgG antibodies in 379 (94.5%) of the patients, respectively. There was no statistical difference regarding the detectability of B19V-specific IgG, with 58.7% ± 28.7% in the study group versus 47.3% ± 21.5% in the control group ($p = 0.63$). Furthermore, no statistical difference was calculated for the reported B19V-specific IgM, with 2.8% ± 4.8% in the study group versus 1.8% ± 2.5% in the control group ($p = 0.79$).

For the immunohistological detection of B19V proteins (VP1 and VP2), cryosections from frozen EMB were examined in 18 studies and the B19V protein expression was reported in 43.1% of MC-/DCM-specimens. No data were available for the immunohistological detection of B19V proteins in EMB from control patients.

3.3. Distribution of Viruses in Patients with DCM/MC and Control Patients

In all study patients apart from B19V, which was detected in 1688 (49.3%) patients, other viruses were also detected in a smaller percentage: enterovirus, human herpesvirus 6 (HHV-6), adenovirus (ADV), Epstein-Barr virus (EBV), and cytomegalovirus (CMV) (Table 3). Multiple infections with simultaneous detection of various viral genomes was reported in $n = 163$ (12.3%) patients.

Table 3. Distribution of viruses in MC-/DCM-patients and in control patients.

Virus	n (%)
Parvovirus B19 (B19V)	1688 (46.85%)
Enterovirus (EV)	203 (5.36%)
Human Herpes virus-6 (HHV-6)	176 (4.88%)
Adenovirus (EDV)	44 (1.22%)
Epstein-Barr virus (EBV)	30 (0.83%)
Cytomegalovirus (CMV)	28 (0.77%)

3.4. PCR Proof of B19V Genomes Comparing Patients with DCM/MC and Controls

The main attention of this meta-analysis was focused on the question, if a B19V infection can be a risk factor for DCM/MC or if there is no difference in comparison to donor hearts. In order to clarify this, a direct comparison between DCM/MC patients and healthy donor hearts by using PCR was performed in the MA02 cohort comprising $n = 638$ subjects. There was no statistically significant different rate of B19V positivity in myocardial tissues comparing controls (mean: 38.8 ± 24.1%) versus the MC/DCM-patients (45.5 ± 24.3%; $p = 0.58$). There was also no statistical difference between the positivity rate of B19V genomes in myocardial tissues of MA01 (46.0 ± 19.5%) and the two patient groups of MA02 ($p > 0.05$).

The forest plot of the eight studies with a control group shows the comparison of B19V detection with PCR in DCM/MC patients and control patients (Figure 3). No significantly higher detection rate of B19V in the study group was shown in comparison to the control groups of these eight studies ($p = 0.3285$)

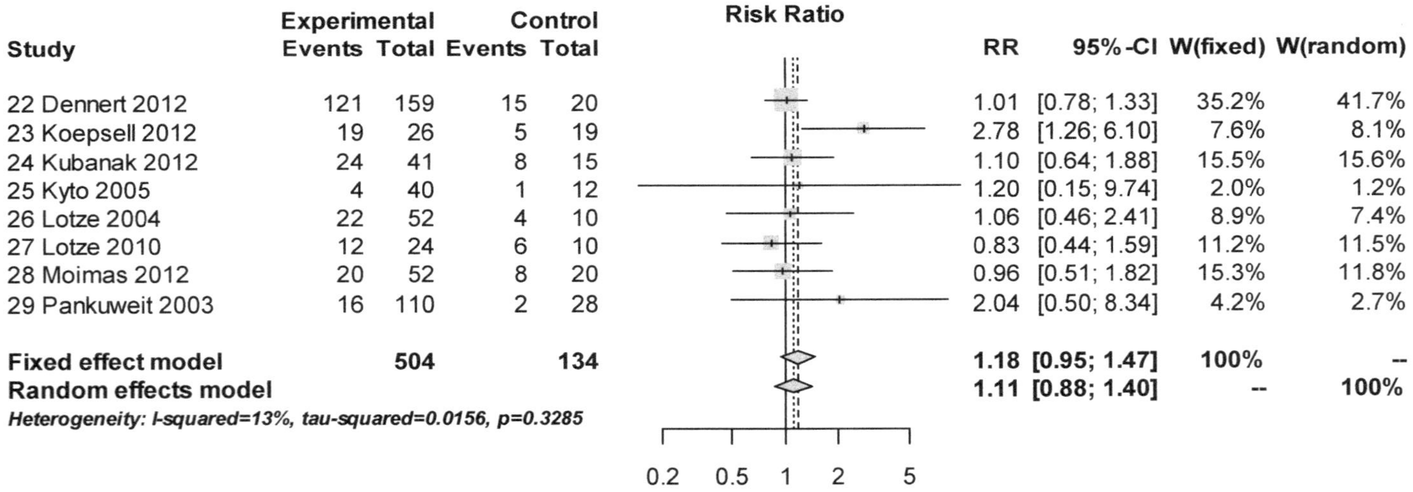
Study
Experimental Events Total
Control Events Total
Risk Ratio
RR 95%-CI W(fixed) W(random)
22 Dennert 2012 121 159 15 20 1.01 [0.78; 1.33] 35.2% 41.7%
23 Koepsell 2012 19 26 5 19 2.78 [1.26; 6.10] 7.6% 8.1%
24 Kubanak 2012 24 41 8 15 1.10 [0.64; 1.88] 15.5% 15.6%
25 Kyto 2005 4 40 1 12 1.20 [0.15; 9.74] 2.0% 1.2%
26 Lotze 2004 22 52 4 10 1.06 [0.46; 2.41] 8.9% 7.4%
27 Lotze 2010 12 24 6 10 0.83 [0.44; 1.59] 11.2% 11.5%
28 Moimas 2012 20 52 8 20 0.96 [0.51; 1.82] 15.3% 11.8%
29 Pankuweit 2003 16 110 2 28 2.04 [0.50; 8.34] 4.2% 2.7%
Fixed effect model 504 134 1.18 [0.95; 1.47] 100% --
Random effects model 1.11 [0.88; 1.40] -- 100%
Heterogeneity: I-squared=13%, tau-squared=0.0156, p=0.3285
0.2
0.5
1
2
5

Figure 3. Plot of the $n = 8$ studies with control group. The mean relative risk (RR) is represented with the grey diamond and the dotted vertical line. The grey squares show the RR for the individual studies, the horizontal lines show the corresponding 95% confidence intervals. Experimental: study group, Control: control group, Events: sum of events, Total: number of patients of the corresponding group, RR: relative risk.

4. Discussion

In patients presenting with MC or DCM, EMB can be performed as a diagnostic procedure [1,44]. Apart from the histological and immunohistological diagnosis, PCR detection of virus genomes is recommended [11]. In this context, B19V genomes are most frequently detected compared with other viral genomes studied [13,21,45].

For the enterovirus/Coxsackievirus B3 there is a causative association between detection of virus genome and appearance of myocardial disease. Apart from the experimental confirmation in murine models, a meta-analysis has also shown the association between enterovirus and MC/DCM compared to controls; a prognostic as well as therapeutic importance has also been shown [15,17,46]. However, such an association has not been proven convincingly for B19V in MC/DCM. The main aim of our study was to systematically review the published studies focusing on this topic, and to perform a meta-analysis of the available data. Similar detection rates with B19V genomes have been documented in various regions of the world, including Europe, North America, and Asia [47]. The range of seropositivity for B19V rises substantially from fetal to advanced age. In Germany, seropositivity for B19V extends from 20.4% in children up to 79.1% in people over 65 years of age [48]. Similar data could also be shown in England/Wales (21%–75%), Belgium (74%), and Italy (79%) [49]. The transmission of B19V occurs through droplets, blood, or close body contact. After seroconversion, lifelong seropositivity ensues. The often asymptomatic course after first B19 infection facilitates the spread of the virus. B19V usually persists mostly lifelong in various tissues, a phenomenon also known as "bioportfolio" [16,47]. For tonsillar tissues, Pyöriä et al. have recently identified B cells as the main cell type of B19V genome persistence [50]. This investigation also supports the maintenance of pathogen-specific humoral immune responses as a consequence of B-cell long-term survival. Thus, the frequent detection of B19V genomes in EMB of DCM/MC patients raises the question of pathogenic relevance, since it might be in parts due to lifelong persistence of B19V DNA in terms of a "bioportfolio" effect as well [51,52].

4.1. PCR Diagnosis of B19V

In the 21 studies without a control group, which assessed 2786 DCM/MC patients, B19V genomes were proven by PCR in 50.3% of the patients. A similar rate of B19V proof of 56.9% was also reported in the DCM/MC patients of the eight studies which included a control group. In total, in the 29 studies including 3290 DCM/MC patients, B19V genomes were detected by PCR in EMB in 49.3% of the patients. In the control group, detection of B19V by PCR was reported in 37.5% of EMB specimens, being not significantly different to the findings in control patients ($p = 0.509$). These data imply pathogenetically insignificant latency of B19V genomes in a proportion of myocardial tissues of both MC-/DCM-patients and controls. Thus, PCR evidence of B19V genomes is not sufficient to indicate a disease relationship between B19V and MC/DCM [51,52]. These data may be compatible with the "bioportfolio" phenomenon, known for the PCR detection of B19V genomes in other human tissues [16]. More information (i.e., replicative status, viral protein expression) is pertinent to achieve a comprehensive workup of myocardial B19V infection [28,29,42,52]. The lack of such additional information could be a pivotal reason for the neutral trial result of an anti-viral interferon treatment study in MC/DCM associated with B19V, which was only based on the PCR proven B19V genome in EMB [18].

4.2. Factors Potentially Influencing EMB Diagnosis

The 29 studies included in this meta-analysis have been performed in different centers with different assessment methods. The heterogeneity of the inclusion criteria of the 29 studies as well as of the diagnostic methods and the measured results might have contributed to heterogeneity. The advances in virus load quantification, differentiation of genotypes and of viral replications status are additional methodological issues which cannot be unified in all studies, since the technical evolution of these methods was incremental over time. Hence, the first investigations did not address these detailed issues. It can be assumed that there were differences in the size and quantity of EMB tissue specimens among the 29 studies, as well as multiple sources of methodological differences regarding DNA extraction and PCR protocols. Depending on the individual center, different primers and probes were used for the PCR. Besides, the number of obtained EMB samples per patient, from which DNA is extracted, varied significantly among the different studies from 1 to 6 EMB for evaluation of viral genomes [12,13,22]. Another important issue may be the sampling error, which is well known to impair the diagnostic accuracy of histological EMB evaluation [53], but is not precisely known for the virological analyses of EMB [54]. Finally, the problem of the preferred ventricle for the obtainment of EMB in the context of myocarditis or DCM has not been solved yet [7,55]. Another important factor is the timing of EMB in the natural course of the disease, with higher amounts of virus load in the acute compared to the chronic phase [45,56]. Additionally, the prognostic relevance of differentiating the B19V genotype is incompletely understood [30,36]. Taken together, these data highlight the importance of standardized, uniform methodological approaches for the proof of relevant myocardial B19V infections.

4.3. Control Group

The data on myocardial samples from the control group are extremely important, since these are the only available data comparing B19V infections in non-MC and non-DCM patients. Nonetheless, the ideal myocardial samples would have been EMB from cardiovascular healthy, age- and sex-matched controls, which however is not possible due to obvious ethical constraints. A further issue is the not well-standardized sampling region among the eight studies.

4.4. Prognostic Relevance of PCR Proven B19V Genomes in the Endomyocardium

In a prospective single center study with clinically suspected myocarditis, the PCR proof of viral genomes in EMB, including B19V, was not associated with prognosis, as opposed to the adverse outcome in patients with immunohistological proof of intramyocardial inflammation [6]. The adverse prognostic impact of intramyocardial inflammation was also confirmed in investigations focusing on cardiac magnetic resonance (CMR) based detection of late gadolinium enhancement (LGE) in patients presenting with both MC and DCM [57,58]. Further publications did not confirm an adverse impact of B19V genomes in EMB of patients with clinically suspected MC or DCM [27,35]. Only in one study, focusing on highly selected DCM patients with diverse courses of spontaneous viral elimination versus viral persistence, a potential prognostic impact was reported for viral genomes persisting over 6 months of follow up EMB investigations, including B19V, either as monoinfection or as part of multiple viral genomes present in EMB [5]. These insights were not confirmed in a comparable analysis [59]. So far, we are lacking detailed data on comprehensive B19V investigations including the kinetics of viral loads, the differentiation of the B19V replication status, the B19V genotypes, the B19V protein expression pattern, and the cellular and humoral antiviral immune responses in selected patients with biologically relevant myocardial B19V infections.

4.5. Future Management Strategies

Evidence based management strategies of MC/DCM patients are based on general heart failure guidelines [60]. In rare cases of giant cell or eosinophilic myocarditis, immunosuppressive treatment has a class I indication for the improvement of the outcome [44]. For the time being, there is no widely accepted, evidence based anti-viral or pathogen directed therapy for a viral MC/DCM [18,61]. Antiviral interferon-beta treatment has shown positive clinical and prognostic effects in enteroviral/Coxsackievirus B persistence in single center and multicenter studies, including some evidence for effective viral elimination, however, this antiviral treatment has not proved as effective in B19V associated MC/DCM [17,61]. Selection of B19V positive patients with high B19V loads might be a relevant approach to identify subgroups of B19V patients who might benefit from immunomodulatory treatment [62]. Comprehensive, standardized diagnostic differentiation of MC/DCM patients with endomyocardial B19V infections with biological and prognostic relevance (possibly including viral replication, myocardial B19V protein expression, and ongoing active cellular and/or humoral anti-B19V immune response) might be a key approach for both an updated diagnostic classification of B19V associated viral cardiomyopathy [14], and a more meaningful selection of candidates for future antiviral immunomodulatory treatment trials.

4.6. Limitations of the Study

All potential limitation issues known for meta-analyses also apply to this study [63]. This meta-analysis enables a standardized aspect of the available evidence of virus diagnosis in DCM/MC patients; it portrays no general recommendation for the further procedure in a viral infection coexistent with myocardial disease. For the evaluation of individual measured data from the studies it was not always possible, because of missing statements about the results, to show mean values. For the determined virus load of B19V using PCR no mean value could be reported, because in the few studies in which the virus load was reported, either an individual value or a total measurement range was given. For the assessment of B19V load by using PCR in the control group no mean value could be calculated, as only two studies reported such values. An overview of the values of B19V loads in EMB from patients versus healthy study participants would be of paramount importance, because significant differences between MC and DCM patients were reported [45]. Nevertheless, it must be stated, that the comparison of patient groups in this publication was merely based on the presumed clinical diagnosis that was reported to the pathology institute when sending in the EMB samples. Thus, a reliable verification of the clinical parameters in this publication is impossible, and the evaluation of these data cannot be regarded as representative.

5. Conclusions

This meta-analysis shows that the mere PCR proof of B19V genomes in EMB has no significant association with the clinical diagnosis of MC/DCM, since this finding is equally present in control hearts. The lack of disease specificity is compatible with the "bioportfolio" phenomenon known for other non-cardiac organs [16]. The appreciation of these insights improve our understanding of the missing significant clinical effects of immunomodulatory strategies in MC-/DCM-patients associated with B19V genomes EMB proven by PCR. In order to identify biologically relevant B19V myocardial infections, additional characteristics of a B19V infection and of the anti-B19V immune response might be helpful, such as the B19V virus load, the differentiation of B19V genotype, the B19V replication status, the characterization of myocardial B19V protein expression patterns, and the differentiation between an active humoral and cellular anti-B19V response versus the pathogenetically insignificant latent persistence of B19V genomes [28,29,52,56]. This comprehensive, standardized characterization could lead to the development of specific features for the selection of well characterized B19V positive MC-/DCM-patients who may ultimately profit from tailored anti-viral immunomodulatory treatment strategies [51].

Author Contributions: Conceptualization, M.N.; methodology, M.N., B.K., A.A. and M.M.; software, M.N., B.K. and M.M.; validation, M.N., B.K., S.M. and A.G.R.; formal analysis, M.N., B.K., M.M., A.A., S.M. and A.G.R.; investigation, M.N., B.K., M.M., A.A., S.M. and A.G.R.; writing—original draft preparation, A.G.R., B.K., M.M. and M.N.; writing—review and editing, A.G.R., B.K., M.M., A.A., S.M. and M.N.; visualization, M.N., B.K., M.M., A.A. and A.G.R; supervision, M.N.

Funding: This research received no external funding.

Conflicts of Interest: M.N. has received grants by the Deutsche Forschungsgemeinschaft (DFG) through the Sonderforschungsbereich Transregio 19 "Inflammatory Cardiomyopathy" (SFB TR19) (TP B2), and by the University Hospital Giessen and Marburg Foundation Grant "T cell functionality" (UKGM 10/2009). M.N. has been consultant to the IKDT (Institute for Cardiac Diagnosis and Therapy GmbH, Berlin) 2004–2008.

Abbreviations

B19V	parvovirus B19
CMR	cardiac magnetic resonance
DCM	dilated cardiomyopathy
DCMi	inflammatory cardiomyopathy
EMB	endomyocardial biopsy or biopsies
EV	enterovirus: enteroviral
IHC	immunohistochemical
LGE	late gadolinium enhancement
LVEF	left ventricular ejection fraction
LVEDD	left ventricular end-diastolic diameter
MC	myocarditis
PCR	polymerase chain reaction

References

1. Noutsias, M.; Maisch, B. Myocarditis and pericarditis. In *The ESC Textbook of Acute and Intensive Cardiac Care*, 2nd ed.; Tubaro, M., Vranckx, P., Price, S., Vrints, C., Eds.; Oxford University Press: Oxford, UK, 2014; Volume 2, pp. 547–560.
2. D'Ambrosio, A.; Patti, G.; Manzoli, A.; Sinagra, G.; di Lenarda, A.; Silvestri, F.; di Sciascio, G. The fate of acute myocarditis between spontaneous improvement and evolution to dilated cardiomyopathy: A review. *Heart* **2001**, *85*, 499–504. [CrossRef] [PubMed]
3. Noutsias, M.; Seeberg, B.; Schultheiss, H.P.; Kühl, U. Expression of cell adhesion molecules in dilated cardiomyopathy: Evidence for endothelial activation in inflammatory cardiomyopathy. *Circulation* **1999**, *99*, 2124–2131. [CrossRef] [PubMed]
4. Angelini, A.; Calzolari, V.; Calabrese, F.; Boffa, G.M.; Maddalena, F.; Chioin, R.; Thiene, G. Myocarditis mimicking acute myocardial infarction: Role of endomyocardial biopsy in the differential diagnosis. *Heart* **2000**, *84*, 245–250. [CrossRef] [PubMed]
5. Kühl, U.; Pauschinger, M.; Seeberg, B.; Lassner, D.; Noutsias, M.; Poller, W.; Schultheiss, H.P. Viral persistence in the myocardium is associated with progressive cardiac dysfunction. *Circulation* **2005**, *112*, 1965–1970. [CrossRef] [PubMed]
6. Kindermann, I.; Kindermann, M.; Kandolf, R.; Klingel, K.; Bultmann, B.; Muller, T.; Lindinger, A.; Bohm, M. Predictors of outcome in patients with suspected myocarditis. *Circulation* **2008**, *118*, 639–648. [CrossRef] [PubMed]
7. Mahrholdt, H.; Goedecke, C.; Wagner, A.; Meinhardt, G.; Athanasiadis, A.; Vogelsberg, H.; Fritz, P.; Klingel, K.; Kandolf, R.; Sechtem, U. Cardiovascular magnetic resonance assessment of human myocarditis: A comparison to histology and molecular pathology. *Circulation* **2004**, *109*, 1250–1258. [CrossRef]
8. Mavrogeni, S.; Spargias, C.; Bratis, C.; Kolovou, G.; Markussis, V.; Papadopoulou, E.; Constadoulakis, P.; Papadimitropoulos, M.; Douskou, M.; Pavlides, G.; et al. Myocarditis as a precipitating factor for heart failure: Evaluation and 1-year follow-up using cardiovascular magnetic resonance and endomyocardial biopsy. *Eur. J. Heart Fail.* **2011**, *13*, 830–837. [CrossRef]
9. Gutberlet, M.; Spors, B.; Thoma, T.; Bertram, H.; Denecke, T.; Felix, R.; Noutsias, M.; Schultheiss, H.P.; Kühl, U. Suspected chronic myocarditis at cardiac MR: Diagnostic accuracy and association with immunohistologically detected inflammation and viral persistence. *Radiology* **2008**, *246*, 401–409. [CrossRef]
10. Mahfoud, F.; Gartner, B.; Kindermann, M.; Ukena, C.; Gadomski, K.; Klingel, K.; Kandolf, R.; Bohm, M.; Kindermann, I. Virus serology in patients with suspected myocarditis: Utility or futility? *Eur. Heart J.* **2011**, *32*, 897–903. [CrossRef]
11. Caforio, A.L.; Pankuweit, S.; Arbustini, E.; Basso, C.; Gimeno-Blanes, J.; Felix, S.B.; Fu, M.; Helio, T.; Heymans, S.; Jahns, R.; et al. European Society of Cardiology Working Group on M.; Pericardial, D. Current state of knowledge on aetiology, diagnosis, management, and therapy of myocarditis: A position statement of the European Society of Cardiology Working Group on Myocardial and Pericardial Diseases. *Eur. Heart J.* **2013**, *34*, 2636–2648.

12. Pankuweit, S.; Moll, R.; Baandrup, U.; Portig, I.; Hufnagel, G.; Maisch, B. Prevalence of the parvovirus B19 genome in endomyocardial biopsy specimens. *Hum. Pathol.* **2003**, *34*, 497–503. [CrossRef]
13. Kühl, U.; Pauschinger, M.; Noutsias, M.; Seeberg, B.; Bock, T.; Lassner, D.; Poller, W.; Kandolf, R.; Schultheiss, H.P. High prevalence of viral genomes and multiple viral infections in the myocardium of adults with "idiopathic" left ventricular dysfunction. *Circulation* **2005**, *111*, 887–893. [CrossRef] [PubMed]
14. Westphal, J.G.; Rigopoulos, A.G.; Bakogiannis, C.; Ludwig, S.E.; Mavrogeni, S.; Bigalke, B.; Doenst, T.; Pauschinger, M.; Tschope, C.; Schulze, P.C.; et al. The MOGE(S) classification for cardiomyopathies: Current status and future outlook. *Heart Fail. Rev.* **2017**, *22*, 743–752. [CrossRef] [PubMed]
15. Baboonian, C.; Treasure, T. Meta-analysis of the association of enteroviruses with human heart disease. *Heart* **1997**, *78*, 539–543. [CrossRef] [PubMed]
16. Norja, P.; Hokynar, K.; Aaltonen, L.M.; Chen, R.; Ranki, A.; Partio, E.K.; Kiviluoto, O.; Davidkin, I.; Leivo, T.; Eis-Hubinger, A.M.; et al. Bioportfolio: Lifelong persistence of variant and prototypic erythrovirus DNA genomes in human tissue. *Proc. Natl. Acad. Sci. USA* **2006**, *103*, 7450–7453. [CrossRef]
17. Kuhl, U.; Lassner, D.; von Schlippenbach, J.; Poller, W.; Schultheiss, H.P. Interferon-Beta improves survival in enterovirus-associated cardiomyopathy. *J. Am. Coll Cardiol.* **2012**, *60*, 1295–1296. [CrossRef]
18. Zimmermann, O.; Rodewald, C.; Radermacher, M.; Vetter, M.; Wiehe, J.M.; Bienek-Ziolkowski, M.; Hombach, V.; Torzewski, J. Interferon beta-1b therapy in chronic viral dilated cardiomyopathy–is there a role for specific therapy? *J. Card Fail.* **2010**, *16*, 348–356. [CrossRef]
19. Liberati, A.; Altman, D.G.; Tetzlaff, J.; Mulrow, C.; Gotzsche, P.C.; Ioannidis, J.P.; Clarke, M.; Devereaux, P.J.; Kleijnen, J.; Moher, D. The PRISMA statement for reporting systematic reviews and meta-analyses of studies that evaluate health care interventions: Explanation and elaboration. *PLoS Med.* **2009**, *6*, e1000100. [CrossRef]
20. Neupane, B.; Richer, D.; Bonner, A.J.; Kibret, T.; Beyene, J. Network meta-analysis using R: a review of currently available automated packages. *PLoS ONE* **2014**, *9*, e115065. [CrossRef]
21. Kühl, U.; Pauschinger, M.; Bock, T.; Klingel, K.; Schwimmbeck, C.P.; Seeberg, B.; Krautwurm, L.; Noutsias, M.; Poller, W.; Schultheiss, H.P.; et al. Parvovirus B19 infection mimicking acute myocardial infarction. *Circulation* **2003**, *108*, 945–950. [CrossRef]
22. Lotze, U.; Egerer, R.; Tresselt, C.; Gluck, B.; Dannberg, G.; Stelzner, A.; Figulla, H.R. Frequent detection of parvovirus B19 genome in the myocardium of adult patients with idiopathic dilated cardiomyopathy. *Med. Microbiol. Immunol. (Berl.)* **2004**, *193*, 75–82. [CrossRef] [PubMed]
23. Vallbracht, K.B.; Schwimmbeck, P.L.; Kuhl, U.; Seeberg, B.; Schultheiss, H.P. Endothelium-dependent flow-mediated vasodilation of systemic arteries is impaired in patients with myocardial virus persistence. *Circulation* **2004**, *110*, 2938–2945. [CrossRef] [PubMed]
24. Kyto, V.; Vuorinen, T.; Saukko, P.; Lautenschlager, I.; Lignitz, E.; Saraste, A.; Voipio-Pulkki, L.M. Cytomegalovirus infection of the heart is common in patients with fatal myocarditis. *Clin. Infect. Dis.* **2005**, *40*, 683–688. [CrossRef]
25. Tschöpe, C.; Bock, C.T.; Kasner, M.; Noutsias, M.; Westermann, D.; Schwimmbeck, P.L.; Pauschinger, M.; Poller, W.C.; Kühl, U.; Kandolf, R.; et al. High prevalence of cardiac parvovirus B19 infection in patients with isolated left ventricular diastolic dysfunction. *Circulation* **2005**, *111*, 879–886. [CrossRef] [PubMed]
26. Mahrholdt, H.; Wagner, A.; Deluigi, C.C.; Kispert, E.; Hager, S.; Meinhardt, G.; Vogelsberg, H.; Fritz, P.; Dippon, J.; Bock, C.T.; et al. Presentation, patterns of myocardial damage, and clinical course of viral myocarditis. *Circulation* **2006**, *114*, 1581–1590. [CrossRef] [PubMed]
27. Kuethe, F.; Sigusch, H.H.; Hilbig, K.; Tresselt, C.; Gluck, B.; Egerer, R.; Figulla, H.R. Detection of viral genome in the myocardium: Lack of prognostic and functional relevance in patients with acute dilated cardiomyopathy. *Am. Heart J.* **2007**, *153*, 850–858. [CrossRef]
28. Escher, F.; Kühl, U.; Sabi, T.; Suckau, L.; Lassner, D.; Poller, W.; Schultheiss, H.P.; Noutsias, M. Immunohistological detection of Parvovirus B19 capsid proteins in endomyocardial biopsies from dilated cardiomyopathy patients. *Med. Sci. Monit.* **2008**, *14*, CR333–CR338. [CrossRef]
29. Escher, F.; Modrow, S.; Sabi, T.; Kuhl, U.; Lassner, D.; Schultheiss, H.P.; Noutsias, M. Parvovirus B19 profiles in patients presenting with acute myocarditis and chronic dilated cardiomyopathy. *Med. Sci. Monit.* **2008**, *14*, CR589–CR597.
30. Kühl, U.; Lassner, D.; Pauschinger, M.; Gross, U.M.; Seeberg, B.; Noutsias, M.; Poller, W.; Schultheiss, H.P. Prevalence of erythrovirus genotypes in the myocardium of patients with dilated cardiomyopathy. *J. Med. Virol.* **2008**, *80*, 1243–1251. [CrossRef]

31. Schenk, T.; Enders, M.; Pollak, S.; Hahn, R.; Huzly, D. High prevalence of human parvovirus B19 DNA in myocardial autopsy samples from subjects without myocarditis or dilative cardiomyopathy. *J. Clin. Microbiol.* **2009**, *47*, 106–110. [CrossRef]
32. Yilmaz, A.; Mahrholdt, H.; Athanasiadis, A.; Vogelsberg, H.; Meinhardt, G.; Voehringer, M.; Kispert, E.M.; Deluigi, C.; Baccouche, H.; Spodarev, E.; et al. Coronary vasospasm as the underlying cause for chest pain in patients with PVB19 myocarditis. *Heart* **2008**, *94*, 1456–1463. [CrossRef]
33. Zimmermann, O.; Bienek-Ziolkowski, M.; Wolf, B.; Vetter, M.; Baur, R.; Mailander, V.; Hombach, V.; Torzewski, J. Myocardial inflammation and non-ischaemic heart failure: Is there a role for C-reactive protein? *Basic. Res. Cardiol.* **2009**, *104*, 591–599. [CrossRef] [PubMed]
34. Moulik, M.; Breinholt, J.P.; Dreyer, W.J.; Kearney, D.L.; Price, J.F.; Clunie, S.K.; Moffett, B.S.; Kim, J.J.; Rossano, J.W.; Jefferies, J.L.; et al. Viral endomyocardial infection is an independent predictor and potentially treatable risk factor for graft loss and coronary vasculopathy in pediatric cardiac transplant recipients. *J. Am. Coll Cardiol.* **2010**, *56*, 582–592. [CrossRef] [PubMed]
35. Lotze, U.; Egerer, R.; Gluck, B.; Zell, R.; Sigusch, H.; Erhardt, C.; Heim, A.; Kandolf, R.; Bock, T.; Wutzler, P.; et al. Low level myocardial parvovirus B19 persistence is a frequent finding in patients with heart disease but unrelated to ongoing myocardial injury. *J. Med. Virol.* **2010**, *82*, 1449–1457. [CrossRef] [PubMed]
36. Ruppert, V.; Meyer, T.; Balbach, A.; Richter, A.; Muller, H.H.; Maisch, B.; Pankuweit, S. Genotype-specific effects on left ventricular function in parvovirus B19-positive patients with dilated cardiomyopathy. *J. Med. Virol.* **2011**, *83*, 1818–1825. [CrossRef] [PubMed]
37. Stewart, G.C.; Lopez-Molina, J.; Gottumukkala, R.V.; Rosner, G.F.; Anello, M.S.; Hecht, J.L.; Winters, G.L.; Padera, R.F.; Baughman, K.L.; Lipes, M.A. Myocardial parvovirus B19 persistence: Lack of association with clinicopathologic phenotype in adults with heart failure. *Circ. Heart Fail.* **2011**, *4*, 71–78. [CrossRef] [PubMed]
38. Dennert, R.; van Paassen, P.; Wolffs, P.; Bruggeman, C.; Velthuis, S.; Felix, S.; van Suylen, R.J.; Crijns, H.J.; Cohen Tervaert, J.W.; Heymans, S. Differences in Virus Prevalence and Load in the Hearts of Patients with Idiopathic Dilated Cardiomyopathy with and without Immune-Mediated Inflammatory Diseases. *Clin. Vaccine Immunol.* **2012**, *19*, 1182–1187. [CrossRef] [PubMed]
39. Koepsell, S.A.; Anderson, D.R.; Radio, S.J. Parvovirus B19 is a bystander in adult myocarditis. *Cardiovasc. Pathol.* **2012**, *21*, 476–481. [CrossRef] [PubMed]
40. Kubanek, M.; Sramko, M.; Berenova, D.; Hulinska, D.; Hrbackova, H.; Maluskova, J.; Lodererova, A.; Malek, I.; Kautzner, J. Detection of Borrelia burgdorferi sensu lato in endomyocardial biopsy specimens in individuals with recent-onset dilated cardiomyopathy. *Eur. J. Heart Fail.* **2012**, *14*, 588–596. [CrossRef]
41. Moimas, S.; Zacchigna, S.; Merlo, M.; Buiatti, A.; Anzini, M.; Dreas, L.; Salvi, A.; Di Lenarda, A.; Giacca, M.; Sinagra, G. Idiopathic dilated cardiomyopathy and persistent viral infection: Lack of association in a controlled study using a quantitative assay. *Heart Lung Circ.* **2012**, *21*, 787–793. [CrossRef]
42. Kuhl, U.; Lassner, D.; Dorner, A.; Rohde, M.; Escher, F.; Seeberg, B.; Hertel, E.; Tschope, C.; Skurk, C.; Gross, U.M.; et al. A distinct subgroup of cardiomyopathy patients characterized by transcriptionally active cardiotropic erythrovirus and altered cardiac gene expression. *Basic. Res. Cardiol.* **2013**, *108*, 372. [CrossRef] [PubMed]
43. Miranda, J.O.; Costa, L.; Rodrigues, E.; Teles, E.L.; Baptista, M.J.; Areias, J.C. Paediatric dilated cardiomyopathy: Clinical profile and outcome. The experience of a tertiary centre for paediatric cardiology. *Cardiol. Young* **2015**, *25*, 333–337. [CrossRef] [PubMed]
44. Cooper, L.T.; Baughman, K.L.; Feldman, A.M.; Frustaci, A.; Jessup, M.; Kühl, U.; Levine, G.N.; Narula, J.; Starling, R.C.; Towbin, J.; et al. The role of endomyocardial biopsy in the management of cardiovascular disease: A scientific statement from the American Heart Association, the American College of Cardiology, and the European Society of Cardiology. *Circulation* **2007**, *116*, 2216–2233. [CrossRef] [PubMed]
45. Bock, C.T.; Klingel, K.; Kandolf, R. Human parvovirus B19-associated myocarditis. *N. Engl. J. Med.* **2010**, *362*, 1248–1249. [CrossRef] [PubMed]
46. Noutsias, M.; Liu, P. Coxsackievirus Induced Murine Myocarditis and Immunomodulatory Interventions. In *Inflammatory Cardiomyopathy (DCMi)—Pathogenesis and Therapy*; Schultheiss, H.P., Noutsias, M., Eds.; Birkhäuser Verlag: Basel, Switzerland, 2010; Volume 1, pp. 51–70.
47. Young, N.S.; Brown, K.E. Parvovirus B19. *N. Engl. J. Med.* **2004**, *350*, 586–597. [CrossRef] [PubMed]

48. Rohrer, C.; Gartner, B.; Sauerbrei, A.; Bohm, S.; Hottentrager, B.; Raab, U.; Thierfelder, W.; Wutzler, P.; Modrow, S. Seroprevalence of parvovirus B19 in the German population. *Epidemiol. Infect.* **2008**, *1*, 1–12. [CrossRef] [PubMed]
49. Brown, K.E. Detection and quantitation of parvovirus B19. *J. Clin. Virol.* **2004**, *31*, 1–4. [CrossRef]
50. Pyoria, L.; Toppinen, M.; Mantyla, E.; Hedman, L.; Aaltonen, L.M.; Vihinen-Ranta, M.; Ilmarinen, T.; Soderlund-Venermo, M.; Hedman, K.; Perdomo, M.F. Extinct type of human parvovirus B19 persists in tonsillar B. cells. *Nat. Commun.* **2017**, *8*, 14930. [CrossRef]
51. Modrow, S. Parvovirus B19: The causative agent of dilated cardiomyopathy or a harmless passenger of the human myocard? *Ernst. Scher. Res. Found. Workshop* **2006**, *1*, 63–82.
52. Lindner, J.; Noutsias, M.; Lassner, D.; Wenzel, J.; Schultheiss, H.P.; Kuehl, U.; Modrow, S. Adaptive immune responses against parvovirus B19 in patients with myocardial disease. *J. Clin. Virol.* **2009**, *44*, 27–32. [CrossRef]
53. Hauck, A.J.; Kearney, D.L.; Edwards, W.D. Evaluation of postmortem endomyocardial biopsy specimens from 38 patients with lymphocytic myocarditis: Implications for role of sampling error. *Mayo. Clin. Proc.* **1989**, *64*, 123545. [CrossRef]
54. Noutsias, M. Myocarditis. In *Algorithms in Heart Failure*; Maisel, A.S., Filippatos, G., Eds.; Jaypee Brothers Medical Publishers (P.) Ltd.: New Delhi, India, 2016; Volume 1, pp. 323–345.
55. Yilmaz, A.; Kindermann, I.; Kindermann, M.; Mahfoud, F.; Ukena, C.; Athanasiadis, A.; Hill, S.; Mahrholdt, H.; Voehringer, M.; Schieber, M.; et al. Comparative evaluation of left and right ventricular endomyocardial biopsy: Differences in complication rate and diagnostic performance. *Circulation* **2010**, *122*, 900–909. [CrossRef] [PubMed]
56. Streitz, M.; Noutsias, M.; Volkmer, R.; Rohde, M.; Brestrich, G.; Block, A.; Klippert, K.; Kotsch, K.; Ay, B.; Hummel, M.; et al. NS1 specific CD8+ T-cells with effector function and TRBV11 dominance in a patient with parvovirus B19 associated inflammatory cardiomyopathy. *PLoS ONE* **2008**, *3*, e2361. [CrossRef] [PubMed]
57. Grun, S.; Schumm, J.; Greulich, S.; Wagner, A.; Schneider, S.; Bruder, O.; Kispert, E.M.; Hill, S.; Ong, P.; Klingel, K.; et al. Long-term follow-up of biopsy-proven viral myocarditis: Predictors of mortality and incomplete recovery. *J. Am. Coll Cardiol.* **2012**, *59*, 1604–1615. [CrossRef] [PubMed]
58. Lehrke, S.; Lossnitzer, D.; Schob, M.; Steen, H.; Merten, C.; Kemmling, H.; Pribe, R.; Ehlermann, P.; Zugck, C.; Korosoglou, G.; et al. Use of cardiovascular magnetic resonance for risk stratification in chronic heart failure: Prognostic value of late gadolinium enhancement in patients with non-ischaemic dilated cardiomyopathy. *Heart* **2011**, *97*, 727–732. [CrossRef] [PubMed]
59. Nowalany-Kozielska, E.; Koziel, M.; Domal-Kwiatkowska, D.; Wojciechowska, C.; Jachec, W.; Kawecki, D.; Tomasik, A.; Przywara-Chowaniec, B.; Weglarz, L.; Reichman-Warmusz, E.; et al. Clinical Significance of Viral Genome Persistence in the Myocardium of Patients with Dilated Cardiomyopathy. *Intervirology* **2015**, *58*, 350–356. [CrossRef] [PubMed]
60. Ponikowski, P.; Voors, A.A.; Anker, S.D.; Bueno, H.; Cleland, J.G.; Coats, A.J.; Falk, V.; Gonzalez-Juanatey, J.R.; Harjola, V.P.; Jankowska, E.A.; et al. Authors/Task Force, M. 2016 ESC Guidelines for the diagnosis and treatment of acute and chronic heart failure: The Task Force for the diagnosis and treatment of acute and chronic heart failure of the European Society of Cardiology (ESC)Developed with the special contribution of the Heart Failure Association (HFA) of the ESC. *Eur. Heart J.* **2016**, *37*, 2129–2200. [PubMed]
61. Schultheiss, H.P.; Piper, C.; Sowade, O.; Waagstein, F.; Kapp, J.F.; Wegscheider, K.; Groetzbach, G.; Pauschinger, M.; Escher, F.; Arbustini, E.; et al. Betaferon in chronic viral cardiomyopathy (BICC) trial: Effects of interferon-beta treatment in patients with chronic viral cardiomyopathy. *Clin. Res. Cardiol.* **2016**, *105*, 763–773. [CrossRef]

62. Dennert, R.; Velthuis, S.; Schalla, S.; Eurlings, L.; van Suylen, R.J.; van Paassen, P.; Tervaert, J.W.; Wolffs, P.; Goossens, V.J.; Bruggeman, C.; et al. Intravenous immunoglobulin therapy for patients with idiopathic cardiomyopathy and endomyocardial biopsy-proven high PVB19 viral load. *Antivir. Ther.* **2010**, *15*, 193–201. [CrossRef]
63. Ak, A.; Porokhovnikov, I.; Kuethe, F.; Schulze, P.C.; Noutsias, M.; Schlattmann, P. Transcatheter vs. surgical aortic valve replacement and medical treatment: Systematic review and meta-analysis of randomized and non-randomized trials. *Herz* **2018**, *43*, 325–337. [CrossRef]

viruses

MDPI

Article

Human Bocavirus Infection Markers in Peripheral Blood and Stool Samples of Children with Acute Gastroenteritis

Zaiga Nora-Krukle [1,*], Anda Vilmane [1], Man Xu [2], Santa Rasa [1], Inga Ziemele [3,4], Elina Silina [4], Maria Söderlund-Venermo [2], Dace Gardovska [3,4] and Modra Murovska [1]

1 Institute of Microbiology and Virology, Rīga Stradiņš University, 5 Ratsupites St., LV-1067 Riga, Latvia; zaiga.nora@rsu.lv (Z.N.K.); anda.vilmane@rsu.lv (A.V.); santa.rasa@rsu.lv (S.R.); modra@latnet.lv (M.M.)
2 Department of Virology, University of Helsinki, 3 (PL21), 00014 Helsinki, Finland; man.xu@helsinki.fi (M.X.); maria.soderlund-venermo@helsinki.fi (M.S.-V.)
3 Children's Clinical University Hospital, 45 Vienibas Avenue, LV-1004 Riga, Latvia; inga.ziemele@gmail.com (I.Z.); dace.gardovska@rsu.lv (D.G.)
4 Department of Paediatrics, Rīga Stradiņš University, 16 Dzirciema St., LV-1067 Riga, Latvia; sil.elina.23@gmail.com (E.S.)
* Correspondence: zaiga.nora@rsu.lv; Tel.: +371-67060837

Received: 5 October 2018; Accepted: 13 November 2018; Published: 15 November 2018

Abstract: Human bocaviruses (HBoVs) 1–4 belong to the Parvoviridae family, and they infect the respiratory or gastrointestinal tracts in children. We investigated the prevalence of HBoV1–4 DNAs in the blood and stool samples, and of HBoV1–4 IgG and IgM in the plasma samples, of children presenting with acute gastroenteritis (AGE). In addition, we identified HBoV co-infections with the five most frequent gastrointestinal pathogens. A total of 83 paired blood and stool samples were collected from children aged five years or less. Infection markers of HBoV1, 2, or 3 (viral DNA in blood and/or stool and/or antibodies) were detected in 61 out of 83 (73.5%) patients. HBoV1, 2, or 3 DNA as a monoinfection was revealed in 18.1%, 2.4%, and 1.2%, respectively, and 21.7% in total. In 56.1% of the HBoV DNA-positive patients, the presence in stool of another virus—most frequently norovirus or rotavirus—was observed. In conclusion, this study, for the first time, illustrates the prevalence and genetic diversity of HBoVs in Latvian children with gastroenteritis, and shows a widespread distribution of these viruses in the community. HBoV1 and 2 are commonly found as single infectious agents in children with AGE, suggesting that the viruses can be as pathogenic by themselves as other enteric agents are.

Keywords: human bocavirus; children; acute gastroenteritis

1. Introduction

Acute gastroenteritis (AGE) is common and affects all age groups around the world, and is the second-leading cause of child morbidity among pediatric infectious diseases. Globally, nearly 1.7 billion episodes of childhood diarrheal disease, and 525,000 deaths, occur annually in children less than five years of age [1].

Latvian Centre for Disease Prevention and Control data show that AGE is the fifth leading cause of morbidity overall, causing 3.7% of all illnesses in children during their first year of life. In children under one year of age, the incidence of AGE in the past five years (from 2012 to 2016) has increased, from 804 episodes in 2012 to 1059 episodes in 2016 [2].

Viruses such as rotavirus (RoV), noroviruses (HNoV), enteric adenoviruses (HAdV), and astroviruses (HAstV) are the major causes of AGE, but in many patients, despite various diagnostic methods, the etiological agent of the disease remains unidentified [3,4].

There are four HBoVs in the Parvoviridae family, and the Parvovirinae subfamily, belonging to the *Bocaparvovirus* genus, of which HBoV1 causes mild to severe respiratory tract infections mainly in children under the age of five. HBoV1 was first revealed in pooled nasopharyngeal aspirates of children in 2005, but can be found also in stool samples [5–7]. A few years later, in 2009, HBoV2 and HBoV3, and in 2010 also HBoV4, were discovered in stool samples of children [8–10]. HBoV2 is more frequently found in stool samples than in respiratory tract samples, but its association with AGE is disputed [8,9,11,12]. HBoV2 has only occasionally been found in the respiratory tract [13,14]. To date there is no confirmed association between HBoV3 or HBoV4 and AGE or respiratory tract infections [10,12,14,15].

The aim of this study was to investigate the detection rates of the respiratory and enteric HBoVs, as well as to determine co-infections with the five most frequent gastrointestinal pathogens in children presenting with gastroenteritis, in order to identify the possible role of HBoVs in the etiology of the disease in Latvia. This is the largest study of HBoVs in AGE where viral DNA findings in stool and blood samples have been compared with serology.

2. Materials and Methods

2.1. Patients and Samples

This study was performed in the Infectious Diseases Department of the Children's Clinical University Hospital of Riga, Latvia from November 2013 to April 2017. Children who were hospitalized and who fulfilled the criteria for AGE (with diarrhea and/or vomiting, febrile temperature (i.e., axillary temperature higher or equal to 37.5 °C), with the duration of acute illness of less than 10 days) were included in this prospective study. The median duration of hospitalization was two days. On inspection, symptoms of acute respiratory tract infection (ARTI) in combination with AGE were also determined in some of the patients. Exclusion criteria were: Patients with chronic diseases and patients with bacterial gastroenteritis.

Altogether, 83 children were enrolled in the study. Of these 83 children, 51 (61.4%) were male and 32 (38.6%) were female ($p = 0.0051$). The median age was 19 months; 8 patients (9.6%) were less than 6 months old, 15 (18.1%) were 6–12 months old, 35 (43.2%) patients were 12–24 months old, and 25 (30.1%) were 2–5 years old. Pediatricians divided the patients into two groups: The AGE group (patients with gastrointestinal symptoms only) of 61 patients and the AGE–ARTI group (patients with symptoms of both AGE and ARTI) of 22 patients.

Stool and blood samples were obtained from all 83 children and studied for the presence of HBoVs and five gastro-intestinal viruses (HNoV genogroup I (HNoVGI) and II (HNoVGII), RoV, HAdV, HAstV, and sapovirus (HSaV)).

All procedures performed in the study involving human participants were in accordance with the ethical standards of the institutional and/or national research committee and with the 1964 Helsinki declaration and its later amendments or comparable ethical standards. The study protocol was approved by the Ethics Committee of the Rīga Stradiņš University (ethical approval issued on 30 May 2013; permission code: 25/30.05.2013). Written informed consent was received from all parents or guardians of participating children.

2.2. Nucleic Acid Extraction and PCR Analysis

DNA from whole blood was extracted using phenol-chloroform extraction, and from stool specimens using commercially available QIAamp DNA Stool Mini Kit (Qiagen, Valencia, CA, USA) according to the manufacturer's protocol. The quantity of DNA was measured spectrophotometrically, and the quality of the DNA was proved using β-globin gene polymerase chain reaction (PCR). HBoVs were detected by nested PCR (nPCR), using primers amplifying the VP1/2 gene sequence of all four HBoVs, as described previously [10], followed by electrophoretic analysis of the PCR products in a 1.7% agarose gel. The positive qualitative nPCR results were verified and the HBoV loads were evaluated by a commercially available real-time quantitative PCR detection kit for HBoV genomes according to the manufacturer's protocol (human bocavirus viral protein (VP) gene genesig standard kit, Genesig, Primerdesign Ltd., Southampton, UK). All stool samples were screened for five human viruses (HNoVGI and HNoVGII, RoV, HAdV, HAstV, HSaV) using a multiplex real-time PCR gastrointestinal virus assay (GI-Virus Assay, Seegene, Seoul, Korea).

2.3. Nucleotide Sequence Analysis

The HBoV-positive nPCR products were purified by MinElute PCR Purification Kit (Qiagen, Germany) and sequenced with ABI Prism 3100 Genetic Analyzer (Applied Biosystems, Foster City, CA, USA). Sequences were analyzed initially using program Chromas 2.5.1. and after that compared to the reference strains using the Basic Local Alignment Search Tool (BLAST).

2.4. VLP-Based Enzyme Immunoassay

HBoV1–4 IgG and IgM class antibodies were measured in all plasma samples from the children with AGE or AGE–ARTI, by in-house enzyme immunoassays (EIA) based on biotinylated virus-like particles (VLPs) of recombinant major capsid protein (VP3) at the Department of Virology, University of Helsinki, as described previously [16,17]. To verify that the IgG result was specific to each HBoV, a blocking reaction with VLPs of the heterologous HBoVs was performed in the plasma samples, for example, in HBoV1 IgG EIA, blocking in plasma was done with HBoV2 and HBoV3 non-biotinylated VLPs, and in HBoV2 IgG EIA, with HBoV1 and HBoV3 non-biotinylated VLPs [17,18]. The positivity cut-offs in competitive and non-competitive IgG EIA were 0.095 (mean +3SD) and 0.151 (mean +3SD), respectively, and in non-competitive IgM EIA, it was 0.131 (mean +3SD).

2.5. Statistical Methods

The statistical analysis was performed by GraphPad Prism 7.0 software, La Jolla, CA, USA (Fisher's exact test, Mann–Whitney test, ANOVA). A p value < 0.05 was considered statistically significant.

3. Results

In total, HBoV-specific antibodies and/or DNA was detected in 61 out of the 83 (73.5%) patients included in the study. HBoV DNA in blood and/or stool samples was detected in 42 out of 83 (50.6%) patients, whereas nine out of 83 (10.8%) patients were IgM-positive and 51 out of 83 (61.4%) patients were IgG positive.

In the AGE group 33 out of 61 (54.1%) children were positive for HBoV DNA; 15 out of 33 (45.5%) children in blood samples only, seven out of 33 (21.2%) children in stool samples only, and 11 out of 33 (33.3%) children in both blood and stool samples. Sequencing results revealed that blood harbored only HBoV1 DNA, which was found in 26 patients; however, in stool samples HBoV1 DNA was detected in 11 patients, HBoV2 DNA in five patients, HBoV3 DNA in two patients, and HBoV4 DNA in none of the patients (Table 1).

Table 1. Human bocavirus PCR and EIA results of children with acute gastroenteritis, or acute gastroenteritis with acute respiratory tract infection.

PCR Findings in Blood/Stool	*n*	IgM+			IgG+				IgM−/IgG−
		HBoV1	HBoV2	HBoV1 & HBoV2	HBoV1	HBoV2	HBoV1 & HBoV2	HBoV1 & HBoV3	
AGE group, *n* = 61									
HBoV1+/HBoV1+	6	2 [a]			3				3
HBoV1+/HBoV2+	4	1 [a]			1	2			1
HBoV1+/HBoV3+	1				1				
HBoV1+/HBoVs−	15	2 [a]			9	2	1		3
HBoVs−/HBoV1+	5				4	1			
HBoVs−/HBoV2+	1					1			
HBoVs−/HBoV3+	1							1	
HBoVs−/HBoVs−	28				6	2	1	1	
AGE–ARTI group, *n* = 22									
HBoV1+/HBoV1+	3	1 [a]		1 [a]	1		1		1
HBoV1+/HBoV2+	0								
HBoV1+/HBoV3+	0								
HBoV1+/HBoVs−	6	1 [a]	1 [a]		3		1		2
HBoVs−/HBoV1+	0								
HBoVs−/HBoV2+	0								
HBoVs−/HBoV3+	0								
HBoVs−/HBoVs−	13				7	1	1		

+/− presence/absence of viral DNA in corresponding sample; AGE—acute gastroenteritis; ARTI—acute respiratory tract infection; PCR—polymerase chain reaction; IgG—immunoglobulin G [average absorbances ± standard deviation (range): HBoV1 1.560 ± 1.153 (0.107–3.950); HBoV2 0.460 ± 0.449 (0.134–1.794); HBoV3 0.852 ± 0.676 (0.162–1.65)]; IgM—immunoglobulin M [average absorbances ± standard deviation (range): HBoV1 0.582 ± 0.417 (0.151–1.382); HBoV2 0.146 and 0.185]; HBoV—human bocavirus; HBoV1 and HBoV2—antibodies against HBoV1 and 2 simultaneously; [a] patients with also the presence of IgG; *n*—number of patients.

In the AGE–ARTI group, of the nine out of 22 (40.9%) HBoV DNA-positive patients, HBoV DNA was detected in blood samples only in six out of nine (66.7%) patients, and in both blood and stool samples in three out of nine (33.3%) cases. None of the children in the AGE–ARTI group harbored viral DNA only in stool samples. Sequencing data affirmed that all detected virus-specific sequences, in both blood and stool samples, of the AGE–ARTI group belonged to HBoV1. There was no statistically significant difference between viral DNA findings in the two specimen types of the two groups ($p > 0.05$).

In the whole patient cohort, viral loads of ≥1 copies/µg DNA was detected in 15 (42.9%) out of 35 HBoV1 DNA-positive blood samples, with a median (IQR) of 58.69 (202.3–4.88) copies/µg DNA, and in 16 (72.7%) out of 22 HBoV DNA-positive stool samples, with a median (IQR) of 10.12 (144.7–3.95) copies/µg DNA.

3.1. HBoV-Specific Antibodies and DNA in Blood and Stool Samples

In the AGE group, HBoV-specific IgG antibodies were found in 36 out of 61 (59.0%) patients. Among them, 24 out of 36 (66.7%) patients were specific for HBoV1, of which two (5.6%) patients also had IgG against HBoV2 and two other patients against HBoV3. In turn, HBoV2-specific IgG antibodies alone were revealed in eight (22.2%) patients but none had only HBoV3 IgG. Five of the 24 IgG-positive patients (20.8%) also had HBoV1-specific IgM antibodies. None of the examined plasma samples in the AGE group was seropositive for HBoV4 (Table 1).

Ten (16.4%) out of the 61 AGE patients were HBoV-IgG-positive without having viral DNA in their blood or stool samples, whereas in seven out of 61 (11.5%) patients both HBoV IgG antibodies as well as DNA were detected in stool samples (Table 1). In four out of these seven patients, the IgG antibodies were specific to HBoV1. Two of these four patients were also IgG-positive for HBoV2 and one patient-for HBoV3. In 12 out of 61 (19.7%) patients, HBoV1 viremia as well as HBoV-specific IgG was found, but in nine patients the IgG was HBoV1-specific. Interestingly, two of these 12 patients had IgG against HBoV2 only and one against both HBoV1 and 2. Seven of the 61 (8.2%) patients were HBoV-seropositive and had HBoV DNA in both blood and stool samples. Five of those seven patients were IgG-positive for HBoV1 and two patients for HBoV2. Finally, in seven out of the 61 (11.5%) other patients, HBoV DNA in blood and/or stool samples occurred in seronegative individuals. Five children with HBoV1 DNA in blood and/or stool samples had HBoV1-specific IgG and IgM (Table 1).

In the AGE–ARTI group, nine (40.9%) out of 22 patients had HBoV-specific IgG antibodies, but no viremia or DNA in stool samples. In seven out of those nine patients, the IgG was specific to HBoV1, in one to HBoV2, and in one to both HBoV1 and HBoV2. Four out of 22 patients had both HBoV1 viremia and HBoV1-specific IgG antibodies, one of which was also seropositive for HBoV2. Three (13.6%) out of 22 patients had HBoV DNA both in blood and stool samples, and in two of them HBoV1- and 2-specific antibodies were also found (Table 1). Four patients from the AGE–ARTI group had IgM antibodies to either HBoV1 or HBoV2, whereas three patients were seronegative, but viremia had HBoV DNA in blood samples, or in both blood and stool samples.

In the whole study group, the seroprevalences of HBoV1, 2, and 3 were 50.6%, 16.9%, and 2.4%, respectively, the differences being statistically significant ($p < 0.0001$; $p < 0.0001$; $p = 0.0027$, respectively).

3.2. Co-Infections

All 83 stool samples were re-tested for five gastrointestinal viruses (HNoV GI and HNoVGII, RoV, HAdV, HAstV, and HSaV) by a multiplex real-time PCR. One or more of these enteric viruses were detected in 44 of the 83 patient stools; 33 out of 61 among the AGE children and 11 out of 22 among the AGE–ARTI children.

In the AGE group, 15 out of 43 (34.9%) patients had HBoV DNA and/or antibodies and also one more of analyzed enteric viruses, whereas eight (18.6%) patients had a genomic sequence of two additional enteric viruses (Table 2). The most frequently co-detected virus was HNoVGII, which was present in 16 out of 43 (37.2%) stool samples, followed by RoV in 12 out of 43 (27.9%), HAdV in two out of 43 (4.7%), and HAstV in one out of 43 (2.3%) stool samples. HNoVGII and RoV was detected significantly more frequently than HAdV or HAstV ($p = 0.0003$ and $p < 0.0001$, and $p = 0.0068$ and $p = 0.0016$, respectively) (Table 2). HBoV DNAs in stool samples were detected in 19 out of 61 (31.1%) patients, among whom HBoV monoinfection was revealed in eight patients, others had co-infection with one or two enteric viruses. In eight out of 61 (13.1%) patients of the AGE group, no viruses were detected in their stool samples.

Table 2. Presence of human bocaviruses and other enteric pathogens.

Virus Patient Groups	*n*	HAdV	HNoVGII	RoV	HAdV/HNoVGII	HNoVGII/RoV	HNoVGII/HAstV	WCI
AGE, HBoVs+	43	1	8	6	1	6	1	20
AGE, HBoVs−	18	1	3	5		1		8
AGE–ARTI, HBoVs+	18	1	8	1				8
AGE–ARTI, HBoVs−	4		1					3

+/− presence/absence of HBoV in corresponding sample; AGE—acute gastroenteritis; ARTI—acute respiratory tract infection; HAdV—adenovirus; HAstV—astrovirus; HBoV—human bocavirus; HNoVGII—norovirus genogroup II; RoV—rotavirus; WCI—without co-infection; *n*—number of patients.

In the AGE–ARTI group, HBoV DNA in stool samples was revealed in three out of 22 patients, from them one patient had HBoV monoinfection. Ten out of 18 (55.6%) patients had HBoV DNA and/or antibodies as well as one of five more analyzed enteric viruses genomic sequences, and none with two or more viruses. The co-presence of HBoV1 DNA with HNoVGII or RoV RNA was detected in eight and one stool sample(s), respectively ($p = 0.0178$). HNoVGII was revealed more often than HAdV, which was also found in one stool sample ($p = 0.0178$) (Table 2).

All 83 patients were divided into four age groups to analyze HBoV monoinfection and co-infections with tested enteric viruses (Table 3). Patients aged 0–6 months had HBoV monoinfections only, but patients in the age groups from 6–60 months had co-infection with HNoV GII significantly more often than with RoV ($p = 0.0438$). Co-infection with HAdV was significantly less common than with HNoVGII ($p < 0.0001$).

Table 3. Presence of human bocaviruses and other enteric pathogens in patients in different age groups.

Viruses Age (Months)	*n*	HNoVGII	RoV	HAdV	HAstV
0–6 (HBoV+)	5				
0–6 (HBoV−)	3	1			
6–12 (HBoV+)	10	5	1	1	
6–12 (HBoV−)	5		1		
12–24 (HBoV+)	22	8	5		1
12–24 (HBoV−)	13	4	5	1	
24–60 (HBoV+)	24	11	7	2	
24–60 (HBoV−)	1				

+/− presence/absence of HBoV in corresponding sample; HBoV–human bocavirus; HNoVGII—norovirus genogroup II; RoV—rotavirus; HAdV—adenovirus; HAstV—astrovirus; *n*—number of patients. There was no statistically significant difference between the HBoV viral load in blood samples in the case of single and co-infections ($p = 0.2721$).

4. Discussion

This study was set up to elucidate the association of HBoVs with pediatric gastroenteritis and to determine the occurrence of co-infection with five of the most frequent acute gastroenteritis-causing viruses. The recruited patients were divided into two groups—children with AGE and children with AGE and ARTI. It is a common clinical experience that symptoms of both those clinical conditions may occur simultaneously.

The detection rate of HBoV infection markers in our study cohort was 73.5%. One of the explanations for such a high percentage is that our study reflects the results from both viral DNA and antibody findings, which were not always overlapping in each patient. However, a longitudinal study of weekly oral fluid samples from infants, analyzed by PCR for HBoV1 DNA, in America revealed that 76% of the children experienced a primary HBoV1 infection during the first 18 months of their life [19]. Another point is the inclusion criteria for patients participating in the study. Accordingly, we included only those patients in whom several bacterial and/or viral causative agents for AGE or AGE–ARTI were not identified in the clinic. The patients were thus pre-selected.

This is the first study so far where the methods of molecular biology and serology are combined, analyzing blood, plasma, and stool samples from all the recruited patients. In the AGE group, HBoV DNA was detected in blood or in stool samples, or in both simultaneously, but in the AGE–ARTI group there were no cases in which any HBoV was detected in stool samples only. The sequencing of the positive PCR products was used to identify the genotype of HBoV. Sequencing results were compared to the reference sequence from the National Center for Biotechnology Information database, revealing 99–100% similarity (Suppl. 1). In the current study, sequencing results showed that only the HBoV1 genomic sequence was found in the patients' blood samples, though in stool samples HBoV2 and HBoV3 were also detected. Moreover, in the AGE–ARTI group, HBoV1 was also found in stool samples, demonstrating that HBoV1 is more a respiratory pathogen.

HBoV DNA in stool samples was detected in 25.3% of all patients, which is much higher than in other studies that have reported occurrence from 5.7% to 9.2% [12,20–22]. No statistically significant difference in frequency of HBoV1 DNA prevalence between the AGE and AGE–ARTI groups was found [i.e., 42.6% and 40.9%, respectively ($p = 1$)]. Conversely, HBoV2 or HBoV3 was detected only in seven out of 61 (11.5%) stool samples from the AGE patient group but none in the AGE–ARTI group ($p = 0.1812$). In a similar study from Finland, researchers analyzed nasal swab and stool samples from

955 children with ARTI, with both AGE–ARTI and AGE showing that HBoV2 and HBoV3, just like in our study, were more commonly found in stool samples [12].

In our study, a viral load higher or equal to one copy/µg DNA was detected in 42.9% of the HBoV-positive blood samples and in 76.2% of the positive stool samples. Results showed that a high viral load correlates with acuteness of the virus infection, because six out of nine HBoV1 and/or HBoV2 IgM-positive patients had elevated viral loads compared with HBoV IgM negative patients. There was no clinical difference between patients with high or low HBoV loads revealed in blood or stool samples. However, other studies, where respiratory samples were analyzed, showed correlations of high viral load with increasing disease duration or severity [7,23,24].

It has been shown that a combination of serological and PCR-based methodology is necessary for an accurate diagnosis of HBoV1 respiratory tract infection [16,25].

In 59.0% of patients from the AGE group and in 68.2% of patients from the AGE–ARTI group, HBoV-specific IgG antibodies were detected ($p = 0.610$). In the whole study cohort, the HBoV1 IgG seroprevalence is statistically higher than those of HBoV2 or HBoV3; in 50.6%, 16.9%, and 2.4%, respectively ($p < 0.0001$ for both). Additionally, the HBoV2 IgG prevalence is higher than that of HBoV3 IgG ($p = 0.0027$). HBoV4 DNA or specific antibodies were not found in this study, nor in our previous study [26], which allows us to conclude that HBoV4 is absent, or circulates rarely, in the Latvian child population.

Out of 21 patients with HBoV DNA-positive stool samples in the study cohort, five (23.8%) had an acute HBoV1 and two (9.5%) an acute HBoV2 infection, based on the presence of HBoV viremia and IgM, in addition to virus DNA, in stool samples.

There is much discussion among scientists and clinicians regarding whether HBoV1 co-infections may exacerbate the illness and have a meaningful role in the etiopathogenesis of the disease. To find out if there is a monoinfection of HBoV1–4, or if the patient is co-infected with other viruses, patients' stool samples were examined for the presence of the most widespread causative viral agents of AGE: RoV, HNoV (GI and GII), enteric HAdV, HAstV, and HSaV. In our study cohort, HNoVGII was the most commonly detected virus in stool samples, followed by HBoV and RoV. These were detected in 34.9%, 25.3%, and 22.9% of the cohort, respectively. Taking into account only HBoV DNA findings in stool samples, HBoV as a monoinfection was revealed in 10.8% of 83 patients, whereas another virus as a co-infection was detected in 15.7% of the patients from the cohort. The number of co-infecting viruses in HBoV-positive cases ranged from one to two.

Results of the study show that most of the HBoV2-positive cases were patients with AGE without symptoms of respiratory tract infections. Also, HBoV2 positive cases were most frequently monoinfections, which was statistically significant ($p = 0.0365$), demonstrating its nature of being predominantly an enteric virus. Similar results have been reported by other research groups [19,27]. Previous studies have mostly detected HBoV1 in respiratory specimens and HBoV2 in stool samples [11–13]. However, HBoV1 is also often detected in stool samples and in some regions HBoV1 is the most frequently detected HBoV in stool samples [27]. This is consistent with the results of our study. It has been shown that HBoV1 first causes respiratory tract infection and then persists without any symptoms for several months, and a hypothesis is that thereafter the virus would infect the gastrointestinal tract, perhaps causing symptoms of gastroenteritis [28]. Alternatively, HBoV1 can be swallowed during acute respiratory disease and then appear in stools; however, it is known that diarrhea in small children might be an additional symptom in HBoV1 respiratory infection [12,29].

The present study, for the first time, illustrates the prevalence and genetic diversity of HBoVs in the Latvian child population with gastroenteritis, and demonstrates the widespread distribution of these viruses in the community. HBoV1 is commonly found as a single infectious agent in children with AGE, suggesting that the virus can be as pathogenic by itself as other enteric agents are. This study revealed that, in the AGE group, HBoV1 is the most common bocavirus detected in stools, leaving open the question regarding HBoV1's ability to survive in the passage through the gastrointestinal tract, or acting as a causal agent of the disease.

Supplementary Materials: The following are available online at http://www.mdpi.com/1999-4915/10/11/639/s1, Supplement 1: Sequencing results.

Author Contributions: Conceptualization, Z.N.-K.; investigation, Z.N.-K., M.X., and A.V.; resources, I.Z. and E.S.; data curation, S.R. and Z.N.-K.; writing—original draft preparation, Z.N.-K.; writing—review and editing, A.V., M.X., S.R., I.Z., E.S., M.S.-V., D.G., and M.M.; supervision, M.S.-V., M.M., and D.G.; project administration, Z.N.-K., M.S.-V., and M.M.; funding acquisition, Z.N.-K., M.S.-V., M.X., D.G., and M.M.

Funding: This study was supported in parts by the Rīga Stradiņš University research project "Epidemiology, pathogenicity of human bocavirus (HBoV) types and their possible connection to lower respiratory tract diseases and acute gastroenteritis in children" RSU ZP 17/2013; the National Research Program "BIOMEDICINE", project No. 5.6.2; the 7FP project "Unlocking infectious diseases research potential at Riga Stradiņš University", Baltinfect, agreement number 316275; the China Scholarship Council; the Sigrid Jusélius Foundation; and the Life and Health Medical Grant Association, Helsinki, Finland.

Acknowledgments: We thank Derek Pheby, Visiting Professor of Epidemiology at Buckinghamshire New University, UK, for advising on the use of English in this paper.

Conflicts of Interest: The authors declare no conflicts of interest.

References

1. World Health Organization. Diarrhoeal Disease Fact Sheet N°330. Available online: http://www.who.int/mediacentre/factsheets/fs330/en/ (accessed on 2 May 2017).
2. Disease Prevention and Control Centre of Latvia. State Statistics Survey, Children's Health. Available online: https://www.spkc.gov.lv/en/statistics (accessed on 25 April 2018).
3. Wilhelmi, I.; Roman, E.; Sanchez-Fauquier, A. Viruses causing gastroenteritis. *Clin. Microbiol. Infect.* **2003**, *9*, 247–262. [CrossRef] [PubMed]
4. Wikswo, M.E.; Hall, A.J. Outbreaks of acute gastroenteritis transmitted by person-to-person contact—United States, 2009–2010. *MMWR Surveill Summ.* **2012**, *61*, 1–12. [PubMed]
5. Allander, T.; Tammi, M.T.; Eriksson, M.; Bjerkner, A.; Tiveljung-Lindell, A.; Andersson, B. Cloning of a human parvovirus by molecular screening of respiratory tract samples. *Proc. Natl. Acad. Sci. USA* **2005**, *102*, 12891–12896. [CrossRef] [PubMed]
6. Kesebir, D.; Vazquez, M.; Weibel, C.; Shapiro, E.D.; Ferguson, D.; Landry, M.L.; Kahn, J.S. Human bocavirus infection in young children in the United States: Molecular epidemiological profile and clinical characteristics of a newly emerging respiratory virus. *J. Infect. Dis.* **2006**, *194*, 1276–1282. [CrossRef] [PubMed]
7. Zhao, B.; Yu, X.; Wang, C.; Teng, Z.; Wang, C.; Shen, J.; Gao, Y.; Zhu, Z.; Wang, J.; Yuan, Z.; et al. High Human Bocavirus Viral Load Is Associated with Disease Severity in Children under Five Years of Age. *PLoS ONE* **2013**, *8*, e62318. [CrossRef] [PubMed]
8. Kapoor, A.; Slikas, E.; Simmonds, P.; Chieochansin, T.; Naeem, A.; Shaukat, S.; Alam, M.M.; Sharif, S.; Angez, M.; Zaidi, S.; et al. A newly identified bocavirus species in human stool. *J. Infect. Dis.* **2009**, *199*, 196–200. [CrossRef] [PubMed]
9. Arthur, J.L.; Higgins, G.D.; Davidson, G.P.; Givney, R.C.; Ratcliff, R.M. A novel bocavirus associated with acute gastroenteritis in Australian children. *PLoS Pathog.* **2009**, *5*, e1000391. [CrossRef] [PubMed]
10. Kapoor, A.; Simmonds, P.; Slikas, E.; Li, L.; Bodhidatta, L.; Sethabutr, O.; Triki, H.; Bahri, O.; Oderinde, B.S.; Baba, M.M.; et al. Human bocaviruses are highly diverse, dispersed, recombination prone, and prevalent in enteric infections. *J. Infect. Dis.* **2010**, *201*, 1633–1643. [CrossRef] [PubMed]
11. Chieochansin, T.; Kapoor, A.; Delwart, E.; Poovorawan, Y.; Simmonds, P. Absence of detectable replication of human bocavirus species 2 in respiratory tract. *Emerg. Infect. Dis.* **2009**, *15*, 1503–1505. [CrossRef] [PubMed]
12. Paloniemi, M.; Lappalainen, S.; Salminen, M.; Kätkä, M.; Kantola, K.; Hedman, L.; Hedman, K.; Söderlund-Venermo, M.; Vesikari, T. Human bocaviruses are commonly found in stools of hospitalized children without causal association to acute gastroenteritis. *Eur. J. Pediatr.* **2014**, *173*, 1051–1057. [CrossRef] [PubMed]
13. Han, T.H.; Kim, C.H.; Park, S.H.; Kim, E.J.; Chung, J.Y.; Hwang, E.S. Detection of human bocavirus-2 in children with acute gastroenteritis in South Korea. *Arch. Virol.* **2009**, *154*, 1923–1927. [CrossRef] [PubMed]

14. Koseki, N.; Teramoto, S.; Kaiho, M.; Gomi-Endo, R.; Yoshioka, M.; Takahashi, Y.; Nakayama, T.; Sawada, H.; Konno, M.; Ushijima, H.; et al. Detection of human bocaviruses 1 to 4 from nasopharyngeal swab samples collected from patients with respiratory tract infections. *J. Clin. Microbiol.* **2012**, *50*, 2118–2121. [CrossRef] [PubMed]
15. Wang, Y.; Gonzalez, R.; Zhou, H.; Li, J.; Li, Y.; Paranhos-Baccalà, G.; Vernet, G.; Guo, L.; Wang, J. Detection of human bocavirus 3 in China. *Eur. J. Clin. Microbiol. Infect. Dis.* **2011**, *30*, 799–805. [CrossRef] [PubMed]
16. Söderlund-Venermo, M.; Lahtinen, A.; Jartti, T.; Hedman, L.; Kemppainen, K.; Lehtinen, P.; Allander, T.; Ruuskanen, O.; Hedman, K. Clinical assessment and improved diagnosis of bocavirus-induced wheezing in children, Finland. *Emerg. Infect. Dis.* **2009**, *15*, 1423–1430. [CrossRef] [PubMed]
17. Kantola, K.; Hedman, L.; Tanner, L.; Simell, V.; Mäkinen, M.; Partanen, J.; Sadeghi, M.; Veijola, R.; Knip, M.; Ilonen, J.; et al. B-Cell Responses to Human Bocaviruses 1–4: New Insights from a Childhood Follow-Up Study. *PLoS ONE* **2015**, *10*, e0139096. [CrossRef] [PubMed]
18. Kantola, K.; Hedman, L.; Arthur, J.; Alibeto, A.; Delwart, E.; Lau, T.; Ruuskanen, O.; Hedman, K.; Söderlund-Venermo, M. Seroepidemiology of human bocaviruses 1–4. *J. Infect. Dis.* **2011**, *204*, 1403–1412. [CrossRef] [PubMed]
19. Lasure, N.; Gopalkrishna, V. Molecular epidemiology and clinical severity of Human Bocavirus (HBoV) 1-4 in children with acute gastroenteritis from Pune, Western India. *J. Med. Virol.* **2017**, *89*, 17–23. [CrossRef] [PubMed]
20. Cashman, O.; O'Shea, H. Detection of human bocaviruses 1, 2 and 3 in Irish children presenting with gastroenteritis. *Arch. Virol.* **2012**, *157*, 1767–1773. [CrossRef] [PubMed]
21. Nawaz, S.; Allen, D.J.; Aladin, F.; Gallimore, C.; Iturriza-Gómara, M. Human bocaviruses are not significantly associated with gastroenteritis: Results of retesting archive DNA from a case control study in the UK. *PLoS ONE* **2012**, *7*, e41346. [CrossRef] [PubMed]
22. Martin, E.T.; Kuypers, J.; McRoberts, J.P.; Englund, J.A.; Zerr, D.M. Human Bocavirus 1 Primary Infection and Shedding in Infants. *J. Infect. Dis.* **2015**, *212*, 516–524. [CrossRef] [PubMed]
23. Deng, Y.; Gu, X.; Zhao, X.; Luo, J.; Luo, Z.; Wang, L.; Fu, Z.; Yang, X.; Liu, E. High viral load of human bocavirus correlates with duration of wheezing in children with severe lower respiratory tract infection. *PLoS ONE* **2012**, *7*, e34353. [CrossRef] [PubMed]
24. Zhou, L.; Zheng, S.; Xiao, Q.; Ren, L.; Xie, X.; Luo, J.; Wang, L.; Huang, A.; Liu, W.; Liu, E. Single detection of human bocavirus 1 with a high viral load in severe respiratory tract infections in previously healthy children. *BMC Infect. Dis.* **2014**, *14*, 424. [CrossRef] [PubMed]
25. Xu, M.; Arku, B.; Jartti, T.; Koskinen, J.; Peltola, V.; Hedman, K.; Söderlund-Venermo, M. Comparative Diagnosis of Human Bocavirus 1 Respiratory Infection With Messenger RNA Reverse-Transcription Polymerase Chain Reaction (PCR), DNA Quantitative PCR, and Serology. *J. Infect. Dis.* **2017**, *215*, 1551–1557. [CrossRef] [PubMed]
26. Nora-Krukle, Z.; Rasa, S.; Vilmane, A.; Gravelsiņa, S.; Kalis, M.; Ziemele, I.; Naciute, M.; Petraitiene, S.; Mieliauskaite, D.; Klimantaviciene, M.; et al. Presence of human bocavirus 1 in hospitalised children with acute respiratory tract infections in Latvia and Lithuania. *Proc. Latv. Acad. Sci. Sect. B* **2016**, *70*, 198–204. [CrossRef]
27. Chow, B.D.; Ou, Z.; Esper, F.P. Newly recognized bocaviruses (HBoV, HBoV2) in children and adults with gastrointestinal illness in the United States. *J. Clin. Virol.* **2010**, *47*, 143–147. [CrossRef] [PubMed]
28. Campos, G.S.; Silva Sampaio, M.L.; Menezes, A.D.; Tigre, D.M.; Moura Costa, L.F.; Chinalia, F.A.; Sardi, S.I. Human bocavirus in acute gastroenteritis in children in Brazil. *J. Med. Virol.* **2016**, *88*, 166–170. [CrossRef] [PubMed]
29. Vicente, D.; Cilla, G.; Montes, M.; Pérez-Yarza, E.G.; Pérez-Trallero, E. Human bocavirus, a respiratory and enteric virus. *Emerg. Infect. Dis.* **2007**, *13*, 636–637. [CrossRef] [PubMed]

viruses

MDPI

Article

Establishment of a Parvovirus B19 NS1-Expressing Recombinant Adenoviral Vector for Killing Megakaryocytic Leukemia Cells

Peng Xu [1,2,*,†], Xiaomei Wang [1,2,†], Yi Li [1] and Jianming Qiu [2,*]

1 Hubei Engineering Research Center of Viral Vector, Wuhan University of Bioengineering, Wuhan 430415, China
2 Department of Microbiology, Molecular Genetics and Immunology, University of Kansas Medical Center, Kansas City, KS 66160, USA
* Correspondence: xupenghuashi@163.com (P.X.); jqiu@kumc.edu (J.Q.); Tel.: +1-913-588-4329 (P.X. & J.Q.); Fax: +1-913-588-7295 (P.X. & J.Q.)
† P.X. and X.W. contribute equally to the study.

Received: 30 July 2019; Accepted: 3 September 2019; Published: 4 September 2019

Abstract: Adenoviral viral vectors have been widely used for gene-based therapeutics, but commonly used serotype 5 shows poor transduction efficiency into hematopoietic cells. In this study, we aimed to generate a recombinant adenovirus serotype 5 (rAd5) vector that has a high efficiency in gene transfer to megakaryocytic leukemic cells with anticancer potential. We first modified the rAd5 backbone vector with a chimeric fiber gene of *Ad5* and *Ad11p* (rAd5F11p) to increase the gene delivery efficiency. Then, the nonstructural protein NS1 of human parvovirus B19 (B19V), which induces cell cycle arrest at the G2/M phase and apoptosis, was cloned into the adenoviral shuttle vector. As the expression of parvoviral NS1 protein inhibited Ad replication and production, we engineered the cytomegalovirus (CMV) promoter, which governs NS1 expression, with two tetracycline operator elements ($TetO_2$). Transfection of the rAd5F11p proviral vectors in Tet repressor-expressing T-REx-293 cells produced rAd in a large quantity. We further evaluated this chimeric rAd5F11p vector in gene delivery in human leukemic cells, UT7/Epo-S1. Strikingly, the novel rAd5F11p-B19NS1-GFP vector, exhibited a transduction efficiency much higher than the original vector, rAd5-B19NS1-GFP, in UT7/Epo-S1 cells, in particular, when they were transduced at a relatively low multiplicity of infection (100 viral genome copies/cell). After the transduction of rAd5F11p-B19NS1-GFP, over 90% of the UT7/Epo-S1 cells were arrested at the G2/M phase, and approximately 40%–50% of the cells were undergoing apoptosis, suggesting the novel rAd5F11P-B19NS1-GFP vector holds a promise in therapeutic potentials of megakaryocytic leukemia.

Keywords: parvovirus B19; adenoviral vector; cell cycle arrest; apoptosis; anti-cancer

1. Introduction

Adenovirus (Ad) is a nonenveloped icosahedral virus and has a double-stranded DNA genome of 30 to 38 kbp. Ad has been studied intensively for over 50 years in models of virus–cell interactions, cellular processing, and latterly as a gene delivery vector. To date, over 60 serotypes of human Ad have been described, most of which infect the respiratory or gastrointestinal tracts and the eye [1]. Recombinant Ad (rAd) is one of the most popular gene delivery vectors and has been used constantly for phase I to III clinical trials in the development of vaccines and therapeutic gene transfer in the last 20 years [2]. The reasons for why rAd is widely used for gene vectors are that Ad has a wide range of tropism to cells and tissues, and infections are not associated with serious pathogenicity in general [3]. rAd vectors have been proved to efficiently deliver transgenes to the nucleus of a wide range of cell types and then mediate a high level of expression of the transgenes. Moreover, rAd vectors transduce both proliferating and differentiated cells [4]. After infection, rAd vectors remain episomal and do not integrate into the host cell genome, which minimizes the risk of insertional mutagenesis. Furthermore, rAd vectors have a remarkable DNA packaging capacity, offering possibilities for genetic manipulations. Last, rAd vectors are easy to produce, requiring very limited 'hands on' time from shuttle/backbone plasmid cotransfection to the isolation of virus particles.

However, the commonly used Adenovirus serotype 5 (*Ad5*) has a poor transduction efficiency in hematopoietic cells, mainly because of the low expression of *Ad5* receptors on the cells [5]. For Ad entering the cells, the key step is the interaction between viral fiber knob and its cellular receptor. So, a method for changing the knob domain or even the entire fiber gene of *Ad5* is used to improve the gene delivery efficiency to target cells. Different Ad serotypes exhibit different tissue tropism because of the different fiber proteins. *Ad11p*, which belongs to the human species B adenoviruses, was reported to have the ability to infect human $CD34^+$ hematopoietic cells [6]. Therefore, the chimeric Ad vector containing a chimeric fiber protein between *Ad5* and *Ad11p* fibers may have higher transduction efficiency to hematopoietic cells than the *Ad5* vector.

Parvovirus B19 (B19V) belongs to the *Erythroparvovirus* genus within the *Parvoviridae* family [7]. B19V has a high tropism for the human erythroid progenitor cells (EPCs) from the bone marrow and fetal liver [8]. B19V has a linear single stranded DNA (ssDNA) genome of approximately 5.6 kb, which has identical inverted terminal repeats (ITRs) of 383 nucleotides at both ends [9]. The double-stranded replicative-form (RF) DNA of the B19V genome encodes a large nonstructural protein (NS1). B19V NS1, 671 amino acids (aa) in length, has a molecular weight of approximately 78 kDa. NS1 predominantly localizes in the nucleus of infected cells, as it contains nuclear localization signals at amino acid residues 177 to 180 (KKPR) and 316 to 321 (KKCGKK) [10]. B19V NS1 not only plays important roles in viral DNA replication and transcription activation [11], but also executes a cytotoxic effect on human erythroid cells. B19V-infected cells have ultrastructural features associated with apoptosis, and the NS1 has been identified as the apoptosis-inducer [12,13]. Besides, we have previously found that B19V NS1 induces cell cycle arrest at the G2/M phase [14].

Leukemias are a group of life-threatening malignant disorders of the blood and bone marrow. Despite significant progress achieved in the past decade in the chemotherapy-based and targeted treatments of several leukemia subsets, relapse remains common after an initial response, indicating the resistance of leukemia cells to current therapies.

In this study, we modified the *Ad5* fiber gene in rAd5 with the *Ad11P* fiber gene to increase the transduction efficiency into UT7/Epo-S1 cell line, which was generated by Kazuo Sugamura and is susceptible to B19V infection [15]. UT7/Epo-S1 is a subline derived from UT7/Epo, which is an erythropoietin (Epo)-dependent cell line, and originating from UT7, a megakaryocytic leukemia cell line [16]. We demonstrated that the transduction of the chimeric rAd that expresses B19V NS1-induced cell cycle arrest and apoptosis. Thus, our novel rAd5F11P-B19NS1 vector, which can be subjected to further genetic manipulations, holds promise for gene-based therapeutic medicine of leukemia treatment.

2. Material and Methods

2.1. Cell Lines

HEK293 cells (CRL-1573) were purchased from the American Type Culture Collection (ATCC) (Manassas, VA, USA) and were cultured in Dulbecco's modified Eagle's medium (DMEM; GE Healthcare Biosciences, Piscataway, NJ, USA) with 10% fetal calf serum (Sigma-Aldrich, St. Louis, MO, USA).

T-REx-293 cells were purchased from Invitrogen (Carlsbad, CA, USA) and were cultured in DMEM plus 10% fetal calf serum and 10 μg/mL blasticidin.

UT7/Epo-S1 cells were obtained from Dr. Kevin Brown at the Hematology Branch, NHLBI, NIH, with permission from Dr. Kazuo Sugamura at Tohoku University, Japan, and were cultured under normoxic conditions in DMEM containing 10% fetal calf serum (FCS) and 2 U/mL erythropoietin (Amgen, Thousand Oaks, CA, USA).

2.2. Plasmids

The DNA sequences coding B19V NS1 were codon-optimized and purchased at GenScript USA Inc. (Piscataway, NJ, USA) as previously described [17].

The pacAd5 CMV-GFP transfer plasmid was made by digesting the pacAd5 U6-GFP (purchased from Cell Biolabs (San Diego, CA, USA)) with XhoI to remove the mU6 promoter and multiple cloning site (MCS). Then the CMV promoter, MCS, and a bGH poly(A) signal were inserted.

The CMV promoter of the pacAd5 CMV-GFP vector was modified by inserting two repeated tetracycline operator elements (5′-TCC CTA TCA GTG ATA GAG ATC TCC CTA TCA GTG ATA GAG A-3′) at 9 bases behind the TATA box, resulting in pacAd5 CMVTetO_2-GFP. C-terminally Strep-tagged optimized (opt) B19V NS1 was inserted into pacAd5 CMVTetO_2-GFP to generate the transfer plasmid, pacAd5 CMVTetO_2-B19NS1-GFP.

pacAd5 9.2-100 was purchased from Cell Biolabs, Inc. (San Diego, CA, USA) The fiber gene in the pacAd5 9.2-100 was replaced with a chimeric fiber gene encoding the *Ad5* fiber tail domain and *Ad11p* fiber shaft and knob domains described as before [18]. Firstly, pacAd5 9.2-100 was digested into two fragments by EcoRI. The large fragment of 26,438 bp was saved for use, the small fragment of 8509 bp which contains *Ad5* fiber gene was ligated to EcoRI-digested pGEX-3Z to generate pGEX-3Z-Ad5F. Secondly, chimeric fiber gene Ad5F11P was synthesized using an overlapping PCR strategy, with AgeI or Alf II site at each end. Thirdly, AgeI/Alf II fragment that encodes *Ad5* fiber gene from pGEX-3Z-Ad5F was replaced with the synthesized Ad5F11P digested by the same enzymes to form a new plasmid, pGEX-3Z-Ad5F11P. Finally, pGEX-3Z-Ad5F11P was digested with EcoRI, and ligated with the large fragment of the EcoRI-digested pacAd5 9.2-100 to generate pacAd5F11P 9.2-100.

All plasmids were sequenced to confirm their constructions at MCLAB (South San Francisco, CA, USA).

2.3. Recombinant Adenoviral (rAd) Vector Construction and Purification

rAd was made following the instructions provided by Cell Biolabs (San Diego, CA, USA). Briefly, linearized shuttle vector pacAd5 CMVTetO_2-GFP or pacAd5 CMVTetO_2-B19NS1-GFP were transfected into T-REx-293 cells with linearized Ad genome backbone, pacAd5 9.2-100 or pacAd5F11P 9.2-100. After one week, when plaques were formed, cells were collected and resuspended in phosphate buffered saline (PBS), pH 7.4, and lysed by three cycles of freezing and thawing. Crude viral lysates were collected for virus propagation. The final viral lysates were spun at 10,000 rpm for 30 min, and then the supernatant was collected and dissolved in CsCl at a density of 1.36 g/mL for centrifugation in a Sorvall TH641 rotor at 36,000 rpm for 36 h at 20 °C Fractions of 500 μL were collected using a Piston Gradient Fractionator (BioComp, Fredericton, NB, Canada).

2.4. Q-PCR

The primers and FAM (6-carboxyfluorescein)-labeled probe used for quantification of rAd DNA were designed to target the *GFP* gene: Forward primer (5′-CTG CTG CCC GAC AAC CA-3′), Reverse primer (5′-TGT GAT CGC GCT TCT CGT T-3′), and the probe (5′-FAM-TAC CTG AGC ACC CAG TCC GCC CT-BHQ1-3′). Quantitative PCR was performed as described previously [19] on a 7500 Fast real-time PCR system (Applied Biosystems, Foster City, CA, USA).

2.5. Fluorescence Images

GFP fluorescence images were taken at a magnification of 10 × (objective lens), with a Nikon Eclipse Ti-S inverted microscope (Nikon, Tokyo, Japan).

2.6. Flow Cytometry Analysis

(i) Cell cycle analysis: Cell cycle analysis was performed using the 4′,6-diamidino-2-phenylindole (DAPI) staining described as before [20]. Briefly, rAd-transduced UT7/Epo-S1 cells were washed with PBS, fixed by 1% Paraformaldehyde (PFA), then permeabilized with 0.4% tween-20 and stained with DAPI at a concentration of 1 μg/mL for 30 min in dark. Samples were analyzed by flow cytometry within 1 h.

(ii) Fluorescent-Labeled Inhibitors of Caspases (FLICA): FLICA Caspase-9 assay kit was purchased from ImmunoChemistry Technologies (Bloomington, MN, USA) and the assay was performed following the manufacturer's protocol. Briefly, 290 μL of rAd-transduced UT7/Epo-S1 cells was incubated with 10 μL of the working solution of the reagent and then incubated for approximately 1 h, and then analyzed with a flow cytometer.

(iii) Apoptosis analysis: FITC-conjugated Annexin V and Propidium Iodide (PI) double staining was performed following the manufacturer's protocol. Briefly, rAd-transduced UT7/Epo-S1 cells were washed twice with cold PBS and then resuspended in 1 × Binding Buffer at a concentration of 1×10^6 cells/mL. A volume of 100 μL of the solution (1×10^5 cells) was transferred to a 1.5 mL tube, with 5 μL of FITC Annexin V and 5 μL of PI. After gentle vertexing, the cells were incubated for 15 min at RT (25 °C) in dark, with 400 μL of 1 × Binding Buffer, and were analyzed by flow cytometry within 1 h.

All processed samples were analyzed on a three-laser flow cytometer (LSR II; BD Biosciences (San Jose, CA, USA)) at the Flow Cytometry Core at the University of Kansas Medical Center. All flow cytometry data were analyzed using FACS DIVA software (BD Biosciences).

2.7. Western Blot

Cells were transfected or transduced as indicated in each figure. The cells were harvested and lysed 2 days post-transfection/transduction. Western blotting was performed to analyze the lysates as previously described [21], using anti-strep and β-actin antibodies.

3. Results

3.1. Modification of the rAd Vector System

In order to generate a rAd vector that has high tropism to leukemia cells, we made a rAd vector that has a chimeric fiber of *Ad5* and *Ad11p* [18]. As the rAd backbone vector pacAd5 9.2-100 is too large to manipulate, we digested pacAd5 9.2-100 with EcoRI and ligated the Ad 8.5 Kb fragment, which contains the *Ad5* fiber gene, into pGEX-3Z plasmid, then mutated the *Ad5* fiber gene to be a chimeric gene of *Ad5* and *Ad11p*. Finally, we subcloned the Ad 8.5 Kb fragment back to the rAd backbone vector pacAd5 9.2-100, resulting in pacAd5F11P 9.2-100 (Figure 1).

It has been reported that autonomous parvoviruses, such as rat parvovirus H-1 (H-1PV), interfere with Ad replication due to the NS1 protein [22]. Therefore, we modified the CMV promoter in the shuttle plasmid, which transcribes B19V NS1-encoding mRNA, by inserting two tetracycline operator elements (Figure 2A,B). As a result, CMV promoter-driven NS1 expression was inhibited in the packaging cells, T-REx-293 cells, which constitutively expressed the tetracycline repressor [23], allowing a high-yield rAd production. As a control, the CMVTetO$_2$ promoter still had activities in normal HEK293 cells (Figure 2C).

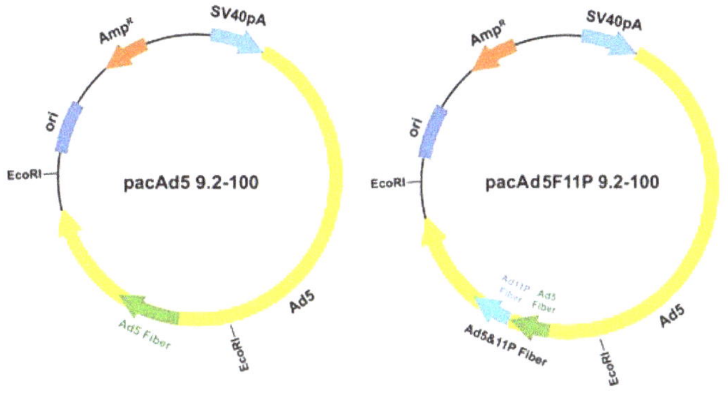

Figure 1. Modifications of the adenoviral backbone vector pacAd5 9.2-100. The proviral gene of units 9.2-100 of the *Ad5* and chimeric fiber Ad are diagramed. The chimeric *Ad5* and *Ad11P* fiber gene is indicated.

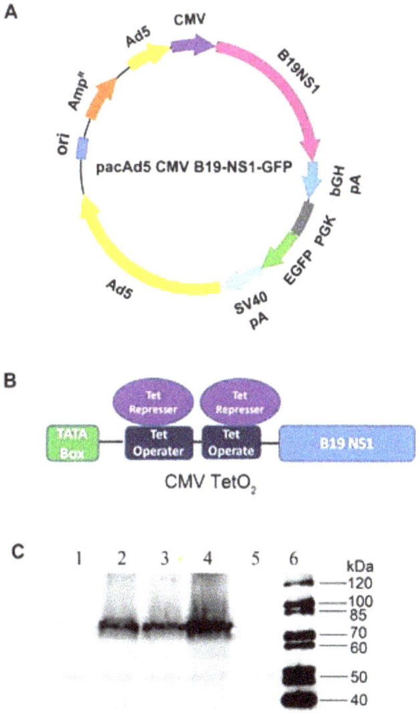

Figure 2. Modifications of the adenoviral shuttle vectors. (**A**,**B**) Modification of the CMV promoter. The transfer plasmid pacAd5 CMV-B19NS1-EGFP is diagrammed. Two tetracycline operator elements were inserted into the CMV promoter, which govern B19V NS1 expression. (**C**) Validation of the CMVTetO_2 promoter activity. HEK293 cells and T-REx-293 cells were transfected with pacAd5 CMV-B19NS1-GFP and pacAd5 CMVTetO_2-B19NS1-GFP, respectively. At 48 h post-transfection, cells were collected for Western blotting using anti-strep antibody to check B19V NS1 expression. Lane 1: HEK293 cells control; Lane 2: HEK293 cells transfected with pacAd5 CMV-B19NS1-GFP; Lane 3: HEK293 cells transfected with pacAd5 CMVTetO_2-B19NS1-GFP; Lane 4: T-REx-293 cells transfected with pacAd5 CMV-B19NS1-GFP; Lane 5: T-REx-293 cells transfected with pacAd5 CMVTetO_2-B19NS1-GFP; Lane 6: protein ladder.

3.2. Production of B19V NS1-Expressing rAd

T-REx-293 cells were co-transfected with linearized pacAd5 CMVTetO_2-GFP or pacAd5 CMVTetO_2-B19NS1-GFP and linearized pacAd5F11P 9.2-100 (Figure 3A). After one week, we found a high percentage (>80%) of GFP-expressing cells and a few plaques appeared, which were likely caused by rAd5F11P-GFP and rAd5F11P-B19NS1-GFP (Figure 3B). We then harvested the rAd-producing cells, released the viruses from cells, and saved the crude viral lysates (initial viral stocks). The initial viral stocks were used to amplify the virus in T-REx-293 cells, and the final viral lysates were then purified using CsCl gradient ultracentrifugation. The purified viruses were titrated by quantitative-PCR (qPCR) using a TaqMan probe targeting the *GFP* gene, which had titers of 5×10^{12} vgc/mL (viral genome copies (vgc) per mL).

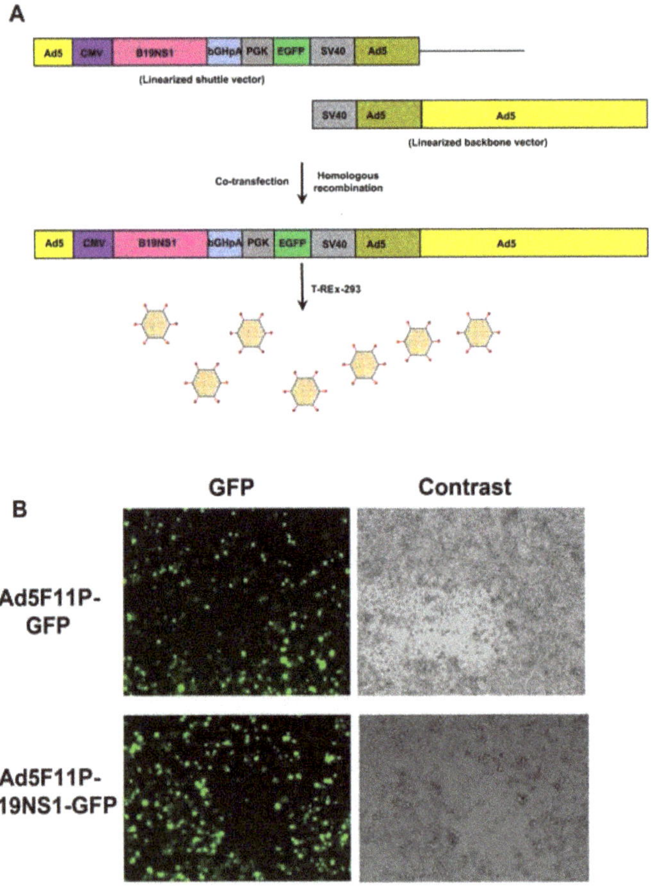

Figure 3. Production of recombinant adenovirus expressing GFP and B19NS1-GFP. (**A**) The schematic flowchart of recombinant Ad production. Both the Ad shuttle and proviral backbone plasmids are transfected into cells. After homologous recombination, a rAd proviral genome is generated, which further replicates to produce rAd virions as diagramed. (**B**) Recombinant adenovirus production. T-REx-293 cells were co-transfected using linearized pacAd5 CMVTetO_2-GFP or pacAd5 CMVTetO_2-B19NS1-GFP with linearized pacAd5F11P 9.2-100. After one week, GFP expression was monitored under a Nikon Eclipse Ti-S inverted microscope at 10× magnification.

3.3. Ad5F11p-B19NS1-GFP Is More Effective in the Transduction of Leukemia Cells at a Relatively Low Multiplicity of Infection (MOI)

We next transduced the UT7/Epo-S1 cells with rAd5F11p-B19NS1-GFP and rAd5-B19NS1-GFP, respectively, at various MOIs (viral genome copies (vgc) per cell). We found that at an MOI of 100, the rAd5F11p-B19NS1-GFP transduced >90% of UT7/Epo-S1 cells while rAd5-B19NS1-GFP transduced only <30%; at MOI of 500 and 1000, the transduction efficiency was over 90%, similar between transductions using rAd5F11p-B19NS1-GFP and rAd5-B19NS1-GFP (Figure 4). This result suggests that the rAd5F11p-B19NS1-GFP vector transduces UT7/Epo-S1 cells more efficiently than the rAd5-B19NS1-GFP vector, when they were used at a relatively low MOI.

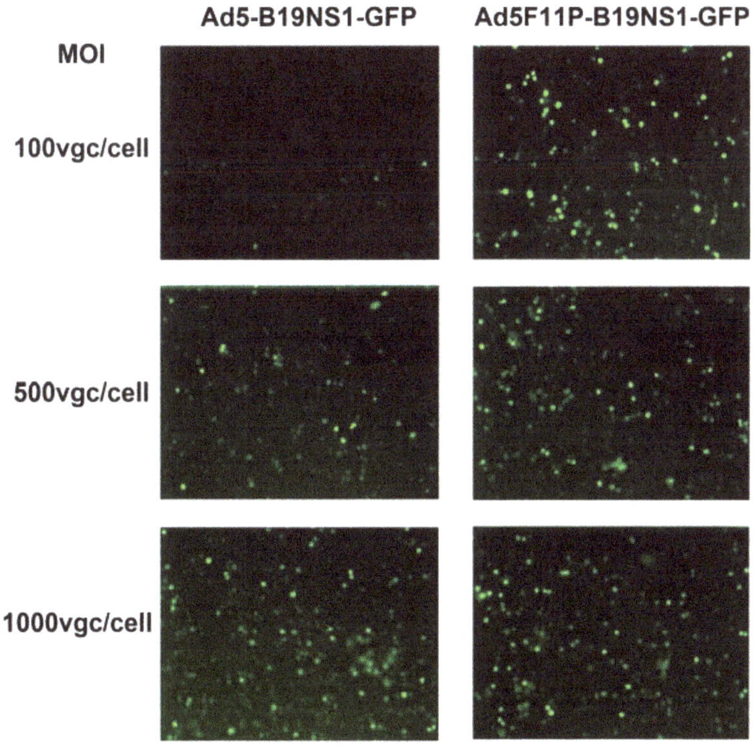

Figure 4. rAd5F11p-B19NS1-GFP is more effective than the parent rAd5 in the transduction of leukemia cells UT7/Epo-S1 at a relatively low MOI. UT7/Epo-S1 cells were transduced with rAd5-B19NS1-GFP or rAd5F11p-B19NS1-GFP at three different MOIs (100, 500, and 1000 vgc/cell), respectively. At 48 h post-transduction, GFP expression was monitored under a Nikon Eclipse Ti-S inverted microscope at 10× magnification.

3.4. rAd5F11p-B19NS1-GFP Induces a Cell Cycle Arrest at G2 Phase and Apoptosis in Transduced Cells

In order to test our hypothesis to use B19V NS1 to kill leukemia cells, we transduced UT7/Epo-S1 cells with Ad5F11P-GFP (as a control) and Ad5F11p-B19NS1-GFP at an MOI of 100, respectively, to ensure over 90% of the cells were transduced. Western blotting was performed to detect the NS1 expression (Figure 5A). Cells were harvested at 48 h post-transduction and stained with DAPI to detect the cell cycle. We found that over 90% of the cells were arrested at G2/M (Figure 5B,C). This is consistent with our previous study that B19V NS1 protein is a key factor for disrupting the cell cycle at the G2/M phase [14].

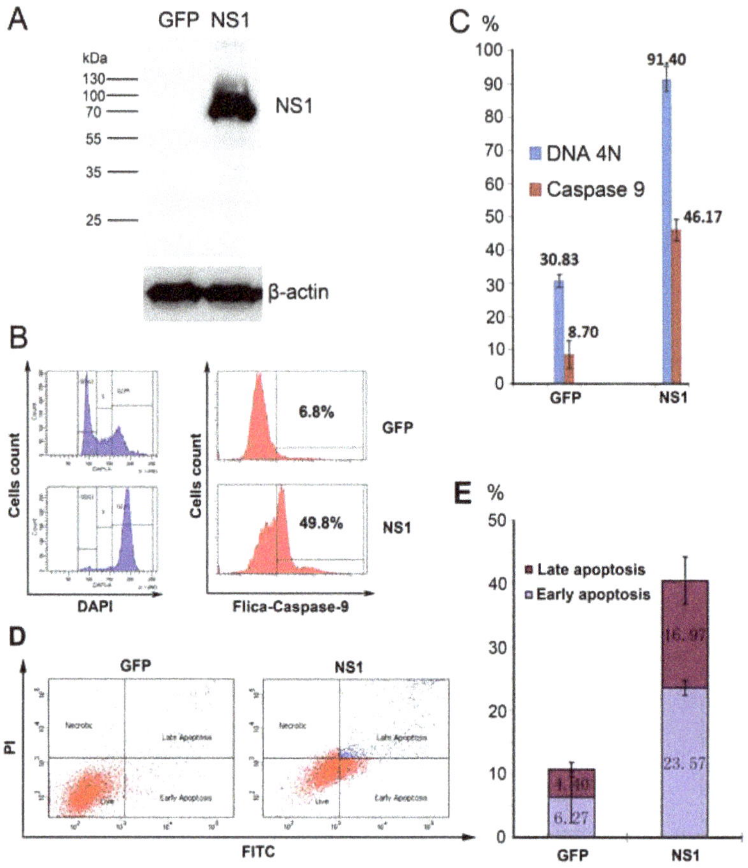

Figure 5. rAd5F11p-B19NS1-GFP induces cell cycle arrest at the G2/M phase and apoptosis in UT7/Epo-S1 cells. UT7/Epo-S1 cells were transduced with rAd5F11p-GFP or rAd5F11p-B19NS1-GFP at an MOI of 100 vgc/cell. After 48 h post-transduction, (**A**) Western blotting. Transduced cells were collected for Western blot analysis using an anti-strep antibody. The same membrane was reprobed by using anti-β-actin antibody. (**B**,**C**) Cell cycle analysis and Fluorescent-Labeled Inhibitors of Caspases (FLICA). Transduced cells were fixed and stained using 4′,6-diamidino-2-phenylindole (DAPI) or FLICA caspase-9. Cell cycle and caspase-9 activity were detected by flow cytometry. (**D**,**E**) Transduced cells were stained with Annexin-V FITC and Propidium Iodide (PI), followed by flow cytometry analysis. The percentages of both early and late apoptotic cells are presented with averages and standard deviations, which were obtained from at least three independent experiments.

Next, we looked into apoptosis induced by NS1 as previously reported [12]. Caspase-9 is an important member of the Caspase family and caspase-9 further processes other caspase members, including caspase-3 and caspase-7, to initiate a caspase cascade, which leads to apoptosis [24]. We chose caspase-9 activity as a marker to measure apoptosis. We found that compared with only 8.7% GFP-expressing cells, NS1 expression increased caspase-9 activity to 46.17% (Figure 5B,C). We also carried out Annexin V-FITC and PI double staining to confirm the NS1-induced apoptosis. The results showed, for GFP control, the apoptosis (early and late) percentage was 6.27% and 4.40%, respectively (a total 10.67%). For B19V NS1, the apoptosis (early and late) percentage was 23.57% and 16.97%, respectively (a total 40.54 %) (Figure 5D,E).

Taken together, all of these results showed that chimeric fiber increased the tropism of the B19V NS1-expressing rAd to leukemia cells UT7/Epo-S1. The expressed NS1 induced over 90% of the leukemia cells arrested at the G2/M phase and the approximately 50% undergoing apoptosis.

4. Discussion

In this study, we modified the *Ad5* fiber gene into a chimeric *Ad5* and *Ad11P* fiber gene to increase the transduction efficiency into leukemia cells UT7/Epo-S1. The fiber gene-modified rAd5F11P-B19NS1-GFP transduces UT7/Epo-S1 more effectively than the rAd5-B19NS1-GFP. More importantly, the transduction of NS1-expressing rAd vector induced nearly all the cells arrested at the G2/M phase. Cancer cells are considered as cells that cannot control their cell cycle progression. During tumorigenesis, due to genetic and epigenetic changes, the regulation of cell cycle is malfunctioned, resulting in uncontrolled cell proliferation [25]. Our novel rAd5F11P-B19NS1-GFP could be a promising gene-based therapeutic approach with anti-leukemia potential.

The cellular receptor for commonly used *Ad5* is coxsackie virus and adenovirus receptor (CAR) on the cell membrane. After the initial interaction between *Ad5* fiber with CAR, the second interaction between the RGD motif of the penton bases with $\alpha_v\beta_3$ and $\alpha_v\beta_5$ integrins facilitates *Ad5* internalization by endocytosis [26]. However, both CAR and $\alpha_v\beta_3$ and $\alpha_v\beta_5$ integrins are poorly expressed on the cell membrane of hematopoietic cells, thus rAd5 has a poor transduction efficiency into hematopoietic cells [5]. The interaction of the fiber knob with the cellular receptor is the key step by which Ad enters the cell. Different adenoviral serotypes exhibit different tissue tropism because their fiber proteins recognize and interact with different cellular receptors [27,28]. *Ad11p*, which belongs to adenovirus group B, has been reported to infect human $CD34^+$ hematopoietic cells [6]. Thus, we replaced *Ad5* fiber with a chimeric fiber gene encoding the *Ad5* fiber tail domain and the *Ad11p* fiber shaft and knob domains. In our case, the chimeric *Ad5* and *Ad11P* fiber recognizes its cellular receptor on UT7/Epo-S1 cells more efficiently than the parent *Ad5* fiber, which could explain why the Ad5F11p-B19NS1-GFP is more effective in the transduction of UT7/Epo-S1 cells at a relatively low MOI than the rAd5-B19NS1-GFP.

Our previous study has found that NS1 induces cell cycle arrest at the G2/M phase through its C-terminal transactivation domain, and NS1 transactivates signaling from ATR to CDC25C. Phosphorylated CDC25C prevents the dephosphorylation of CDK1 at tyrosine 15. Thus, an inactive cyclin B1–CDK1 complex is imported to the nucleus, thereby blocking progression from the G2- to the M-phase. We believe that the cell cycle arrest induced by NS1 in UT7/Epo-S1 is caused by the NS1-inactivated CDC25C. The CDC25C protein is a phosphatase responsible for the dephosphorylation and activation of CDK1 to promote the transition of cells to mitosis, so NS1-inactivated CDC25C could inhibit cancer cell proliferation. Apoptosis is a programmed cell death involving the sequential activation of caspases. The NS1-induced apoptosis activates caspase-9, indicating the intrinsic pathway, which is also called the mitochondrion-mediated pathway, which is different from the NS1-induced apoptosis during B19V infection [29].

In our study, we use modified rAd expressing B19V NS1 to induce cell cycle arrest and apoptosis in UT7/Epo-S1 cells at the G2/M phase, which shows a promising tool to kill the megakaryocytic leukemic cells. Our next step is to modify the promoter which controls NS1 expression into the hTERT promoter, which has activity specifically in cancer cells. Using this strategy, we could more specifically induce the cell cycle arrest and apoptosis of cancer cells. Thus, the rAd5F11P-B19NS1-GFP vector holds promise in gene-based therapeutics for anticancer potential to human leukemia.

Author Contributions: Conceptualization, J.Q.; Formal analysis, P.X. and X.W.; Funding acquisition, X.W., Y.L. and J.Q.; Investigation, P.X. and X.W.; Methodology, P.X., X.W. and Y.L.; Resources, J.Q.; Supervision, Y.L. and J.Q.; Writing—original draft, P.X. and J.Q.; Writing—review & editing, P.X. and J.Q.

Funding: This work was supported by the National Natural Science Foundation of China [grant numbers 31470268, 31700873]; Natural Science Foundation of Hubei [grant number 2017CFB240].

Conflicts of Interest: The authors declare no competing financial interests.

References

1. Russell, W.C. Adenoviruses: Update on structure and function. *J. Gen. Virol.* **2009**, *90*, 1–20. [CrossRef] [PubMed]
2. Ginn, S.L.; Amaya, A.K.; Alexander, I.E.; Edelstein, M.; Abedi, M.R. Gene therapy clinical trials worldwide to 2017: An update. *J. Gene Med.* **2018**, *20*, e3015. [CrossRef] [PubMed]
3. Yamamoto, Y.; Nagasato, M.; Yoshida, T.; Aoki, K. Recent advances in genetic modification of adenovirus vectors for cancer treatment. *Cancer Sci.* **2017**, *108*, 831–837. [CrossRef] [PubMed]
4. Ehrke-Schulz, E.; Zhang, W.; Gao, J.; Ehrhardt, A. Recent Advances in Preclinical Developments Using Adenovirus Hybrid Vectors. *Hum. Gene Ther.* **2017**, *28*, 833–841. [CrossRef] [PubMed]
5. Nilsson, M.; Ljungberg, J.; Richter, J.; Kiefer, T.; Magnusson, M.; Lieber, A.; Widegren, B.; Karlsson, S.; Fan, X. Development of an adenoviral vector system with adenovirus serotype 35 tropism; efficient transient gene transfer into primary malignant hematopoietic cells. *J. Gene Med.* **2004**, *6*, 631–641. [CrossRef]
6. Mei, Y.F.; Segerman, A.; Lindman, K.; Hörnsten, P.; Wahlin, A.; Wadell, G. Human hematopoietic ($CD34^+$) stem cells possess high-affinity receptors for adenovirus type 11p. *Virology* **2004**, *328*, 198–207. [CrossRef]
7. Qiu, J.; Söderlund-Venermo, M.; Young, N.S. Human Parvoviruses. *Clin. Microbiol. Rev.* **2017**, *30*, 43–113. [CrossRef]
8. Chen, A.Y.; Kleiboeker, S.; Qiu, J. Productive Parvovirus B19 Infection of Primary Human Erythroid Progenitor Cells at Hypoxia Is Regulated by STAT5A and MEK Signaling but not HIFa. *PLoS Pathog.* **2011**, *7*, e1002088. [CrossRef]
9. Zhi, N.; Zadori, Z.; Brown, K.E.; Tijssen, P. Construction and sequencing of an infectious clone of the human parvovirus B19. *Virology* **2004**, *318*, 142–152. [CrossRef]
10. Wan, Z.; Zhi, N.; Wong, S.; Keyvanfar, K.; Liu, D.; Raghavachari, N.; Munson, P.J.; Su, S.; Malide, D.; Kajigaya, S.; et al. Human parvovirus B19 causes cell cycle arrest of human erythroid progenitors via deregulation of the E2F family of transcription factors. *J. Clin. Investig.* **2010**, *120*, 3530–3544. [CrossRef]
11. Ganaie, S.S.; Qiu, J. Recent Advances in Replication and Infection of Human Parvovirus B19. *Front. Cell. Infect. Microbiol.* **2018**, *8*, 166. [CrossRef] [PubMed]
12. Poole, B.D.; Zhou, J.; Grote, A.; Schiffenbauer, A.; Naides, S.J. Apoptosis of liver-derived cells induced by parvovirus B19 nonstructural protein. *J. Virol.* **2006**, *80*, 4114–4121. [CrossRef] [PubMed]
13. Thammasri, K.; Rauhamäki, S.; Wang, L.; Filippou, A.; Kivovich, V.; Marjomaki, V.; Naides, S.J.; Gilbert, L. Human parvovirus B19 induced apoptotic bodies contain altered self-antigens that are phagocytosed by antigen presenting cells. *PLoS ONE* **2013**, *8*, e67179. [CrossRef] [PubMed]
14. Xu, P.; Zhou, Z.; Xiong, M.; Zou, W.; Deng, X.; Ganaie, S.S.; Kleiboeker, S.; Peng, J.; Liu, K.; Wang, S.; et al. Parvovirus B19 NS1 protein induces cell cycle arrest at G2 -phase by activating the ATR-CDC25C-CDK1 pathway. *PLoS Pathog.* **2017**, *13*, e1006266. [CrossRef] [PubMed]
15. Morita, E.; Tada, K.; Chisaka, H.; Asao, H.; Sato, H.; Yaegashi, N.; Sugamura, K. Human parvovirus B19 induces cell cycle arrest at G2 phase with accumulation of mitotic cyclins. *J. Virol.* **2001**, *75*, 7555–7563. [CrossRef] [PubMed]
16. Shimomura, S.; Komatsu, N.; Frickhofen, N.; Anderson, S.; Kajigaya, S.; Young, N.S. First continuous propagation of B19 parvovirus in a cell line. *Blood* **1992**, *79*, 18–24. [PubMed]
17. Zhi, N.; Wan, Z.; Liu, X.; Wong, S.; Kim, D.J.; Young, N.S.; Kajigaya, S. Codon optimization of human parvovirus B19 capsid genes greatly increases their expression in nonpermissive cells. *J. Virol.* **2010**, *84*, 13059–13062. [CrossRef]
18. Lu, Z.Z.; Ni, F.; Hu, Z.B.; Wang, L.; Wang, H.; Zhang, Q.W.; Huang, W.R.; Wu, C.T.; Wang, L.S. Efficient gene transfer into hematopoietic cells by a retargeting adenoviral vector system with a chimeric fiber of adenovirus serotype 5 and 11p. *Exp. Hematol.* **2006**, *34*, 1171–1182. [CrossRef]
19. Huang, Q.; Deng, X.; Yan, Z.; Cheng, F.; Luo, Y.; Shen, W.; Lei-Butters, D.C.; Chen, A.Y.; Li, Y.; Tang, L.; et al. Establishment of a reverse genetics system for studying human bocavirus in human airway epithelia. *PLoS Pathog.* **2012**, *8*, e1002899. [CrossRef]
20. Lou, S.; Luo, Y.; Cheng, F.; Huang, Q.; Shen, W.; Kleiboeker, S.; Tisdale, J.F.; Liu, Z.; Qiu, J. Human parvovirus B19 DNA replication induces a DNA damage response that is dispensable for cell cycle arrest at phase G2/M. *J. Virol.* **2012**, *86*, 10748–10758. [CrossRef]

21. Xu, P.; Chen, A.Y.; Ganaie, S.S.; Cheng, F.; Shen, W.; Wang, X.; Kleiboeker, S.; Li, Y.; Qiu, J. The 11-Kilodalton Nonstructural Protein of Human Parvovirus B19 Facilitates Viral DNA Replication by Interacting with Grb2 through Its Proline-Rich Motifs. *J. Virol.* **2018**, *93*, e01464-18. [CrossRef] [PubMed]
22. El-Andaloussi, N.; Bonifati, S.; Kaufmann, J.K.; Mailly, L.; Daeffler, L.; Deryckère, F.; Nettelbeck, D.M.; Rommelaere, J.; Marchini, A. Generation of an adenovirus-parvovirus chimera with enhanced oncolytic potential. *J. Virol.* **2012**, *86*, 10418–10431. [CrossRef] [PubMed]
23. Yao, F.; Svensjö, T.; Winkler, T.; Lu, M.; Eriksson, C.; Eriksson, E. Tetracycline repressor, tetR, rather than the tetR-mammalian cell transcription factor fusion derivatives, regulates inducible gene expression in mammalian cells. *Hum. Gene Ther.* **1998**, *9*, 1939–1950. [CrossRef] [PubMed]
24. Li, P.; Zhou, L.; Zhao, T.; Liu, X.; Zhang, P.; Liu, Y.; Zheng, X.; Li, Q. Caspase-9: Structure, mechanisms and clinical application. *Oncotarget* **2017**, *8*, 23996–24008. [CrossRef] [PubMed]
25. Evan, G.I.; Vousden, K.H. Proliferation, cell cycle and apoptosis in cancer. *Nature* **2001**, *411*, 342–348. [CrossRef] [PubMed]
26. Wickham, T.J.; Mathias, P.; Cheresh, D.A.; Nemerow, G.R. Integrins alpha v beta 3 and alpha v beta 5 promote adenovirus internalization but not virus attachment. *Cell* **1993**, *73*, 309–319. [CrossRef]
27. Knaan-Shanzer, S.; Van Der Velde, I.; Havenga, M.J.; Lemckert, A.A.; De Vries, A.A.; Valerio, D. Highly efficient targeted transduction of undifferentiated human hematopoietic cells by adenoviral vectors displaying fiber knobs of subgroup B. *Hum. Gene Ther.* **2001**, *12*, 1989–2005. [CrossRef]
28. Rea, D.; Havenga, M.J.; van Den Assem, M.; Sutmuller, R.P.; Lemckert, A.; Hoeben, R.C.; Bout, A.; Melief, C.J.; Offringa, R. Highly efficient transduction of human monocyte-derived dendritic cells with subgroup B fiber-modified adenovirus vectors enhances transgene-encoded antigen presentation to cytotoxic T cells. *J. Immunol.* **2001**, *166*, 5236–5244. [CrossRef]
29. Sol, N.; Le Junter, J.; Vassias, I.; Freyssinier, J.M.; Thomas, A.; Prigent, A.F.; Rudkin, B.B.; Fichelson, S.; Morinet, F. Possible interactions between the NS-1 protein and tumor necrosis factor alpha pathways in erythroid cell apoptosis induced by human parvovirus B19. *J. Virol.* **1999**, *73*, 8762–8770.

viruses

MDPI

Review

H-1 Parvovirus as a Cancer-Killing Agent: Past, Present, and Future

Clemens Bretscher [1] and Antonio Marchini [1,2,*]

[1] Laboratory of Oncolytic Virus Immuno-Therapeutics, F011, German Cancer Research Center, Im Neuenheimer Feld 242, 69120 Heidelberg, Germany; c.bretscher@dkfz.de

[2] Laboratory of Oncolytic Virus Immuno-Therapeutics, Luxembourg Institute of Health, 84 Val Fleuri, L-1526 Luxembourg, Luxembourg

* Correspondence: antonio.marchini@lih.lu or a.marchini@dkfz.de; Tel.: +352-26-970-856 or +49-6221-42-4969

Received: 16 May 2019; Accepted: 14 June 2019; Published: 18 June 2019

Abstract: The rat protoparvovirus H-1PV is nonpathogenic in humans, replicates preferentially in cancer cells, and has natural oncolytic and oncosuppressive activities. The virus is able to kill cancer cells by activating several cell death pathways. H-1PV-mediated cancer cell death is often immunogenic and triggers anticancer immune responses. The safety and tolerability of H-1PV treatment has been demonstrated in early clinical studies in glioma and pancreatic carcinoma patients. Virus treatment was associated with surrogate signs of efficacy including immune conversion of tumor microenvironment, effective virus distribution into the tumor bed even after systemic administration, and improved patient overall survival compared with historical control. However, monotherapeutic use of the virus was unable to eradicate tumors. Thus, further studies are needed to improve H-1PV's anticancer profile. In this review, we describe H-1PV's anticancer properties and discuss recent efforts to improve the efficacy of H-1PV and, thereby, the clinical outcome of H-1PV-based therapies.

Keywords: oncolytic virus immune therapy; rodent protoparvoviruses; H-1PV; combination therapies; second generation parvovirus treatments

1. Oncolytic Viruses: A General Introduction

Oncolytic viruses (OVs) are a novel class of self-propagating anticancer agents that act in a multimodal fashion to kill cancer cells [1]. The basis of their mechanism of action is the ability to selectively target, replicate in, and eventually lyse cancer cells without harming normal cells, tissues, or organs. This oncotropism can be either a natural property of the virus or the result of virus engineering at the level of virus cell entry (e.g., modification of the virus capsid to redirect the OV more specifically to receptors overexpressed in cancer cells) or virus replication (e.g., insertion of cancer-specific miRNAs into the viral promoters, which restricts replication within transformed cells).

In addition to this direct killing activity, OVs can engage the immune system in the fight against cancer [2]. Within the tumor microenvironment, a variety of different mechanisms prevent the immune system from attacking cancer cells [3,4]. OVs have the ability to reshape the tumor microenvironment and re-establish immune surveillance, thus acting as vaccine adjuvants [5]. Indeed, in addition to disseminating new progeny viral particles, OV-induced cancer cell lysis is associated with the release of danger-associated molecular patterns, pathogen-associated molecular patterns, and tumor-associated antigens, which triggers inflammatory immune responses directed against not only the virus (via the production of virus-neutralizing antibodies) but also the tumor. The immune system therefore becomes the best ally of the virus in the elimination of cancer cells, even those not directly infected by the virus (e.g., small disseminated metastasis).

Furthermore, some OVs have a natural ability to disrupt tumor vasculature, thus inducing necrosis of tumor cells due to deprivation of oxygen and nutrients [6–8].

Treatment of thousands of cancer patients with various OVs has demonstrated that their safety and tolerability are excellent, and that OVs are associated with only minor side effects, which are limited to flu-like symptoms such as fatigue, fever, and chills [9,10].

Talimogene laherparepvec (T-Vec or Imlygic) was the first OV approved by the US Food and Drug Administration and the European Medicines Agency, at the end of 2015, for the treatment of malignant metastatic melanoma [11,12]. It is a genetically engineered herpes simplex virus (HSV) carrying the granulocyte-macrophage colony-stimulating factor (GM-CSF), which is intended to strengthen the immune response. T-Vec reveals another interesting property of OVs: their anticancer potential can be reinforced by inserting a therapeutic transgene into their genome, for example, an apoptosis inducer with bystander effects to kill cancer cells that eventually become virus-resistant, or immune-modulators (e.g., GM-CSF) to promote more sustained antitumor immunity.

As a result of their anticancer properties, no fewer than forty OVs from at least ten families are currently being tested in clinical trials against a number of malignant indications, alone or in combination with other anticancer modalities (e.g., chemotherapy, radiotherapy, and immunotherapy) [13]. In addition to HSV, the list includes adenovirus (Ad), vaccinia virus, measles virus, coxsackie virus, poliovirus, reovirus, Newcastle disease virus, vesicular stomatitis virus, Seneca Valley virus and protoparvovirus (PV) [13]. Each of these OVs has a distinct mechanism of action, tumor tropism, immunogenicity, possibility of expressing therapeutic transgenes, potential risk of pathogenicity, stability, and specific advantages and limitations associated with the production process. These variations justify the continued development of these different virus platforms. Some of these viruses have entered late-phase clinical development and will hopefully soon become a therapeutic option for cancer patients.

Clinical studies have shown that OV treatment is often effective only in a small percentage of patients, which emphasizes the importance of developing new strategies to improve clinical outcome. As with other anticancer treatments, the combination of OVs with other therapies is believed to improve treatment efficacy. Therefore, the design of novel OV-based combination therapies is the subject of intense research for all OVs under clinical development [14]. Particularly promising are the combinations of OVs with other forms of immunotherapy (e.g., checkpoint blockade) [2,15–17].

In the next section, we present one of the clinically relevant OVs, the rat protoparvovirus H-1PV. We discuss its main features and clinical applications, along with recent advances in improving its anticancer activities. It is important to mention that parallel studies have been carried out also using other rodent protoparvoviruses as anticancer agents [18–22]. Given the focus of the review to H-1PV, these studies will not be discussed in full here.

2. The Rat Protoparvovirus (PV) H-1PV: A Biosketch

H-1PV was first discovered by Toolan and co-workers in the late 1950s (first publication in 1960) from transplantable human tumors [23]. It was soon realized that the infection was not causative of the tumor, but rather opportunistic, and that the virus displayed a natural tropism for human cancer cells [24]. In the 1960s and later in 1982, Toolan's laboratory further showed that H-1PV suppressed viral- and chemical-induced tumors as well as reduced the incidence of spontaneous tumors in animal models [25–27]. These discoveries were seminal in establishing the concept that H-1PV's ability to infect human tumor cells might be used therapeutically.

H-1PV is a member of the *Parvoviridae* family, genus *Protoparvovirus* (Figure 1), which also includes the Kilham rat virus, rat minute virus, LuIII virus, mouse parvovirus, minute virus of mice (MVM), and tumor virus X [28]. Some of these viruses are presently the subject of preclinical investigations aimed at evaluating their potential as anticancer therapeutics. H-1PV is among the smallest known viruses, with a diameter of 25 nm, roughly the size of a ribosome. The natural hosts of H-1PV are rats. H-1PV is shed from the animals through the feces, and transmission occurs via the oronasal route. Under normal conditions, the virus is stable for several months in the environment.

The H-1PV viral capsid contains a linear, single-stranded DNA molecule with a length of about 5100 bases. The original isolate of H-1PV was derived from an adventitious infection of the human Hep-1 hepatoma cell line, transplanted in cortisone-immunosuppressed rats [23]. Since then, the virus was further propagated in human transformed cell lines. Therefore, the current H-1PV may differ from authentic field isolates. Small differences in the length and sequence of the genome may occur naturally as a result of the virus adapting to different host cells by acquiring missense mutations or small deletions in the coding and noncoding regions of the viral genome (see below). The viral genome includes two promoters: the early P4 promoter controls the expression of the non-structural (NS) transcription unit, which encodes the nonstructural proteins NS1 and NS2; and the late P38 promoter regulates the expression of the viral particle (VP) transcription unit, which encodes the VP1 and VP2 capsid proteins and the nonstructural small alternatively translated (SAT) protein. At its extremities, the viral genome contains palindromic sequences that form hairpin structures, which serve as self-priming origins during viral DNA replication [29,30].

The 83 kDa nonstructural protein NS1 is expressed early after infection and plays multiple essential roles during the virus life cycle. NS1 activities are modulated by post-translational modifications such as phosphorylation and acetylation (see below) [31]. Owing to its ATPase and helicase activities, NS1 is the major regulator of viral DNA replication. It also plays a pivotal role in viral gene transcription, given its ability to modulate the transcription of its own P4 promoter and to activate the P38 promoter by binding specifically to DNA [32] (for a detailed review of the NS1 mechanisms of action, see Nüesch and Rommelaere, 2014 [33]). NS1 is also the major effector of virus cytotoxicity (see below), and its expression is sufficient to trigger cell cycle arrest and apoptosis—similar to expression of the whole virus [34]. The role of H-1PV NS2 is less understood, but, based on studies on the closely related parvovirus MVM, it is thought to involve the modulation of viral DNA replication, viral mRNA translation, capsid assembly, and virus cytotoxicity [35].

The H-1PV capsid, like that of other parvoviruses, consists of 60 protein subunits: 10 copies of VP1 and 50 copies of VP2 [36]. VP1 (81 kDa) and VP2 (65 kDa) are translated from the same RNA via alternative splicing, but they differ in their N-terminus. VP1 is 142 amino acids longer than VP2 (735 vs. 593 amino acids). The VP1-N-terminal region has been associated with phospholipase A2 (PLA2)-like activity and contains nuclear localization signals. Both properties are important for the transfer of the viral genome from the endocytic compartment to the cell nucleus [37–40]. In fully infectious, mature virions, but not in empty capsids lacking viral DNA, VP2 undergoes proteolytic cleavage of 18–21 amino acids at its N-terminus to form VP3, which becomes the major component of the viral capsid [36].

Structural crystallographic analysis of the H-1PV capsid has revealed the typical capsid of parvoviruses: a cylindrical structure surrounded by a canyon-like depression at the fivefold axes, spike protrusions at the icosahedral threefold axes, and a dimple-like depression at the twofold axes that appears to be involved in cell-surface recognition and binding [36].

The H-1PV-specific cellular receptor(s) remain to be identified, although terminal sialic acid has been shown to play an essential role in H-1PV cell surface binding and entry [41]. Indeed, treatment with neuraminidase, which cleaves sialic acid from the cellular surface, strongly reduces H-1PV infection by impairing virus cell attachment. The essential role of sialic acid in H-1PV cell surface recognition was confirmed in Chinese hamster ovary (CHO) cells. Whereas the parental CHO Pro-5 cells, which express sialic acid on their surface, are fully susceptible to H-1PV infection, the two isogenic CHO Lec 1 and Lec 2 mutants, which lack sialic acid, are resistant. Two residues at the twofold depression, I368 and H374, are essential for binding to sialic acid [41].

Based on homology with other members of the *Parvoviridae* family, H-1PV cell entry is believed to occur after virus cell membrane binding, via clathrin-mediated endocytosis (for a comprehensive review of PV entry mechanisms, see the review from Ros et al., 2017 [42]). However, the H-1PV cell entry pathways remain to be elucidated. After trafficking into the cytosol, H-1PV penetrates the nucleus. For its viral DNA replication, the virus needs proliferating cells but is itself unable to induce a quiescent cell to enter S-phase. Once the cell enters S-phase, the single-stranded genome is converted to the active double-stranded forms that are accessible for transcription [42,43]. As soon as empty capsids are assembled into the cell nucleus, the single-stranded viral genome is transferred to the shells, and the progeny viruses are transported to the cytoplasm. At the completion of its life cycle, the virus induces cell lysis, which is associated with the extracellular release of progeny viral particles. These new virions can initiate second rounds of lytic infection in neighbouring cells [42].

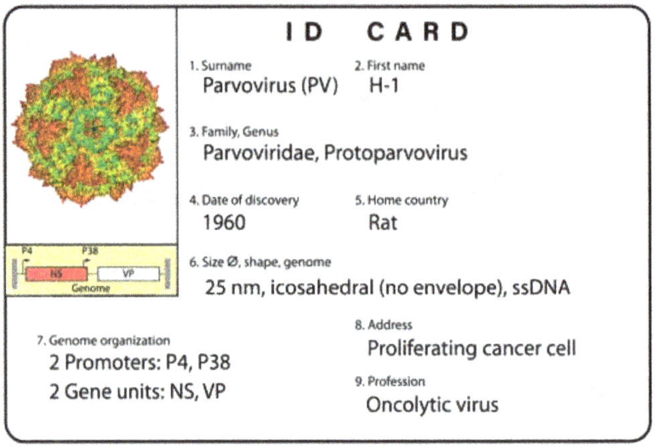

Figure 1. H-1PV's ID card. An overview of H-1PV classification and main features. The virus genome is a single-stranded DNA (ssDNA) molecule including two promoters. The P4 promoter controls the nonstructural unit (NS), which encodes the NS1 and NS2 nonstructural proteins; and the P38 promoter regulates the expression of the VP gene unit, which encodes the VP1 and VP2 capsid proteins. At its extremities, the viral genome contains palindromic sequences (depicted in grey) that are important for virus DNA amplification. An in silico model of the virus capsid is shown [41]. See text for a more detailed description.

3. H-1PV at the Preclinical Level: Acquiring License to Kill Cancer Cells

In this paragraph we discuss the main features that make H-1PV an attractive oncolytic virus (OV).

3.1. Non-Pathogenicity in Humans

The natural host of the H-1PV is the rat. Humans are naturally not infected with the virus. No link has been established between the virus and human diseases, and no pre-existing immunity to H-1PV has been demonstrated in humans. The latter represents an advantage of H-1PV over OVs based on human pathogens (e.g., HSV and Ad), as H-1PV may have a larger therapeutic window before the appearance of neutralizing antibodies. Laboratory studies have demonstrated that although H-1PV can penetrate normal, non-transformed cells, this infection fails to produce new virus particles (i.e., it is an abortive infection) and to induce cell lysis [44]. Clinical studies have shown that H-1PV treatment is safe, well tolerated, and not associated with unwanted side effects (see below).

3.2. Natural Oncotropism

Because of H-1PV's limited genomic information, its life cycle is strictly dependent on the host cell. Some of the factors needed for a productive virus infection are more abundant or more specifically active in the cancer cell than in its normal counterpart. Thus, the cancer cell provides a more favourable milieu than the normal cell for sustaining the virus life cycle. The determinants of H-1PV oncoselectivity have been the focus of several recent reviews and are not discussed in detail here [18,31,44]. Some of these interactions have been described for the closely related MVM and are believed to take place for other PVs, including H-1PV. Briefly, PVs take advantage of some of the (epi)genetic defects that distinguish cancer cells (listed below) at many stages of their life cycle.

3.2.1. Uncontrolled Proliferation

PV DNA replication and, in particular, the conversion of the single-stranded genome into the active double-stranded form rely on cellular factors (e.g., the cyclin A/CDK2 complex) that are S-phase-specific and typically expressed in proliferating cells [45,46].

3.2.2. Dysregulated Signaling Pathways

Various factors that are overexpressed in cancer cells are active in controlling PV nuclear transfer (e.g., CDK1/PKCα-mediated rupture of the nuclear envelope [47]), NS1 activities (e.g., PDK1/PKB/PKC involvement in the phosphorylation of NS1 [48]), viral gene expression (e.g., members of the E2F, Ets, and ATF families of transcription factors are needed to activate the P4 promoter [44,47,49]), virus replication (e.g., interaction with components of the DNA damage response, such as RPA-P32, γH2AX, NBS1-P, ATR, ATRIP, and ATM, which are recruited in the subnuclear PV replication centres, the so-called APAR bodies [50]), viral progeny capsid assembly and nuclear transport (e.g., MAP3K-mediated phosphorylation of capsid intermediates [51]), and virus egress (e.g., XPO1, PKB, PKCη, and Radexin, which regulate various steps involved in trafficking of the virus outside the cell [52–54]).

3.2.3. Impairments of Innate Antiviral Immunity

Defects in the innate immune system are common in cancer cells, which often makes them unable to counteract a virus infection efficiently. H-1PV infection, similarly to MVM infection, triggers an antiviral innate immune response that is associated with the production of type I interferons (IFNs) in normal cells but not in cancer cells. This antiviral response efficiently blocked H-1PV multiplication only in normal cells [21]. However, the sensitivity of rodent PVs to type I IFNs is presently a matter of scientific discussion [20,55–58].

All these interactions (and probably many others still to be characterized) define whether a certain cancer cell is susceptible or not to H-1PV infection. The discovery of new H-1PV cellular modulators is extremely important, as these signatures may serve as markers to predict if a certain patient is likely to respond favorably or not to H-1PV treatment (see also below).

3.3. Oncolytic Activities

Cancer cell lines and primary cultures derived from various tumor entities, including brain, pancreas, breast, lung, cervical and colorectal cancers, melanoma, and osteosarcoma, are susceptible to H-1PV infection and oncolysis (reviewed in [18]). H-1PV was also shown to efficiently infect and kill cancer cell lines derived from hematological diseases such as Burkitt lymphoma, diffuse large B-cell lymphoma, T-cell acute lymphoblastic leukaemia, and cutaneous T-cell lymphoma [59]. Both apoptosis and non-apoptotic cell death have been reported to be induced by H-1PV [34]. Furthermore, in glioma cells, H-1PV induces lysosome-dependent cell death with relocation of active cathepsins B and L (CTSB and CTSL) from lysosomes into the cytosol and concomitant repression of two cathepsin inhibitors, cystatin B and C [60]. By inducing this alternative cell death pathway, H-1PV is able to overcome glioma cell resistance to conventional cytotoxic agents like cisplatin or to soluble death ligands such as the pro-apoptosis inducer TNF-related apoptosis-inducing ligand (TRAIL).

The reasons why H-1PV induces lysosome-dependent cell death in glioma cells, but apoptosis or other forms of cell death (e.g., necrosis) in other cancer cell lines, were recently investigated by our laboratory. We discovered that pro-survival members of the BCL2 family (e.g., BCL2, BCL2L2, BCL2L1, and MCL1), which are overexpressed in glioma (and other tumor) cells and contribute to their resistance to apoptosis inducers, acted as negative modulators of H-1PV-induced apoptosis. Indeed, the addition of BH3 mimetics such as ABT-737 (which inhibits pro-survival BCL2 proteins) rescued the ability of H-1PV to induce apoptosis in these cells, thereby strongly potentiating H-1PV glioma cell oncolysis [61].

H-1PV-induced cell death is mediated by NS1 through the accumulation of reactive oxygen species, which leads to oxidative stress, mitochondrial outer membrane permeabilization, DNA damage, cell cycle arrest, and, finally, caspase activation [34].

H-1PV-induced cell death is also associated with several markers of immunogenic cell death, such as release of the high-mobility group box protein B1 [62] and the immunogenic heat shock protein HSP72 [63]. In a co-culture experiment in which melanoma cells were grown together with dendritic cells (DCs), H-1PV-induced cell lysis stimulated DC maturation and activation [64], accompanied by the production of proinflammatory cytokines such as IL-6 and TNF-α. Mature DCs were able to activate antigen-specific cytotoxic T cells, which resulted in IFNγ production (discussed in the issue by Angelova and Rommelaere [58]).

3.4. *Oncosuppressive Activities*

The oncosuppressive activities of H-1PV have been demonstrated in various animal models (reviewed in [18,44]). Oncosuppression is a result not only of H-1PV tumor oncolysis, but also of the activation of immune responses. The immunostimulatory activities of H-1PV are discussed in the issue by Angelova and Rommelaere [58]. As examples of the oncosuppressive activities of H-1PV, here we summarize experiments carried out in animal models of glioma and pancreatic ductal adenocarcinoma (PDAC) [58].

3.4.1. Glioma Models

In an immunocompetent rat model in which RG2 rat glioma cells were implanted into the brain of allogenic Wistar rats, intratumoral treatment with a single dose of H-1PV (1×10^7 plaque forming units/animal) significantly increased the overall survival of tumor-bearing animals, with one-third of the treated animals undergoing complete tumor remission [65]. Similar anticancer activity was achieved after systemic or intranasal delivery of H-1PV, although higher concentrations of virus were required in comparison to local injection [65,66]. These experiments show the ability of H-1PV to cross the blood-brain barrier in order to reach tumor cells. The NS1 viral protein was detected in tumors but not in normal surrounding tissues, confirming the oncoselectivity of H-1PV. The expression of the oncotoxic viral protein was associated with higher levels of CTSB, confirming previous results obtained in cell culture models [60]. Furthermore, progeny viruses were isolated from the animals, providing evidence of efficient virus multiplication in tumors [65] but not in other organs or tissues [67,68]. Virus treatment was not associated with weight loss or other adverse toxic events [65,66,68], even when the virus was directly injected into the brain of naive rats at high concentrations [67].

Importantly, involvement of the immune system in the elimination of cancer cells was also demonstrated, as antibody depletion of CD8+ T cells strongly reduced virus-mediated oncosuppression [69].

The oncosuppressive activity of H-1PV was also confirmed using the U87 xenograft model of human gliomas in immunodeficient rnu rats [65]. Rnu rats lack a normal thymus and, thus, cannot form T cells. In this model, T cells seem to be dispensable for H-1PV oncosuppression. However, it is not possible to exclude that other immune components such as macrophages and natural killer (NK) cells, which are still functional in rnu rats, may have participated in the elimination of cancer cells, thus compensating for the absence of T cells. In support of this hypothesis, H-1PV was shown to stimulate NK anticancer activity [70].

3.4.2. Pancreatic Ductal Adenocarcinoma (PDAC) Models

H-1PV was used alone or in combination with gemcitabine, the first-line treatment for PDAC. In a syngeneic orthotopic rat model of PDAC, H-1PV treatment alone prolonged animal overall survival. However, a stronger anticancer activity was observed when the virus was combined with gemcitabine [71]. H-1PV's ability to replicate in PDAC cell lines positively correlated with SMAD4 expression levels. Indeed, it was seen that SMAD4 bound to the P4 promoter, thereby modulating its activity [72]. A large set of experiments confirmed in PDAC models the central role of the immune system in H-1PV-mediated oncosuppression. H-1PV has the ability to evoke both innate and adaptive immune responses, as discussed in detail by Angelova and Rommelaere [58].

4. H-1PV Goes to Patients: Meeting the First Endpoints

First clinical use of H-1PV for the treatment of cancer goes back to 1965 [73]. These studies provided first evidence that H-1PV treatment was safe, although, at the regimes used, it did not alter the course of the patients' cancers. This evidence, together with the subsequent preclinical results described above, laid the foundations for the launch in 2011 of a phase I/IIa clinical trial (named ParvOryx) using H-1PV for the treatment of patients suffering from recurrent glioblastoma (GBM) (see also Angelova and Rommelaere, this issue [58]). GBM is the most aggressive and common type of primary malignant brain tumor in the adult brain. GBM remains uniformly fatal, with a dismal median overall survival of only 12–15 months and with only 4.5% of patients surviving more than 5 years. Hence, new therapeutic options are urgently needed [74]. ParvOryx was the first clinical trial in Germany to use OVs. The study involved 18 patients, subdivided into two arms that were treated with escalating doses of H-1PV administered intratumorally or intravenously. The results of the study are summarized in Figure 2. The trial met its endpoints by demonstrating that monotherapy with H-1PV is safe and generally well tolerated. H-1PV showed the ability to cross the blood–brain barrier, to distribute widely in the tumor microenvironment, and to trigger inflammatory responses, confirming previous results obtained at the preclinical level. Compared to historical controls, progression-free and overall survival of the patients was improved, although all patients ultimately died from the disease. A randomized, double-blind study needs to be performed to unequivocally demonstrate the efficacy of H-1PV treatment.

A second clinical study (ParvOryx02), launched in 2015, used H-1PV to treat patients with PDAC. PDAC is one of the most lethal forms of human cancer, with a five-year survival rate of about 6% and a median patient survival rate of less than six months after diagnosis [75]. ParvOryx02 involved a total of seven PDAC patients with at least one liver metastasis. Escalating doses of H-1PV were given intravenously (40% of the dose subdivided in four equal daily fractions) and locally into liver metastases (60% in one single treatment) [76]. Recruitment has been completed, and the study is presently in its evaluation stage. Safety and tolerability are the main endpoints of the study, while evaluation of antitumor activity and clinical efficacy are the secondary objectives.

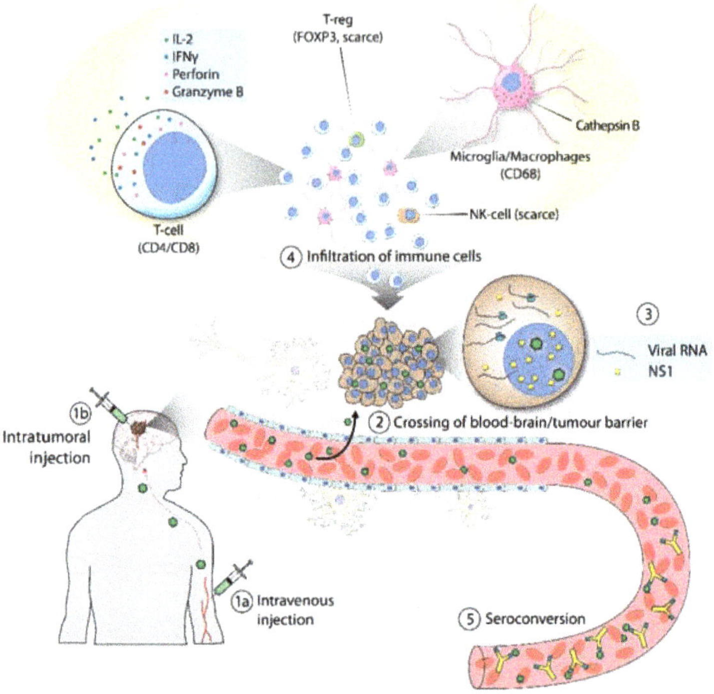

Figure 2. Clinical trial of H-1PV in patients with glioblastoma. (1) H-1PV was administered intratumorally (a) or intravenously (b). (2) H-1PV injected intravenously reached the brain tumor by crossing the blood–brain barrier. (3) H-1PV successfully infected cancer cells, which were positive for viral RNA and NS1 protein (although NS1 expression was below detection limits when the virus was given intravenously). (4) H-1PV induced immunoconversion of the tumor microenvironment (TME), which was characterized by infiltration of CD4+ and CD8+ T cells. T cells were found in their active state, as deduced from the expression of perforin and granzyme B. Microglia/microphages were also observed in the TME. These cells expressed high levels of cathepsin B. By contrast, only a small number of regulatory T cells (T-reg), which tested positive for FOXP3, and few natural killer (NK) cells were detected. (5) Seroconversion occurred after a few days, with the production of virus-neutralizing antibodies.

5. H-1PV Back to the Bench: Further Improving Its Anticancer Profile

As discussed in the previous sections, preclinical and clinical results using wild-type H-1PV as a monotherapy are promising and support its use as an anticancer agent. Nevertheless, these results also show that, as seen for other OVs, there is a discrepancy between H-1PV anticancer efficacy achieved at the preclinical level (e.g., in animal models) and that observed in patients. The fact that H-1PV treatment did not eradicate the tumors clearly indicates the need to improve its efficacy.

The field of oncolytic virus therapy in the last years shifted from considering the OVs as self-amplifying drugs able to directly kill cancer cells by inducing their lysis, to a form of immunotherapy acting indirectly through the induction of anticancer immune responses. However, it remains unclear how many rounds of lytic cycles are needed to harness the immune system to act against the cancer. The clinical experience gathered in these years indicated that, with the exception of few anecdotic cases, treatment with OVs was unable to eliminate all cancer cells. Even in the cases where virus treatment resulted in shrinkage of the tumor and induction of anticancer immune responses, tumors were not completely cured and eventually relapsed. It is possible that the high heterogeneity of tumors and the immunosuppressive nature of the TME have helped some tumor cells to survive the treatment.

We believe that, like for other OVs H-1PV efforts should also be further directed not only to enhance the immune modulatory activities of the virus but also to increase virus multiplication, spread, and oncolysis in the tumor bed. If a larger number of cancer cells are targeted and killed by the virus in the first place, the induction of anticancer immune responses is likely to be more robust.

Also of primary importance is the identification of reliable biomarkers that could be used to identify those patients most likely to benefit from H-1PV-based anticancer treatments. Currently, several approaches are being pursued in an attempt to improve the anticancer potential of H-1PV (Figure 3). Preclinical proofs of concept for some of these approaches have already been acquired, warranting clinical translation of these novel therapies.

5.1. H-1PV-Based Combination Therapies

Cancer heterogeneity often limits the efficacy of a single anticancer treatment, rendering it unable to eliminate all cancer cells. A common trend in anticancer therapy is, therefore, the rational design of novel combinatorial treatments that combine two or more agents with complementary mechanisms of action, leading to additive or better synergistic anticancer effects without increasing adverse events. Similarly, a logical approach to improve the efficacy of H-1PV (and, in general, any OV) is to search for other anticancer modalities that increase virus potency while preserving the safety profile (Figure 3).

5.1.1. H-1PV in Combination with Conventional Treatments

For the sake of expediting clinical translation, OVs have been combined with first-line treatments such as radiotherapy and chemotherapy, often with encouraging results [77,78]. Geletneky and colleagues showed that radiotherapy sensitized low-passage cultures of human glioma to H-1PV treatment [79]. In particular, pre-irradiation 24 h before H-1PV infection increased the fraction of glioma cells in S-phase, thereby rendering the cells more susceptible to H-1PV replication. This effect led to increased cell killing even in radiation-resistant glioma cells. However, this promising protocol has yet to be validated in animal models. As radiotherapy also has immunostimulatory activity [80], it would be interesting to verify whether co-treatment also results in more sustained anticancer immune reactions.

Gemcitabine is a chemotherapeutic drug that acts as a cytidine analogue. However, its use is often accompanied with high toxicity and limited efficacy due to quick acquisition of drug resistance by the cancer cell [81]. H-1PV/gemcitabine co-treatment showed an additive killing activity in vitro that was associated with higher levels of cathepsin B, suggesting that co-treatment triggered a lysosomal cell death pathway. Higher levels of HMGB1 danger signalling were also observed, providing some indications that the killing activity induced more sustained anticancer immune responses [62].

H-1PV efficiently infected and killed gemcitabine-resistant PDAC cells, thus circumventing the drug resistance of the cancer cells. By contrast, gemcitabine pretreatment seemed to potentiate H-1PV anticancer activity through still uncharacterized mechanisms. In a syngeneic orthotopic rat model of PDAC, the consecutive combination of gemcitabine and H-1PV increased the overall survival of tumor-bearing animals with no apparent unwanted cytotoxic effects [71], warranting clinical translation of such a protocol. Further studies are required to optimize these protocols and find the most opportune specific regimes, sequence of addition, and temporal schedule of treatment.

5.1.2. H-1PV in Combination with Epigenetic Modulators

The histone deacetylase inhibitor (HDI), valproic acid (VPA), significantly increases the oncolytic activity of H-1PV. VPA and other HDIs have been shown to induce cell cycle arrest and apoptosis in cancer cells [82]. VPA, which is currently in clinical use for the treatment of epilepsy, is being tested in various clinical trials as an anticancer agent, alone or in combination with other drugs (source: https://clinicaltrials.gov). At doses within the clinical range used for long-term treatment of epileptic patients and sublethal for cancer cells, VPA boosted the oncolytic activity of H-1PV in a synergistic manner in cancer cell lines derived from cervical and pancreatic carcinomas but not in normal, non-transformed cell cultures [83]. Synergistic anticancer activity was attributed to the ability of VPA to increase the acetylation status of the NS1 protein. Two lysine residues, K85 and K257, were found by mass spectrometry to be acetylated within NS1, and their acetylation levels were enhanced by the addition of VPA. Acetylated NS1 has increased DNA binding and transcriptional activities, which resulted in enhanced virus replication in tumor cells. Co-treatment with H-1PV and VPA was associated with a significant increase in oxidative stress associated with accumulation of intracellular reactive oxygen species and DNA damage. Enhanced H-1PV replication and oxidative stress contributed to the synergistic killing activity. However, because of the pleiotropic action of VPA, the role of other uncharacterized mechanisms (e.g., VPA-mediated modulation of the innate immune response) could not be excluded. Validation of the protocol in animal models showed that VPA strongly enhanced the oncosuppression activity of H-1PV, which resulted in complete and long-lasting tumor remission in all co-treated animals under conditions in which single treatment had no, or only slight, benefits for animal survival. This outcome was accompanied by higher virus multiplication, oxidative stress, and DNA damage, thus confirming the results obtained in cell culture experiments [83].

5.1.3. H-1PV in Combination with Apoptosis Inducers

More recently, the BH3 mimetic ABT-737 has also been found to act synergistically with H-1PV [61]. ABT-737 is an inhibitor of pro-survival/anti-apoptotic Bcl-2 proteins, which are involved in the regulation of apoptosis. Defects in the apoptotic pathways occur frequently in cancer cells. One of the most common mechanisms by which cancer cells counteract apoptotic stimuli is the overexpression of Bcl-2 proteins [84]. The addition of the drug significantly potentiated H-1PV oncolysis against a large panel of cancer cell lines derived from solid tumors including gliomas, pancreatic carcinomas, and cervical carcinomas as well as lung, head and neck, breast, and colon cancers. This strong anticancer effect was also observed in cancer cell lines that were poorly susceptible to H-1PV oncolysis. More recently, the co-treatment was validated in xenograft rat models of human glioma and pancreatic carcinoma. In these animal models, ABT-737 significantly boosted H-1PV-mediated oncosuppression, resulting in a significant increase in animal overall survival (unpublished results). Further studies are required to determine the mechanisms underlying the synergistic anticancer effect and to verify whether increased oncolysis leads to more robust stimulation of anticancer immune responses.

5.1.4. H-1PV in Combination with Antiangiogenic and Immune-Modulating Drugs

Because of their immunostimulatory activities and ability to convert an immunosuppressive cold tumor microenvironment (TME) into an inflamed one, OVs are presently under evaluation as boosters of other forms of immunotherapy with very promising results obtained at both preclinical and clinical levels [2,12,85]. The combination of H-1PV with other immune therapeutics (e.g., checkpoint blockade) holds great promise, as discussed in the issue by Angelova and Rommelaere [58] and in other recent reviews [69,86]. This promise was exemplified by a recent report describing nine patients with primary or recurrent glioblastoma who were treated as part of a compassionate use program with a combination of H-1PV, the antiangiogenic antibody bevacizumab, and the PD-1 checkpoint blockade, nivolumab [87]. This study strongly supports the combination of H-1PV with antiangiogenic drugs and checkpoint blockade and warrants further investigation to define optimal treatment regimes. Unfortunately, preclinical evaluation of combined treatments involving H-1PV and immune checkpoint blockade (e.g., with antibodies against PD-1, PD-L1) is hampered by the lack of a mouse cancer cell line that is permissive to H-1PV infection, which precludes the use of syngeneic mouse tumor models. However, as the cancer immunotherapy field is progressing rapidly, antibodies against rat immune-checkpoint proteins may become available in the near future, rendering possible the use of rat models that are susceptible to H-1PV treatment.

5.2. Second-Generation Propagation-Competent H-1PV-Based Vectors

The strategies pursued thus far to improve the anticancer properties of H-1PV are listed below and summarized in Figure 3B.

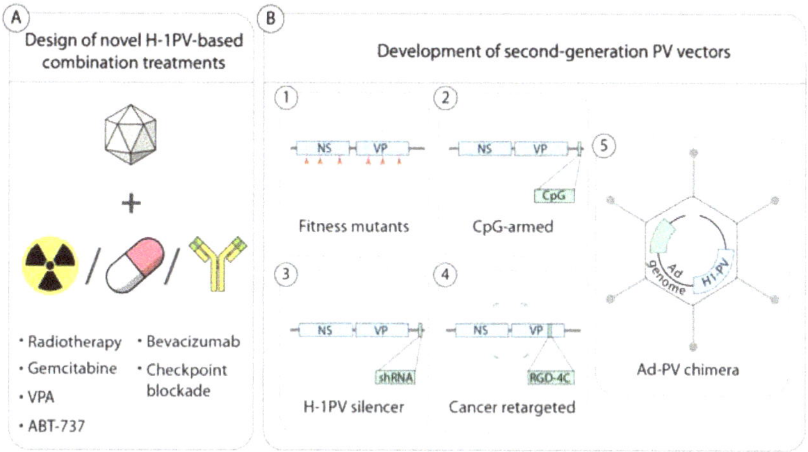

Figure 3. Improving H-1PV-based therapies. (**A**) Combination with drugs. H-1PV anticancer activity can be improved by combining the virus with other anticancer modalities. (**B**) Development of second-generation PV vectors. (1) H-1PV was successfully genetically modified by directed molecular evolution. By serially passaging H-1PV in semipermissive cancer cells, the virus acquired random mutations (orange arrowheads) that improved virus replication and spreading. (2 and 3) Functional elements (CpG motifs or an shRNA expression cassette) were inserted into the H-1PV genome without affecting its replication ability. These elements enhanced virus-mediated immune modulation and oncolysis, respectively. (4) Virus retargeting. The viral capsid was genetically modified by inserting an arginine-glycine-aspartic acid (RGD-4C) peptide, which improved cancer specificity at the level of virus cell entry. (5) Construction of Ad–PV chimeras. An engineered version of the H-1PV genome was inserted into a nonreplicative adenovirus (Ad) genome. The Ad–PV chimera brought the H-1PV genome into cancer cells and produced fully infectious H-1PV particles. The anticancer properties of Ad–PV chimera can be increased by inserting a therapeutic transgene into the Ad component of the Ad–PV hybrid genome (in green).

5.2.1. H-1PV Fitness Mutants

H-1PV is a fast-evolving virus that can adapt to a specific host cell environment by acquiring spontaneous genetic modifications. A naturally occurring H-1PV variant was isolated in a newborn human kidney cell line NB-E in the course of routine plaque purification [88]. The virus featured a 114 nucleotide (nt) in-frame deletion (nt 2022–2135 of the viral genome) encompassing the NS region and a duplication of a 58 nt repeated sequence within the right-hand palindrome. As a consequence of the deletion, NS1 and NS2 proteins lost 38 amino acids at the C-terminus and internally, respectively. The deletion conferred to the virus a superior fitness at the level of nuclear export and spreading compared to wild-type H-1PV [89]. In a subsequent study, Hashemi et al. explored the effects of mutations within the H-1PV NS encoding region. By introducing into the H-1PV genome single nucleotide changes that have been shown to improve the fitness of the closely related lymphotropic strain of MVM, the authors generated H-1PV fitness variants with enhanced infectivity and transduction efficiency [35].

In another study, Nuesch et al. generated a number of adapted variants by serially passaging H-1PV in semipermissive, low-passage human glioma cell cultures. The variants contained small deletions and/or point mutations leading to single amino acid substitutions within both the coding (NS and VP gene units) and the untranslated regions of the viral genome [90]. Similar to previous studies, small deletions were found between nts 2000 and 2200 of the viral genome, suggesting that this part of the genome may represent a hotspot of variability for adapting the virus to a certain cell host. The adapted viruses displayed greater capacity to replicate in glioma cells and increased infectivity. The evaluation of the oncolytic activity of these fitness mutants, both in cell culture and animal models, together with the assessment of their safety profile is an interesting area of future research.

5.2.2. H-1PVs Armed with Immune Stimulators

The limited packaging capacity of PVs allows the insertion of only small heterologous DNA sequences (max. 250 bases) into their genome (the insertion of larger transgenes can only be at the expense of the VP region, rendering the recombinant PVs replication deficient [91]).

Raykov et al. inserted CpG motifs into the untranslated region of the H-1PV genome downstream of the VP gene unit [92]. These sequences are frequently found in the genomes of microbes and have immunostimulatory activities. Insertion of CpG elements into the virus genome did not affect virus replication and infectivity. CpG-armed viruses were endowed with enhanced immunogenicity and adjuvant capacity in both cell culture and animal models [58,92,93].

5.2.3. H-1PVs Armed with RNA Interference Triggers

Tumors are often highly heterogeneous in nature. Within a certain tumor, a fraction of cells may be moderately susceptible to H-1PV infection and survive virus treatment, leading to tumor relapse. RNA interference technology is used to silence the expression of genes involved in carcinogenesis in order to revert the malignant phenotype. To potentiate H-1PV oncotoxicity and provide the virus with an additional mode of action for killing those cancer cells that are poorly sensitive to its infection, we inserted single hairpin RNA (shRNA) expression cassettes into the untranslated region of the H-1PV genome. In a proof of concept study, we showed that the new virus, which we called H-1PV silencer, was able to express shRNAs at high levels and was efficient in gene silencing while retaining its ability to replicate and propagate efficiently [94]. More recently, we constructed an H-1PV silencer expressing shRNAs targeting CDK9 (H-1PV sil-shCDK9), whose expression and activity are often dysregulated in cancer cells, thus contributing to cancer development. H-1PV sil-shCDK9 has superior oncolytic activity in semipermissive pancreatic- and prostate-derived cancer cell lines in comparison with wild-type virus. Validation of these results in xenograft nude rat models of human pancreatic (AsPC-1) and prostate (PC3) carcinomas confirmed the stronger anticancer activity of H-1PV sil-shCDK9, which led to a significant increase in the overall survival of treated animals. These results warrant further development of this promising approach.

5.2.4. Cancer Retargeted H-1PVs

Although H-1PV preferentially expresses and replicates its genome in (pre)neoplastic cells, it is also able to infect normal cells in a nonproductive way in which it is harmless for the cells. However, uptake of the virus by normal cells sequesters a significant portion of the administered viral dose away from the tumor target, thus reducing its efficacy [95]. It would be beneficial to limit H-1PV entry specifically to cancer cells, especially in view of the systemic delivery of the virus in therapeutic applications. Allaume et al. showed that it is possible to genetically engineer the H-1PV capsid and modify the tropism of the virus at the level of virus entry [41]. Based on an in silico model (Figure 1), the authors identified two putative residues involved in the binding to sialic acid at the twofold axis of symmetry of the virus capsid. Amino acid exchange at one of these sites (H174R) strongly reduced cell surface binding and entry without affecting virus capsid formation. This mutant was used as a template for the insertion of an arginine-glycine-aspartic acid (RGD)-4 cyclic peptide, known to bind $\alpha_V\beta_3$ and $\alpha_V\beta_5$, two integrins that are often overexpressed in cancer cells and angiogenic blood vessels [96]. Insertion of the peptide in one of the most protruding loops of the threefold spike of the virus capsid rescued virus infectivity and conferred to the virus improved specificity for cancer cells.

5.2.5. Adenovirus (Ad)–PV Chimera

To combine the high titre and efficient gene transfer capacity of Ad with the anticancer potential of H-1PV (PV), an engineered version of the H-1PV genome was inserted into a replication-defective (E1- and E3-deleted) Ad5 vector genome to create an Ad–PV chimera [97]. The Ad carrier serves as a Trojan horse to bring the H-1PV genome into cancer cells, where the PV DNA is excised from the Ad backbone and autonomously initiates a genuine PV cycle, resulting in the production of PV particles. These PV particles retain the ability to infect neighbouring cancer cells, kill them, and induce secondary rounds of lytic infection, thereby amplifying the initial cytotoxic activity of the chimera (Figure 4). As a consequence, the Ad–PV chimera exerts stronger cytotoxic activities against various cancer cell lines than those of the PV and Ad parental viruses while still being innocuous to a panel of normal primary human cells. The Ad–PV chimera also offers the advantage of overcoming the limited cargo capacity of the PV. Indeed, the Ad backbone can accommodate therapeutic transgene(s) encoding pro-apoptotic or immunostimulating factors, whose activity may reinforce the anticancer effect of PV. Therefore, the chimera offers the advantage of combining in only one vector, effectors for both cancer gene therapy (non-propagating Ad-mediated delivery and expression of therapeutic transgenes in cancer cells) and oncolytic viro-immunotherapy (PV particles retaining oncolytic and anticancer adjuvant properties as well as the capacity for propagating in the tumor bed).

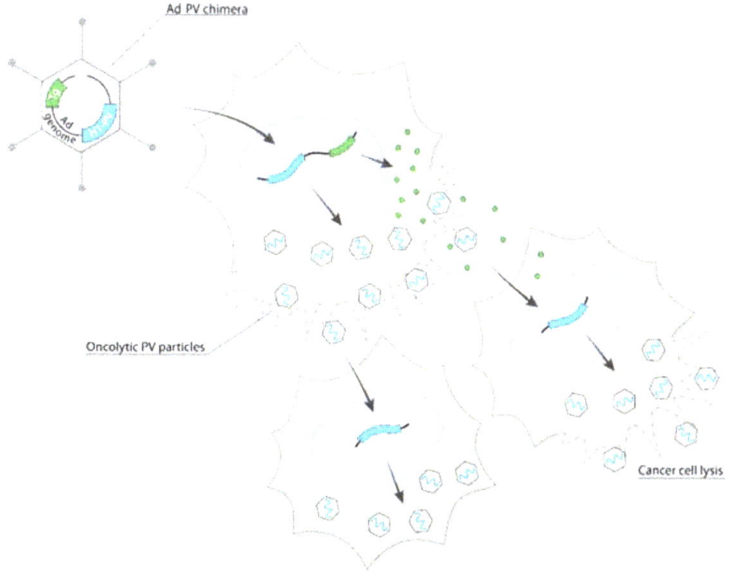

Figure 4. The Ad–PV chimera strategy. The entire oncolytic H-1PV genome (light blue) was inserted into a replication-defective E1 and E3-deleted Ad5 vector genome (Ad, in black). The chimera effectively delivers the PV genome into cancer cells, from which progeny PV particles are generated. Additionally, a transgene (in green) is expressed from the vector genome and can act intracellularly or extracellularly. These PV particles can infect neighbouring cancer cells, kill them, and induce secondary rounds of lytic infection, thus amplifying the initial cytotoxic activity of the chimera [97].

5.3. *Recombinant Propagation-Deficient H-1PV-Based Vectors*

As reported above, protoparvoviruses have a limited packaging capacity. As a result, only small heterologous DNA sequences can be inserted in the parvoviral genome, without impairing the ability of the virus to self-propagate. Arming protoparvoviruses with larger transgenes is still possible by replacing a part of the VP gene unit with a therapeutic gene [95,98]. These recombinant

PVs (recPVs) retain the NS1/2 coding sequences (controlled by the parvoviral P4 promoter) and the parvoviral genome telomeres, which are necessary for viral DNA amplification and packaging. Expression of the transgene is generally kept under control of the genuine parvoviral late promoter P38, whose activity is upregulated by NS1. Production of recPV takes place in producer cell lines upon co-transfection of the recombinant viral genome (containing the transgene) with a second plasmid harbouring the VP gene unit (Figure 5). The latter provides in trans the VP proteins needed for virus assembly, thus compensating for the disruption of the structural genes in the recombinant viral genome. The recombinant parvoviral particles generated in this way are DNA replication competent but propagation-defective and achieve transgene expression only in primarily infected cells as a one-hit event. The deletion of a portion of the structural genes gives the opportunity to insert transgenes up to approximately 1200 nt, while the insertion of larger transgenes strongly impairs virus production. Recombinant rodent parvoviruses have been constructed using MVM and H-1PV infectious plasmids as backbones. Examples of transgene products expressed by means of recombinant H-1PV vectors include pro-apoptotic apoptin [99], immunostimulatory cytokines/chemokines (e.g., human *IL2*, *CCL7*, and *CCL2*) [100], and antiangiogenic modulators (e.g., CXCL10 and CXCL4L1) [101,102]. Some of these recPVs are therapeutically promising, as they proved to have an enhanced anticancer activity in preclinical animal models. However, efficient production of these recombinants remains a major obstacle in their way to the clinic [98]. Co-transfection of the above helper system with a plasmid containing the adenoviral E2a, E4(orf6), and the VA RNA genes (e.g., pXX6 plasmid) improved the production of recPVs by more than 10-fold [91]. Based on these results, an Ad harbouring the VP gene unit was constructed and used as a helper. This VP expressing Ad further improved the recPV yields because it allowed cell lines that were difficult to transfect but efficient at producing recPVs (e.g., NB324K) to be used according to a protocol that relied entirely on virus infection [103]. Further research and development activities are worth conducting to optimize and scale-up recPV production.

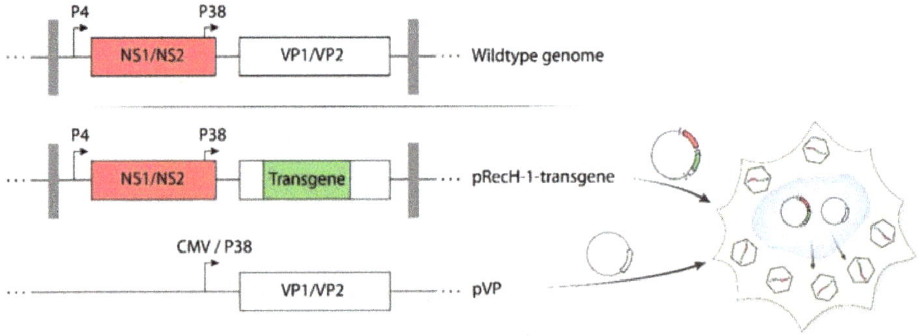

Figure 5. Production of recombinant H-1PV. For the production of recombinant H-1PV, a part of the VP1/VP2 region of the wild-type genome is removed and replaced with a transgene (in green). The VP gene unit under the control of a cytomegalovirus (CMV) or P38 promoter is provided in trans by a helper plasmid (pVP). Upon co-transfection of the plasmids, the producer cell line generates fully infectious, yet propagation-deficient, parvovirus particles containing the recombinant viral genome.

6. Where Next for H-1PV?

Research on H-1PV as an oncolytic agent goes back to the 1960s. Since then, many efforts have been devoted to elucidating the virus life cycle, its strict interactions with the cancer cell host, and its anticancer properties. After more than 50 years of preclinical research, these efforts culminated with the aforementioned launch of the first clinical study in patients with recurrent glioblastoma. The results of the clinical study showed that H-1PV treatment is safe, well tolerated, and associated with first signs of anticancer efficacy. These results provide new impetus for novel research and development activities aimed at further strengthening the H-1PV anticancer profile and bringing into the clinic more potent H-1PV-based therapies that could improve clinical outcome.

In Section 5, we provided examples of how this could be achieved through the rational design of H-1PV-based combination therapies and/or the development of novel, more potent, second-generation H-1PV vectors. These studies are particularly important and should guarantee a portfolio of novel, more efficient PV-based treatments to be tested in clinical trials. All these strategies should aim to increase oncolysis not only in quantitative but also in qualitative terms. Indeed, how a certain treatment kills cancer cells determines the success of the therapy, as the treatments vary in their immunogenicity and, thus, engage the immune system to act against the cancer at different degrees. To maximize the role of the immune system in destroying cancer cells, combinations of H-1PV with other forms of immunotherapy are particularly promising strategies. This was observed within the frame of a compassionate use program in patients with glioblastoma (see Section 5).

To increase the success rate of the virus treatment, it is also very important to identify biomarkers that could predict the outcome of the therapy. Currently, we are still missing basic knowledge on the determinants that make a tumor susceptible or resistant to H-1PV infection. For instance, it remains elusive why some cancer cells sustain virus replication more efficiently than others. Also, the entry pathways used by H-1PV and the mechanisms underlying virus trafficking into the nucleus are largely uncharacterized. Studies in these areas may reveal key cellular modulators (either activators or repressors) of the virus life cycle that could help us to predict whether a certain patient is likely to benefit from virus treatment. This information may be used as part of a more personalized virus treatment in which a certain therapy is selected according to patient tumor genetic makeup. At the same time, these studies may provide the key to improving virus treatment, for instance by guiding us in the identification of new drugs that could reinforce virus replication and oncolysis in tumor cells or of new means to improve next-generation PV vectors (e.g., shRNA targeting negative modulators of the virus life cycle). These new developments may overcome current molecular restrictions that limit efficacy and thereby extend the success of H-1PV-based therapies.

Author Contributions: C.B. and A.M. wrote the manuscript and designed the figures.

Funding: This work was partly supported by research grants from Luxembourg Cancer Foundation, Télévie and DKFZ-MOST German-Israeli Cooperation in Cancer Research to A.M.

Acknowledgments: We thank Assia Angelova, Jean Rommelaere, and Caroline Hadley (INLEXIO) for critical reading.

Conflicts of Interest: A.M. is an inventor in several H-1PV-related patents/patent applications. No other conflict of interest are declared by the authors.

References

1. Kaufman, H.L.; Kohlhapp, F.J.; Zloza, A. Oncolytic viruses: A new class of immunotherapy drugs. *Nat. Rev. Drug Discov.* **2015**, *14*, 642–662. [CrossRef] [PubMed]
2. Achard, C.; Surendran, A.; Wedge, M.E.; Ungerechts, G.; Bell, J.; Ilkow, C.S. Lighting a Fire in the Tumor Microenvironment Using Oncolytic Immunotherapy. *EBioMedicine* **2018**, *31*, 17–24. [CrossRef] [PubMed]
3. Najafi, M.; Goradel, N.H.; Farhood, B.; Salehi, E.; Solhjoo, S.; Toolee, H.; Kharazinejad, E.; Mortezaee, K. Tumor microenvironment: Interactions and therapy. *J. Cell. Physiol.* **2019**, *234*, 5700–5721. [CrossRef] [PubMed]
4. Balkwill, F.R.; Capasso, M.; Hagemann, T. The tumor microenvironment at a glance. *J. Cell Sci.* **2012**, *125 Pt 23*, 5591–5596. [CrossRef]
5. Breitbach, C.J.; Lichty, B.D.; Bell, J.C. Oncolytic Viruses: Therapeutics With an Identity Crisis. *EBioMedicine* **2016**, *9*, 31–36. [CrossRef] [PubMed]
6. Breitbach, C.J.; Arulanandam, R.; De Silva, N.; Thorne, S.H.; Patt, R.; Daneshmand, M.; Moon, A.; Ilkow, C.; Burke, J.; Hwang, T.H.; et al. Oncolytic vaccinia virus disrupts tumor-associated vasculature in humans. *Cancer Res.* **2013**, *73*, 1265–1275. [CrossRef]

7. Benencia, F.; Courreges, M.C.; Conejo-Garcia, J.R.; Buckanovich, R.J.; Zhang, L.; Carroll, R.H.; Morgan, M.A.; Coukos, G. Oncolytic HSV exerts direct antiangiogenic activity in ovarian carcinoma. *Hum. Gene Ther.* **2005**, *16*, 765–778. [CrossRef]
8. Cinatl, J., Jr.; Michaelis, M.; Driever, P.H.; Cinatl, J.; Hrabeta, J.; Suhan, T.; Doerr, H.W.; Vogel, J.U. Multimutated herpes simplex virus g207 is a potent inhibitor of angiogenesis. *Neoplasia* **2004**, *6*, 725–735. [CrossRef]
9. Chiocca, E.A.; Rabkin, S.D. Oncolytic viruses and their application to cancer immunotherapy. *Cancer Immunol. Res.* **2014**, *2*, 295–300. [CrossRef]
10. Russell, S.J.; Peng, K.W.; Bell, J.C. Oncolytic virotherapy. *Nat. Biotechnol.* **2012**, *30*, 658–670. [CrossRef]
11. Ledford, H. Cancer-fighting viruses win approval. *Nature* **2015**, *526*, 622–623. [CrossRef] [PubMed]
12. Conry, R.M.; Westbrook, B.; McKee, S.; Norwood, T.G. Talimogene laherparepvec: First in class oncolytic virotherapy. *Hum. Vaccin Immunother.* **2018**, *14*, 839–846. [CrossRef] [PubMed]
13. Fountzilas, C.; Patel, S.; Mahalingam, D. Review: Oncolytic virotherapy, updates and future directions. *Oncotarget* **2017**, *8*, 102617–102639. [CrossRef] [PubMed]
14. Marchini, A.; Scott, E.M.; Rommelaere, J. Overcoming Barriers in Oncolytic Virotherapy with HDAC Inhibitors and Immune Checkpoint Blockade. *Viruses* **2016**, *8*, 9. [CrossRef] [PubMed]
15. Bommareddy, P.K.; Shettigar, M.; Kaufman, H.L. Integrating oncolytic viruses in combination cancer immunotherapy. *Nat. Rev. Immunol.* **2018**, *18*, 498–513. [CrossRef] [PubMed]
16. LaRocca, C.J.; Warner, S.G. Oncolytic viruses and checkpoint inhibitors: Combination therapy in clinical trials. *Clin. Transl. Med.* **2018**, *7*, 35. [CrossRef] [PubMed]
17. Samson, A.; Scott, K.J.; Taggart, D.; West, E.J.; Wilson, E.; Nuovo, G.J.; Thomson, S.; Corns, R.; Mathew, R.K.; Fuller, M.J.; et al. Intravenous delivery of oncolytic reovirus to brain tumor patients immunologically primes for subsequent checkpoint blockade. *Sci. Transl. Med.* **2018**, *10*, eaam7577. [CrossRef]
18. Marchini, A.; Bonifati, S.; Scott, E.M.; Angelova, A.L.; Rommelaere, J. Oncolytic parvoviruses: From basic virology to clinical applications. *Virol. J.* **2015**, *12*, 6. [CrossRef]
19. Vollmers, E.M.; Tattersall, P. Distinct host cell fates for human malignant melanoma targeted by oncolytic rodent parvoviruses. *Virology* **2013**, *446*, 37–48. [CrossRef]
20. Paglino, J.C.; Andres, W.; van den Pol, A.N. Autonomous parvoviruses neither stimulate nor are inhibited by the type I interferon response in human normal or cancer cells. *J. Virol.* **2014**, *88*, 4932–4942. [CrossRef]
21. Grekova, S.; Zawatzky, R.; Horlein, R.; Cziepluch, C.; Mincberg, M.; Davis, C.; Rommelaere, J.; Daeffler, L. Activation of an antiviral response in normal but not transformed mouse cells: A new determinant of minute virus of mice oncotropism. *J. Virol.* **2010**, *84*, 516–531. [CrossRef] [PubMed]
22. Vollmers, E.M.; D'Abramo, A., Jr.; Cotmore, S.F.; Tattersall, P. Genome sequence of tumor virus x, a member of the genus protoparvovirus in the family parvoviridae. *Genome Announc.* **2014**, *2*, e00758-14. [CrossRef] [PubMed]
23. Toolan, H.W.; Dalldore, G.; Barclay, M.; Chandra, S.; Moore, A.E. An Unidentified, Filtrable Agent Isolated from Transplanted Human Tumors. *Proc. Natl. Acad. Sci. USA* **1960**, *46*, 1256–1258. [CrossRef] [PubMed]
24. Toolan, H.W. A virus associated with transplantable human tumors. *Bull. N. Y. Acad. Med.* **1961**, *37*, 305–310. [PubMed]
25. Toolan, H.W. Lack of oncogenic effect of the H-viruses for hamsters. *Nature* **1967**, *214*, 1036. [CrossRef]
26. Toolan, H.W.; Ledinko, N. Inhibition by H-1 virus of the incidence of tumors produced by adenovirus 12 in hamsters. *Virology* **1968**, *35*, 475–478. [CrossRef]
27. Toolan, H.W.; Rhode, S.L., 3rd; Gierthy, J.F. Inhibition of 7,12-dimethylbenz(a)anthracene-induced tumors in Syrian hamsters by prior infection with H-1 parvovirus. *Cancer Res.* **1982**, *42*, 2552–2555.
28. Cotmore, S.F.; Agbandje-McKenna, M.; Chiorini, J.A.; Mukha, D.V.; Pintel, D.J.; Qiu, J.; Soderlund-Venermo, M.; Tattersall, P.; Tijssen, P.; Gatherer, D.; et al. The family Parvoviridae. *Arch. Virol.* **2014**, *159*, 1239–1247. [CrossRef]
29. Cotmore, S.F.; Tattersall, P. Parvoviruses: Small Does Not Mean Simple. *Annu. Rev. Virol.* **2014**, *1*, 517–537. [CrossRef]
30. Li, L.; Cotmore, S.F.; Tattersall, P. Parvoviral left-end hairpin ears are essential during infection for establishing a functional intranuclear transcription template and for efficient progeny genome encapsidation. *J. Virol.* **2013**, *87*, 10501–10514. [CrossRef]

31. Nuesch, J.P.; Lacroix, J.; Marchini, A.; Rommelaere, J. Molecular pathways: Rodent parvoviruses—Mechanisms of oncolysis and prospects for clinical cancer treatment. *Clin. Cancer Res.* **2012**, *18*, 3516–3523. [CrossRef] [PubMed]
32. Cotmore, S.F.; Christensen, J.; Nuesch, J.P.; Tattersall, P. The NS1 polypeptide of the murine parvovirus minute virus of mice binds to DNA sequences containing the motif [ACCA]2-3. *J. Virol.* **1995**, *69*, 1652–1660. [PubMed]
33. Nuesch, J.P.; Rommelaere, J. Tumor Suppressing Properties of Rodent Parvovirus NS1 Proteins and Their Derivatives. *Adv. Exp. Med. Biol.* **2014**, *818*, 99–124.
34. Hristov, G.; Kramer, M.; Li, J.; El-Andaloussi, N.; Mora, R.; Daeffler, L.; Zentgraf, H.; Rommelaere, J.; Marchini, A. Through Its Nonstructural Protein NS1, Parvovirus H-1 Induces Apoptosis via Accumulation of Reactive Oxygen Species. *J. Virol.* **2010**, *84*, 5909–5922. [CrossRef]
35. Hashemi, H.; Condurat, A.L.; Stroh-Dege, A.; Weiss, N.; Geiss, C.; Pilet, J.; Cornet Bartolome, C.; Rommelaere, J.; Salome, N.; Dinsart, C. Mutations in the Non-Structural Protein-Coding Sequence of Protoparvovirus H-1PV Enhance the Fitness of the Virus and Show Key Benefits Regarding the Transduction Efficiency of Derived Vectors. *Viruses* **2018**, *10*, 150. [CrossRef] [PubMed]
36. Halder, S.; Nam, H.J.; Govindasamy, L.; Vogel, M.; Dinsart, C.; Salome, N.; McKenna, R.; Agbandje-McKenna, M. Structural characterization of H-1 parvovirus: Comparison of infectious virions to empty capsids. *J. Virol.* **2013**, *87*, 5128–5140. [CrossRef] [PubMed]
37. Harbison, C.E.; Chiorini, J.A.; Parrish, C.R. The parvovirus capsid odyssey: From the cell surface to the nucleus. *Trends Microbiol.* **2008**, *16*, 208–214. [CrossRef]
38. Cotmore, S.F.; D'Abramo, A.M., Jr.; Ticknor, C.M.; Tattersall, P. Controlled conformational transitions in the MVM virion expose the VP1 N-terminus and viral genome without particle disassembly. *Virology* **1999**, *254*, 169–181. [CrossRef]
39. Mani, B.; Baltzer, C.; Valle, N.; Almendral, J.M.; Kempf, C.; Ros, C. Low pH-dependent endosomal processing of the incoming parvovirus minute virus of mice virion leads to externalization of the VP1 N-terminal sequence (N-VP1), N-VP2 cleavage, and uncoating of the full-length genome. *J. Virol.* **2006**, *80*, 1015–1024. [CrossRef]
40. Zadori, Z.; Szelei, J.; Lacoste, M.C.; Li, Y.; Gariepy, S.; Raymond, P.; Allaire, M.; Nabi, I.R.; Tijssen, P. A viral phospholipase A2 is required for parvovirus infectivity. *Dev. Cell* **2001**, *1*, 291–302. [CrossRef]
41. Allaume, X.; El-Andaloussi, N.; Leuchs, B.; Bonifati, S.; Kulkarni, A.; Marttila, T.; Kaufmann, J.K.; Nettelbeck, D.M.; Kleinschmidt, J.; Rommelaere, J.; et al. Retargeting of rat parvovirus H-1PV to cancer cells through genetic engineering of the viral capsid. *J. Virol.* **2012**, *86*, 3452–3465. [CrossRef] [PubMed]
42. Ros, C.; Bayat, N.; Wolfisberg, R.; Almendral, J.M. Protoparvovirus Cell Entry. *Viruses* **2017**, *9*, 313. [CrossRef] [PubMed]
43. Cotmore, S.F.; Tattersall, P. Parvoviral host range and cell entry mechanisms. *Adv. Virus Res.* **2007**, *70*, 183–232. [PubMed]
44. Angelova, A.L.; Geletneky, K.; Nuesch, J.P.; Rommelaere, J. Tumor Selectivity of Oncolytic Parvoviruses: From in vitro and Animal Models to Cancer Patients. *Front. Bioeng. Biotechnol.* **2015**, *3*, 55. [CrossRef] [PubMed]
45. Deleu, L.; Pujol, A.; Faisst, S.; Rommelaere, J. Activation of promoter P4 of the autonomous parvovirus minute virus of mice at early S phase is required for productive infection. *J. Virol.* **1999**, *73*, 3877–3885. [PubMed]
46. Bashir, T.; Rommelaere, J.; Cziepluch, C. In vivo accumulation of cyclin A and cellular replication factors in autonomous parvovirus minute virus of mice-associated replication bodies. *J. Virol.* **2001**, *75*, 4394–4398. [CrossRef]
47. Porwal, M.; Cohen, S.; Snoussi, K.; Popa-Wagner, R.; Anderson, F.; Dugot-Senant, N.; Wodrich, H.; Dinsart, C.; Kleinschmidt, J.A.; Pante, N.; et al. Parvoviruses cause nuclear envelope breakdown by activating key enzymes of mitosis. *PLoS Pathog.* **2013**, *9*, e1003671. [CrossRef] [PubMed]
48. Bar, S.; Rommelaere, J.; Nuesch, J.P. PKCeta/Rdx-driven phosphorylation of PDK1: A novel mechanism promoting cancer cell survival and permissiveness for parvovirus-induced lysis. *PLoS Pathog.* **2015**, *11*, e1004703. [CrossRef]

49. Fuks, F.; Deleu, L.; Dinsart, C.; Rommelaere, J.; Faisst, S. ras oncogene-dependent activation of the P4 promoter of minute virus of mice through a proximal P4 element interacting with the Ets family of transcription factors. *J. Virol.* **1996**, *70*, 1331–1339.
50. Majumder, K.; Etingov, I.; Pintel, D.J. Protoparvovirus Interactions with the Cellular DNA Damage Response. *Viruses* **2017**, *9*, 323. [CrossRef]
51. Riolobos, L.; Valle, N.; Hernando, E.; Maroto, B.; Kann, M.; Almendral, J.M. Viral oncolysis that targets Raf-1 signaling control of nuclear transport. *J. Virol.* **2010**, *84*, 2090–2099. [CrossRef] [PubMed]
52. Bar, S.; Daeffler, L.; Rommelaere, J.; Nuesch, J.P. Vesicular egress of non-enveloped lytic parvoviruses depends on gelsolin functioning. *PLoS Pathog.* **2008**, *4*, e1000126. [CrossRef] [PubMed]
53. Nuesch, J.P.; Bar, S.; Lachmann, S.; Rommelaere, J. Ezrin-radixin-moesin family proteins are involved in parvovirus replication and spreading. *J. Virol.* **2009**, *83*, 5854–5863. [CrossRef] [PubMed]
54. Eichwald, V.; Daeffler, L.; Klein, M.; Rommelaere, J.; Salome, N. The NS2 proteins of parvovirus minute virus of mice are required for efficient nuclear egress of progeny virions in mouse cells. *J. Virol.* **2002**, *76*, 10307–10319. [CrossRef] [PubMed]
55. Grekova, S.; Aprahamian, M.; Giese, N.; Schmitt, S.; Giese, T.; Falk, C.S.; Daeffler, L.; Cziepluch, C.; Rommelaere, J.; Raykov, Z. Immune cells participate in the oncosuppressive activity of parvovirus H-1PV and are activated as a result of their abortive infection with this agent. *Cancer Biol. Ther.* **2010**, *10*, 1280–1289. [CrossRef] [PubMed]
56. Mattei, L.M.; Cotmore, S.F.; Tattersall, P.; Iwasaki, A. Parvovirus evades interferon-dependent viral control in primary mouse embryonic fibroblasts. *Virology* **2013**, *442*, 20–27. [CrossRef] [PubMed]
57. Schlehofer, J.R.; Rentrop, M.; Mannel, D.N. Parvoviruses are inefficient in inducing interferon-beta, tumor necrosis factor-alpha, or interleukin-6 in mammalian cells. *Med. Microbiol. Immunol.* **1992**, *181*, 153–164. [CrossRef]
58. Angelova, A.; Rommelaere, J. Immune System Stimulation by Oncolytic Rodent Protoparvoviruses. *Viruses* **2019**, *11*, 415. [CrossRef]
59. Angelova, A.L.; Witzens-Harig, M.; Galabov, A.S.; Rommelaere, J. The Oncolytic Virotherapy Era in Cancer Management: Prospects of Applying H-1 Parvovirus to Treat Blood and Solid Cancers. *Front. Oncol.* **2017**, *7*, 93. [CrossRef]
60. Di Piazza, M.; Mader, C.; Geletneky, K.; Herrero y Calle, M.; Weber, E.; Schlehofer, J.; Deleu, L.; Rommelaere, J. Cytosolic Activation of Cathepsins Mediates Parvovirus H-1-Induced Killing of Cisplatin and TRAIL-Resistant Glioma Cells. *J. Virol.* **2007**, *81*, 4186–4198. [CrossRef]
61. Marchini, A.; Li, J.; Schroeder, L.; Rommelaere, J.; Geletneky, K. Cancer therapy with a parvovirus combined with a Bcl-2 inhibitor. U.S. Patent 9,889,169, 13 February 2018.
62. Angelova, A.L.; Grekova, S.P.; Heller, A.; Kuhlmann, O.; Soyka, E.; Giese, T.; Aprahamian, M.; Bour, G.; Ruffer, S.; Cziepluch, C.; et al. Complementary induction of immunogenic cell death by oncolytic parvovirus H-1PV and gemcitabine in pancreatic cancer. *J. Virol.* **2014**, *88*, 5263–5276. [CrossRef] [PubMed]
63. Moehler, M.; Zeidler, M.; Schede, J.; Rommelaere, J.; Galle, P.R.; Cornelis, J.J.; Heike, M. Oncolytic parvovirus H1 induces release of heat-shock protein HSP72 in susceptible human tumor cells but may not affect primary immune cells. *Cancer Gene Ther.* **2003**, *10*, 477–480. [CrossRef] [PubMed]
64. Moehler, M.H.; Zeidler, M.; Wilsberg, V.; Cornelis, J.J.; Woelfel, T.; Rommelaere, J.; Galle, P.R.; Heike, M. Parvovirus H-1-Induced Tumor Cell Death Enhances Human Immune Response In Vitro via Increased Phagocytosis, Maturation, and Cross-Presentation by Dendritic Cells. *Hum. Gene Ther.* **2005**, *16*, 996–1005. [CrossRef] [PubMed]
65. Geletneky, K.; Kiprianova, I.; Ayache, A.; Koch, R.; Herrero Y Calle, M.; Deleu, L.; Sommer, C.; Thomas, N.; Rommelaere, J.; Schlehofer, J.R. Regression of advanced rat and human gliomas by local or systemic treatment with oncolytic parvovirus H-1 in rat models. *Neuro-Oncology* **2010**, *12*, 804–814. [CrossRef] [PubMed]
66. Kiprianova, I.; Thomas, N.; Ayache, A.; Fischer, M.; Leuchs, B.; Klein, M.; Rommelaere, J.; Schlehofer, J.R. Regression of glioma in rat models by intranasal application of parvovirus h-1. *Clin. Cancer Res.* **2011**, *17*, 5333–5342. [CrossRef] [PubMed]
67. Geletneky, K.; Leoni, A.L.; Pohlmeyer-Esch, G.; Loebhard, S.; Leuchs, B.; Hoefer, C.; Jochims, K.; Dahm, M.; Huber, B.; Rommelaere, J.; et al. Bioavailability, biodistribution, and CNS toxicity of clinical-grade parvovirus H1 after intravenous and intracerebral injection in rats. *Comp. Med.* **2015**, *65*, 36–45.

68. Geletneky, K.; Leoni, A.L.; Pohlmeyer-Esch, G.; Loebhard, S.; Baetz, A.; Leuchs, B.; Roscher, M.; Hoefer, C.; Jochims, K.; Dahm, M.; et al. Pathology, organ distribution, and immune response after single and repeated intravenous injection of rats with clinical-grade parvovirus H1. *Comp. Med.* **2015**, *65*, 23–35.
69. Geletneky, K.; Nuesch, J.P.; Angelova, A.; Kiprianova, I.; Rommelaere, J. Double-faceted mechanism of parvoviral oncosuppression. *Curr. Opin. Virol.* **2015**, *13*, 17–24. [CrossRef]
70. Bhat, R.; Dempe, S.; Dinsart, C.; Rommelaere, J. Enhancement of NK cell antitumor responses using an oncolytic parvovirus. *Int. J. Cancer* **2011**, *128*, 908–919. [CrossRef]
71. Angelova, A.L.; Aprahamian, M.; Grekova, S.P.; Hajri, A.; Leuchs, B.; Giese, N.A.; Dinsart, C.; Herrmann, A.; Balboni, G.; Rommelaere, J.; et al. Improvement of gemcitabine-based therapy of pancreatic carcinoma by means of oncolytic parvovirus H-1PV. *Clin. Cancer Res.* **2009**, *15*, 511–519. [CrossRef]
72. Dempe, S.; Stroh-Dege, A.Y.; Schwarz, E.; Rommelaere, J.; Dinsart, C. SMAD4: A predictive marker of PDAC cell permissiveness for oncolytic infection with parvovirus H-1PV. *Int. J. Cancer* **2010**, *126*, 2914–2927. [CrossRef] [PubMed]
73. Toolan, H.W.; Saunders, E.L.; Southam, C.M.; Moore, A.E.; Levin, A.G. H-1 virus viremia in the human. *Proc. Soc. Exp. Biol. Med.* **1965**, *119*, 711–715. [CrossRef]
74. Johnson, D.R.; O'Neill, B.P. Glioblastoma survival in the United States before and during the temozolomide era. *J. Neurooncol.* **2012**, *107*, 359–364. [CrossRef]
75. Malvezzi, M.; Bertuccio, P.; Levi, F.; La Vecchia, C.; Negri, E. European cancer mortality predictions for the year 2014. *Ann. Oncol.* **2014**, *25*, 1650–1656. [CrossRef] [PubMed]
76. Hajda, J.; Lehmann, M.; Krebs, O.; Kieser, M.; Geletneky, K.; Jager, D.; Dahm, M.; Huber, B.; Schoning, T.; Sedlaczek, O.; et al. A non-controlled, single arm, open label, phase II study of intravenous and intratumoral administration of ParvOryx in patients with metastatic, inoperable pancreatic cancer: ParvOryx02 protocol. *BMC Cancer* **2017**, *17*, 576. [CrossRef] [PubMed]
77. Ottolino-Perry, K.; Diallo, J.S.; Lichty, B.D.; Bell, J.C.; McCart, J.A. Intelligent design: Combination therapy with oncolytic viruses. *Mol. Ther.* **2010**, *18*, 251–263. [CrossRef] [PubMed]
78. Wennier, S.T.; Liu, J.; McFadden, G. Bugs and drugs: Oncolytic virotherapy in combination with chemotherapy. *Curr. Pharm. Biotechnol.* **2012**, *13*, 1817–1833. [CrossRef] [PubMed]
79. Geletneky, K.; Hartkopf, A.D.; Krempien, R.; Rommelaere, J.; Schlehofer, J.R. Improved killing of human high-grade glioma cells by combining ionizing radiation with oncolytic parvovirus H-1 infection. *J. Biomed. Biotechnol.* **2010**, *2010*, 350748. [CrossRef] [PubMed]
80. Wennerberg, E.; Vanpouille-Box, C.; Bornstein, S.; Yamazaki, T.; Demaria, S.; Galluzzi, L. Immune recognition of irradiated cancer cells. *Immunol. Rev.* **2017**, *280*, 220–230. [CrossRef] [PubMed]
81. Burris, H.A., 3rd; Moore, M.J.; Andersen, J.; Green, M.R.; Rothenberg, M.L.; Modiano, M.R.; Cripps, M.C.; Portenoy, R.K.; Storniolo, A.M.; Tarassoff, P.; et al. Improvements in survival and clinical benefit with gemcitabine as first-line therapy for patients with advanced pancreas cancer: A randomized trial. *J. Clin. Oncol.* **1997**, *15*, 2403–2413. [CrossRef] [PubMed]
82. Minucci, S.; Pelicci, P.G. Histone deacetylase inhibitors and the promise of epigenetic (and more) treatments for cancer. *Nat. Rev. Cancer* **2006**, *6*, 38–51. [CrossRef]
83. Li, J.; Bonifati, S.; Hristov, G.; Marttila, T.; Valmary-Degano, S.; Stanzel, S.; Schnolzer, M.; Mougin, C.; Aprahamian, M.; Grekova, S.P.; et al. Synergistic combination of valproic acid and oncolytic parvovirus H-1PV as a potential therapy against cervical and pancreatic carcinomas. *EMBO Mol. Med.* **2013**, *5*, 1537–1555. [CrossRef] [PubMed]
84. Andersen, M.H.; Svane, I.M.; Kvistborg, P.; Nielsen, O.J.; Balslev, E.; Reker, S.; Becker, J.C.; Straten, P.T. Immunogenicity of Bcl-2 in patients with cancer. *Blood* **2005**, *105*, 728–734. [CrossRef] [PubMed]
85. Twumasi-Boateng, K.; Pettigrew, J.L.; Kwok, Y.Y.E.; Bell, J.C.; Nelson, B.H. Oncolytic viruses as engineering platforms for combination immunotherapy. *Nat. Rev. Cancer* **2018**, *18*, 419–432. [CrossRef] [PubMed]
86. Moehler, M.; Goepfert, K.; Heinrich, B.; Breitbach, C.J.; Delic, M.; Galle, P.R.; Rommelaere, J. Oncolytic Virotherapy as Emerging Immunotherapeutic Modality: Potential of Parvovirus H-1. *Front. Oncol.* **2014**, *4*, 92. [CrossRef] [PubMed]
87. Geletneky, K.; Bartsch, A.; Weiss, C.; Bernhard, H.; Marchini, A.; Rommelaere, J. ATIM-40. High rate of objective anti.tumor response in 9 patients with glioblastoma after viro-immunotherapy with oncolytic parvovirus H-1 in combination with bavacicumab and PD-1 checkpoint blockade. *Neuro-Oncology* **2018**, *20* (Suppl. 6), vi10. [CrossRef]

88. Faisst, S.; Faisst, S.R.; Dupressoir, T.; Plaza, S.; Pujol, A.; Jauniaux, J.C.; Rhode, S.L.; Rommelaere, J. Isolation of a fully infectious variant of parvovirus H-1 supplanting the standard strain in human cells. *J. Virol.* **1995**, *69*, 4538–4543.
89. Weiss, N.; Stroh-Dege, A.; Rommelaere, J.; Dinsart, C.; Salome, N. An in-frame deletion in the NS protein-coding sequence of parvovirus H-1PV efficiently stimulates export and infectivity of progeny virions. *J. Virol.* **2012**, *86*, 7554–7564. [CrossRef]
90. Nüesch, J.; Thomas, N.; Plotzky, C.; Jean, R. Modified Rodent Parvovirus Capable of Propagating and Spreading through Human Gliomas. Patent No. EP2384761B1, 4 September 2013.
91. El-Andaloussi, N.; Endele, M.; Leuchs, B.; Bonifati, S.; Kleinschmidt, J.; Rommelaere, J.; Marchini, A. Novel adenovirus-based helper system to support production of recombinant parvovirus. *Cancer Gene Ther.* **2011**, *18*, 240–249. [CrossRef]
92. Raykov, Z.; Grekova, S.; Leuchs, B.; Aprahamian, M.; Rommelaere, J. Arming parvoviruses with CpG motifs to improve their oncosuppressive capacity. *Int. J. Cancer* **2008**, *122*, 2880–2884. [CrossRef]
93. Grekova, S.P.; Aprahamian, M.; Giese, N.A.; Bour, G.; Giese, T.; Grewenig, A.; Leuchs, B.; Hörlein, R.; Heller, A.; Angelova, A.L.; et al. Genomic CpG Enrichment of Oncolytic Parvoviruses as a Potent Anticancer Vaccination Strategy for the Treatment of Pancreatic Adenocarcinoma. *J. Vaccines Vaccin* **2014**, *5*. [CrossRef]
94. Illarionova, A.; Rommelaere, J.; Leuchs, B.; Marchini, A. Modified Parvovirus Useful for Gene Silencing. Patent No. EP2620503, 31 July 2013.
95. Cornelis, J.J.; Salome, N.; Dinsart, C.; Rommelaere, J. Vectors based on autonomous parvoviruses: Novel tools to treat cancer? *J. Gene Med.* **2004**, *6* (Suppl. 1), S193–S202. [CrossRef] [PubMed]
96. Zitzmann, S.; Ehemann, V.; Schwab, M. Arginine-glycine-aspartic acid (RGD)-peptide binds to both tumor and tumor-endothelial cells in vivo. *Cancer Res.* **2002**, *62*, 5139–5143.
97. El-Andaloussi, N.; Bonifati, S.; Kaufmann, J.K.; Mailly, L.; Daeffler, L.; Deryckere, F.; Nettelbeck, D.M.; Rommelaere, J.; Marchini, A. Generation of an adenovirus-parvovirus chimera with enhanced oncolytic potential. *J. Virol.* **2012**, *86*, 10418–10431. [CrossRef] [PubMed]
98. Cornelis, J.J.; Lang, S.I.; Stroh-Dege, A.Y.; Balboni, G.; Dinsart, C.; Rommelaere, J. Cancer gene therapy through autonomous parvovirus–mediated gene transfer. *Curr. Gene Ther.* **2004**, *4*, 249–261. [CrossRef]
99. Olijslagers, S.; Dege, A.Y.; Dinsart, C.; Voorhoeve, M.; Rommelaere, J.; Noteborn, M.H.; Cornelis, J.J. Potentiation of a recombinant oncolytic parvovirus by expression of Apoptin. *Cancer Gene Ther.* **2001**, *8*, 958–965. [CrossRef]
100. Dempe, S.; Lavie, M.; Struyf, S.; Bhat, R.; Verbeke, H.; Paschek, S.; Berghmans, N.; Geibig, R.; Rommelaere, J.; Van Damme, J.; et al. Antitumoral activity of parvovirus-mediated IL-2 and MCP-3/CCL7 delivery into human pancreatic cancer: Implication of leucocyte recruitment. *Cancer Immunol. Immunother.* **2012**, *61*, 2113–2123. [CrossRef]
101. Lavie, M.; Struyf, S.; Stroh-Dege, A.; Rommelaere, J.; Van Damme, J.; Dinsart, C. Capacity of wild-type and chemokine-armed parvovirus H-1PV for inhibiting neo-angiogenesis. *Virology* **2013**, *447*, 221–232. [CrossRef]
102. Dinsart, C.; Pervolaraki, K.; Stroh-Dege, A.; Lavie, M.; Ronsse, I.; Rommelaere, J.; Van Damme, J.; Van Raemdonck, K.; Struyf, S. Recombinant Parvoviruses Armed to Deliver CXCL4L1 and CXCL10 Are Impaired in Their Antiangiogenic and Antitumoral Effects in a Kaposi Sarcoma Tumor Model Due To the Chemokines' Interference with the Virus Cycle. *Hum. Gene Ther.* **2017**, *28*, 295–306. [CrossRef]
103. El-Andaloussi, N.; Leuchs, B.; Bonifati, S.; Rommelaere, J.; Marchini, A. Efficient recombinant parvovirus production with the help of adenovirus-derived systems. *J. Vis. Exp.* **2012**, *62*, e3518. [CrossRef] [PubMed]

viruses

MDPI

Review

Immune System Stimulation by Oncolytic Rodent Protoparvoviruses

Assia Angelova and Jean Rommelaere *

German Cancer Research Center (DKFZ), 69120 Heidelberg, Germany; a.angelova@dkfz-heidelberg.de
* Correspondence: j.rommelaere@dkfz-heidelberg.de; Tel.: +49-6221-42-4960

Received: 18 April 2019; Accepted: 2 May 2019; Published: 4 May 2019

Abstract: Rodent protoparvoviruses (PVs), parvovirus H-1 (H-1PV) in particular, are naturally endowed with oncolytic properties. While being historically described as agents that selectively replicate in and kill cancer cells, recent yet growing evidence demonstrates that these viruses are able to reverse tumor-driven immune suppression through induction of immunogenic tumor cell death, and the establishment of antitumorigenic, proinflammatory milieu within the tumor microenvironment. This review summarizes the most important preclinical proofs of the interplay and the cooperation between PVs and the host immune system. The molecular mechanisms of PV-induced immunostimulation are also discussed. Furthermore, initial encouraging in-human observations from clinical trials and compassionate virus uses are presented, and speak in favor of further H-1PV clinical development as partner drug in combined immunotherapeutic protocols.

Keywords: rodent protoparvoviruses; oncolytic activity; tumor microenvironment; immunomodulation; preclinical; clinical trials

1. Bystander Antitumor Effect of Protoparvovirus-Induced Oncolysis

As reviewed recently [1,2], rodent protoparvoviruses are endowed with oncolytic properties. The molecular basis of protoparvovirus cancer cell specificity and killing activity is the subject of another review in this special issue [3]. In some cancer animal models, this direct viral oncolytic effect is potent enough to fully eradicate infected tumors, correlating with virus spread and viral oncotoxic protein NS1 expression throughout the neoplastic tissue [4]. In most models, however, intratumoral virus multiplication and propagation are limited. Protoparvovirus-induced tumor suppression can still take place in such systems, where only a minor fraction of tumor cells gets lytically infected [5,6]. An extreme case is the one of animals implanted with double tumors, in which the protoparvovirus-induced lysis of the infected tumor leads to regression of the non-infected distant tumor, in the absence of virus transfer [7,8]. These data speak for the involvement of an immune bystander effect taking over from the initial direct viral oncolytic effect to complete tumor elimination. The tight cooperation between protoparvoviruses and the immune system to synergistically achieve tumor suppression is evidenced by a number of phenomenological observations and mechanistic investigations, as reviewed below. Most of these studies concern the rodent protoparvovirus H-1PV and (tumor) cells of either rat (the natural host of this virus) or human origin. Since H-1PV is not infectious for mouse cells, a few cited works were carried out in murine models with closely related mouse protoparvoviruses, in particular the prototype strain of the minute virus of mice (MVMp). H-1PV and its close relatives will be collectively designated PVs in this review.

2. Phenomenological Evidence of PV-Immune System Cooperation

Animals cured of their cancer as a result of PV treatment develop tumor-specific memory responses protecting them against subsequent challenges with the same tumor cells, in the absence of detectable viral imprints [5,9–11]. This long-term vaccination effect is somewhat expected from the viral oncolysis-dependent release of tumor-associated antigens (TAAs) triggering tumor-specific adaptive cellular immune responses. Besides protecting animals from cancer recurrence, these responses also contribute to PV-induced elimination of primary tumors, as indicated by the ability of H-1PV to enhance the efficiency of an autologous tumor cell-based therapeutic vaccine [7].

Direct indications of the role of the immune system in PV-mediated tumor destruction were obtained through different complementary approaches.

- PV antineoplastic efficacy is higher in immunocompetent, as compared to immunodeficient animals. The impairment of the acquired cell-mediated arm of the host immune system by genetic means [11,12], or by experimental cell depletion [7,13], was indeed found to correlate with reduced PV capacity for tumor suppression.
- Adoptive transfer of splenocytes from rats undergoing H-1PV-mediated tumor regression into naïve animals bearing the same tumor protects the recipients against cancer development, in absence of detectable virus transmission [14].
- Animals undergoing tumor suppression upon PV treatment show distinct changes in tumors and lymphoid tissues, pointing to the induction of Th1-type cellular immune responses. This induction was revealed through the elevated production of cytokines (notably interferon (IFN)-γ and tumor necrosis factor (TNF)-α), the infiltration of tumors with activated helper and cytotoxic T lymphocytes (CTLs), and the proliferation of cytotoxic and/or helper T cells in spleen and tumor-draining lymph nodes [7,8,12,14,15]. While this response is likely to be directed mostly against viral epitopes, its stimulation by uninfected tumor cells under in vivo and/or in vitro conditions argues for at least some level of tumor specificity [11,16].
- Upon H-1PV infection, human pancreatic carcinoma cells can prime human immune cells to inhibit tumor development. This was shown in a humanized patient-derived xenograft model, using ex vivo primed human dendritic and T cells for immunodeficient mice reconstitution and growth suppression of pancreatic cancer cells derived from the same patient [15].
- There is a first hint of H-1PV oncosuppressive capacity enhancement through co-treatment with immunostimulants. In a model of late (peritoneal carcinomatosis-associated) pancreatic cancer, co-application of IFN-γ improved H-1PV-mediated control of the disease [16]. This improvement correlated with enhanced activability of isolated peritoneal macrophages (TNF-α production) and splenocytes (proliferation).
- PV propensity for inducing Th1 environment is substantiated by the bias of the virus-neutralizing humoral response elicited after infection towards Th1/IFN-γ-dependent IgG2a isotype antibodies [17,18]. Furthermore, some PVs were found to potentiate autoimmune reactions through the modulation of T cell effector functions [19,20].

A straightforward mechanism of PV priming of antitumor immune reactions would be the release of cellular TAAs and/or viral antigens as a result of the lytic infection of tumor cells, leading to induction of tumor-specific responses and the generation of a proimmune milieu. Yet another non-exclusive possibility deserves to be considered. PVs may act on the immune system, either directly, by infecting various immune cells, or indirectly, by causing infected (tumor) cells to produce viral and/or cellular signals (the so-called pathogen- and damage-associated molecular patterns, PAMPs and DAMPs, respectively), which are recognized by immune cells, and regulate their activity. Two pieces of in vivo evidence support the latter possibility.

- In mice infected with MVMp, extratumoral viral gene expression has been detected in lymphoid tissues [18] and assigned to rare subpopulations of cells known to play a role in cancer immune surveillance, namely myeloid dendritic cells (DCs) and B1 lymphocytes [21]. Interestingly, MVMp-infected animals show striking upregulation of the expression of IP-10, a chemoattractant known to be produced by these cells and to have antitumoral properties. In a rat model of pancreatic carcinoma, an initial burst of extratumoral H-1PV expression has also been observed in lymphoid organs [6].

- A first indication of H-1PV intrinsic immunostimulatory activity has been obtained for virus mutants that are endowed with higher anticancer potency, while keeping the same oncolytic efficacy as the wild-type virus. These mutants were obtained by arming the PV genome with known immunostimulating PAMPs, namely unmethylated CpG motifs. The CpG mutants proved superior to the original virus at inducing the above-mentioned immunological changes in tumors and lymphoid tissues, in particular DC activation in tumor-draining lymph nodes [15,22].

3. Mechanistic Evidence of PV Capacity for Modulating the Immune System

The ability of PVs to upregulate the immune system has been demonstrated through a number of in vitro studies using immune cell cultures or co-cultures with tumor cells.

PV immunostimulating activity is mediated in part by tumor cell factors whose expression is modulated by virus infection. PVs have been found to kill tumor cells through multiple mechanisms (for reviews, see [1,2,23]). Besides being multimodal, PV-induced tumor cell death has been proved to be immunogenic.

- A first hint of the interconnection between H-1PV and immunogenic cell death (ICD) has been given by the observation that human myeloid leukemia cell variants selected for their resistance to the virus also resisted TNF-α, a known inducer of the release of a plethora of proinflammatory DAMPs and cytokines [24].
- H-1PV infection makes human melanoma cells able to trigger the activation/maturation of innate immune cells, DCs in particular [25]. Similarly, microglia and DC subsets get activated after co-culture with MVMp-infected mouse glioma cells [11]. PVs are much more potent than other inducers of tumor cell death in having this immunostimulating effect. H-1PV-dependent DC activation has been found to correlate with strong and long-lasting release of the DAMP heat shock protein (HSP) 72 by infected human melanoma cells [25]. DCs incubated with H-1PV-induced melanoma cell lysates show increased expression of both specific Toll-like receptors (TLRs) and NF-kB, arguing for a role of TLR signaling in virus-mediated maturation of DCs [26].
- In keeping with their relaying role between innate and adaptive immunity, human DCs activated by H-1PV-induced tumor cell lysates are able to phagocytose these lysates and cross-present TAAs, leading to the stimulation of CTL clones specific for these epitopes [27,28].
- H-1PV infection confers to human pancreatic and colon carcinoma cells an enhanced capacity for stimulating natural killer cells (NKCs) to release cyto/chemokines and kill tumor cells [29,30]. This H-1PV-mediated increase in NKC oncotoxic activity has been traced back to both the overexpression of ligands specific for various NKC activation receptors and the down-modulation of MHC class I molecules on virus-infected tumor cells.
- In agreement with the above data, incubation with H-1PV-infected human pancreatic carcinoma cells induces Th1/M1 immune signature in human peripheral blood mononuclear cells (PBMCs), as revealed in particular by the enhanced production of IFN-γ and TNF-α [14]. These changes are intriguing, given their known association with tumor immune rejection. This modulation was achieved by infected pancreatic cancer cells, which are unable to support virus production, and is therefore likely to result from immunogenic signals produced by infected tumor cells instead of PBMC infection by progeny virions. It is worth noting that H-1PV can exert, in addition, direct effects on PBMCs, as discussed below.

The immunostimulating activity of PV-induced tumor cell lysates can be boosted by co-application of immunomodulators, or by virus manipulation

- H-1PV cooperates with other inducers of ICD, resulting in the production of a broader spectrum of DAMPs by co-treated tumor cells. This can be exemplified by an H-1PV/gemcitabine chemovirotherapeutic treatment, whose capacity for inducing human pancreatic cancer cells to release two main markers of ICD, the DAMPs high mobility group box (HMGB) 1 and ATP, relies on the virus and the drug, respectively [31]. In agreement with these data, H-1PV and gemcitabine act synergistically to induce pancreatic carcinoma cells to activate co-cultured human PBMCs, as revealed by the production of IFN-γ [15].

- Another intriguing strategy for improving the immunostimulating activity of PV-induced tumor cell lysates consists of combinations of immune checkpoint blockers to remove inhibitory signals of T cell activation. First credit to this application was given by the potentiating effect of sunitinib, a receptor tyrosine kinase inhibitor with immune checkpoint blockade properties, on the ability of H-1PV-infected human melanoma cell lysates to induce DC cross-presentation-dependent activation of tumor antigen-specific CTLs [28]. Furthermore, the immune checkpoint-blocking antibody tremelimumab may stimulate human DC maturation mediated by H-1PV-induced colon carcinoma cell lysates [32].
- Arming the H-1PV genome with immunostimulating CpG elements boosts virus capacity for inducing the above-mentioned tumor surveillance-predictive IFN-γ/TNF-α signature, upon infection of co-cultures of human PBMCs and pancreatic cancer cells [15].

Besides inducing tumor cells to produce immunostimulating signals, PVs can also infect distinct immune cells and activate them in a direct way. This appears to be true in spite of the remarkable oncotropism, which restricts the effects of PVs on normal tissues [1]. PVs can indeed enter many normal cells, and while being abortive, infection may still have physiological impacts, particularly on the immune system. Infection of human PBMCs with H-1PV is abortive, leading to no detectable production/release of progeny virions [14,33]. Analysis of H-1PV life-cycle in distinct immune cells shows that virus entry takes place in T, B and NK lymphocyte subpopulations, monocytes and DCs, but replication gets blocked at various subsequent steps, with no or limited production of the viral cytotoxic protein NS1 [14,25,29,33,34]. Human neutrophils also prove to be non-permissive for H-1PV [33]. A similar abortion of MVMp life-cycle has been observed after infection of human PBMCs [34], mouse splenocytes [21], DCs [11] and glial cells [35]. The abortive PV infection of isolated immunocytes causes no or little harm to these cells [25,29,33,35]. However, H-1PV infection of human PBMCs is associated with significant toxic effects for which B lymphocytes or NKCs may be targets [14,33]. This cytotoxicity appears, at least in part, not to be a direct consequence of virus infection, but to be mediated by cellular factors that accumulate in vitro after being released from distinct immune cells as a result of their activation by H-1PV.

- Some normal human immune cells appear to respond to PV infection by producing type I IFNs, as detected in human PBMCs exposed to H-1PV or MVMp [34,36]. Distinct human immune cells, most likely plasmacytoid DCs, appear to sense PV infection through TLRs and possibly also through other receptors [34]. The activation of type I IFN response in these cells may contribute to their resistance to PV infection due to abortion of virus replication (see above). This response may still be host range-dependent, as MVMp failed to induce similar type I IFN production in mouse plasmacytoid DCs [37]. It is noteworthy, however, that some non-immune normal cells may also be induced to produce type I IFNs upon PV infection, depending on the host cell origin. While the capacity of MVMp for triggering type I IFN production has been demonstrated in normal fibroblasts derived from mice, the natural host of this virus [38–40], PVs have failed to evoke detectable type I IFN response in a number of normal human cell types [36]. Altogether, these observations indicate that although many human cells may fail to develop type I IFN response after being exposed to rodent PVs, a distinct subset of immune cells are able to sense PV infection and sustain significant type I IFN production. Besides having antiviral functions, type I IFNs exert a wide range of stimulatory activities on both the innate and acquired arm of the immune system. It therefore seems justified to include these cytokines in the series of potential mediators of PV immunostimulation.

- PV infection of immune cells can have other phenotypic impacts besides type I IFN induction. The analysis of the functional impact of H-1PV infection on isolated subsets of human immune cells has revealed virus capacity for activating T helper cells (expression of activation markers and secretion of Th interleukins (ILs)) [33], macrophages (TNF-α release) [14] and DCs (TNF-α and proinflammatory IL production, expression of type I IFN-stimulated genes) [15]. A weak stimulating effect of MVMp infection on mouse DCs has also been reported [11]. Direct PV infection appears to be less efficient at activating DCs than incubation with PV-infected tumor cells [27]. In contrast to the stimulation of the above-mentioned immune cells, a down-regulating effect of H-1PV has been observed for regulatory T cells whose suppressive activity is inhibited by infection [33]. It is worth noting that the immunostimulatory signals induced by direct PV infection overlap those induced by incubation with infected tumor cells (see previous sections), suggesting that some of the activating effects of the latter cells may be mediated by PAMPs, as well as the above-mentioned cellular DAMPs. In agreement with the phenotypic changes induced in individual immune cells, H-1PV infection of PBMCs generates a TNF-α/IFN-γ/IL-2 signature that is accompanied by activation and focal proliferation of T cells, with the prevalence of $CD4^+$ Th cells [14,15,33]. Similarily, conditioned immunocytes from mouse spleen and lymph nodes sustain enhanced IFN-γ production after MVMp infection [21]. Altogether, these observations are indicative of PV direct capacity for Th1-biased immune upregulation. In agreement with the above-mentioned TLR involvement in PV induction of type I IFN production by PBMCs, an H-1PV mutant armed with CpG motifs proves to be more effective than the wild-type virus in triggering antigen-presenting and T cell activation, and IFN-γ, IL-2 and type I IFN release after infection of human PBMCs [15].

4. Conclusions: Use of H-1PV and Its Relatives to Fine-Tune Immune Responses

The above data give credit to the ability of PVs to (in) directly interact with the immune system and generate a microenvironment favorable to the development of both innate and acquired cell-mediated immune responses (Figure 1). While resulting in part from phenotypic changes directly induced by PVs in immunocytes, immune upregulation is exacerbated in the presence of tumors. This tumor dependence reflects the fact that infected neoplastic cells are factories for the production, not only of progeny virions, but also of PAMPs and DAMPs, which act to alert the immune system. In consequence, PV-mediated immunostimulation proves to be directed, at least in part, against tumors in various model systems. The potential application of this property to cancer therapy raises the question of whether the immunomodulating activity of PVs poses any risk to the host. Two lines of evidence speak for H-1PV and MVMp being friendly immunostimulators.

- The PV-mediated immunological activation observed in in vitro models takes place in the absence of major toxicity for immune cells, which undergo an abortive infection with no or few direct cytopathic effects (see above). It should, however, be stated that this conclusion cannot be extended to all rodent PVs, some of which target cells of the hematopoietic system and can lead to immune dysfunctions [41].
- Animal studies show that infection of natural hosts with H-1PV and MVMp, even at very high doses and repeated treatment, is not associated with any immunotoxicity or threatening overactive immune responses, such as cytokine storms, autoimmunity or overt inflammation [18,42]. Furthermore, PV adjuvant effects described above in cancer animal models were not accompanied by any harmful immunological side effects [6,12]. Therefore, these viruses have a generally low proinflammatory profile and depend on the presence of neoplastic tissues to exert immune adjuvant effects that are targeted at infected tumors and surrounding lymphoid organs. This tumor specificity of danger signaling by H-1PV and MVMp speaks for the inclusion of PV-based treatments in the developing arsenal of cancer immunotherapies.

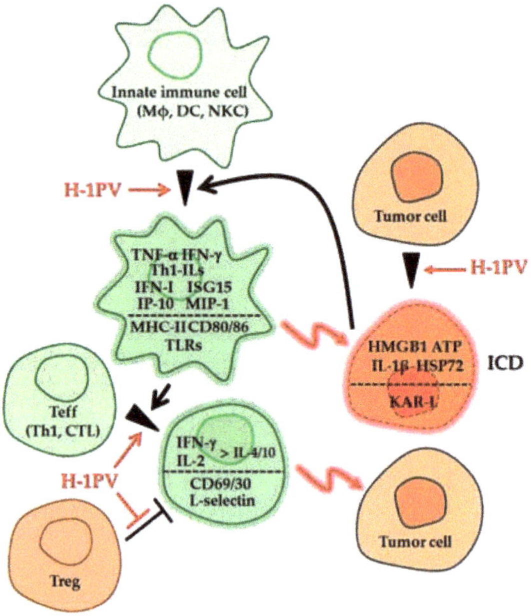

Figure 1. Preclinical evidence of H-1PV impact on the crosstalk between immune and tumor cells. Innate and adaptive immune cells are stimulated as a result of both their contact with H-1PV-infected tumor cells and their direct infection with the virus. This immunostimulatory effect of H-1PV is revealed through the induction of markers of immunogenic death in infected tumor cells and of phenotypic activation in immune cells. The mediators involved include a number of cytokines/extracellular signaling molecules and cell membrane receptors/ligands, as listed for the corresponding cell types (above and below the dotted line, respectively). For details and references, see main text. ATP, adenosine triphosphate; CD, cluster of differentiation; CTL, cytotoxic T lymphocyte; DC, dendritic cell; HMGB, high mobility group box; HSP, heat shock protein; ICD, immunogenic cell death; IFN, interferon; IL, interleukin; IP, interferon-gamma-induced protein; ISG, interferon-stimulated gene; KAR-L, killer activation receptor ligand; Mφ, macrophage; MHC, major histocompatibility complex; MIP, macrophage inflammatory protein; NKC, natural killer cell; Teff, effector T cell; Th, T helper; TLR, Toll-like receptor; Treg, regulatory T cell.

5. First Clinical Hints of H-1PV Capacity for Tumor Microenvironment Immunomodulation in Cancer Patients

The above described preclinical evidence of H-1PV capacity to exert immunostimulatory effects in various cancer models raises the question of whether similar observations could also be made in a clinical context, i.e., in H-1PV-treated cancer patients. In 2011, the first-in-man PV clinical trial (ParvOryx01) was launched in recurrent glioblastoma patients [43]. Trial initiation was prompted by preclinical reports of Geletneky et al., demonstrating striking PV-induced tumor regression in intratumorally and systemically treated glioma-bearing animals [10]. First clinical experience brought much essential knowledge, which laid the ground for further H-1PV clinical developments. ParvOryx01 demonstrated that the virus exhibits a reliable safety and tolerability profile in both local and systemic applications, and poses no risk of environmental contamination or undesired transmission to third persons. Furthermore, intratumoral H-1PV expression was also documented in virus local injection site-distant tumor areas, and in intravenously treated patients. H-1PV capacity to cross the blood-brain/tumor barrier, already described in animal glioma models [10], was therefore confirmed in men. The progression-free and overall survival of ParvOryx01 patients compared favorably with published meta-analyses of recurrent glioblastoma cases [44]. Notably, ParvOryx01 provided observations in support of H-1PV's double-faceted mode of action as both an oncolytic and immunostimulatory anticancer agent. Virus-specific T cells were detected in the peripheral blood of the majority of ParvOryx01 patients [44]. Although antiviral immune responses are generally considered restrictive for the efficacy of OV therapy, growing evidence suggests that they can reverse the tumor-driven host immune suppression by inducing ICD, facilitating the initial priming of antitumor immune responses, and establishing a niche suitable for the development of tumor-specific immunity [45]. It is indeed noteworthy that glioma-specific peripheral T cell responses were detected in half of the tested H-1PV-treated glioblastoma patients [44].

The availability of resected glioblastoma tissues allowed the analysis of the tumor microenvironment (TME) nine days after H-1PV treatment administration. In comparison with historical controls, in patients who received H-1PV treatment, activated granzyme B and perforin-positive CTLs and Th cells massively infiltrated the tumor. Both perivascular and diffuse intratumoral immune infiltrates were observed [44,46]. In contrast, only scarce, single scattered Treg cells were seen. IFN-γ and IL-2 expression was also detected in these tumors. Glioblastoma-associated microglia/macrophages (GAM) displayed pronounced CD68 and cathepsin B (CTSB) upregulation, characteristic of an activated state (Figure 2). Of note, apoptosis of glioma cells induced by microglia-derived secreted CTSB has been shown in vitro [47].

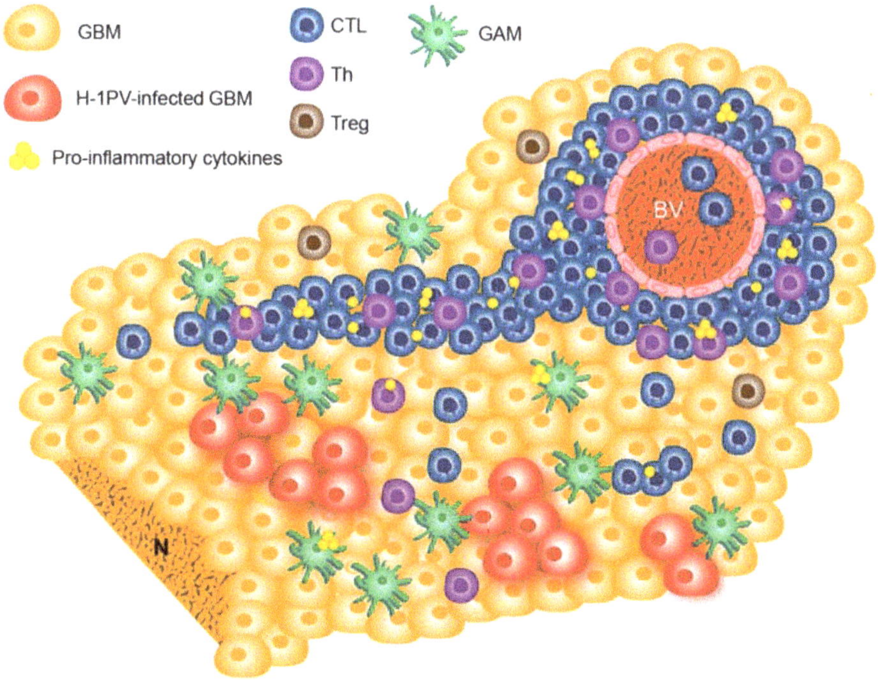

Figure 2. Tumor microenvironment immune landscape as identified in resected tumors from H-1PV-treated recurrent glioblastoma patients. Microglia/macrophage activation, diffuse and perivascular tumor infiltration with activated Th and cytotoxic T cells, and proinflammatory cytokine expression were observed in patient-derived tumor tissue sections. Only scarce Treg cells were present. H-1PV transcripts as well as the oncotoxic NS1 protein were detected in clustered tumor cells. For details and references, see [44,46] and main text. BV, blood vessel; CTL, cytotoxic T lymphocyte; GAM, glioblastoma-associated microglia/macrophages; GBM, glioblastoma; N, necrosis; Th, T helper; Treg, regulatory T cell.

The above data hint at the establishment in H-1PV-treated glioblastoma patients of a "hot", proinflammatory TME, which may facilitate tumor targeting by host antitumor immune responses. This offers the possibility to synergistically increase TME "warming up" by combining H-1PV with other immunotherapeutic strategies. Indeed, H-1PV was recently combined with bevacizumab [48] or bevacizumab and checkpoint inhibition [49,50] within the frame of a compassionate virus use program. This H-1PV-based viro-immunotherapeutic approach achieved high rates of objective antitumor responses in glioblastoma patients, raising increased expectations towards the efficiency of the concept. It is noteworthy that bevacizumab, although originally developed as an antiangiogenic drug, exerts in addition a certain degree of immunomodulation. Bevacizumab reduces vascular endothelial growth factor (VEGF)-induced defects in DC functions, and inhibits tumor infiltration by immune regulatory cells, such as Treg and myeloid-derived suppressor cells (MDSCs) [51]. Bevacizumab and H-1PV therefore converge on the possession of several immune system boosting effects, which is likely to be the reason behind the favorable response obtained in glioblastoma patients subjected to combined treatment with both agents.

Following the successful completion of ParvOryx01, a second H-1PV clinical trial (ParvOryx02) was launched, which aimed to assess virus combination with gemcitabine for the treatment of inoperable metastatic pancreatic cancer [52]. The immunomodulating properties of gemcitabine have not yet been clearly documented. Nonetheless, Suzuki et al. [53,54] reported that this chemotherapeutic drug selectively eliminates splenic MDSCs and exerts significant immune stimulation in murine tumor models. In the ParvOryx02 trial setting, H-1PV oncolytic and immunomodulating capacities are expected to synergize with the cytotoxic (and immunostimulatory?) effects of gemcitabine. ParvOryx02 outcome evaluation is currently ongoing and will provide further experience of value in the development of H-1PV-based cancer viro-immunotherapies.

Author Contributions: A.A. and J.R. wrote the manuscript.

Funding: H-1PV (ParvOryx) clinical trials and compassionate use programs are sponsored by Oryx GmbH & Co.KG (Baldham, Germany).

Acknowledgments: All present and past members of the Tumor Virology Division (F010) at the German Cancer Research Center are greatly acknowledged for their contribution to the work described in this review. We would like to thank Jutta Jung (Corporate Design and Marketing, DKFZ, Heidelberg) for artwork assistance.

Conflicts of Interest: The authors declare no conflict of interest.

References

1. Angelova, A.L.; Geletneky, K.; Nüesch, J.P.F.; Rommelaere, J. Tumor selectivity of oncolytic parvoviruses: From in vitro and animal models to cancer patients. *Front. Bioeng. Biotechnol.* **2015**, *3*, 55. [CrossRef]
2. Marchini, A.; Bonifati, S.; Scott, E.M.; Angelova, A.L.; Rommelaere, J. Oncolytic parvoviruses: From basic virology to clinical applications. *Virol. J.* **2015**, *12*, 6. [CrossRef] [PubMed]
3. Bretscher, C.; Marchini, A. H-1PV parvovirus as a cancer-killing agent: Recent developments in the field. *Viruses* **2019**, under review.
4. Angelova, A.; Aprahamian, M.; Balboni, G.; Delecluse, H.J.; Feederle, R.; Kiprianova, I.; Grekova, S.; Galabov, A.S.; Witzens-Harig, M.; Ho, A.D.; et al. Oncolytic rat parvovirus H-1PV, a candidate for the treatment of human lymphoma: In vitro and in vivo studies. *Mol. Ther.* **2009**, *17*, 1164–1172. [CrossRef]
5. McKisic, M.D.; Paturzo, F.X.; Smith, A.L. Mouse parvovirus infection potentiates rejection of tumor allografts and modulates T cell effector functions. *Transplantation* **1996**, *61*, 292–299. [CrossRef] [PubMed]
6. Angelova, A.; Aprahamian, M.; Grekova, S.; Hajri, A.; Leuchs, B.; Giese, N.; Herrmann, A.; Dinsart, C.; Balboni, G.; Rommeleare, J.; et al. Improvement of gemcitabine-based therapy of pancreatic carcinoma by means of oncolytic parvovirus H-1PV. *Clin. Cancer Res.* **2009**, *15*, 511–519. [CrossRef]
7. Raykov, Z.; Grekova, S.; Galabov, A.S.; Balboni, G.; Koch, U.; Aprahamian, M.; Rommelaere, J. Combined oncolytic and vaccination activities of parvovirus H-1 in a metastatic tumor model. *Oncol. Rep.* **2007**, *17*, 1493–1499. [CrossRef] [PubMed]

8. Rommelaere, J.; Geletneky, K.; Angelova, A.L.; Daeffler, L.; Dinsart, C.; Kiprijanova, I.; Schlehofer, J.R.; Raykov, Z. Oncolytic parvoviruses as cancer therapeutics. *Cytokine Growth Factor. Rev.* **2010**, *21*, 185–195. [CrossRef]
9. Guetta, E.; Graziani, Y.; Tal, J. Suppression of Ehrlich ascites tumors in mice by minute virus of mice. *JNCI* **1986**, *76*, 1177–1180. [PubMed]
10. Geletneky, K.; Kiprianova, I.; Ayache, A.; Koch, R.; Herrero, Y.; Calle, M.; Deleu, L.; Sommer, C.; Thomas, N.; Rommelaere, J.; et al. Regression of advanced rat and human gliomas by local or systemic treatment with oncolytic parvovirus H-1 in rat models. *Neuro-Oncology* **2010**, *12*, 804–814. [CrossRef]
11. Grekova, S.P.; Raykov, Z.; Zawatzky, R.; Rommelaere, J.; Koch, U. Activation of a glioma-specific immune response by oncolytic minute virus of mice infection. *Cancer Gene. Ther.* **2012**, *19*, 468–475. [CrossRef] [PubMed]
12. Giese, N.A.; Raykov, Z.; De Martino, L.; Vecchi, A.; Sozzani, S.; Dinsart, C.; Cornelis, J.J.; Rommelaere, J. Suppression of metastatic hemangiosarcoma by a parvovirus MVMp vector transducing the IP-10 chemokine into immunocompetent mice. *Cancer Gene. Ther.* **2002**, *9*, 432–442. [CrossRef]
13. Geletneky, K.; Nüesch, J.P.F.; Angelova, A.; Kiprianova, I.; Rommelaere, J. Double-faceted mechanism of parvoviral oncosuppression. *Curr. Opin. Virol.* **2015**, *13*, 17–24. [CrossRef] [PubMed]
14. Grekova, S.P.; Aprahamian, M.; Giese, N.A.; Schmitt, S.; Giese, T.; Falk, C.S.; Daeffler, L.; Cziepluch, C.; Rommelaere, J.; Raykov, Z. Immune cells participate in the oncosuppressive activity of parvovirus H-1PV and are activated as a result of their abortive infection with this agent. *Cancer Biol. Ther.* **2010**, *10*, 1280–1289. [CrossRef]
15. Grekova, S.P.; Aprahamian, M.; Giese, N.A.; Bour, G.; Giese, T.; Grewenig, A.; Leuchs, B.; Hörlein, R.; Heller, A.; Angelova, A.L.; et al. Genomic CpG enrichment of oncolytic parvoviruses as a potent anticancer vaccination strategy for the treatment of pancreatic adenocarcinoma. *J. Vaccines Vaccin.* **2014**, *5*, 227. [CrossRef]
16. Grekova, S.; Aprahamian, M.; Daeffler, L.; Leuchs, B.; Angelova, A.; Giese, T.; Galabov, A.S.; Heller, A.; Giese, N.A.; Rommelaere, J.; et al. Interferon-gamma improves the vaccination potential of oncolytic parvovirus H-1PV for the treatment of peritoneal carcinomatosis in pancreatic cancer. *Cancer Biol. Ther.* **2011**, *12*, 889–895. [CrossRef] [PubMed]
17. Ball-Goodrich, L.J.; Paturzo, F.X.; Johnson, E.A.; Steger, K.; Jacoby, R.O. Immune responses to the major capsid protein during parvovirus infection of rats. *J. Virol.* **2002**, *76*, 10044–10049. [CrossRef] [PubMed]
18. Lang, S.I.; Giese, N.A.; Rommelaere, J.; Dinsart, C.; Cornelis, J.J. Humoral immune responses against minute virus of mice vectors. *J. Gene Med.* **2006**, *8*, 1141–1150. [CrossRef]
19. McKisic, M.D.; Macy, J.D., Jr.; Delano, M.L.; Jacoby, R.O.; Paturzo, F.X.; Smith, A.L. Mouse parvovirus infection potentiates allogeneic skin graft rejection and induces syngeneic graft rejection. *Transplantation* **1998**, *65*, 1436–1446. [CrossRef]
20. Chung, Y.H.; Jun, H.S.; Son, M.; Bao, M.; Bae, H.Y.; Kang, Y.; Yoon, J.W. Cellular and molecular mechanism for Kilham rat virus-induced autoimmune diabetes in DR-BB rats. *J. Immunol.* **2000**, *165*, 2866–2876. [CrossRef]
21. Raykov, Z.; Savelieva, L.; Balboni, G.; Giese, T.; Rommelaere, J.; Giese, N.A. B1 lymphocytes and myeloid dendritic cells in lymphoid organs are preferential extratumoral sites of parvovirus MVMp expression. *J. Virol.* **2005**, *79*, 3517–3524. [CrossRef] [PubMed]
22. Raykov, Z.; Grekova, S.; Leuchs, B.; Aprahamian, M.; Rommelaere, J. Arming parvoviruses with CpG motifs to improve their oncosuppressive capacity. *Int. J. Cancer* **2008**, *122*, 2880–2884. [CrossRef]
23. Nüesch, J.P.F.; Lacroix, J.; Marchini, A.; Rommelaere, J. Molecular pathways: Rodent parvoviruses: Mechanisms of oncolysis and prospects for clinical cancer treatment. *Clin. Cancer Res.* **2012**, *18*, 3516–3523. [CrossRef] [PubMed]
24. Rayet, B.; Lopez-Guerrero, J.A.; Rommelaere, J.; Dinsart, C. Induction of programmed cell death by parvovirus H-1 in U937 cells: Connection with the TNFα signalling pathway. *J. Virol.* **1998**, *72*, 8893–8903. [PubMed]
25. Moehler, M.; Zeidler, M.; Schede, J.; Rommelaere, J.; Galle, P.R.; Cornelis, J.J.; Heike, M. Oncolytic parvovirus H-1 induces release of heat-shock protein HSP72 in susceptible human tumor cells but may not affect primary immune cells. *Cancer Gene Ther.* **2003**, *10*, 477–480. [CrossRef] [PubMed]
26. Sieben, M.; Schaefer, P.; Dinsart, C.; Galle, P.R.; Moehler, M. Activation of the human immune system via toll-like receptors by the oncolytic parvovirus H-1. *Int. J. Cancer* **2013**, *132*, 2548–2556. [CrossRef] [PubMed]

27. Moehler, M.H.; Zeidler, M.; Wilsberg, V.; Cornelis, J.J.; Woelfel, T.; Rommelaere, J.; Galle, P.R.; Heike, M. Parvovirus H1-induced tumor cell death enhances human immune response in vitro via increased phagocytosis, maturation and cross-presentation by dendritic cells. *Hum. Gene Ther.* **2005**, *16*, 996–1005. [CrossRef] [PubMed]
28. Moehler, M.; Sieben, M.; Roth, S.; Springsguth, F.; Leuchs, B.; Zeidler, M.; Dinsart, C.; Rommelaere, J.; Galle, P.R. Activation of the human immune system by chemotherapeutic or targeted agents combined with the oncolytic parvovirus H-1. *BMC Cancer* **2011**, *11*, 464. [CrossRef] [PubMed]
29. Bhat, R.; Dempe, S.; Dinsart, C.; Rommelaere, J. Enhancement of NK cell anti-tumour responses using an oncolytic parvovirus. *Int. J. Cancer* **2011**, *128*, 908–919. [CrossRef]
30. Bhat, R.; Rommelaere, J. NK cell-dependent killing of colon carcinoma cells is mediated by natural cytotoxicity receptors (NCRs) and stimulated by an oncolytic virus. *BMC Cancer* **2013**, *13*, 367. [CrossRef]
31. Angelova, A.; Grekova, S.; Heller, A.; Kuhlmann, O.; Soyka, E.; Giese, T.; Aprahamian, M.; Bour, G.; Rüffer, S.; Cziepluch, C.; et al. Complementary induction of immunogenic cell death by oncolytic parvovirus H-1PV and gemcitabine in pancreatic cancer. *J. Virol.* **2014**, *88*, 5263–5276. [CrossRef]
32. Heinrich, B.; Goepfert, K.; Delic, M.; Galle, P.R.; Moehler, M. Influence of the oncolytic parvovirus H-1, CTLA-4 antibody tremelimumab and cytostatic drugs on the human immune system in a human in vitro model of colorectal cancer cells. *Oncol. Targets Ther.* **2013**, *6*, 1119–1127. [CrossRef]
33. Moralès, O.; Richard, A.; Martin, N.; Mrizak, D.; Sénéchal, M.; Pancré, V.; Rommelaere, J.; Caillet-Fauquet, P.; de Launoit, Y.; Delhem, N. Activation of a helper and not regulatory human $CD4^+$ T cell response by oncolytic H-1 parvovirus. *PLoS ONE* **2012**, *7*, e32197. [CrossRef]
34. Raykov, Z.; Grekova, S.; Hörlein, R.; Leuchs, B.; Giese, T.; Giese, N.A.; Rommelaere, J.; Zawatzky, R.; Daeffler, L. TLR-9 contributes to the antiviral innate immune sensing of rodent parvoviruses MVMp and H-1PV by normal human immune cells. *PLoS ONE* **2013**, *8*, e55086. [CrossRef]
35. Abschuetz, A.; Kehl, T.; Geibig, R.; Leuchs, B.; Rommelaere, J.; Regnier-Vigouroux, A. The oncolytic murine autonomous parvovirus, a candidate vector for glioma gene therapy, is innocuous to normal and immunocompetent mouse glial cells. *Cell Tissue Res.* **2006**, *325*, 423–436. [CrossRef]
36. Paglino, J.C.; Andres, W.; van den Pol, A.N. Autonomous parvoviruses neither stimulate nor are inhibited by the type I interferon response in human normal or cancer cells. *J. Virol.* **2014**, *88*, 4932–4942. [CrossRef] [PubMed]
37. Mattei, L.M.; Cotmore, S.F.; Li, L.; Tattersall, P.; Iwasaki, A. Toll-like receptor 9 in plasmacytoid dendritic cells fails to detect parvoviruses. *J. Virol.* **2013**, *87*, 3605–3608. [CrossRef] [PubMed]
38. Grekova, S.; Zawatzky, R.; Hoerlein, R.; Cziepluch, C.; Mincberg, M.; Davis, C.; Rommelaere, J.; Daeffler, L. Activation of an antiviral response in normal but not transformed mouse cells: A new determinant of minute virus of mice (MVMp) oncotropism. *J. Virol.* **2010**, *84*, 516–531. [CrossRef] [PubMed]
39. Mattei, L.M.; Cotmore, S.F.; Tattersall, P.; Iwasaki, A. Parvovirus evades interferon-dependent viral control in primary mouse embryonic fibroblasts. *Virology* **2013**, *442*, 20–27. [CrossRef] [PubMed]
40. Ventoso, I.; Berlanga, J.J.; Almendral, J.M. Translation control by protein kinase R restricts minute virus of mice infection: Role in parvovirus oncolysis. *J. Virol.* **2010**, *84*, 5043–5051. [CrossRef] [PubMed]
41. Cornelis, J.J.; Deleu, L.; Koch, U.; Rommelaere, J. Parvovirus oncosuppression. In *Parvoviruses*; Kerr, J.R., Cotmore, S.F., Bloom, M.E., Linden, R.M., Parrish, C.R., Eds.; Edward Arnold Ltd.: London, UK, 2006; pp. 365–378.
42. Geletneky, K.; Leoni, A.L.; Pohlmeyer-Esch, G.; Loebhard, S.; Baetz, A.; Leuchs, B.; Roscher, M.; Hoefer, C.; Jochims, K.; Dahm, M.; et al. Pathology, organ distribution and immune response after single and repeated intravenous injection of rats with clinical-grade parvovirus H-1. *Comp. Med.* **2015**, *65*, 23–35. [PubMed]
43. Geletneky, K.; Huesing, J.; Rommelaere, J.; Schlehofer, J.; Leuchs, B.; Dahm, M.; Krebs, O.; von Knebel Doeberitz, M.; Huber, B.; Hajda, J. Phase I/IIa study of intratumoral/intracerebral or intravenous/intracerebral administration of Parvovirus H-1 (ParvOryx) in patients with progressive primary or recurrent glioblastoma multiforme: ParvOryx01 protocol. *BMC Cancer* **2012**, *12*, 99. [CrossRef] [PubMed]
44. Geletneky, K.; Hajda, J.; Angelova, A.L.; Leuchs, B.; Capper, D.; Bartsch, A.J.; Neumann, J.O.; Schöning, T.; Hüsing, J.; Beelte, B.; et al. Oncolytic H-1 parvovirus shows safety and signs of immunogenic activity in a first I/IIa glioblastoma trial. *Mol. Ther.* **2017**, *25*, 2620–2634. [CrossRef] [PubMed]
45. Gujar, S.; Pol, J.G.; Kim, Y.; Lee, P.W.; Kroemer, G. Antitumor benefits of antiviral immunity: An underappreciated aspect of oncolytic virotherapies. *Trends Immunol.* **2018**, *39*, 209–221. [CrossRef]

46. Angelova, A.L.; Barf, M.; Geletneky, K.; Unterberg, A.; Rommelaere, J. Immunotherapeutic potential of oncolytic H-1 parvovirus: Hints of glioblastoma microenvironment conversion towards immunogenicity. *Viruses* **2017**, *9*, 382. [CrossRef]
47. Hwang, S.Y.; Yoo, B.C.; Jung, J.W.; Oh, E.S.; Hwang, J.S.; Shin, J.A.; Kim, S.Y.; Cha, S.H.; Han, I.O. Induction of glioma apoptosis by microglia-secreted molecules: The role of nitric oxide and cathepsin B. *Biochim. Biophys. Acta.* **2009**, *1793*, 1656–1668. [CrossRef] [PubMed]
48. Geletneky, K.; Angelova, A.; Leuchs, B.; Bartsch, A.; Capper, D.; Hajda, J.; Rommelaere, J. Favorable response of patients with glioblastoma at second or third recurrence to repeated injection of oncolytic parvovirus H-1 in combination with bevacicumab. *Neuro-Oncology* **2015**, *17*, v10–v17. [CrossRef]
49. Geletneky, K.; Weiss, C.; Bernhard, H.; Capper, D.; Leuchs, B.; Marchini, A.; Rommelaere, J. First clinical observation of improved anti-tumor effects of viro-immunotherapy with oncolytic parvovirus H-1 in combination with PD-1 checkpoint blockade and bevacicumab in patients with recurrent glioblastoma. *Neuro-Oncology* **2016**, *18*, vi24. [CrossRef]
50. Geletneky, K.; Bartsch, A.; Weiss, C.; Bernhard, H.; Marchini, A.; Rommelaere, J. High rate of objective anti-tumor response in 9 patients with glioblastoma after viro-immunotherapy with oncolytic parvovirus H-1 in combination with bevacicumab and PD-1 checkpoint blockade. *Neuro-Oncology* **2018**, *20*, vi10. [CrossRef]
51. Elamin, Y.Y.; Rafee, S.; Toomey, S.; Hennesy, B.T. Immune effects of bevacizumab: Killing two birds with one stone. *Cancer Microenviron.* **2015**, *8*, 15–21. [CrossRef]
52. Hajda, J.; Lehmann, M.; Krebs, O.; Kieser, M.; Geletneky, K.; Jäger, D.; Dahm, M.; Huber, B.; Schöning, T.; Sedlaczek, O.; et al. A non-controlled, single arm, open label, phase II study of intravenous and intratumoral administration of ParvOryx in patients with metastatic, inoperable pancreatic cancer: ParvOryx02 protocol. *BMC Cancer* **2017**, *17*, 576. [CrossRef]
53. Suzuki, E.; Kapoor, V.; Jassar, A.S.; Kaiser, L.R.; Albelda, S.M. Gemcitabine selectively eliminates splenic Gr-1+/CD11b+ myeloid suppressor cells in tumor-bearing animals and enhances antitumor immune activity. *Clin. Cancer Res.* **2005**, *11*, 671321. [CrossRef]
54. Suzuki, E.; Sun, J.; Kapoor, V.; Jassar, A.S.; Albelda, S.M. Gemcitabine has significant immunomodulatory activity in murine tumor models independent of its cytotoxic effects. *Cancer Biol. Ther.* **2007**, *6*, 880–885. [CrossRef] [PubMed]

viruses

MDPI

Article

A New Prevalent Densovirus Discovered in *Acari*. Insight from Metagenomics in Viral Communities Associated with Two-Spotted Mite (*Tetranychus urticae*) Populations

Sarah François [1], Doriane Mutuel [1], Alison B. Duncan [2], Leonor R. Rodrigues [3], Celya Danzelle [1,2], Sophie Lefevre [2], Inês Santos [3], Marie Frayssinet [1], Emmanuel Fernandez [4,5], Denis Filloux [4,5], Philippe Roumagnac [4,5], Rémy Froissart [6] and Mylène Ogliastro [1,*]

[1] DGIMI, Univ Montpellier, INRA, F-34095 Montpellier, France; sarah.francois.dgimi@gmail.com (S.F.); Doriane.mutuel@inra.fr (D.M.); celya.danzelle@icloud.com (C.D.); marie.frayssinet@inra.fr (M.F.)
[2] ISEM, Univ Montpellier, CNRS, IRD, EPHE, F-34095 Montpellier, France; alison.duncan@umontpellier.fr (A.B.D.); sophie.lefevre@umontpellier.fr (S.L.)
[3] Centre for Ecology, Evolution and Environmental Changes (cE3c), Univ Lisbon, Faculty of Science, P-1749016 Lisbon, Portugal; leonor.rodrigues89@gmail.com (L.R.R.); inesflsantos@gmail.com (I.S.)
[4] CIRAD, UMR BGPI, F-34398 Montpellier, France; emmanuel.fernandez@cirad.fr (E.F.); denis.filloux@cirad.fr (D.F.); philippe.roumagnac@cirad.fr (P.R.)
[5] BGPI, Univ Montpellier, INRA, CIRAD, Montpellier SupAgro, F-34398 Montpellier, France
[6] MIVEGEC, Univ Montpellier, CNRS, IRD, F-34394 Montpellier, France; remy.froissart@ird.fr
* Correspondence: marie-helene.ogliastro@inra.fr

Received: 29 December 2018; Accepted: 28 February 2019; Published: 7 March 2019

Abstract: Viral metagenomics and high throughput sequence mining have revealed unexpected diversity, and the potential presence, of parvoviruses in animals from all phyla. Among arthropods, this diversity highlights the poor knowledge that we have regarding the evolutionary history of densoviruses. The aim of this study was to explore densovirus diversity in a small arthropod pest belonging to *Acari*, the two-spotted spider mite *Tetranychus urticae*, while using viral metagenomics based on virus-enrichment. Here, we present the viromes obtained from *T. urticae* laboratory populations made of contigs that are attributed to nine new potential viral species, including the complete sequence of a novel densovirus. The genome of this densovirus has an ambisens genomic organization and an unusually compact size with particularly small non-structural proteins and a predicted major capsid protein that lacks the typical PLA2 motif that is common to all ambidensoviruses described so far. In addition, we showed that this new densovirus had a wide prevalence across populations of mite species tested and a genomic diversity that likely correlates with the host phylogeny. In particular, we observed a low densovirus genomic diversity between the laboratory and natural populations, which suggests that virus within-species evolution is probably slower than initially thought. Lastly, we showed that this novel densovirus can be inoculated to the host plant following feeding by infected mites, and circulate through the plant vascular system. These findings offer new insights into densovirus prevalence, evolution, and ecology.

Keywords: parvovirus; viral metagenomics; virus diversity; virus phylogeny; agricultural pests; arthropod; mite; viral communities; viral ecology

---

1. Introduction

Arthropod-infecting parvoviruses, termed densoviruses, have been mostly discovered with a pathology-driven approach, which probably explains the relatively poor number of viral species (i.e., less than 60) that the International Committee for the Taxonomy of Viruses (ICTV) have referenced so far, and the strong bias that exists towards viruses infecting arthropods of health or economic importance [1].

Breakthrough techniques in viral metagenomics and mining high throughput sequencing (HGS) datasets have highlighted the extraordinary diversity and persistence of parvoviruses and parvovirus-related sequences in an unexpected array of animals, including invertebrates [2–4]. These discoveries support the now generally accepted view that viruses are integral components of the microbiome and participate in the functioning of ecosystems of differing size and complexity, i.e., an individual organism or a population of organisms. In the context of the general loss of biodiversity, which is particularly worrisome among arthropods, the question of the prevalence and diversity of their associated microorganisms, including viruses, is of particular interest [5].

Mites and ticks are small arachnids that belong to the *Acari* sub-class that are mostly known for their detrimental impact on human, animal, and plant health [6]. While ticks represent a relatively small number of taxa (around 900 species), all share a parasitic, blood-feeding alimentary regime; mites are extraordinarily diversified (more than 40,000 species) and exhibit a large diversity of lifestyles, including plant feeders, mite-predators, or arthropod ectoparasites, with only a few species presenting direct threats to plant or animal health. Among harmful mites, the two-spotted spider mite (*Tetranychus urticae*) is an agricultural pest that can cause significant damage to more than 1100 species of food-producing or flower cultures [7,8]. Treatment against *T. urticae* with synthetic acaricides has resulted in one of the highest incidences of pesticide resistance being recorded in arthropods [9]. In this context, the development of alternative solutions to chemicals is strongly encouraged; one promising way could be to diversify the use of spider mites' natural enemies, and particularly to include their pathogens.

Despite their environmental success and the threat that they represent for agriculture, due to their small size and the poor description of their associated pathologies, spider-mites have been long neglected by virologists. Only one non-occluded, rod-shaped virus, related to a baculovirus, has so far been described following infections in laboratory populations of mites [10,11]. More recently, viral metagenomics and database mining being applied to *Acari* was developed to explore the viral communities (so-called the viromes) that are associated with blood-feeding ticks [12–15]. These studies revealed an extraordinary wealth of viruses, including parvovirus related sequences, and they validated this approach for virus discovery in these small arthropods. A similar approach was also developed to analyze viruses that are associated with *Varroa destructor*, an ectoparasitic mite of honey bees that also transmits several viruses to the bees and are suspected to contribute to colony collapse [16,17]. This work revealed that several viruses from different families can be found in Varroa at the population level, including mite associated viruses that are common in arthropods (e.g., *Baculoviridae*, *Circoviridae*, *Dicistroviridae*, and *Iflaviridae*).

Herein, we used viral metagenomics and in depth sequencing of virion-associated nucleic acids (VANA) [18] to explore the viral communities that are associated with *T. urticae* from two laboratory populations of different geographic origins and rearing host plants. We found eight new putative virus species belonging to taxa that are associated with arthropods and one with fungi, with five of those viral sequences being shared by both mite populations. More specifically, we discovered that the most abundant reads found in both viromes correspond to a new densovirus and probably a new divergent species in the *Ambidensovirus* genus. RACE, PCR, and sequencing confirmed the genome of this new densovirus and the expression of the viral genes in mites. This new densovirus displayed a very compact genome, and the predicted sequence of its major capsid protein lacked the phospholipase A2 motif that is shared so far by all the members of this genus. This virus, initially named Tetranychus urticae-associated ambidensovirus (TuaDV), was also prevalent in different species of spider mites from laboratory populations worldwide and sampled from natural environments. Comparing TuaDV sequence diversity reveals that the virus is highly conserved within each species, but that there is distinct variation between species that are indicative of some virus-host coevolution [19,20]. Finally, we analyzed TuaDV transmission and found that infection can potentially occur via horizontal and vertical routes. In particular, we showed that mites, when feeding, could transfer viral particles to host plants, which could then be further circulated *in planta*, probably through the vascular system. This mechanism, already shown for the aphid densovirus MpDV, suggests that the plant may be used to spread infection to conspecifics and/or to other species [21].

These discoveries expand our knowledge of densovirus prevalence and diversity in an arthropod taxon that has long been neglected by virologists.

2. Materials and Methods

2.1. Spider-Mite Populations and Rearing

Two laboratory *T. urticae* populations from Portugal and France were first analyzed using the VANA metagenomics-based approach to identify the potential virus species. The first population, the so-called the Portuguese (P) population corresponds to a mix of *T. cinnabarinus* and *T. urticae* populations established at the University of Lisbon. This mix comprised a *T. cinnabarinus* population collected in January 2014 in Spain (Almeria) on rose plants (so-called Almeria population), and two *T. urticae* strains; the "London strain", originating from the Vineland region, Ontario, Canada [8] and the "EtoxR" strain originating from Japan and maintained for five years in the laboratory at Bayer CropScience [22]. All of the populations and strains were maintained on bean plants in the laboratory. It should be noted that this mix was established before the distinction was made between *T. urticae* and *T. cinnabarinus* as possibly being separate species and not two morphs of the same species. The second population, so-called the French (F) population was reared in Montpellier and it also constitutes a mix of populations. The majority of these originate from a *T. urticae* collection in May 1994 in the Netherlands (NL, Pijnacker) from cucumber, which were subsequently transferred to Montpellier in 2007, at which time they were split into two populations (still maintained on cucumber plants). In 2011, these two populations were mixed, and subsequently transferred to either tomato, bean, or kept on cucumber plants (four populations being created per host plant type). Note that two of these populations (HH4 and HH3) that were transferred to bean in 2011 were used to characterize TuaDV transmission. A second batch of mites (hereafter called "Mix-Tu") that were used to characterize transmission contained a mix of 11 different mite populations; eight collected in Portugal, two in Spain (including the population collected in Almeria mentioned above), and one in France. All of the laboratory populations were maintained at 25 °C with an 8: 16 Light: Dark (L:D) cycle.

Once the TuaDV virus was identified in the mixes, we measured its prevalence in spider mite populations by analyzing a total of twenty-seven populations from three species of mites (*T. urticae*, *T. cinnabarinus*, and *T. evansi*), out of which TuaDV from eleven populations were partially or fully sequenced (Table S1). Specifically, the mites came from rearing facilities in France (Nice-Valbonne), Greece (Crete), the Netherlands (Santpoort), Belgium (Ghent), and Portugal (Lisbon), and from natural populations across Portugal sampled in the summer of 2017.

2.2. Preparation of Viromes and Sequencing

The samples were made from pools of around 200 individual mites, from which viral particles were purified using the method that was described by Francois et al. [18]. Briefly, the mites were ground in HBSS buffer with beads using a tissue homogenizer. The homogenized extracts were filtered through a 0.45 μm filter and centrifuged at 148.000 × g for 2.5 h at 4 °C to concentrate viral particles. Next, non-encapsidated nucleic acids were eliminated by DNase and RNase digestion for 1.5 h at 37 °C, although some of the non-encapsidated nucleic acids and cellular contamination may remain. Encapsidated DNA and RNA were then extracted using Nucleospin 96 virus Core Kit (Macherey Nagel, Düren, Germany) and RNA was converted to cDNA using a 26 nt primer (Dodeca Linker) composed of a 14 nt linker linked at the 3′ end to N_{12}. Double-stranded DNA was synthetized from single-stranded DNA using Large (Klenow) fragment DNA polymerase and the Dodeca Linker. Double-stranded DNA was further amplified using one 24 nt PCR multiplex identifier primer that was composed of the 14 nt linker used during the RT step linked at the 5′ end to a 10 nt tag that allowed for sample identification. The PCR products were cleaned with QIAquick PCR Purification kit (Qiagen, Courtaboeuf, France) and the libraries were sequenced on Illumina MiSeq pair-end 300 nt (Genewiz, South Plainfield, NJ, USA).

2.3. Bioinformatics Analyses and Database Screening

Demultiplexing was done with the agrep command-line tool to assign reads to the samples from which they originated [23]. Adaptors were removed and the reads were filtered for quality (q30 quality and read length >45 nt) using Cutadapt 1.9 [24]. The cleaned reads were assembled de novo into contigs using SPAdes 3.6.2 (k-mer lengths 21,33,55,77,125) [25] and mapping was performed on contigs of aligned clean reads with Bowtie 2.1.0 (options local very sensitive) [26]. Taxonomic assignment was achieved through searches against the NCBI RefSeq viral database and against the non-redundant (nr) GenBank database using BLASTx with an e-value cutoff of $<10^{-3}$ [27]. Viral contigs were classified as viral operational taxonomic units (vOTU). The most abundant vOTUs were subsequently characterized using an arbitrary abundance cutoff of < 0.1% that was applied for each vOTU in all of the samples to remove the inter-sample contamination that occurred during the preparation and the sequencing of the samples. This abundance threshold was chosen to be twice above to the most abundant virus taxa that were found in the negative control (HBSS buffer). The predicted sequence of full-length viral proteins were aligned and compared with their closest related viruses (found in GenBank database) using MUSCLE 3.7 (16 iterations) [28], according to the species demarcation thresholds that were recommended within the online reports of the ICTV (www.ictv.global/report/parvoviridae).

For database screening, sequences from all viral contigs were used as queries, as well as the genomes contained in NCBI Viral genome database to perform BLASTn searches within the *T. urticae* genome: RefSeq genomic database (GCF_000239435.1, 641 sequences), WGS (CAEY00000000.1, 2035 sequences) and transcriptomes: EST (txid32264, 80855 sequences) and TSA (BioProject 78685, 9614 sequences; BioProject 78689, 17739 sequences; BioProject 6829 sequences), with and an e-value cutoff of $<10^{-3}$.

2.4. Validation of the TuaDV Full-Length Genomic Sequence

To confirm the presence of TuaDV in mites and confirm its complete coding sequence, pools of mites (n~100) from several populations were tested using PCR. Total DNA was extracted with Wizard Genomic kit (Promega Corp., Madison, WI, USA) and then recovered in a final volume 100 µL (100–135 ng/µL). PCR was performed from 100 ng DNA with specific overlapping sets of primers covering the full length of the genome (Table S2) and while using the GoTaq reaction mix (Promega). The amplicons were sequenced with the Sanger method. To determine the extremities of the TuaDV genome, we performed 5′/3′ RACE with specifically designed primers (Table S2). Total RNA was extracted from pools of mites from the HH4 population with the RNeasy minikit (Qiagen). 3′ and 5′RACE PCR were performed using the 5′/3′ RACE kit, 2nd Generation (Roche, Germany), according to the manufacturer's instructions.

2.5. Phylogenetic Analyses

The putative amino acid sequences of *Tetranychus* associated vOTUs were used for phylogenetic analyses. All of the ORFs were translated in silico using the ORF finder (cut off >300 nt, ATG start codon) on Geneious 1.7 [29] and aligned with the corresponding protein fragments of related viruses being deposited on the GenBank nr database using MUSCLE 3.7 (16 iterations) with default settings [28]. The aligned sequences were manually edited to remove gaps. Maximum likelihood phylogenetic trees were produced from these alignments using PhyML 3.1 [30,31] with substitution models being chosen as the best-fit using Prottest 2.4 [32]. One-thousand bootstrap replicates were used to assign the strength of support for branches. Trees were visualized with FigTree 1.4 (http://tree.bio.ed.ac.uk/software%20/figtree/). Outgroups were used when possible, otherwise the trees were mid-point rooted.

2.6. Densovirus Presence and Transmission

The prevalence of TuaDV was assayed from pools of mites from the different populations using PCR, as described above. PCR was run using the following conditions: 95 °C for 2 min, 25 cycles of 95 °C for 45 sec, 57 °C for 45 sec, 72 °C for 1 min, and then 72 °C for 5 min and two sets of specific primers (61F and 693R (NS) and 1125 and 1793R (VP)). Amplicons were run in an agarose gel and stained with ethidium bromide. We also tested for the within-population prevalence of TuaDV in the laboratory population HH4. Extracting DNA from 20 individual mites from this population achieved this and running PCRs, as described above, to test for the presence of the virus.

When considering the universal presence of the virus, a separate experiment tested whether *T. urticae* associated densovirus was vertically transmitted from mothers to their offspring. To do this, 10 females from the HH4 population were isolated on individual bean leaves placed on water saturated cotton, and left to lay eggs for two days at 25 °C with a 8: 16 L: D cycle. Each female laid eggs that were recovered individually with a clean pair of tweezers and transferred to a new individual leaf patch that was placed on water saturated cotton, allowed to hatch, and offspring to develop into adult. Offspring (n = 10) that became adults and their mother were individually tested for viral infection. Total DNA was extracted from each individual mite, as described above, and recovered in 25 µL (8–12 ng/µL per mite). PCR reactions were set as above and run with 40 cycles. Amplicons were run in an agarose gel and stained with ethidium bromide. The detection limit of the method is estimated ~10ng.

To test for TuaDV inoculation and circulation in the host plant, we placed 50 infected mites on an individual leaf of a whole bean plant (8–10 leaves stage). Paraffin jelly was placed at the base of the petiole of each leaf in order to prevent mites from dispersing from the infested leaf to other leaves on the plant. Five days later, the mites were carefully removed from the infected leaf (named L0) and two uninfected leaves from the same plant, one ~8 cm and the other ~20 cm away from the infected leaf, were collected (named L8 and L20, respectively). We performed six independent transmission experiments with the HH4, HH3, and Mix-Tu populations. Three leaves from six non-infested plants were similarly taken and processed as negative controls. Total DNA was extracted from infested plants and negative controls using DNeasy blood and tissue kit (Qiagen) and recovered in 100 µL (40–60 ng/µL for leaves) and 25 µL (15–25 ng/µL for mites). The TuaDV inoculated to plant leaves was assessed by PCR, as described above, while viral loads in mites and leaves was achieved by qPCR with a reaction mixture containing 15–20 ng and 100 ng of mites or plant DNA, respectively, and a pair of TuaDV specific primers (1125F and 1230R, Table S2) using the Sensifast PCR kit (Bioline, UK). qPCR was run on a Roche LC480 cycler (qPHD facility, Univ Montpellier) using the following conditions: 95 °C for 2 min, 25 cycles of 95 °C for 30 sec, 60 °C for 30 sec, 72 °C for 50 sec, and then 72 °C for 5 min, which resulted in a 78 bp amplicon from ORF2 (NS). As the viral genome of TuaDV remains to be cloned, PCR Standardization was achieved with a standard curve that was made with the serial dilution of DNA of the Junonia coenia ambidensovirus (JcDV) as a proxy.

Statistical analyses were performed with the JMP®Version 11 software (SAS Institute Inc., Cary, NC, USA). The analysis of viral load (ng μL^{-1}) within each leaf was performed using a general linear model with leaves (infected, uninfected 8cm or 20 cm away) and mite populations (HH3, HH4 and Mix-Tu) being included in the model as fixed factors. The plant from where the leaves were taken was included in the model as a random factor nested within population.

Accession numbers: The virus sequences reported herein have been deposited in the GenBank database under accession numbers MK533146 to MK533158 and MK543949.

3. Results

3.1. Overview of the Spider Mite Virome

To explore the viral diversity of *T. urticae* populations, we prepared viral particles according to the VANA protocol, from two laboratory populations from France (Montpellier, F population) and Portugal (Lisbon, P population), having different geographical origins and rearing history. Pools of mites from both of the populations were processed for virus-enrichment (VANA) metagenomics and high throughput sequencing. A total of 680,600 cleaned reads were obtained, including 219,982 reads from the French (F) population and 460 618 reads from the Portuguese (P) population.

De novo assembly of the VANA reads in both populations obtained fourteen viral contigs (1.6 to 8.6 kb in length) (Table 1). Thirteen out of the fourteen contigs were mostly related to non-enveloped DNA and RNA viruses belonging to clades infecting arthropods, including *Dicistroviridae*, *Parvoviridae*, *Birnaviridae*, *Nodaviridae*, and unclassified picornavirales. In addition, one viral contig (2481 nt) was similar to yeast and fungi-infecting viruses of the *Narnaviridae* family, which might come from environmental contamination (e.g., food), even though we cannot exclude its replication in spider mites [33]. While nine viral contigs were isolated in the P population only, five viral contigs were common to both of the populations (Figure 1), which was surprising given their different origins and rearing history.

Among the five viral contigs that are common to both viromes, the one that is assigned to the *Parvoviridae* family was largely dominant in terms of reads abundance (>28% of viral reads in both populations), with the others being found at much lower frequencies (0.1% to 10.6%) (Figure 1). Sequence analysis and open reading frame (ORF) prediction showed that this parvovirus has an ambisense genomic organization with a predicted small Non Structural protein-1 (NS1) that shared 39% aa identity with the NS1 of its closest relative, the Lupine feces-associated densovirus 2, which was discovered from viral gut metagenomics of the iberian wolf and has no associated arthropod host so far (accession number: ASM93489). Accordingly, the phylogenetic tree that is based on the NS1 protein clustered this densovirus with Lupine feces-associated densovirus 2 among the *Ambidensovirus* genus (Figure 2). According to the new species demarcation threshold in the *Densovirinae* sub-family that was proposed by the ICTV (i.e., < 85% related by NS1 amino acid sequence identity [34]), this new densovirus might represent a new divergent species in the *Ambidensovirus* genus and the first densovirus isolated from *Acari* (Figure 2, Table 1). Hereafter, this virus is referred to as Tetranychus urticae-associated ambidensovirus (TuaDV).

Although the *Birnaviridae* family has been poorly investigated, the phylogenetic analyses showed that the polymerase protein of Tetranychus urticae-associated birnavirus that was found in *T. urticae* viromes (representing 3.8% of reads) clustered with Drosophila melanogaster birnavirus (Figure 3) within an unclassified lineage. The polymerase and capsid proteins of this putative novel entomobirnavirus also shared 30% aa identity with the Infectious bursal disease virus (accession number AAS10174.1) and 33% aa identity with the Blotched snakehead virus (accession number YP_052864.1), respectively. Therefore, this putative novel birnavirus could represent the first birnavirus isolated from Arachnids (Table 1).

Table 1. Description of the fourteen virus contigs found in *T. urticae* viromes and protein identity comparison with their closest relatives.

Baltimore Classification	Viral Family	Viral Contig	Contig Length (nt)	Putative Protein	Best Hit (BLASTx)	Accession Number	Protein Identity (%)
ssDNA	*Parvoviridae*	Tetranychus urticae-associated ambidensovirus	3411	polymerase (NS1)	*Lupine feces-associated densovirus 2*	ASM93489.1	39%
				capsid		ASM93488.1	30%
dsRNA	*Birnaviridae*	Tetranychus urticae-associated birnavirus Segment A	2899	polymerase	*Infectious bursal disease virus*	AAS10174.1	30%
		Tetranychus urticae-associated birnavirus Segment B	2501	polyprotein	*Blotched snakehead virus*	YP_052864.1	33%
ss+RNA	*Nodaviridae*	Tetranychus urticae-associated nodavirus Segment A 1	3230	polymerase	*Hubei noda-like virus 9*	APG76321.1	58%
		Tetranychus urticae-associated nodavirus Segment A 2	2538	polymerase	*Hubei noda-like virus 8*	YP_009337881.1	62%
		Tetranychus urticae-associated nodavirus Segment B 1	1661	capsid	*Hubei noda-like virus 9*	YP_009337880.1	21%
		Tetranychus urticae-associated nodavirus Segment B 2	1658	capsid			53%
		Tetranychus urticae-associated nodavirus Segment B 3	1570	capsid			58%
	Dicistroviridae	Tetranychus urticae-associated dicistrovirus 1	8290	polymerase	*Beihai picorna-like virus 70*	APG78061.1	24%
				capsid		APG78062.1	20%
		Tetranychus urticae-associated dicistrovirus 2	8449	polymerase		APG78061.1	23%
				capsid		APG78062.1	20%
	Unclassified *Picornavirales*	Aphis glycines virus 1	8592	polymerase	*Aphis glycines virus 1*	AHC72013.1	96%
				capsid		AHC72012.1	99%
		Tetranychus urticae-associated picorna-like virus 1	8151	polymerase		AHC72013.1	71%
				capsid		AHC72012.1	75%
		Tetranychus urticae-associated picorna-like virus 2	6432	polypotein	*Hubei picorna-like virus 80*	YP_009337381.1	53%
	Narnaviridae	Tetranychus urticae-associated narnavirus	2481	polymerase	*Hubei narna-like virus 3*	YP_009337787.1	45%

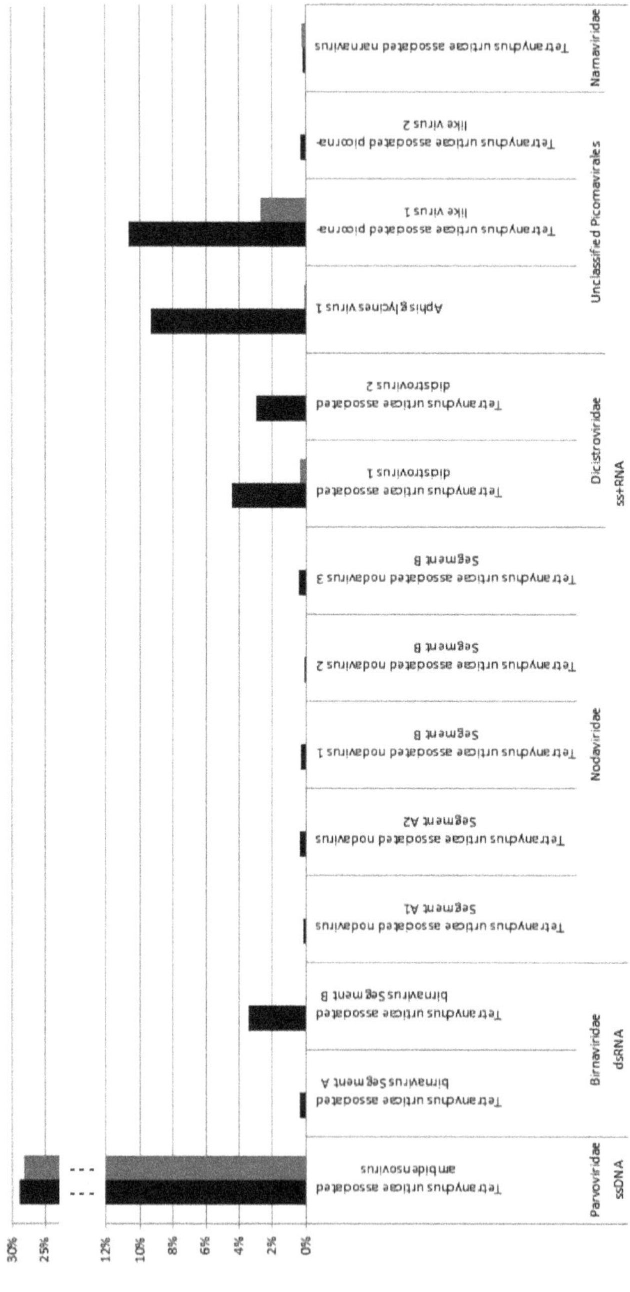

Figure 1. Relative abundance of putative viral species in the viromes of Portuguese (black) and French (grey) *T. urticae* colonies.

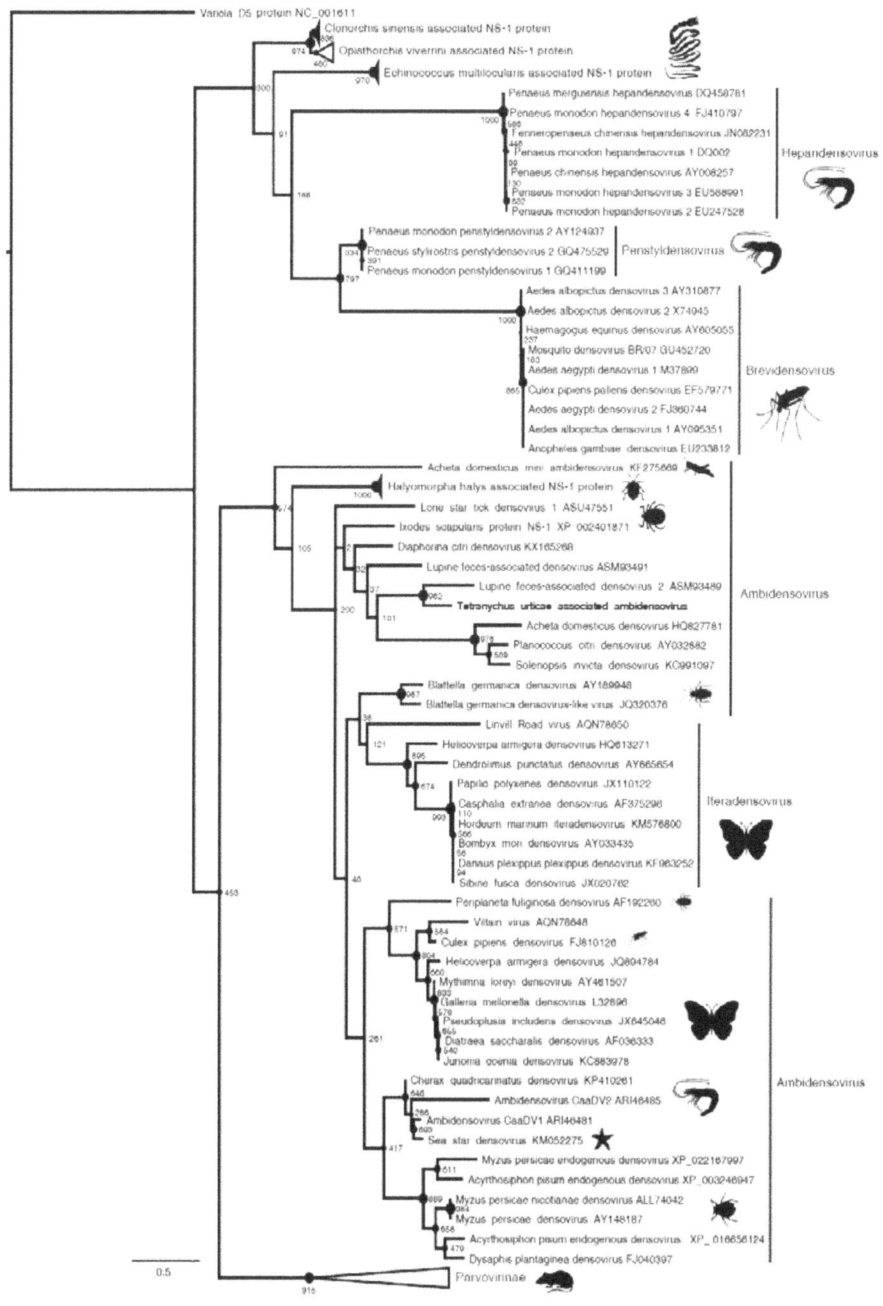

Figure 2. *Cont.*

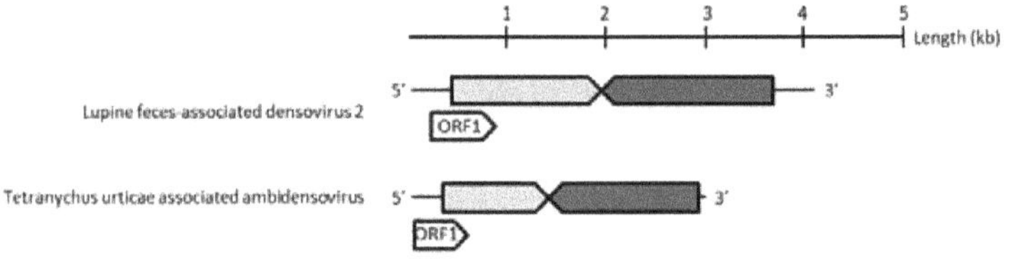

Figure 2. Maximum *Parvoviridae* likelihood phylogenetic tree based on a part of the NS1 protein containing the SF3 domain, including 105 parvovirus sequences and Tetranychus urticae-associated ambidensovirus (in bold). The alignment of 155 amino acids in length was produced using MUSCLE 3.7 (16 iterations) and was ungapped by hand. The tree was rooted with the SF3 domain of the Variola virus D5 protein. Bootstrap values are indicated at each node. Scale bar corresponds to amino acid substitutions per site. Genera of the *Parvoviridae* family are indicated in brackets. Genomic organization of Tetranychus urticae-associated ambidensovirus is also indicated. Grey arrows and rectangles: predicted open reading frames (ORF), Light grey: putative NS; dark grey: putative capsid protein (CP or VP). Arrow: complete ORF.

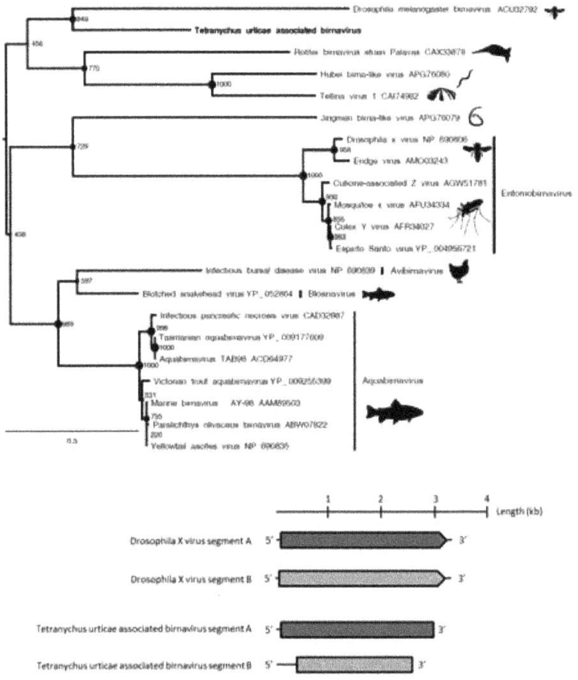

Figure 3. Maximum *Birnaviridae* likelihood phylogenetic tree based on part of the polyprotein, including 20 birnavirus species and Tetranychus urticae-associated birnavirus (in bold). The alignment of 602 amino acids in length was produced using MUSCLE 3.7 (16 iterations) and was ungapped by hand. The tree was mid-point rooted. Bootstrap values are indicated at each node. Scale bar corresponds to amino acid substitutions per site. Genera of the *Birnaviridae* family are indicated in brackets. Genomic organization of Tetranychus urticae-associated birnavirus is also indicated. Grey arrows and rectangles: predicted open reading frames (ORF), Light grey: putative NS; dark grey: putative capsid protein (CP). Arrow: complete ORF; Rectangle: truncated ORF.

Regarding two of the three viral contigs clustering within the *Nodaviridae* family (Figure 4, Table 1), coding for the capsid protein, and found in the P population only (representing 1.35% of reads), they share up to 58% aa identity with the Hubei noda-like virus 9 capsid protein (accession number:

YP_009337880.1), an unclassified RNA virus. According to the ICTV species demarcation threshold (<87% of capsid protein aa identity) and to the position of polymerase proteins in the phylogenetic tree, the nodaviruses that were found in *T. urticae* viromes may correspond to novel species-level lineages in a novel genus-level lineage in the *Nodaviridae* family (Figure 4, Table 1).

Five contigs were assigned to the *Picornavirales* order. While two contigs clustered in the *Dicistroviridae* family (hereafter referred to as Tetranychus urticae-associated dicistrovirus 1 and 2 (Tuad1 and Tuad2), the other three clustered with the unclassified Picorna-like viruses. The capsids of Tuad1 and Tuad2 both share 20% aa identity with Beihai picorna-like virus 70(accession number APG78062.1; Table 1). Based on the current species demarcation criteria that are used by the ICTV *Dicistroviridae* study group (<90% of capsid protein identity with closest relatives) and the phylogenetic analyses bases on the conserved polymerase protein (Figure 5, Table 1), it is likely that both of the contigs could belong to two novel species-level lineages of the *Dicistroviridae* family. Interestingly, the CP of one of the three unclassified picorna-like viruses shared >99% aa identity with the unclassified picorna-like Aphis glycines virus 1 (Table 1). In addition, the proteins of the two unclassified picorna-like viruses (hereafter referred to as *Tetranychus urticae*, being associated picorna-like virus 1 and 2) share 53% to 75% aa identity with Aphis glycines virus 1 and Hubei picorna-like virus 80 (Table 1). Their phylogenetic trees showed that they might belong to a highly divergent lineage within the *Picornavirales* order (Figure 5). Moreover, Tetranychus urticae-associated picorna-like virus *1* and *2* could represent a new species according to species demarcation criteria that are defined by the ICTV (<90% of capsid protein identity with closest relatives) (Table 1).

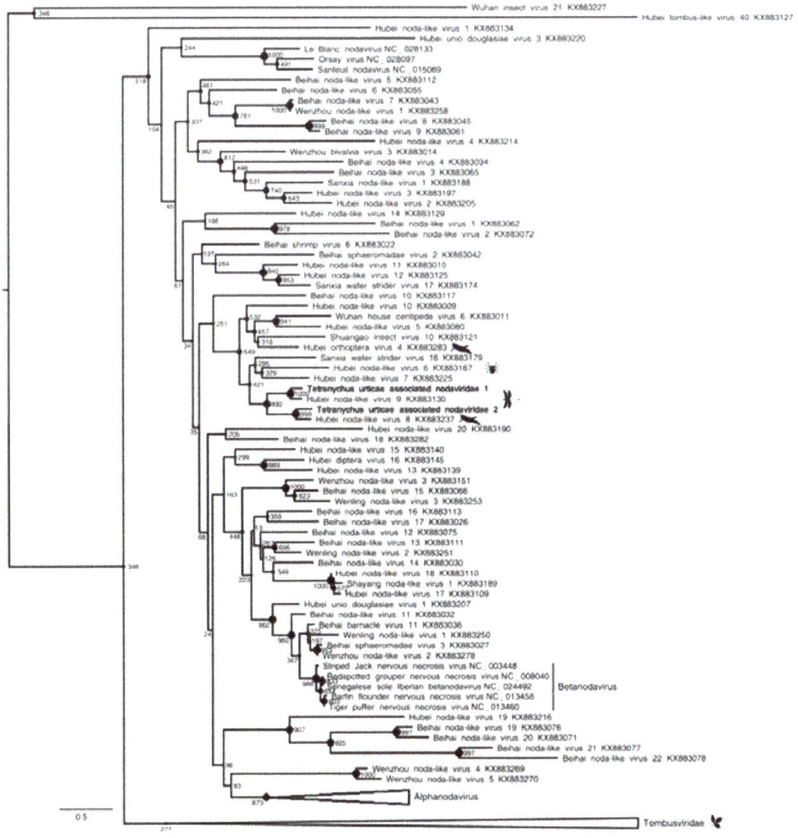

Figure 4. *Cont.*

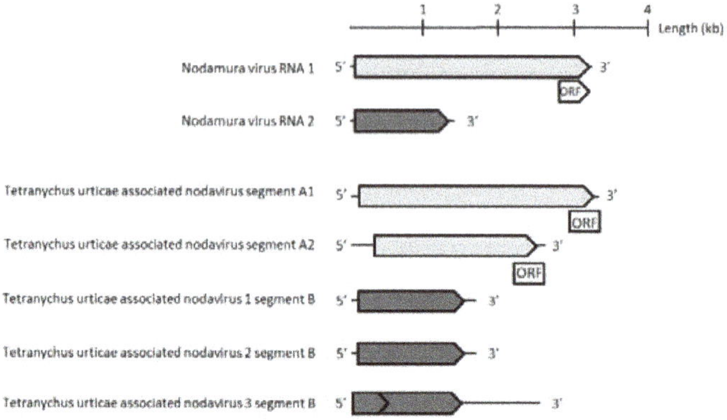

Figure 4. Maximum *Nodaviridae* likelihood phylogenetic tree based on part of the capsid protein, including 239 species and Tetranychus urticae-associated nodaviruses (in bold). The alignment of 229 amino acids in length was produced using MUSCLE 3.7 (16 iterations) and was ungapped by hand. The tree was mid-point rooted. Bootstrap values are indicated at each node. Scale bar corresponds to amino acid substitutions per site. Genomic organization of Tetranychus urticae-associated nodaviruses is also indicated. Grey arrows and rectangles: predicted open reading frames (ORF), Light grey: putative NS; dark grey: putative capsid protein (CP). Arrow: complete ORF; Rectangle: truncated ORF.

Finally, the Tetranychus urticae-associated narnavirus, present in 0.15% and 0.2% of reads in P and F populations, respectively, was the only one found in this study that historically belongs to a family of fungi-infecting viruses. Although very little is known regarding these viruses, the phylogenetic position of its polymerase protein within a clade including associated narnaviruses, as well as members of the *Ourmiavirus* genus, suggests that it might represent a new species-level lineage according to the ICTV species demarcation threshold (<50% of protein sequence identity as compared to the closest relative) (Figure 6, Table 1).

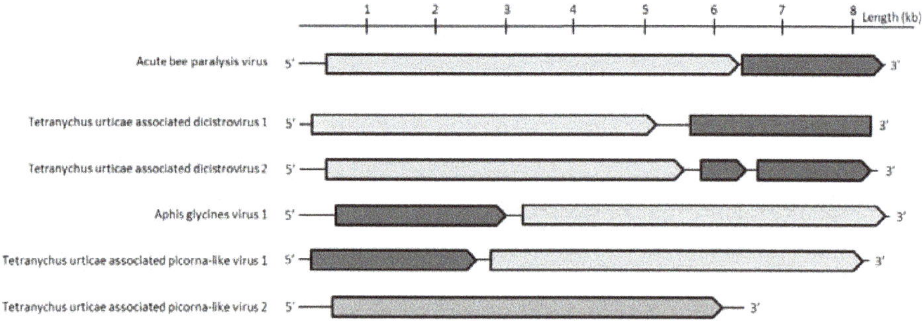

Figure 5. Maximum *Picornavirales* likelihood phylogenetic tree based on part of the polymerase protein, including 504 sequences and Tetranychus urticae-associated picornaviruses (in bold). The alignment of 386 amino acids in length was produced using MUSCLE 3.7 (16 iterations) and was ungapped by hand. The tree was mid-point rooted. Bootstrap values are indicated at each node, values <50% were discarded to not overload the tree. Scale bar corresponds to amino acid substitutions per site. Families of the *Picornavirales* order and genera of the *Dicistroviridae* family are indicated in brackets. Genomic organization of Tetranychus urticae-associated picornaviruses is also indicated. Grey arrows and rectangles: predicted open reading frames (ORF), Light grey: putative NS; dark grey: putative CP. Arrows: complete ORF.

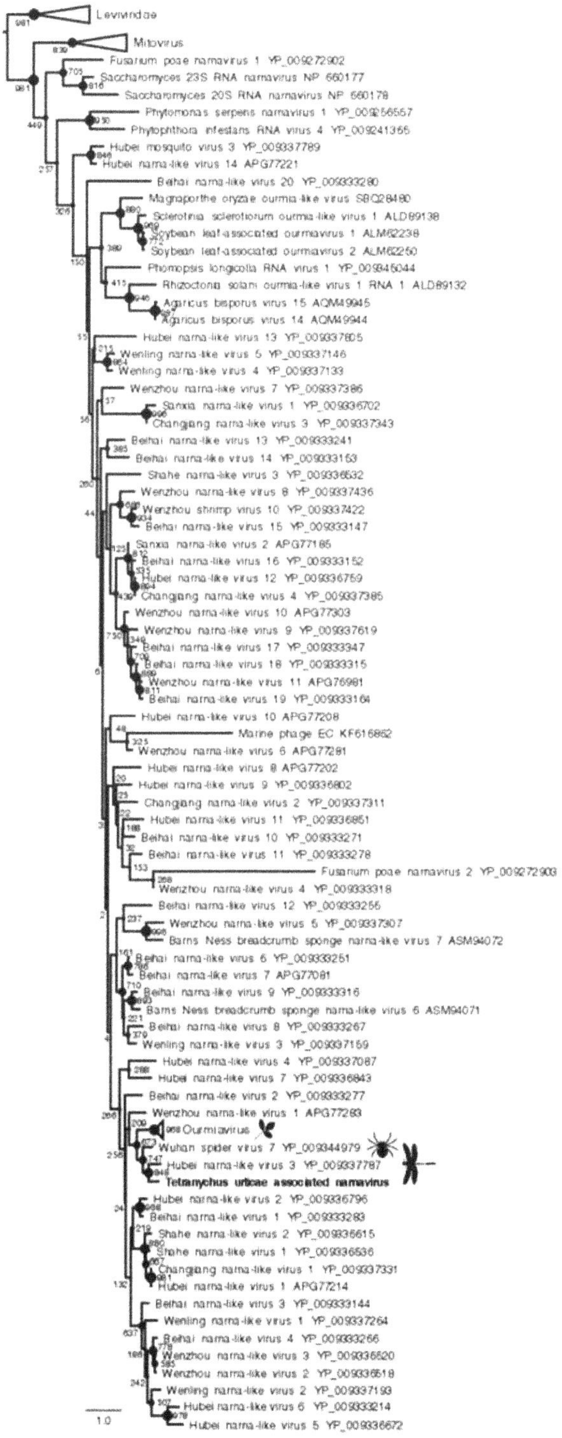

Figure 6. *Cont.*

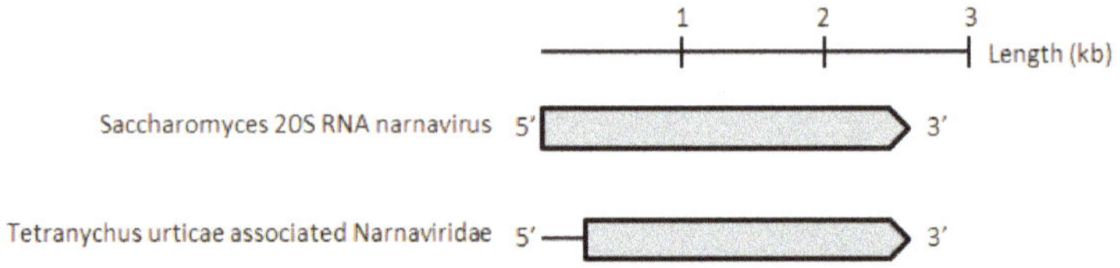

Figure 6. Maximum *Narnaviridae* likelihood phylogenetic tree based on part of the polymerase protein, including 129 species and Tetranychus urticae-associated narnavirus (in bold). The alignment of 121 amino acids in length was produced using MUSCLE 3.7 (16 iterations) and was ungapped by hand. Bootstrap values are indicated at each node. Scale bar corresponds to amino acid substitutions per site. Genomic organization of Tetranychus urticae-associated narnavirus is also indicated. Grey arrows: putative NS.

3.2. Genomic and Transcriptomic Database Screening

To gain insights into the diversity and the distribution of viruses in *T. urticae*, we further screened mite genomic and transcriptomic datasets using all ten viruses that were identified in this study as queries. Our search highlighted that *T. urticae* transcriptomes contained sequences that displayed >95% of nucleotidic identity to Aphis glycines virus 1 and Tetranychus urticae-associated picorna-like virus 1 (Table 2). Interestingly, one sequence that was related to an ambidensovirus was found in the genome of *T. urticae*, but this sequence was different from TuaDV (70% of nucleotidic identity with a sequence of 536 nt length). No sequence corresponding to TuaDV was found in any of the transcriptomes that were analyzed, suggesting that this virus might correspond to a non-endogenized virus, whose origin remains to be clarified.

In addition to these viruses, we found in *T. urticae* genomes and transcriptomes, 16 sequences belonging to large viruses, including giant viruses (*Mimiviridae*, *Phycodnaviridae*, *Poxviridae*, and *Baculoviridae*). These sequences were not found in the viromes that we generated in this study (i.e., using VANA based method) and we cannot exclude that the sequences corresponding to this large dsDNA virus might have a cellular rather than a viral origin. Eight sequences that were related to *Rhabdoviridae* were found in the *T. urticae* genome, which all corresponded to the nucleoprotein N, and we also found these sequences in the EST transcriptome (six sequences > 95% of nucleotide identity). Last, we also found sequences that were related to plant viruses in the TSA transcriptome of *T. urticae* that might originate from diet contamination. One transcriptomic sequence (accession number GW017620.1) matched with the Tetranychus urticae-associated nodavirus segment B1, although its small size did not allow its for assignation with high confidence (Table 2).

Table 2. Summary of the number of sequences found in the *Tetranychus urticae* genomic and/or transcriptomic databases that display homologies with viral species discovered in the viromes generated in this study.

Viral Contig	Contig Length (nt)	ref_seq Genomics	EST	TSA
Tetranychus urticae-associated ambidensovirus	3411	0	0	0
Tetranychus urticae-associated birnavirus Segment A	2899	0	0	0
Tetranychus urticae-associated birnavirus Segment B	2501	0	0	0
Tetranychus urticae-associated nodavirus Segment A 1	3230	0	0	0
Tetranychus urticae-associated nodavirus Segment A 2	2538	0	0	0
Tetranychus urticae-associated nodavirus Segment B 1	1661	0	**1**	0
Tetranychus urticae-associated nodavirus Segment B 2	1658	0	0	0
Tetranychus urticae associated nodavirus Segment B 3	1570	0	0	0
Tetranychus urticae associated dicistrovirus 1	8290	0	0	0
Tetranychus urticae associated dicistrovirus 2	8449	0	0	0
Aphis glycines virus 1	8592	0	**105**	0
Tetranychus urticae associated picorna-like virus 1	8151	0	0	**14**
Tetranychus urticae associated picorna-like virus 2	6432	0	0	0
Tetranychus urticae associated narnavirus	2481	0	0	0

3.3. Characterization of a Novel Densovirus in Spider-Mites

As pointed out above, the size of the densovirus contig found in mites populations was about 3.4 kb, which was much smaller than genomes characterized so far in the *Ambidensovirus* genus, which, when excluding the terminal repeats (ITRs), is around 4 kb for the Acheta domesticus mini ambidensovirus and up to 5kb for Lepidopteran ambidensoviruses [34]. Ambidensoviruses usually display a single ORF encoding for one to four structural proteins (VP1–4) that are produced by splicing or leaky scanning, and three ORFs encoding for non-structural (NS) proteins. Viruses in the *Parvoviridae* family are characterized by two typical domains: i) a phospholipase A2 (PLA2) motif located in VP1 of most parvoviruses, including in all species described so far in the *Ambidensovirus* genus; and, ii) a Super Family 3 (SF3) helicase domain that is located in the NS1 protein and common to all parvoviruses [35].

The contig corresponding to the TuaDV genome predicted three to four open reading frames (ORFs), one encoding a typical VP protein (ORF1), and two to three putative ORFs encoding NS proteins (ORF2–4) (Figure 2). 5′ and 3′ RACEs further verified the 5′ and 3′ ends of the viral genome and we performed overlapping PCRs with specific primers and sequenced the amplicons using the Sanger method (Figure 7). These results further confirmed that both of the populations shared the same TuaDV genomic sequence and that both expressed viral genes.

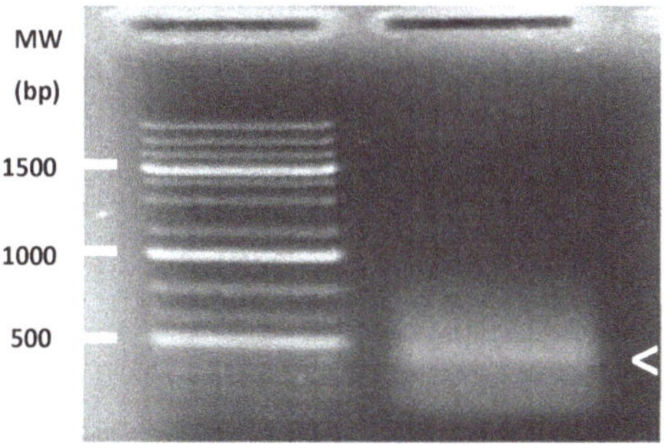

Figure 7. Identification of the transcription starting site of ORF2 (*ns* gene) of the TuaDV by 5′ RACE PCR. Agarose gel showed a major amplicon at ~500 bp (white arrowhead). The amplicon was sequenced to recover the 5′ end sequence.

We did not obtain any complementary sequence for ORF1 (VP), which thus predicted a 505-amino acids (aa) protein of 55 kDa that lacked the typical PLA2 motif that is common to all ambidensoviruses described so far. Concerning the reverse strand, we obtained the complete coding sequence of the NS ORFs with a predicted ORF2 (NS1) sequence of 354 aa protein of 39 kDa, harboring the typical SF3 domain, while a predicted ORF3 (NS2) has a 273 aa protein and a molecular weight of 30 kDa. In addition, a small ORF4 (95 aa) was predicted and it might encode for a putative 10 kDa NS3 protein. With such a compact genome, this virus would be the smallest densovirus that is described so far, including the Acheta domesticus mini ambidensovirus, with both viruses having sizes that are comparable to species from the *Iteradensovirus* genus. The closest relative of TuaDV was the Lupine feces-associated densovirus 2 (accession number KY214445.1), which shares 30% identity with NS1 and 31% identity with VP [36]. The putative NS2 of these viruses shared 25% identity. If correct, these NS predicted ORFs would have an ORF3 initiating upstream ORF2, which is unusual among ambidensoviruses. Based on the current species demarcation criteria that were used by the ICTV, all of these features suggest that TuaDV is a new mini ambidensovirus species among the *Ambidensovirus* genus that shares little sequence identity with the Acheta domesticus mini ambidensovirus.

Given the theoretical rapid evolution of ssDNA viruses [37], the fact that mite populations with different origins and rearing history share identical virus sequences more likely suggests that contamination occurred between laboratories, due to mites and material exchange, which is also supported by the introduction of the Almeria population in the Montpellier laboratory at the time.

3.4. TuaDV Prevalence and Diversity in Mite Populations

To better understand the origin of the TuaDV that infected the P and F reared populations (so-called here after TuaDV_Rearing (R) to discriminate from _Field populations), we investigated its prevalence and diversity in different *Tetranychus* species with different origins. Twenty-seven samples from three species of *Tetranychus* (*T. urticae*, *T. cinnabarinus*, and *T. evansi*) were collected from various fields in Portugal and from rearing facilities worldwide (France, Brazil, Netherlands, Belgium, and Crete), representing 19 and eight samples, respectively (Figure 8). Interestingly, the genome of the Lupine feces densovirus 2 was recently discovered by metagenomics from feces of Iberian wolves that were sampled in Portugal (South Douro region), which suggests that distant relatives of TuaDV are present in the environment, at least on the Iberian Peninsula.

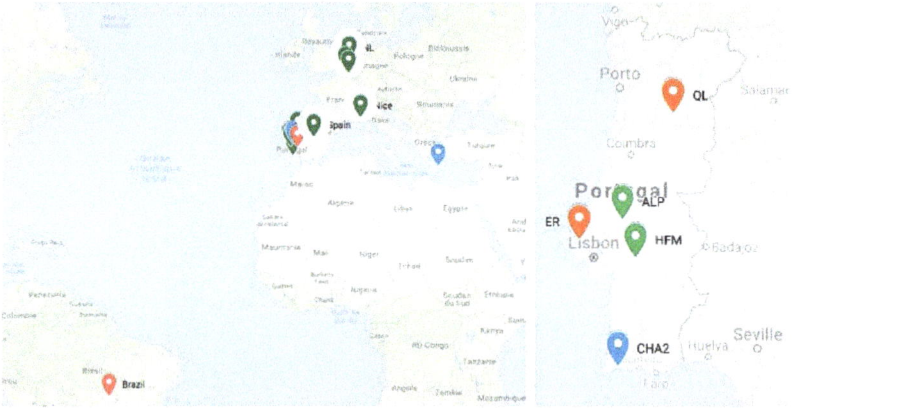

A B

Figure 8. Map representing the origin of spider mites' populations worldwide (**A**) and in Portugal (boxed) (**B**) where the prevalence of TuaDV has been assayed by PCR and sequenced (full or partial genome) and in Portugal (**B**). *T. urticae* (green), *T. cinnabarinus* (blue), and *T. evansi* (red). Maps were made from maps.google.com.

TuaDV presence and its genomic sequences in each population were confirmed by conventional PCRs using various sets of primers and sequencing (see Materials & Methods section). Note that each sample corresponds to a pool of mites from the same species that were collected in the same field/rearing. Amplicons were obtained with all sets of primers and they were of the expected size, for all samples, thus indicating 100% prevalence in the samples, and suggests a wide prevalence of TuaDV in spider mite populations, both in natural environments and from all of the rearing facilities tested. However, we cannot determine whether all of the individual mites were infected or few were highly infected.

To investigate the phylogenetic relationship between the viruses, we sequenced TuaDV amplicons from 11 selected samples, i.e., four *T. urticae* (a second sample from France, Belgium, Netherlands, and Portugal), four *T. cinnabarinus* (Portugal), and three *T. evansi* (Portugal and Brazil); for each species, one sample corresponds to mites that were collected from the field. We used various sets of primers in order to cover the full-length genome or the ORF2 (NS1 gene) only (Table S1).

We reconstructed the TuaDV full length genomes from three species that were recently collected in Portugal by sequence assembly and alignments. The recovered genomes displayed a high identity score (Table 3), with the TuaDV that was isolated from *T. evansi* being the most distantly related (81% identity with the original TuaDV_R genome; 86% when considering only the identity of NS1); although, these viruses belong to the same species according to the species demarcation criteria of the ICTV.

The TuaDV genomes that were sequenced from *T. urticae* and *T. cinnabarinus* were both similar to the initial TuaDV_R (99.8%; 100% identity of NS1), with only three and five synonymous substitutions between TuaDV_R and TuaDV from *T. cinnbarinus* and *T. urticae* from natural populations, respectively; the virus from the two natural populations differed by five substitutions, which further suggests that TuaDV_R originates from *T. cinnabarinus*. This relatedness is congruent with the phylogenetic position of *T. urticae* and *T. cinnabarinus*, often considered as two morphs of the same species, with *T. evansi* being more distantly related [19,20]. Moreover, it suggests that the infection of the population reared in Portugal originated from the Almeria population introduced in the rearing three years ago (see methods section).

Table 3. Percentage identity (DNA; aa) between the TuaDVs. *Upper panel.* VP1 coding sequence (CDS)/protein isolated from field populations. *Lower panel* NS1 CDS/protein isolated from field populations.

	T. cinnabarinus	***T. evansi***	***T. urticae*_Field**	***T. urticae*_R (TuaDV)**
T. cinnabarinus		(79.0; 79.6)%	(99.8; 99.4)%	(99.8; 100)%
T. evansi	(79.0; 79.6)%		(79.0; 79.6)%	(78.9; 79.6)%
*T. urticae*_Field	(99.8; 99.4)%	(79.0; 79.6)%		(99.6; 99.4)%
*T. urticae*_R (TuaDV)	(99.8; 100)%	(78.9; 79.6)%	(99.6; 99,4)%	

	T. evansi	***T. urticae*_Field**	***T. urticae*_R (TuaDV)**
T. evansi		(83.3; 86.0)%	(83.2; 86.5)%
*T. urticae*_Field	(83.3; 86.0)%		(99.9; 99.7)%
*T. urticae*_R (TuaDV)	(83.2; 86.5)%	(99.9; 99.7)%	

To better assess the prevalence and origin of the TuaDV, we partially sequenced ORF2 from 10 other spider mite samples that originated from natural and rearing populations worldwide. The results also revealed high identity scores between all of the populations, with the highest being within species (100% identity at the nucleotidic level) independently of their origin, i.e., from natural populations and rearings in Portugal.

Altogether, these results suggest that TuaDV is prevalent in natural populations of *Tetranychus* in Portugal and it displays a genetic diversity that likely correlates with the mite phylogeny. The poor genetic diversity that exists between the *T. urticae* laboratory and natural populations, with the exception of the Nice population, is striking and it suggests that infections of laboratory populations occurred in Portugal from wild populations and then spread between rearing facilities worldwide with material exchanges between laboratories. A broader geographical sampling of natural populations, including more *Tetranychus* species, needs to be performed in order to test this hypothesis and evaluate the diversity of TuaDV worldwide.

3.5. TuaDV Can be Vertically Transmitted and Circulate in Planta

In the search for the TuaDV route(s) of transmission, first we assayed TuaDV prevalence in individual mites using PCR. We found that 90% (18/20) of the individuals from the population HH4 tested were positive for TuaDV. Due to this high prevalence and the absence of an uninfected population, we did not test for horizontal transmission. We tested vertical transmission (from mothers to offspring), from 10 females from the HH4 population that all layed eggs and then tested 10 offspring per positive female. We found that seven females were positive to TuaDV, out of which four females had positive offspring, with levels of vertical transmission that greatly differed between females. Mean levels of vertical transmission was estimated at 28% ($\pm$ 0.9 SE), and it was highly variable between females with 8/10 for one female and 5/10 for the 3 others (versus 0/10 for females where no vertical transmission was detected). Such variability between offspring probably revealed quantitative variability in the vertical transmission of TuaDV. Although, we cannot exclude to have underestimated the vertical transmission due to the limit of the detection method.

Fecal-oral contamination is a common route of horizontal transmission. Interestingly, an aphid densovirus (MpDV) has been shown to be injected into plants by aphids and circulate *in planta*, which thus participate to its horizontal transmission to conspecifics [21]. Unlike aphids, mites used their stylets to pierce leaf mesophyll cells, where they then inject saliva and suck the cell cytoplasm. Mites are not considered to be vectors, although their feeding behavior injures their host, which can cause the transmission of viruses, in a way that is similar the mite *Varroa destructor* transmit viruses to bees [16]. To test whether TuaDV could be transmitted to the plant during mite feeding, we set up an infestation assay on bean plants (see method section) and assayed virus transmission to plant leaves by PCR. The results obtained from all pairs of primers showed that the leaves on which mites were reared on (L0) were all positive for the three populations tested. This result showed that infected mites have contaminated leaf surfaces, which further suggests that feces and/or saliva are a source of virus (Figure 9). Interestingly, the distant leaves (L8 and L20) were also positive, although the levels decreased with the distance from the primary leaf (L0), suggesting that the virus could circulate within the plant without replicating. Control leaves from the non-infested plants (no mites) and negative controls with no template were negative. We next wanted to quantify the likelihood of TuaDV transmission from the mite to the plant and between the leaves of different distances. Quantification of TuaDV from mites and leaves was performed using a pair of specific primers in ORF2 and a standard curve that was established from serial dilutions of a construct containing the Junonia coenia ambidensovirus genome as a proxy for TuaDV genome quantification. Negative controls (leaves with not mites) displayed Ct values that were similar to negative controls with no template. We estimated that the load of TuaDV per mite was 7.10^6 veg ($\pm$ 8.10^5 SE), and we found 2.10^7 veg ($\pm$ 4.10^6 SE) on L0, which represents the viral shedding from 50 mites for five days. Thus, viral shedding per mite with saliva and feces was estimated at 9.10^4 veg ($\pm$ 1. 10^4 SE)/day, which represents 1.5% ($\pm$ 0.37 SE) of the total amount of virus estimated per mite. Concerning leaves at 8 (L8) and 20 cm (L20) distance from L0, we found 2.10^4 veg ($\pm$ 7.10^3 SE) and 3500 veg/leaf ($\pm$ 3100 SE) in L8 and L20, respectively, with an increasing variation between experiments when increasing the distance from L0. Based on these results, we estimated that 0.08 % ($\pm$ 0.02 SE) of TuaDV contaminating L0 was inoculated into the plant vascular system and recovered in L8, and representing 0.017% ($\pm$ 0.016 SE) in L20. Levels of virus declined with distance from the infested leaf ($F_{2,10}$ = 124.08, $p < 0.0001$), but there was no different between the different populations ($F_{2,3}$ = 3.28, p = 0.1757).

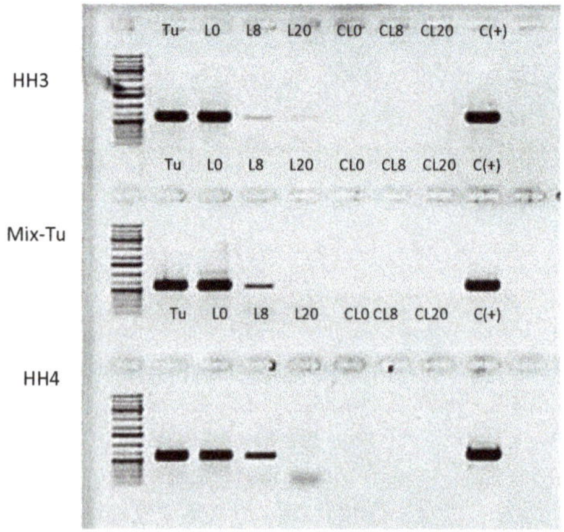

Figure 9. Transmission of TuaDV in plants. PCR from total DNA (100ng) extracted from mites, their isolated feeding leaf (L0) and two non-infested leaves at 8 and 20 cm distance (L8 and L20 respectively). Leaves from non-infested plants (CL0, CL8, and CL20) were used as negative controls, while mites were used as positive controls. Three independent F-populations were assayed (HH3, Mix-Tu, and HH4).

Altogether, these results showed that *T. urticae* could vertically and horizontally transmit TuaDV. Vertical transmission varies greatly between females, suggesting an important variation in the amount of virus that can be transmitted. Horizontal transmission occurred through the contamination of food (i.e., plant tissues) from virus shedding with feces and/or saliva. In addition, mites inoculate TuaDV to the plant vascular system, which then can probably circulate from cell-to-cell through plasmodesmata because of its small size (~20nm), to systemically reach distant leaves.

4. Discussion

In the work that is presented here, we used a viral metagenomic approach to explore the diversity of viruses that are associated with the spider mite *Tetranychus urticae*, a small arthropod that has long been neglected by virologists. We showed that several viruses simultaneously circulate in mites, including a panel of eight putative virus species that belong to small, non-enveloped viruses with a RNA genome, and one ssDNA virus with a predicted ambisense genomic organization and belonging to the *Densovirinae* sub-family [34]. This novel densovirus displays two uncommon features among ambidensoviruses, i.e., the most compact genome identified so far, all densoviruses included, and the absence of the PLA2 motif in the major capsid protein.

An unexpected result was that two mite laboratory populations with different origins shared a set of five viruses, representing 5 taxa. If we independently consider these viral taxa replicate, then the probability is low that five phylogenetically distant viruses were found together in two independent populations (although composed of the same host species) just by chance. Thus, the most parsimonious explanation is to consider that a cross contamination occurred between laboratories, especially when considering the absence of diversity between the common virus genotypes. One possibility is that the Almeria population of *T. cinnabarinus*, which was introduced three years ago in the Portuguese rearing, was at the origin of the contamination of the F population, as it was also maintained in Montpellier laboratory at the time the F-population was sampled.

A second unexpected result was to find that three years after we identified TuaDV (which represents more than 70 mites generations), nearly identical virus genotypes were still found to be circulating in both rearings, while considering the expected occurrence of sequence change in viruses due to error-prone replication (particularly high for RNA and ssDNA viruses [37]). One possibility could be that sequence change of virus genomes was slower than expected. In support of that hypothesis, we found that TuaDV genomic sequence from rearings differed by a few substitutions (3 to 5) from the sequences that were found recently in the natural populations of *T. urticae* and *T. cinnabarinus* sampled in Portugal and in different rearing facilities worldwide. Although the level of relatedness was high, we did observe slight differences, indicating that TuaDVs from the Netherlands (Santpoort) and Belgium (Ghent) were more closely related than they were to the samples from Portugal, and the TuaDV from Greece (Crete) was almost identical to the TuaDV from Portugal (99 to 100%). When considering that the Greek population is actually composed of a mix of populations from different origins, this suggests that a cross contamination probably occurred between the laboratories. More interestingly, we found that the TuaDV from the French population of *T. urticae* that originates from Nice-Valbonne was more distantly related to the other strains (88% with the ORF2 of TuaDV_R versus 94 to 100% that are shared by the other *T. urticae* samples). This population was collected in the Nice area 3–5 years ago and then reared there since then, without any exchange with the other facilities of this study (M. Ferrero, personal communication). This suggests that several strains of TuaDV probably circulate in natural populations. We speculate that TuaDV might be under stabilizing selection when circulating in *T. urticae* and *T. cinnabarinus*, that is that most new mutations would be deleterious and thus be quickly removed from the viral populations [38,39]. Moreover, the high identity score of the TuaDV genome found in two "sister" species, *T. cinnabarinus* and *T. urticae*, and the distance with TuaDV from *T. evansi* further supports that divergence and evolution have co-occurred with their hosts' evolution.

The third unexpected result was the discovery in mites viromes of contigs corresponding to three unclassified picorna-like related to Aphis glycines virus 1, one of them sharing 99% nucleotidic identity with the virus that was discovered in aphids at the University of Illinois and published in Genebank in 2013 (#KF360262), the two others being more distantly related (Table 1). Like for TuaDV, such sequence conservation was striking when considering the time and the geographic distance between sampling but also the phylogenetic distance between aphids and mites. The constraints of the host immune system are among mechanisms conditioning virus changes for adaptation. Interestingly, mites and aphids share a genome that has lost canonical components of the immune system [40]. We speculate that such feature may contribute to provide tolerant environments to viruses. Although, the mechanism remains to be addressed.

Most of the virus genotypes that were found in this study were classified within arthropod-infecting taxa and/or their closest phylogenetic taxa were associated with arthropods. The phylogenetic trees that we obtained for each virus highlighted the poor knowledge that we have on arthropod viruses [41–43], with viruses often being located at the base of the phylogenetic trees of the largest taxa, such as for *Parvoviridae* and *Picornavirales*, or grouped into poorly documented viral families, which indicates that a wealth of viruses from these groups remain to be discovered. The set of viruses that we found in this study mostly corresponds to small, non-enveloped viruses, which contrasts with sequences that are found in nucleotidic databases and corresponding to large viruses. The under-representation of large viruses in viromes prepared with the VANA method may result from a technical bias. Indeed, the filtration step that is used in this method to prepare viral particles could eliminate large viruses [44]. This observation thus pinpoints the need to combine approaches to get an exhaustive view of virus diversity that is associated with arthropods.

In natural or experimental populations, mite density can vary due to variation in mortality levels, which can occur without the knowledge of the causal agent(s)/conditions. Whether and how TuaDV affects the mites phenotype remains to be experimentally addressed. As the level of vertical transmission is relatively low, the establishment of TuaDV-free lines to investigate the role of TuaDV by experimental infection is made possible. Interestingly, persistent densoviruses can be found in aphids where they have been shown to confer protection against secondary infections by other pathogens, including viruses and bacteria [45,46]. Unlike those observed for densoviruses that were discovered in aphids, we could not find evidence of virus genomic integration in the mite genome, suggesting that the TuaDV could correspond to an extant virus [4,47]. However, we cannot exclude that viral sequences were cleaned off during *T. urticae* genome assembly [8].

It is becoming clear that both multi-infections and persistent viruses should be considered in order to better understand the phenotypic outcome of infections and the pathogenicity of specific strains that can change their life cycle, from pathogenic to persistent [48]. Densovirus persistent infections are likely common in aphids, and several densoviruses have been described, with one being transmitted through the plant [21,45,47]. Although we need to improve the viral loads quantification method, our results suggest that potentially large amount of TuaDV can contaminate plants when considering the high densities that mites colonies can reach. In a previous study, we described a new densovirus found from viral metagenomics from sea barley (*Hordeum marinum*), probably contaminating/circulating in the plant as well, since the virus was recovered from different leaves and was not associated with any arthropods host [49]. We hypothesized that plants participate to TuaDV horizontal transmission by concentrating viral particles on leaves, thus favoring the spreading of infection in mite populations. Furthermore, the systemic inoculation of viral particles in the plant vascular system could also provide the virus a protective niche against abiotic factors (particularly ultraviolet radiation from the sun) that can be detrimental for viral particles. Interestingly, our results also suggest that the plant might also mediate infections with a panel of arthropod-infecting viruses.

We hypothesized that virus abundance and/or transmission routes might have been selected for virus communities that occur as a unit within their host populations. Indeed, we find that five viruses co-occur and can be maintained in two separate laboratory populations for three years, even if the source is due to a recent contamination. Our results suggest that transmission can occur by vertical and horizontal routes, including via the host plant, leading to a wide prevalence in their host populations. This begs the question as to whether all of these viruses can occur in a multiple infection within single individual hosts or if they never co-infect but separately circulate in mite populations (i.e., one virus preventing the infection by others). Further investigation is required to evaluate whether these viruses interact in a synergic, antagonist, or neutral manner.

In addition to sharing common ecosystems and similar immunologic environments, mites and aphids also share diverse endosymbionts that may provide protection in compensation [40,50]. Whether and how viruses could also provide protection against immunological stress remain to be addressed. Experimental mite colonies could provide a powerful system to combine descriptive and manipulative experiments to test for virus pathogenicity in individual hosts; and their dynamics (prevalence and persistence), and evolution in host populations.

Supplementary Materials: The following are available online at http://www.mdpi.com/1999-4915/11/3/233/s1, Table S1: *Tetranychus* species screened for the presence of TuaDV, Table S2: Sequences of TuaDV primers.

Author Contributions: Conceived and designed the experiments S.F., A.B.D., P.R., R.F., M.O. Performed the experiments: S.F., D.M., L.R.R., S.L., D.F., I.S., C.D., E.F. Sampling: L.R.R., M.F., I.S. Analyzed the data: S.F., A.B.D., P.R., D.F., L.R.R. Contributed reagents/materials/analysis/tools: A.B.D., L.R.R., D.F., S.L., C.D., I.S. Wrote and review the paper: S.F., A.B.D., L.R.R., P.R., R.F., M.O.

Funding: This work was supported by a grant from the Plant Health and Environment INRA division (SPE) and a H2020-EU VIROPLANT grant (773567) to M.O. It was also supported by a PHC-PESSOA grant (38014YC) to A.D.B. and S. Magalhães.

Acknowledgments: S. F. was supported by a scholarship from the National Institute of Agronomical Research (INRA) and from the University of Montpellier (UM). This work is an ISEM contribution number 2019-042. We warmly thank T. Van Leeuwen (Ghent University, Belgium) for providing the LondonS and EtoxR lines, M. Ferrero (Bioline Agrosciences, France) for providing the *T. urticae* Nice-Valbonne strain, and J. M. Alba (University of Amsterdam, NL) for the Ghent strain. We also warmly thank M. van Munster, M. Uzest, V. Brault and S. Blanc for all the insightful discussions and D. Sarkozy for its critical reading of the manuscript.

Conflicts of Interest: The authors declare no conflict of interest.

References

1. Junglen, S.; Drosten, C. Virus discovery and recent insights into virus diversity in arthropods. *Curr. Opin. Microbiol.* **2013**, *16*, 507–513. [CrossRef] [PubMed]
2. Bovo, S.; Mazzoni, G.; Ribani, A.; Utzeri, V.J.; Bertolini, F.; Schiavo, G.; Fontanesi, L. A viral metagenomic approach on a nonmetagenomic experiment: Mining next generation sequencing datasets from pig DNA identified several porcine parvoviruses for a retrospective evaluation of viral infections. *PLoS ONE* **2017**, *12*, 1–17. [CrossRef] [PubMed]
3. Liu, H.; Fu, Y.; Xie, J.; Cheng, J.; Ghabrial, S.A.; Li, G.; Peng, Y.; Yi, X.; Jiang, D. Widespread Endogenization of Densoviruses and Parvoviruses in Animal and Human Genomes. *J. Virol.* **2011**, *85*, 9863–9876. [CrossRef] [PubMed]
4. François, S.; Filloux, D.; Roumagnac, P.; Bigot, D.; Gayral, P.; Martin, D.P.; Froissart, R.; Ogliastro, M. Discovery of parvovirus-related sequences in an unexpected broad range of animals. *Sci. Rep.* **2016**, *6*, 1–13. [CrossRef] [PubMed]
5. Lister, B.C.; Garcia, A. Climate-driven declines in arthropod abundance restructure a rainforest food web. *Proc. Natl. Acad. Sci.* **2018**, *115*, E10397–E10406. [CrossRef] [PubMed]
6. Walter, D.E.; Proctor, H.C. *Mites: Ecology, Evolution & Behaviour*; Springer: Dordrecht, The Netherlands, 2013.
7. Jeppson, L.R.; Keifer, H.H.; Baker, E.W. *Mites Injurious to Economic Plants*; Univ of California Press: Berkeley, CA, USA, 1975.

8. Grbić, M.; Van Leeuwen, T.; Clark, R.M.; Rombauts, S.; Rouzé, P.; Grbić, V.; Osborne, E.J.; Dermauw, W.; Ngoc, P.C.T.; Ortego, F.; et al. The genome of Tetranychus urticae reveals herbivorous pest adaptations. *Nature* **2011**, *479*, 487–492. [CrossRef] [PubMed]
9. Van Leeuwen, T.; Vontas, J.; Tsagkarakou, A.; Dermauw, W.; Tirry, L. Acaricide resistance mechanisms in the two-spotted spider mite Tetranychus urticae and other important Acari: A review. *Insect Biochem. Mol. Biol.* **2010**, *40*, 563–572. [CrossRef] [PubMed]
10. Beavers, J.B.; Reed, D.K. Susceptibility of seven tetranychids to the nonoccluded virus of the citrus red mite and the correlation of the carmine spider mite as a vector. *J. Invertebr. Pathol.* **1972**, *20*, 279–283. [CrossRef]
11. Reed, D.K.; Desjardins, P.R. Morphology of a non-occluded virus isolated from citrus red mite, *Panonychus citri*. *Experientia* **1982**, *38*, 468–469. [CrossRef]
12. Tokarz, R.; Williams, S.H.; Sameroff, S.; Sanchez Leon, M.; Jain, K.; Lipkin, W.I. Virome analysis of Amblyomma americanum, Dermacentor variabilis, and Ixodes scapularis ticks reveals novel highly divergent vertebrate and invertebrate viruses. *J. Virol.* **2014**, *88*, 11480–11492. [CrossRef] [PubMed]
13. Moutailler, S.; Popovici, I.; Devillers, E.; Vayssier-Taussat, M.; Eloit, M. Diversity of viruses in Ixodes ricinus, and characterization of a neurotropic strain of Eyach virus. *New Microbes New Infect.* **2016**, *11*, 71–81. [CrossRef] [PubMed]
14. Sakamoto, J.M.; Ng, T.F.F.; Suzuki, Y.; Tsujimoto, H.; Deng, X.; Delwart, E.; Rasgon, J.L. Bunyaviruses are common in male and female Ixodes scapularis ticks in central Pennsylvania. *PeerJ* **2016**, *4*, e2324. [CrossRef] [PubMed]
15. Xia, H.; Hu, C.; Zhang, D.; Tang, S.; Zhang, Z.; Kou, Z.; Fan, Z.; Bente, D.; Zeng, C.; Li, T. Metagenomic profile of the viral communities in rhipicephalus spp. ticks from Yunnan, China. *PLoS ONE* **2015**, *10*, 1–16. [CrossRef] [PubMed]
16. Levin, S.; Sela, N.; Chejanovsky, N. Two novel viruses associated with the Apis mellifera pathogenic mite Varroa destructor. *Sci. Rep.* **2016**, *6*, 1–9. [CrossRef] [PubMed]
17. Nazzi, F.; Brown, S.P.; Annoscia, D.; Del Piccolo, F.; Di Prisco, G.; Varricchio, P.; Della Vedova, G.; Cattonaro, F.; Caprio, E.; Pennacchio, F. Synergistic parasite-pathogen interactions mediated by host immunity can drive the collapse of honeybee colonies. *PLoS Pathog.* **2012**, *8*, e1002735. [CrossRef] [PubMed]
18. Palanga, E.; Filloux, D.; Martin, D.P.; Fernandez, E.; Bouda, Z.; Gargani, D.; Ferdinand, R.; Zabre, J.; Neya, B.; Sawadogo, M.; et al. Metagenomic-Based Screening and Molecular Characterization of Cowpea- Infecting Viruses in Burkina Faso. *PLoS ONE* **2016**, *11*, e0165188. [CrossRef] [PubMed]
19. Matsuda, T.; Morishita, M.; Hinomoto, N.; Gotoh, T. Phylogenetic Analysis of the Spider Mite Sub-Family Tetranychinae (Acari: Tetranychidae) Based on the Mitochondrial COI Gene and the 18S and the 59 End of the 28S rRNA Genes Indicates That Several Genera Are Polyphyletic. *PLoS ONE* **2014**, *9*, e108672. [CrossRef] [PubMed]
20. Matsuda, T.; Kozaki, T.; Ishii, K.; Gotoh, T. Phylogeny of the spider mite sub-family Tetranychinae (Acari: Tetranychidae) inferred from RNA-Seq data. *PLoS ONE* **2018**, *13*, e0203136. [CrossRef] [PubMed]
21. Van Munster, M.; Janssen, A.; Clérivet, A.; Van Den Heuvel, J. Can plants use an entomopathogenic virus as a defense against herbivores? *Oecologia* **2005**, *143*, 396–401. [CrossRef] [PubMed]
22. Uesugi, R.; Goka, K.; Osakabe, M. Genetic basis of resistances to chlorfenapyr and etoxazole in the two-spotted spider mite (Acari: Tetranychidae). *J. Econ. Entomol.* **2002**, *95*, 1267–1274. [CrossRef] [PubMed]
23. Wu, S.; Manber, U. Agrep–A fast approximate pattern-matching tool. In *Conference Proceedings: USENIX Winter 1992 Technical Conference*; USENIX Association: Berkeley, CA, USA, 1992; pp. 153–162.
24. Martin, M. Cutadapt removes adapter sequences from high-throughput sequencing reads. *EMB* **2011**, *17*, 10–12. [CrossRef]
25. Zerbino, D.R.; Birney, E. Velvet: algorithms for de novo short read assembly using de Bruijn graphs. *Genome Res.* **2008**, *18*, 821–829. [CrossRef] [PubMed]
26. Langmead, B. Aligning short sequencing reads with Bowtie. *Curr. Protoc. Bioinforma.* **2010**, *32*, 11–17.
27. Altschul, S.F.; Gish, W.; Miller, W.; Myers, E.W.; Lipman, D.J. Basic local alignment search tool. *J. Mol. Biol.* **1990**, *215*, 403–410. [CrossRef]
28. Edgar, R.C. MUSCLE: Multiple sequence alignment with high accuracy and high throughput. *Nucleic Acids Res.* **2004**, *32*, 1792–1797. [CrossRef] [PubMed]

29. Kearse, M.; Moir, R.; Wilson, A.; Stones-Havas, S.; Cheung, M.; Sturrock, S.; Buxton, S.; Cooper, A.; Markowitz, S.; Duran, C.; et al. Geneious Basic: an integrated and extendable desktop software platform for the organization and analysis of sequence data. *Bioinformatics* **2012**, *28*, 1647–1649. [CrossRef] [PubMed]
30. Dereeper, A.; Guignon, V.; Blanc, G.; Audic, S.; Buffet, S.; Chevenet, F.; Dufayard, J.F.; Guindon, S.; Lefort, V.; Lescot, M.; et al. Phylogeny.fr: robust phylogenetic analysis for the non-specialist. *Nucleic Acids Res.* **2008**, *36*, 465–469. [CrossRef] [PubMed]
31. Guindon, S.; Dufayard, J.-F.; Lefort, V.; Anisimova, M.; Hordijk, W.; Gascuel, O. New algorithms and methods to estimate maximum-likelihood phylogenies: Assessing the performance of PhyML 3.0. *Syst. Biol.* **2010**, *59*, 307–321. [CrossRef] [PubMed]
32. Abascal, F.; Zardoya, R.; Posada, D. ProtTest: Selection of best-fit models of protein evolution. *Bioinformatics* **2005**, *21*, 2104–2105. [CrossRef] [PubMed]
33. Dolja, V.V.; Koonin, E.V. Metagenomics reshapes the concepts of RNA virus evolution by revealing extensive horizontal virus transfer. *Virus Res.* **2018**, *244*, 36–52. [CrossRef] [PubMed]
34. Cotmore, S.F.; Agbandje-McKenna, M.; Chiorini, J.A.; Mukha, D.V.; Pintel, D.J.; Qiu, J.; Soderlund-Venermo, M.; Tattersall, P.; Tijssen, P.; Gatherer, D.; et al. The family Parvoviridae. *Arch. Virol.* **2014**, *159*, 1239–1247. [CrossRef] [PubMed]
35. Cotmore, S.F.; Tattersall, P. Parvoviruses: Small Does Not Mean Simple. *Annu. Rev. Virol.* **2014**, *1*, 517–537. [CrossRef] [PubMed]
36. Conceição-Neto, N.; Godinho, R.; Álvares, F.; Yinda, C.K.; Deboutte, W.; Zeller, M.; Laenen, L.; Heylen, E.; Roque, S.; Petrucci-Fonseca, F.; et al. Viral gut metagenomics of sympatric wild and domestic canids, and monitoring of viruses: Insights from an endangered wolf population. *Ecol. Evol.* **2017**, *7*, 4135–4146. [CrossRef] [PubMed]
37. Duffy, S.; Shackelton, L.A.; Holmes, E.C. Rates of evolutionary change in viruses: Patterns and determinants. *Nat. Rev. Genet.* **2008**, *9*, 267–276. [CrossRef] [PubMed]
38. Duffy, S. Why are RNA virus mutation rates so damn high? *PLoS Biol.* **2018**, *16*, 1–6. [CrossRef] [PubMed]
39. Simmonds, P.; Aiewsakun, P.; Katzourakis, A. Prisoners of war—host adaptation and its constraints on virus evolution. *Nat. Rev. Microbiol.* **2018**. [CrossRef] [PubMed]
40. Santos-Matos, G.; Wybouw, N.; Martins, N.E.; Zélé, F.; Riga, M.; Leitão, A.B.; Vontas, J.; Grbić, M.; Van Leeuwen, T.; Magalhães, S.; et al. Tetranychus urticae mites do not mount an induced immune response against bacteria. *Proceedings. Biol. Sci.* **2017**, *284*, 20170401. [CrossRef] [PubMed]
41. Marklewitz, M.; Zirkel, F.; Kurth, A.; Drosten, C.; Junglen, S. Evolutionary and phenotypic analysis of live virus isolates suggests arthropod origin of a pathogenic RNA virus family. *Proc. Natl. Acad. Sci. USA* **2015**, *112*, 7536–7541. [CrossRef] [PubMed]
42. Li, C.-X.; Shi, M.; Tian, J.-H.; Lin, X.-D.; Kang, Y.-J.; Chen, L.-J.; Qin, X.-C.; Xu, J.; Holmes, E.C.; Zhang, Y.-Z. Unprecedented genomic diversity of RNA viruses in arthropods reveals the ancestry of negative-sense RNA viruses. *Elife* **2015**, *4*, 1–26. [CrossRef] [PubMed]
43. Shi, M.; Lin, X.; Vasilakis, N.; Tian, J.; Li, C.; Chen, L.; Eastwood, G.; Diao, X. Divergent Viruses Discovered in Arthropods and Vertebrates Revise the Evolutionary History of the Flaviviridae and Related Viruses. *J. Virol.* **2016**, *90*, 659–669. [CrossRef] [PubMed]
44. Halary, S.; Temmam, S.; Raoult, D.; Desnues, C. Viral metagenomics: are we missing the giants? *Curr. Opin. Microbiol.* **2016**, *31*, 34–43. [CrossRef] [PubMed]
45. Van Munster, M.; Dullemans, A.M.; Verbeek, M.; Van Den Heuvel, J.F.J.M.; Reinbold, C.; Brault, V.; Clérivet, A.; Van Der Wilk, F. Characterization of a new densovirus infecting the green peach aphid Myzus persicae. *J. Invertebr. Pathol.* **2003**, *84*, 6–14. [CrossRef]
46. Xu, P.; Liu, Y.; Graham, R.I.; Wilson, K.; Wu, K. Densovirus Is a Mutualistic Symbiont of a Global Crop Pest (Helicoverpa armigera) and Protects against a Baculovirus and Bt Biopesticide. *PLoS Pathog.* **2014**, *10*, 2–12. [CrossRef] [PubMed]
47. Clavijo, G.; Van Munster, M.; Monsion, B.; Bochet, N.; Brault, V. Transcription of densovirus endogenous sequences in the Myzus persicae genome. *J. Gen. Virol.* **2016**, *97*, 1000–1009. [CrossRef] [PubMed]
48. Alizon, S.; de Roode, J.C.; Michalakis, Y. Multiple infections and the evolution of virulence. *Ecol. Lett.* **2013**, *16*, 556–567. [CrossRef] [PubMed]

49. Francois, S.; Bernardo, P.; Filloux, D.; Roumagnac, P.; Yaverkovski, N.; Froissart, R.; Ogliastro, M. A Novel Itera-Like Densovirus Isolated by Viral Metagenomics from the Sea Barley Hordeum marinum. *Genome Announc.* **2014**, *2*, e01196-14. [CrossRef] [PubMed]
50. Zélé, F.; Weill, M.; Magalhães, S. Identification of spider-mite species and their endosymbionts using multiplex PCR. *Exp. Appl. Acarol.* **2018**, *74*, 123–138. [CrossRef] [PubMed]

viruses

MDPI

Communication

Characterization of the RNA Transcription Profile of *Bombyx mori* Bidensovirus

Rui Li, Pengfei Chang, Peng Lü, Zhaoyang Hu, Keping Chen, Qin Yao * and Qian Yu *

Institute of Life Sciences, Jiangsu University, Zhenjiang 212013, China; 18086525387@163.com (R.L.); 15751000531@163.com (P.C.); penglu@ujs.edu.cn (P.L.); 15189184890@163.com (Z.H.); kpchen@ujs.edu.cn (K.C.)

* Correspondence: yaoqin@ujs.edu.cn (Q.Y.); qianyu@ujs.edu.cn (Q.Y.); Tel.: +86-1395-294-0568 (Q.Y.); +86-1505-085-3270 (Q.Y.)

Received: 19 March 2019; Accepted: 30 March 2019; Published: 3 April 2019

Abstract: *Bombyx mori* bidensovirus (BmBDV) is a single-stranded DNA (ssDNA) virus from the genus *Bidensovirus* of the Bidnaviridae family, which, thus far, solely infects insects. It has a unique genome that contains bipartite DNA molecules (VD1 and VD2). In this study, we explored the detailed transcription mapping of the complete BmBDV genome (VD1 and VD2) by rapid amplification of cDNA ends (RACE), reverse transcription quantitative real-time PCR (RT-qPCR), and luciferase assays. For the first time, we report the transcription map of VD2. Our mapping of the transcriptional start sites reveals that the NS genes in VD1 have separate transcripts that are derived from overlapping promoters, P5 and P5.5. Thus, our study provides a strategy for alternative promoter usage in the expression of BmBDV genes.

Keywords: *Bombyx mori* bidensovirus; RACE; RT-qPCR; transcription mapping; overlapping promoters

1. Introduction

Bombyx mori bidensovirus (BmBDV) is a unique bipartite DNA virus that currently represents the only species in the genus *Bidensovirus* of the Bidnaviridae family [1]. BmBDV exclusively infects the columnar cells of the larvae midgut epithelium, causing chronic densonucleosis disease. The virion of BmBDV has a non-enveloped, spherical, icosahedral structure, 20–24 nm in diameter, and packages a linear single-stranded DNA molecule from the VD1 (~6.5 kb, GenBank accession no. NC_020928) or VD2 (~6 kb, GenBank accession no. NC_020927) genome [2,3]. Furthermore, both VD1 and VD2 genomes are characterized by having inverted terminal repeats (ITRs) at their ends that form a panhandle structure and share a common terminal sequence (CTS) of 53 nts [4]. VD1 contains four open reading frames (ORFs; ORF1 to ORF4), which encode nonstructural protein 2 (NS2) [5], nonstructural protein 1 (NS1) [6], a major structural protein (VP) [7,8], and DNA polymerase (PolB) [9], respectively. VD2 contains two ORFs, encoding a nonstructural protein 3 (NS3) [3] and a minor capsid structural protein (P133) [10]. NS1 is a multifunctional protein, which is similar to the NS1 protein in parvoviruses, likely possesses activities involving ATPases, site-specific DNA binding, endonucleases, and helicases [6,11]. Thus, it is essential for various processes associated with virus replication [12]. NS2 shares no homology with the NS2 found in protoparvoviruses [5]. However, it may be an integral membrane protein, like the adenovirus death protein (ADP) [13], that may promote cell lysis and virus release [5]. The exact function of the NS2 protein is unknown [14]. PolB is homologous to family B DNA polymerase, which is involved in protein-primed replication [15,16]. BmBDV is the only virus that possesses an ssDNA genome and encodes a DNA polymerase [9,17]. The function of NS3 is unknown. Previous studies have shown that NS3 shares homology with the NS3 of *Galleria mellonella* densovirus (GmDV) [18] and the ORF11 in *Plodia interpunctella* granulosis virus (PiGV) [19], which may play an important role in virus replication [20]. P133 is the largest viral structural protein of BmBDV, and it is similar to the VP3 protein of the *Bombyx mori* cytoplasmic polyhedrosis virus (BmCPV), which belongs to the *Reoviridae* family [10,21]. The amino acid sequences of P133 in the leucine zipper region were conserved and protein homologues occur mainly in the outer layer of the viral capsid, so P133 may interact with viral DNA and be related to virus invasion of host [22]. In addition, BmBDV replicates its genome using a unique DNA replication mechanism that does not follow the typical rolling circle replication model initiated by an enzyme replicator, as other known ssDNA viruses do. Thus, the strategy of BmBDV replication is of great interest to investigate.

Previously, the transcription strategy of the VD1 genome of BmBDV has been studied to some extent. Transcript mapping [23] shows that VD1 produces three mRNAs of 1.1 kb, 1.5 kb, and 3.3 kb in size, respectively. The nonstructural proteins (NS1 and NS2) are expressed by alternative initiation codons from a 1.1 kb mRNA transcript [1], and the major structural proteins (VPs) are expressed by a leaky scanning mechanism [7,8] from a 1.5 kb mRNA transcript. The 3.3 kb mRNA transcript contains the ORF4 that encodes DNA polymerase (PolB). Alternative splicing of mRNA transcripts was not observed during BmBDV gene expression and the transcription strategy of VD2 has not been studied.

In this report, we explore the complete transcription strategy of both the VD1 and VD2 genomes. We find that VD1-NS gene has two separate transcripts, which may be controlled by two overlapping promoters (P5/5.5), which differ from previous studies. We present an analysis of the transcription modalities of NS in VD1. We analyze the NS transcripts of VD1 by reverse transcription quantitative real-time polymerase chain reaction (RT-qPCR) as well as the activity of overlapping promoters' (P5/5.5) activities using a dual-luciferase reporter assay system.

2. Materials and Methods

2.1. Insect Rearing and Virus Propagation

A major impediment to bidensovirus studies is the lack of permissive insect cells that support virus replication in vitro [24]. Therefore, we used a variant of *Bombyx mori* silkworm (Jingsong × Haoyue), which is sensitive to BmBDV infection. The preserved silkworm eggs stored at 4 °C were removed from the refrigerator for pickling to hatch the diapause silkworm eggs. After the larvae had hatched from the eggs, we conducted timely feedings of silkworm larvae using moderately clean and fresh mulberry leaves. On the first day of the fifth instar, the BmBDV solution (5 μL per head) was freshly prepared and used to feed silkworms via oral instillation. We obtained the midguts of silkworms from BmBDV-infected larvae at 24, 48, 72, and 96 h post-infection (hpi), respectively, by dissecting silkworms at different phases. Silkworm midguts were kept in RNAlater® Solution (Invitrogen, Carlsbad, CA, USA) at −80 °C prior to RNA preparation.

2.2. Viral mRNA Extraction and RT-PCR

Total RNA was isolated from BmBDV-infected silkworm midguts (24, 48, 72, and 96 hpi) using Trizol® Reagent (Invitrogen, Carlsbad, CA, USA), as previously reported [24]. The quality of RNA was detected by its absorption value at 260 nm and gel electrophoresis on a 1% agarose gel. The mRNA was extracted using the Poly(A)Purist™ MAG Kit (Invitrogen, Carlsbad, CA, USA) according to the manufacturer's instructions. Reverse transcription (RT)-PCR was performed to identify viral mRNA transcripts from infected larvae and to determine the optimal time to analyze viral mRNA. The primers used are listed in Table S1.

2.3. Identification of the 5′ and 3′ Ends of Viral Transcripts

The full length of cDNA of each gene and the 5′ starts and 3′ ends of the viral transcripts were determined by rapid amplification of cDNA ends (RACE) using SMARTer® RACE 5′/3′ Kit (Clontech, Dalian, China) in accordance to the manufacturer's instructions. Primers were synthesized at Generay Biotech Co, Ltd. (Shanghai, China). Primer sequences are shown in genes in Figure S1, and BmBDV-specific primers are shown in Table S1. All PCR products (see Figure S2) used for the RACE experiments were subsequently cloned into pEASY®-T3 cloning vectors (Transgen, Beijing, China) and submitted for sequencing (see Figures S3 and S4) at Sangon Biotech Co, Ltd. (Shanghai, China).

2.4. Analysis of NS Transcripts from VD1 Using RT-qPCR

The NS1 and NS2 gene segments were amplified using RT-PCR, and the PCR products were extracted using the E.Z.N.A.® Cycle-Pure Kit (Omega, GA, USA). Standard curves of NS1 and NS2 mRNAs were drawn (see Table S2) using the 7300 Fast system (Applied Biosystems, Foster City, CA, USA). The locations of primers targeting NS transcripts are shown in Figure S1, and their sequences are shown in Table S1. The forward primer F2 was unique to NS2 transcripts. Primer F2/R was used to specifically amplify the NS2 transcript, and primer F1/R was used to amplify both transcripts.

2.5. Activities of the Overlapping Promoters P5/5.5

We made two constructs (P1 and P5) (see Figure S5) that have the NS1 and NS2 transcription initiation sites (Inr1 and Inr2) to analyze promoter activities (Figure 4A), in which the intact upstream promoter elements were cloned into the luciferase reporter plasmid (PGL3-basic). Various mutants were generated, in which all ATGs were mutated to ACCs, or the Inr1 (CATT) for the NS1 initiation site was mutated to TTTT, and the TATA1 for NS1 TATA box (TATA1) was mutated to GCGC. Different constructs containing the intact luciferase initiation codon (P1 to P6) served as a positive control for transcription, whereas those lacking the luciferase initiation codon (P1- to P6-) served as reporters. The construct, together with pRL-ie1 was co-transfected into two insect cells (BmN and Hi5) using Cellfectin® reagent (Invitrogen, Carlsbad, CA, USA) in accordance with the manufacturer's instruction. Cells were harvested at 48 hpi, and luciferase activity was determined using the Dual-Luciferase® Reporter Assay System (Promega, Madison, WI, USA) as previously described in reference [25], using the pGL3 luciferase reporter vectors and the pRL-ie1 vector. All of the constructs in this study were verified by sequencing.

3. Results

3.1. Mapping of the Transcripts by 5′/3′ RACE

The full-length cDNA of each gene is shown in Figure 1. Each gene corresponding to a full-length cDNA band, except for NS3, is indicated. Two bands were detected in lane 6 (NS3). The lower band was the same size as predicted, and the upper band was verified to be a non-specific amplified band.

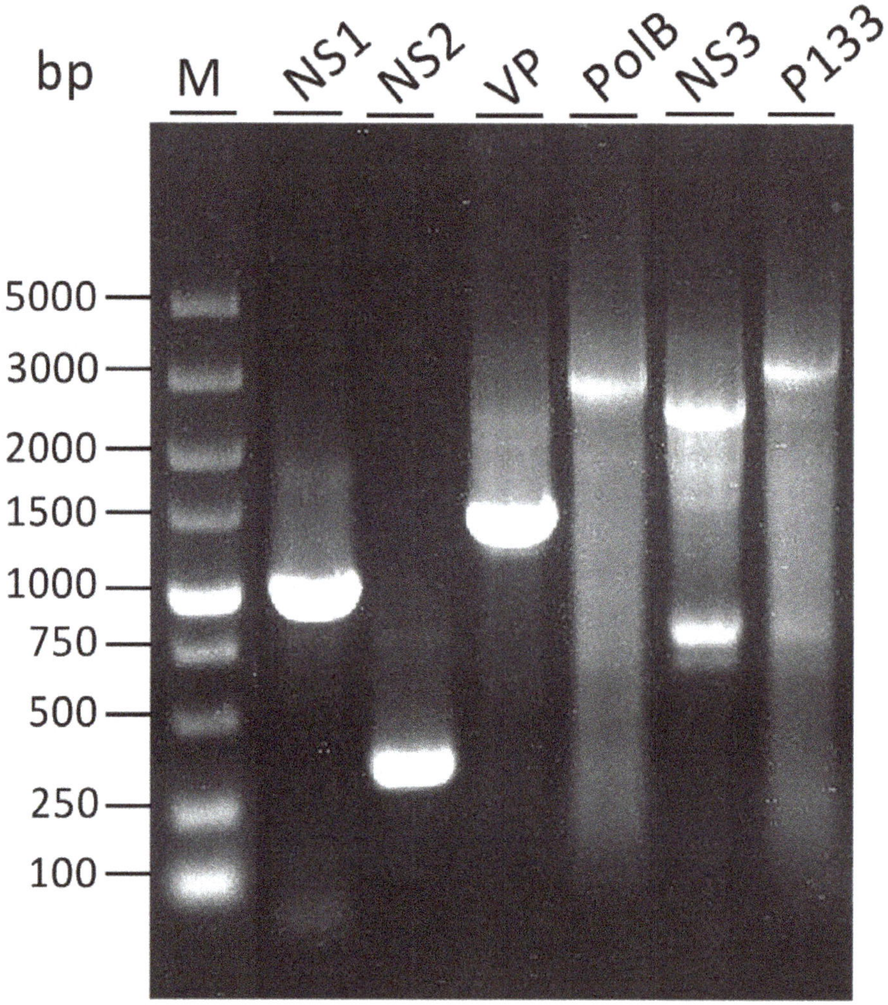

Figure 1. Detection of the full length of cDNA of each gene. Two bands appear in lane 6 (NS3). The lower band was the same size as the predicted, and the upper band has been verified as a non-specific band. The 5′RACE-Ready cDNA was amplified using reverse gene-specific primers (GSPs) (NS1endR, NS2endR, VPendR, PolBendR, NS3endR, P133endR) in Table S1, and universal primer mix (UPM) in the kit.

The results of the RACE experiments showed that each transcript corresponded to an ORF, thus alternative splicing of any mRNA transcripts was not observed. For VD1, in contrast to what was reported previously from one transcript, it was clear that NS1 and NS2 were transcribed from two different transcripts (Figure 2A) [23]. The NS2 transcript started at nt 290, and the NS1 transcript started at nt 316, 3 nts downstream of the NS2 initiation codon. NS2 started at nt 290, which is located at the TATA box of the promoter transcribing NS1. All NS1 and NS2 transcripts terminated at nt 1438 from one canonical AAUAAA polyadenylation signal. The VP transcript started at nt 1350, upstream of the polyadenylation site for NS transcripts, and terminated at nt 2929, which overlapped with the 3′ end of the NS transcript by 89 nts. Notably, the PolB open reading frame (ORF) initiated at

6 nt downstream of the previously presumed ATG, which was 21 nts downstream of the TATA box of the P97 promoter. Consequently, the complementary strand of the PolB transcript overlapped with the VP transcript by 4 nt, which warrants further investigation for any regulatory function.

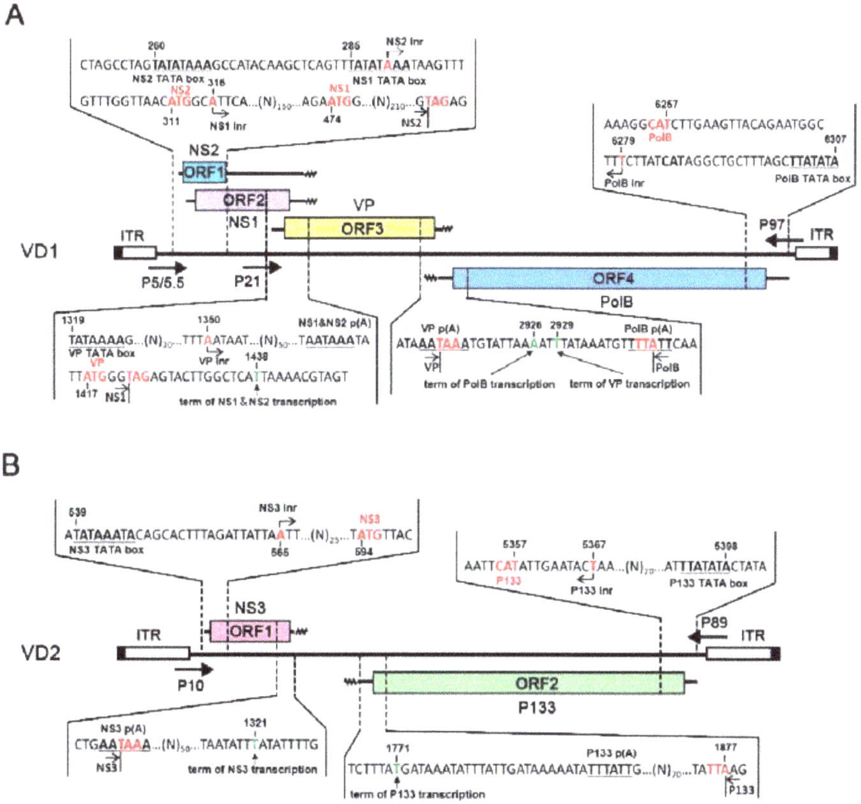

Figure 2. Mapping of 5′ and 3′ ends of *Bombyx mori* bidensovirus (BmBDV) transcripts: (**A**) mapping of 5′ and 3′ ends of VD1, (**B**) mapping of 5′ and 3′ ends of VD2. The bars with inverted terminal repeats (ITRs) at both ends represent the BmBDV genome. Major open reading frames (ORFs) that encode proteins are shown as boxes, whereas mRNA transcripts are indicated in the middle. The wavy lines indicate polyA tails. The arrows indicate the position of the VD1 and VD2 promoters.

For VD2, NS3 started at nt 565, 19 nts downstream of the P10 promoter TATA box at the 5′ end of VD2. The P133 transcript started 24 nt downstream of the P89 promoter TATA box at the 3′ end of VD2 (nt 5367), only 10 nts upstream of the first ATG, and it terminated at nt 1771. In contrast to VD1, NS3 and P133 transcripts terminated at two polyadenylation sites, which were far apart from each other, unlike like VP and PolB mRNAs, which had 4 nts of overlap.

3.2. Analysis of NS Transcripts in VD1

Using 5′ RACE, we observed that two NS transcripts were initiated from different locations on VD1 (Figure 3). This is in contrast to a previous study that showed the NS1 and NS2 transcripts shared the same start site from nt 316 [23]. In order to verify the transcription of NS1 and NS2, we used RT-qPCR to determine the copy numbers of NS1 and NS2 transcripts. Specific primers of the NS2 transcript (F2/R1-2) (Table S1) were used to amplify NS2-specfic transcripts. Surprisingly, specific primers of NS

(F1/R) (Table S1) amplified not only NS1 transcripts but also NS2 transcripts. The NS2 transcription of NS2 was later than that of NS1 because the NS2 transcripts were not observed at 24hpi (Figure 4), but both NS2 and NS1 transcripts were detected from 48 to 96 hpi. Therefore, we conclude that NS1 and NS2 are not transcribed from the same promoter.

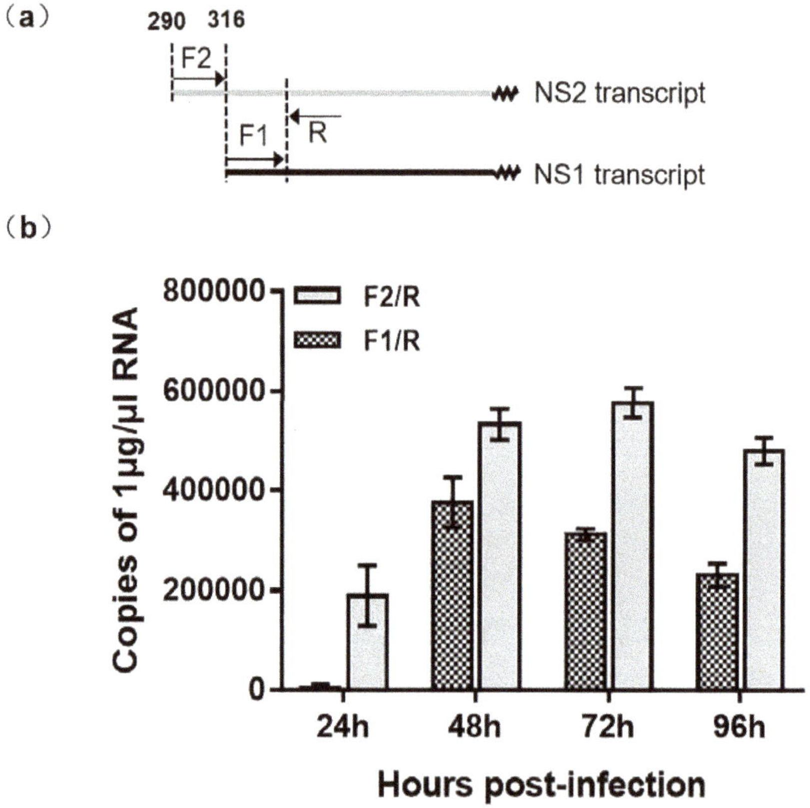

Figure 3. Analysis of NS transcripts of VD1 by RT-qPCR. (**a**) Locations of primers for RT-qPCR. The forward primer F2 is a specific primer for the NS2 transcript, and F1 is shared by the NS2 and NS1 transcripts, which have the same reverse primer, R. (**b**) The copy numbers of the products are amplified. The gray column represents the copy numbers of mRNA products amplified by primer F2/R, and the shadow column indicates the copy numbers of the products amplified by primer F1/R. (n=3), Error bars denote standard deviation.

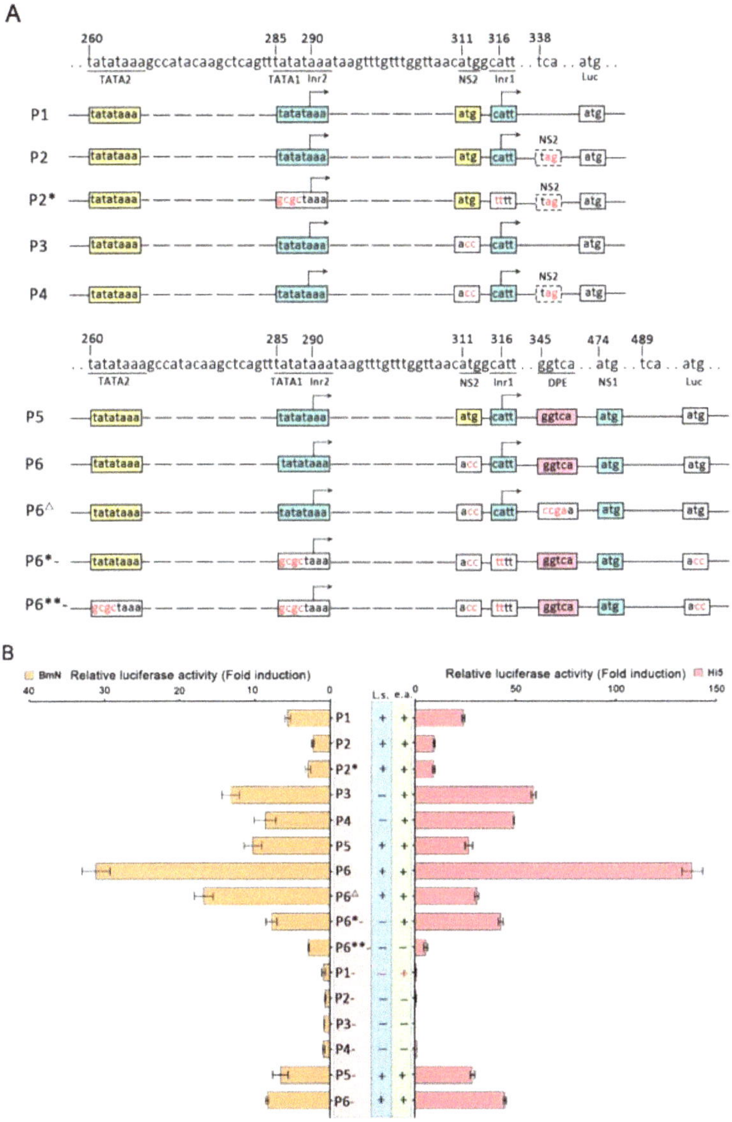

Figure 4. Analysis of P5/5.5 promoter elements using the luciferase reporter system. (**A**) The luciferase reporter plasmids contain NS1 and NS2 transcription initiation sites (Inr1 and Inr2), an NS1 or NS2 initiation codon (ATG), and its intact upstream promoter elements. In the constructs, the boxes represent elements, and the gray boxes represent replaced sequences. In addition, mutants were made for all constructs in which the initiation codon of luciferase was mutated (P1- to P6-), and two constructs, TATA1 and Inr1 (for NS1 transcripts), were mutated (indicated by *). ** represents Inr1. TATA1 and TATA2 all were mutated, and then DPEs were mutated (indicated by $^{\Delta}$). (**B**) The observed luciferase activity. The tendency of activity levels to change in different insect cells (Hi5, BmN) was consistent ("l.s." represents luciferase activity if leaky scanning occurs and "e.p." represents overall expected activities). (n = 3), Error bars denote standard deviation.

3.3. The Function of Overlapping Promoters (P5/5.5)

The results of RACE and RT-qPCR revealed that the NS genes in VD1 expressed separate transcripts. Since there were two TATA box elements upstream of the transcription initiation of NS1, we speculated that the NS1 transcripts may be under the control of two overlapping promoters (P5/5.5). To test this hypothesis, various reporter plasmids were constructed (Figure 4A), and were co-transfected with pRL-ie1 into insect cells (BmN, Hi5), followed by analysis of the function of the two overlapping promoters using luciferase assays. We constructed plasmids (P1 to P4) (Figure 4A) to clearly understand the functions of the two overlapping promoters (P5/5.5). The plasmids (P1 to P4) were expected to express both NS1 and NS2 mRNA. However, we observed low luciferase activity of P1 and P2 (Figure 4B), which came from the NS2-fused protein with luciferase, as direct translation or leaky scanning from the luciferase initiation codon depends on NS1 or NS2 transcripts. Unexpectedly, P1- had no activity when the luciferase initiation codon (ATG) was mutated. This indicated that P5/5.5 had weak activity, which may have been insufficient to start NS2 transcription. In addition, the NS2 initiation codon may not be functional. Therefore, we constructed P3 and P4 by mutating the NS2 initiation codon (ATG) for further examination. Obviously, the results indicated that the activity of P3 and P4 increased, and P3 yielded a 1.3-fold increase and P4 yielded a 2.6-fold increase in luciferase activity, respectively, compared to P1 and P2, in Hi5 cells. Hence, we concluded that the NS2 initiation codon affects the translation of luciferase.

To investigate the function of P5/5.5 in NS1 transcription, we constructed plasmids (P5 to P8) (Figure 4A). We already knew that the NS2 initiation codon negatively regulates luciferase expression. As expected, P5 induced a level of activity that was low but higher than that of P1, suggesting that the promoter may be under the control of a downstream promoter element (DPE). Previous studies have suggested that a DPE consensus, RGWYV(T), is located about 28 to 33 nts downstream of the transcription start site [26]. Particularly, we found a DPE-like sequence, GGTCA, located at 29 nts to 33 nts downstream of Inr1. In order to explore impacts on transcription of NS1 and NS2, the $P6^{\Delta}$ observed through the DPE-like sequence GGTCA in P6 was mutated to CCGA. As expected, the luciferase activity of $P6^{\Delta}$ declined rapidly compared to that of P6.

Transcription initiation is one of the most important control points in the regulation of gene expression [27]. P2* and P6*- only generated NS2 transcripts of NS2 by knocking out TATA1 and Inr1. As indicated from the results, the activity of P2* was similar to that of P2. These results indicate that the two overlapping promoters (P5/5.5) had weak activity levels, which further proved our previous hypothesis. P6*- and P6- had high levels of activity, and the initiation of NS1 and NS2 transcription was closely positioned at either side of the NS2 initiation codon (Figure 2A). Consequently, NS1 could be generated from the NS2 transcript by alternative initiation. In order to investigate the function of NS1 promoter elements for NS2, we made P6**- by knocking out TATA2 in P6*-. The results showed that the activity declined drastically in luciferase activity compared to that of P6*-. However, P6**- also presented a lower level of activity. In conclusion, our deletion analyses suggest that the promoter can induce TATA-box-independent transcription.

4. Discussion

BmBDV was classified as a member of the family *Bidnaviridae* by the International Committee on Taxonomy of Viruses (ICTV) in 2012 [1]. At that time, it was the only species of the *Bidensovirus* genus identified in insects. With the development of metagenomics, more and more viruses have been found in environmental and biological samples [28]. Recently, the presence of ssDNA viruses of the *Bidnaviridae* family in sponges and corals has been reported [29].

In this study, we analyzed the transcription strategies of BmBDV. Transcription mapping was used to show the transcription initiation and termination sites of each gene in BmBDV (see Figure 2). Interestingly, Figure 2A shows that the transcription initiation sites of NS1 and NS2 are closely positioned at either side of the NS2 initiation codon, so NS1 can be generated from the NS2 transcript by alternative initiation. This characteristic is similar to that of *Aedes albopictus* densovirus (AalDV) [30] during transcription. NS1 and NS2 may be encoded from separate transcripts (see Figure 3), which are transcribed by two overlapping promoters. In fact, as shown in Figure 4A, the promoter driving NS2 transcription is the P5 promoter, which contains TATA2 and Inr2. However, since there are two TATA box elements upstream of the transcription initiation of NS1, NS1 transcription may be under the control of P5/5.5. We also found that in VD1, P5/5.5, which drives the transcription of the NS gene is a weak promoter, but its activity is enhanced in the presence of DPE. In BmBDV, both the TATA box and Ins play important roles in the high activity of the promoter driving NS1 and NS2, but are not sufficient to drive the transcription of NS1 genes in BmBDV [25]. Therefore, the transcription of NS2 and NS1 are synergistically driven by overlapping promoters and DPE. Therefore, the expression of NS1 is guaranteed by alternative and overlapping promoters. We know that NS1 is a multifunctional protein that is essential for various processes involved in viral propagation [12]. Obviously, the transcription profile of VD1-NS genes benefits the expression of NS1. Based on the phylogenetic tree analysis of parvovirus NS1, it has been speculated that the *Brevidensovirus* genus is the ancestor of other parvoviruses [31]. AalDV belongs to the *Brevidensovirus* genus and perhaps employs the above transcription strategies to ensure the stable inheritance of AalDV.

Remarkably, despite our finding that NS2 ATG negatively regulates the activity of P5/5.5, P1 has no activity (see Figure 3B) when the NS2 transcription is merely driven by P5 (see Figure 3A); the NS2 initiation codon does not exhibit activity, since P5 is insufficient to initiate NS2 transcription in the absence of DPE. Unexpectedly, the activity of P5/5.5 dramatically increased after the NS2 ATG was mutated (see P3, P4, and P6 in Figure 3B). However, the function of the NS2 initiation codon for P5/5.5 promoters cannot be completely understood using current studies. We hypothesize that NS2 ATG may be in a region that is negatively regulated for the P5/5.5 promoters. The mutation of NS2 ATG can destroy the sequence completion in the original region, causing its regulatory function to cease. We are equally uncertain about whether NS2 ATG has dual functions. This assumption has not been reported before and may be a new finding. Therefore, we need to further investigate into the function of the nearby area of the NS2 ATG.

BmBDV exclusively infects the columnar cells of the larvae midgut epithelium. A major impediment to *Bidensovirus* studies is the lack of permissive insect cells that support virus replication in vitro [32]. BmBDV can be rescued from BmN cells transfected with recombinant plasmids containing the linear full length virus genome [24]. BmBDV has the potential to be a viral vector [33]. To achieve controllable transformation of the viral genome, it is necessary to clarify the transcription strategies of the viral genes. In this study, for the first time, we reported the transcription strategy of VD2 (see Figure 2B). Interestingly, we showed, through mapping, that NS3 and P133 transcripts are terminated at two polyadenylations sites, which are far apart from each other. Therefore, this non-transcribed region could be a suitable locus for the insertion of exogenous genes in a future Bidensoviral vector. In conclusion, our study provides new information that could be used to employ BmBDV as viral vectors and biological control tools in the future.

Supplementary Materials: The following are available online at http://www.mdpi.com/1999-4915/11/4/325/s1, Figure S1: Location of primers designed for RT-PCR and RACE. Figure S2: Analysis of amplicons obtained with different GSPs in 5′ and 3′-RACE (M is 5000 bp marker) of BmBDV transcripts. Figure S3: Sequencing results of 5′-RACE. Figure S4: Sequencing results of 3′-RACE. Figure S5: Mapping of recombinant dual-luciferase reporter vectors identified by restriction enzyme *Kpn*I and *Hind*III. Table S1. Primers used for RT-PCR, and RACE. Table S2. Standard curves equation used qPCR for NS1 and NS2 genes.

Author Contributions: R.L., Q.Y. (Qian Yu) and Q.Y. (Qin Yao) designed the experiment and wrote the paper. R.L. and P.C. performed the experiments. Z.H., P.L. and K.C. provided technical assistance for experiments.

Funding: This research was funded by the National Natural Science Foundation of China, grant number 3157010904 and 31800137, and the Postgraduate Research & Practice Innovation Program of Jiangsu Province, grant number KYCX17_1753, and Natural science foundation of Jiangsu Province, grant number BK20160507, and research funding from Jiangsu University, grant number 17JDG010.

Conflicts of Interest: None of the authors have any conflicts of interest.

References

1. Hu, Z.Y.; Li, G.H.; Li, G.T.; Yao, Q.; Chen, K.P. Bombyx mori bidensovirus: The type species of the new genus Bidensovirus in the new family Bidnaviridae. *Chin. Sci. Bull.* **2013**, *58*, 4528–4532. [CrossRef]
2. Bando, H.; Hayakawa, T.; Asano, S.; Sahara, K.; Nakagaki, M.; Iizuka, T. Analysis of the genetic information of a DNA segment of a new virus from silkworm. *Arch. Virol.* **1995**, *140*, 1147–1155. [CrossRef] [PubMed]
3. Tijssen, P.; Bergoin, M. Densonucleosis viruses constitute an increasingly diversified subfamily among the parvoviruses. *Semin. Virol.* **1995**, *6*, 347–355. [CrossRef]
4. Bando, H.; Choi, H.; Ito, Y.; Nakagaki, M.; Kawase, S. Structural analysis on the single-stranded genomic DNAs of the virus newly isolated from silkworm: The DNA molecules share a common terminal sequence. *Arch. Virol.* **1992**, *124*, 187–193. [CrossRef] [PubMed]
5. Wang, F.; Hu, Z.; He, Y.; Li, G.; Kong, J.; Cao, J.; Chen, K.; Yao, Q. The Non-Structural Protein NS-2 of Bombyx mori Parvo-like Virus is Localized to the Nuclear Membrane. *Curr. Microbiol.* **2011**, *63*, 8–15. [CrossRef] [PubMed]
6. Guohui, L.; Chen, S.; Junhong, Z.; Yuanqing, H.; Huiqing, C.; Jie, K.; Guoping, H.; Keping, C.; Qin, Y. Characterization of Bombyx mori parvo-like virus non-structural protein NS1. *Virus Genes* **2009**, *39*, 396–402.
7. Pan, X.; Peng, L.; Zhang, M.; Hu, Z.; Li, G.; Ma, S.; Fan, F.; Chen, K.; Qin, Y. Expression Analysis of Bombyx mori Bidensovirus Structural Proteins and Assembly of Virus-like Particles in Insect Cells. *Curr. Microbiol.* **2014**, *69*, 567–573. [CrossRef]
8. Peng, L.; Xing, Y.; Hu, Z.; Yang, Y.; Pan, Y.; Chen, K.; Zhu, F.; Zhou, Y.; Chen, K.; Yao, Q. A characterization of structural proteins expressed by Bombyx mori bidensovirus. *J. Invertebr. Pathol.* **2017**, *144*, 18–23.
9. Junhong, Z.; Guohui, L.; Huiqing, C.; Xiaogang, L.; Meng, L.; Keping, C.; Qin, Y. Molecular cloning and expression of key gene encoding hypothetical DNA polymerase from B. mori parvo-like virus. *Genet. Mol. Biol.* **2010**, *33*, 739–744.
10. Jie, K.; Hu, Z.; He, Y.; Li, G.; Jian, C.; Wang, F.; Chen, K.; Qin, Y. Expression analysis of Bombyx mori parvo-like virus VD2-ORF1 gene encoding a minor structural protein. *Biologia* **2011**, *66*, 684–689.
11. Li, G.; Li, M.; Xu, W.; Zhou, Q.; Hu, Z.; Tang, Q.; Chen, K.; Yao, Q. Regulation of BmBDV NS1 by phosphorylation: Impact of mutagenesis at consensus phosphorylation sites on ATPase activity and cytopathic effects. *J. Invertebr. Pathol.* **2016**, *133*, 66–72. [CrossRef]
12. Tijssen, P.; Pénzes, J.J.; Yu, Q.; Pham, H.T.; Bergoin, M. Diversity of small, single-stranded DNA viruses of invertebrates and their chaotic evolutionary past. *J. Invertebr. Pathol.* **2016**, *140*, 83–96. [CrossRef]
13. Scaria, A.; Tollefson, A.E.; Saha, S.K.; Wold, W.S. The E3-11.6K protein of adenovirus is an Asn-glycosylated integral membrane protein that localizes to the nuclear membrane. *Virology* **1992**, *191*, 743–753. [CrossRef]
14. Guohui, L.; Qian, Z.; Zhaoyang, H.; Peng, W.; Qi, T.; Keping, C.; Qin, Y. Determination of the Proteins Encoded by BmBDV VD1-ORF4 and Their Interacting Proteins in BmBDV-Infected Midguts. *Curr. Microbiol.* **2015**, *70*, 623–629.
15. Hayakawa, T.; Kojima, K.; Nonaka, K.; Nakagaki, M.; Sahara, K.; Asano, S.I.; Iizuka, T.; Bando, H. Analysis of proteins encoded in the bipartite genome of a new type of parvo-like virus isolated from silkworm—Structural protein with DNA polymerase motif. *Virus Res.* **2000**, *66*, 101–108. [CrossRef]
16. Li, G.; Hu, Z.; Guo, X.; Li, G.; Tang, Q.; Wang, P.; Chen, K.; Yao, Q. Identification of Bombyx mori Bidensovirus VD1-ORF4 Reveals a Novel;Protein Associated with Viral Structural Component. *Curr. Microbiol.* **2013**, *66*, 527–534. [CrossRef]
17. Gupta, T.; Ito, K.; Kadono-Okuda, K.; Murthy, G.N.; Gowri, E.V.; Ponnuvel, K.M. Characterization and genome comparison of an Indian isolate of bidensovirus infecting the silkworm Bombyx mori. *Arch. Virol.* **2018**, *163*, 125–134. [CrossRef]
18. Yin, H.; Yao, Q.; Guo, Z.; Bao, F.; Yu, W.; Li, J.; Chen, K. Expression of non-structural protein NS3 gene of Bombyx mori densovirus (China isolate). *J. Genet. Genom.* **2008**, *35*, 239–244. [CrossRef]
19. Harrison, R.L.; Rowley, D.L.; Funk, C.J. The Complete Genome Sequence of Plodia Interpunctella Granulovirus: Evidence for Horizontal Gene Transfer and Discovery of an Unusual Inhibitor-of-Apoptosis Gene. *PLoS ONE* **2016**, *11*, e0160389. [CrossRef]
20. Adly, A.A.; Franc¸oise-Xavière, J.; Yi, L.; Gilles, F.; Franc¸ois, C. NS-3 protein of the Junonia coenia densovirus is essential for viral DNA replication in an Ld 652 cell line and Spodoptera littoralis larvae. *J. Virol.* **2004**, *78*, 790–797.

21. Krupovic, M.; Koonin, E.V. Evolution of eukaryotic single-stranded DNA viruses of the Bidnaviridae family from genes of four other groups of widely different viruses. *Sci. Rep.* **2014**, *4*, 5347. [CrossRef] [PubMed]
22. Cotmore, S.F.; Tattersall, P. Parvoviral host range and cell entry mechanisms. *Adv. Virus Res.* **2007**, *70*, 183–232. [PubMed]
23. Wang, Y.J.; Qin, Y. Organization and Transcription Strategy of Genome of Bombyx mori Bidensovirus (China isolate) VD-1. *Chin. J. Biotechnol.* **2006**, *22*, 707–712. [CrossRef]
24. Zhang, P.; Miao, D.; Zhang, Y.; Wang, M.; Hu, Z.; Peng, L.; Yao, Q. Cloning and rescue of the genome of Bombyx mori bidensovirus, and characterization of a recombinant virus. *Virol. J.* **2016**, *13*, 126. [CrossRef] [PubMed]
25. Zhu, S.; Hu, Z.; Chen, K.; Li, G.; Guo, X.; Ma, Y.; Yao, Q. Characterization of the Promoter Elements of Bombyx mori Bidensovirus Nonstructural Gene 1. *Curr. Microbiol.* **2012**, *65*, 643–648. [CrossRef]
26. Juven-Gershon, T.; Kadonaga, J.T. Regulation of gene expression via the core promoter and the basal transcriptional machinery. *Dev. Biol.* **2010**, *339*, 225–229. [CrossRef]
27. Dhar, A.K.; Kaizer, K.N.; Betz, Y.M.; Harvey, T.N.; Lakshman, D.K. Identification of the core sequence elements in Penaeus stylirostris densovirus promoters. *Virus Genes* **2011**, *43*, 367–375. [CrossRef]
28. Mokili, J.L.; Rohwer, F.; Dutilh, B.E. Metagenomics and future perspectives in virus discovery. *Curr. Opin. Virol.* **2012**, *2*, 63–77. [CrossRef] [PubMed]
29. Laffy, P.W.; Wood-Charlson, E.M.; Turaev, D.; Jutz, S.; Pascelli, C.; Botté, E.S.; Bell, S.C.; Peirce, T.; Weynberg, K.D.; Oppen, M.J.H.V. Reef Invertebrate Viromics: Diversity, Host-Specificity & Functional Capacity. *Environ. Microbiol.* **2018**, *20*, 2125–2141. [PubMed]
30. Pham, H.T.; Jousset, F.X.; Perreault, J.; Shike, H.; Szelei, J.; Bergoin, M.; Tijssen, P. Expression strategy of Aedes albopictus densovirus. *J. Virol.* **2013**, *87*, 9928–9932. [CrossRef] [PubMed]
31. Cotmore, S.F.; Mavis, A.M.; Chiorini, J.A.; Mukha, D.V.; Pintel, D.J.; Jianming, Q.; Maria, S.V.; Peter, T.; Peter, T.; Derek, G. The family Parvoviridae. *Arch. Virol.* **2014**, *159*, 1239–1247. [CrossRef] [PubMed]
32. Hu, Z.; Deng, Y.; Zhang, X.; Tang, P.; Sun, W.; Li, G.; Qian, Y.; Qin, Y. Selection and validation of reference genes for reverse transcription quantitative real-time PCR (RT-qPCR) in silkworm infected with Bombyx mori bidensovirus. *Biologia* **2018**, *73*, 897–906. [CrossRef]
33. Guo, R.; Cao, G.; Zhu, Y.; Kumar, D.; Xue, R.; Lu, Y.; Hu, X.; Gong, C. Novel Infection System of Recombinant BmBDV DNA into BmN Cells of Silkworm, Bombyx mori. *Curr. Microbiol.* **2016**, *73*, 587–594. [CrossRef] [PubMed]

viruses

MDPI

Article

Interaction of a Densovirus with Glycans of the Peritrophic Matrix Mediates Oral Infection of the Lepidopteran Pest *Spodoptera frugiperda*

Laetitia Pigeyre [1,2], Malvina Schatz [1,2], Marc Ravallec [2], Leila Gasmi [3], Nicolas Nègre [2], Cécile Clouet [2], Martial Seveno [4], Khadija El Koulali [4], Mathilde Decourcelle [4], Yann Guerardel [5], Didier Cot [6], Thierry Dupressoir [1,2], Anne-Sophie Gosselin-Grenet [2,*] and Mylène Ogliastro [2,*]

1 Ecole Pratique des Hautes Etudes (EPHE), PSL Research Univ, DGIMI, Univ Montpellier, INRA, 34095 Montpellier, France; laetitia.pigeyre@hotmail.com (L.P.); malvina.schatz@ephe.psl.eu (M.S.); thierry.dupressoir@ephe.psl.eu (T.D.)

2 Diversité des Génomes et Interactions Microorganismes Insectes (DGIMI), Univ Montpellier, INRA, 34095 Montpellier, France; marc.ravallec@inra.fr (M.R.); nicolas.negre@umontpellier.fr (N.N.); cecile.clouet@inra.fr (C.C.)

3 Estructura de Recerca Interdisciplinar en Biotecnologia I Biomedicina (ERI-BIOTECMED, Deaprtment of Genetics Faculty of Biological Sciences Univ Valencia, 46100 Burjassot, Spain; gasmi.leila@gmail.com

4 BioCampus, Univ Montpellier, CNRS, INSERM, 34000 Montpellier, France; martial.seveno@fpp.cnrs.fr (M.S.); Khadija.El-Koulali@fpp.cnrs.fr (K.E.K.); Mathilde.Decourcelle@fpp.cnrs.fr (M.D.)

5 Unité de Glycobiologie Structurale et Fonctionnelle (UGSF) Univ Lille, CNRS, UMR 8576—UGSF, 59000 Lille, France; yann.guerardel@univ-lille1.fr

6 Institut Européen des Membranes (IEM), Univ Montpellier, CBRS, ENSCM, 34095 Montpellier, France; didier.cot@umontpellier.fr

* Correspondence: marie-helene.ogliastro@inra.fr (M.O.); anne-sophie.gosselin-grenet@umontpellier.fr (A.-S.G.-G.)

Received: 2 August 2019; Accepted: 11 September 2019; Published: 17 September 2019

Abstract: The success of oral infection by viruses depends on their capacity to overcome the gut epithelial barrier of their host to crossing over apical, mucous extracellular matrices. As orally transmitted viruses, densoviruses, are also challenged by the complexity of the insect gut barriers, more specifically by the chitinous peritrophic matrix, that lines and protects the midgut epithelium; how capsids stick to and cross these barriers to reach their final cell destination where replication goes has been poorly studied in insects. Here, we analyzed the early interaction of the *Junonia coenia* densovirus (JcDV) with the midgut barriers of caterpillars from the pest *Spodoptera frugiperda*. Using combination of imaging, biochemical, proteomic and transcriptomic analyses, we examined in vitro, ex vivo and in vivo the early interaction of the capsids with the peritrophic matrix and the consequence of early oral infection on the overall gut function. We show that the JcDV particle rapidly adheres to the peritrophic matrix through interaction with different glycans including chitin and glycoproteins, and that these interactions are necessary for oral infection. Proteomic analyses of JcDV binding proteins of the peritrophic matrix revealed mucins and non-mucins proteins including enzymes already known to act as receptors for several insect pathogens. In addition, we show that JcDV early infection results in an arrest of *N*-Acetylglucosamine secretion and a disruption in the integrity of the peritrophic matrix, which may help viral particles to pass through. Finally, JcDV early infection induces changes in midgut genes expression favoring an increased metabolism including an increased translational activity. These dysregulations probably participate to the overall dysfunction of the gut barrier in the early steps of viral pathogenesis. A better understanding of early steps of densovirus infection process is crucial to build biocontrol strategies against major insect pests.

Keywords: insect; Lepidoptera; insect parvovirus; chitin; peritrophins; glycans; biocontrol

1. Introduction

The transmission of parvoviruses predominantly occurs by horizontal routes through inhalation or oral exposure, making interaction with mucosal epithelia a crucial part of their pathogenesis (for review [1]). The oral route represents a major challenge for viruses as they need to overcome a diversity of barriers to invade their host. Indeed, most animal epithelia are covered in their apical surface by a carbohydrate-rich meshwork of various complexity and thickness, the glycocalyx, which can be coated by an additional layer of secreted mucus [2]. These structures constitute successive protective surfaces where viruses aggregate and either access to attachment factors and receptors at the surface of the epithelial cells or are eliminated by luminal or cilia movements [3]. This dual fate depends on the virus affinity for glycans, which must allow to escape the trap of the mucus. The diversity of glycans present on the epithelial surfaces vary between and within species and therefore constitute an important component of the innate immunity and of the species barrier [4].

Members of the *Parvoviridae* family are non-enveloped viruses that have a simple capsid with T = 1 icosaedral symmetry protecting a 4–6 kb linear, single stranded (ss) DNA genome [5]. They can cause diseases of various severity in a wide range of animals. Parvovirus interest in human and animal health or in biomedicine as vectors for gene transfer, has long focused research to understand their cell tropism and entry mechanisms. A number of cellular attachment factors and receptors have been characterized, mostly for vertebrates' parvoviruses. They highlight the importance of glycans in capsid recognition and binding specificity [6–8]. However, how capsids interact with epithelia remains poorly known, mainly due to difficulties to reconstitute in cellular models the complexity of animal epithelial systems [9,10].

Insect parvoviruses, named densoviruses, can be highly pathogenic, a feature that can both represent threats for insect mass rearing or opportunities for biocontrol against harmful insects as alternative to chemicals. Developing methods against infections or tools for biocontrol requires a deep understanding of the mechanisms driving host range and pathogenesis.

Like their vertebrate counterparts, densoviruses are mainly transmitted orally, gut recognition and binding constitute the primary step of their pathogenesis. The mechanisms determining densovirus specificity are poorly known. Depending on species, densovirus replication can be either restricted to or exclude the gut, viral particles being then transported across the epithelium by transcytosis to reach internal organs where replication goes [11–14]. Only one cellular receptor has been so far characterized for a "gut restricted" densovirus. It is a mucin of the gut of the silkworm *Bombyx mori*, whose inactivation makes silkworms resistant to infection with the *Bombyx mori* densovirus type 1 (BmDV) [15]. We have previously reported that gut transcytosis of the *Junonia coenia* densovirus (JcDV) involves a gut specific receptor-dependent mechanism in caterpillars [12]. However, the mechanisms used by viral particles to overcome the successive intestinal barriers of different structures and composition remain elusive.

In insects, the intestinal tract is covered by a chitinous acellular layer, which has specific features due to the dual embryonic origin of the gut. Indeed, anterior and posterior extremities of the gut are ectodermal and the acellular layer is covered by an impermeable cuticle. The midgut section is endodermal and has no cuticle but is covered in most insects by a semi-permeable membrane, named the peritrophic matrix (PM) (for review [16]). The PM forms a highly organized lattice of chitin fibrils associated with glycoproteins, mainly peritrophins that have a chitin-binding domain [17,18]. The midgut is thus the portal of entry for most pathogens and their interaction with the PM a critical step of their pathogenesis.

The PM forms pores whose size varies between insect species (e.g., 7–36 nm in Lepidoptera and up to 150 nm in Coleoptera) and developmental stages [19,20]. Large entomopathogenic viruses have developed specific mechanisms to pass through extracellular matrices including virus-encoded enzymes and specific proteins that are associated with the viral particles of baculo-and entomopoxviruses [21–24]. How densoviruses cope with the physical barriers that constitute the gut and in particular the PM is so far unknow. Due to their small size, it was initially thought they could diffuse passively across the pores of the matrix, but measures of the size of pores, the complexity of the PM and the nature of the interactions between components make this hypothesis unlikely [16,20].

We previously reported that following oral infection, viral particles of JcDV, a type species ofthe *Ambidensovirus* genus, aggregate on the PM of *Spodoptera frugiperda* caterpillars as a first step of the infection process [12]. Such rapid virus concentration on a carbohydrate-rich surface suggested a lectin-like activities of the capsids. Although there is no sequence similarity of the unique protein making the surface of the JcDV with lectin domains, its structure displays similarities with cellular carbohydrate binding proteins including lectins, which suggests that capsids could indeed recognize and bind carbohydrates [25].

Herein, we used a combination of approaches, including microscopy, biochemistry, proteomics and transcriptomics, to decipher the interaction of JcDV with PM major components (i.e., chitin, glycans and proteins). We found that capsids affinity for the PM might result from multiple interactions with different glycans including chitin and glycosylated proteins. In addition, we showed that JcDV early infection results in (i) an arrest of *N*-Acetylglucosamine (GlcNAc) secretion by epithelial cells associated with a disorganization of the PM structure mimicking the effect of chitin-binding plant lectin; (ii) substantial changes in the expression of gut genes, which may also contribute to an early gut dysfunction and participate to viral pathogenesis.

2. Materials and Methods

2.1. Insect Rearing and Virus Preparation

Caterpillars were reared under controlled conditions (25 ± 1 °C, 65 to 70% relative humidity [RH], 16-h light, 8-h dark photoperiod) on a wheat germ-based artificial diet. JcDV was amplified by oral infection. At death, larvae were crushed and virus extraction was processed by clarification and filtration on 0.22 μm to constitute a semi-purified virus stock (JcDV). To obtain a purified viral stock (P_JcDV), the semi-purified virus stock was loaded on OptiPrep^{TM} (Sigma-Aldrich, Lyon, France) density gradient and dialyzed against Phosphate-buffered saline (PBS) 1X as previously described in [13]. Viral concentrations were estimated by quantitative PCR (qPCR) as described in [12] and expressed as viral equivalent genomes ([veg]). Virus titers were determined by the tissue culture assay method (50% tissue culture infective dose (TCID50) in the permissive Ld652 cells as previously described [26].

2.2. Calcofluor, Glycans and Lectins

Calcofluor white M2R (Calcofluor; F3543), *N*-Acetyl-D-glucosamine (GlcNAc; A4106), *N*-Acetyl-D-galactosamine (GalNAc; A2795), D-(+)-Fucose (Fucose; F8150), D-(+)-Mannose (Mannose; M6020), Mucin from porcine stomach (Porcine mucin; M2378) and WGA-FITC conjugate (L4895) were all purchased from Sigma-Aldrich (Lyon, France).

2.3. Insect Bioassays

For in vivo bioassays, third-instar (L3) *S. frugiperda* caterpillars were individually infected by feeding with JcDV (10^9 veg/caterpillar) or by intrahemocelic injection (10^9 veg/caterpillar). Each treatment was applied to a cohort of 24 caterpillars and three independent experiments were performed. Calcofluor (0.5% to 3%) was concomitantly administrated with the virus to L3 or L6 caterpillars (as described in the Figures). For competition assays, JcDV was incubated with glycans (GlcNAc, GalNAc, Fucose or Mannose at 5 μM and/or 5 mM; for one hour before feeding or injection. In all experiments, control larvae were fed or injected with PBS. Caterpillars mortality was recorded each day during 10 days and results were presented as survival rates per day. The time to death was assessed by comparing the survival curves using the Kaplan Meier method (GraphPad Prism software, version 7). The significance between groups were analyzed using log-rank (Mantel-cox) tests and Gehan-Breslow-Wilcoxon tests.

2.4. Hemagglutination Assay

Rabbit erythrocytes cells were diluted at 3% (*v*/*v*) with 150 mM NaCl and treated with 0.5 mg/mL of trypsin (Sigma) for 30 min at 37 °C. After 3 washes with 150 mM NaCl, 25 µL serially two-fold dilutions of viral inocula (JcDV or P_JcDV; started from 10^{11} veg/µL) were mixed with 25 µL of erythrocytes in 96 well microtiter plates for 30 min at 37 °C. Positive controls of hemagglutination was performed using 25 µL of WGA (1 mg/mL). Fifty µL of erythrocytes were subsequently added to each well for 30 min at 37 °C. Hemagglutination was read under a light microscope.

2.5. PM Isolation, Ex Vivo Infection and Microscopic Observation

For Calcofluor experiments, PMs were isolated from sixth-instar (L6) *S. frugiperda* caterpillars, previously anesthetized on ice, then opened and washed with Phosphate Buffered Saline (PBS) to remove the food bolus. PMs isolated from caterpillars treated with Calcofluor were fixed 1 h with 4% paraformaldehyde (PFA), then dehydrated with increasing concentrations of ethanol (50% to 100%) and in 1:1 (100% ethanol and hexamethyldisilazane [HMDS]) for 10 min and finally in 100% HMDS for 20 min. After overnight evaporation, samples were ultimately coated with Platinium and observed with a Scanning Electron Microscope (SEM) HITACHI S-4800, with an acceleration voltage of 2 kV and a working distance of 5 mm.

For ex vivo infection experiments, PMs were isolated as described above and incubated for 30 min at room temperature (RT) with JcDV (10^9 veg/µL; 500µL), or with JcDV pre-incubated for 1 h with glycans (GlcNAc, GalNAc, Fucose or Mannose; 5 µM to 5 mM) before infection. The PMs were then washed with PBS and fixed with 4% PFA as above. Immunolabelling of JcDV particles was performed using a specific rabbit anti-capsid antibody (1:1,000; Eurogentec) incubated for 2 h at RT and an anti-rabbit secondary antibody (Alexa Fluor® 568; 1:500; Invitrogen, Carlsbad, CA, USA) incubated for 45 min at RT. Labeled PMs were then mounted in Dako (Sigma) on coverslips for observation. For epifluorescence measurements, we worked on a Zeiss AxioImager Z2, equipped with suitable filters for the dyes, using a 40×/1.3 Plan-Apochromat Oil PH3 and a 63×/1.4 Plan-Apochromat Oil PH3 objectives. For structured illumination images, the Zeiss ApoTome-slider was introduced into the field-stop plane of the microscope to improve resolution of images. We used the ZEN software to operate the microscope and took at least 10 images (10 fields per PM) for each treatment. All images were taken with a CMOS Orca Flash 4.0 B&W camera. Images were processed with Fiji software. The intensity of fluorescence (arbitrary unit) were measured on epifluorescence images. Statistical analyses were performed using the non-parametric Kruskal-Wallis test (GraphPad Prism Software, version 7, GraphPad Software, San Diego, CA, USA). Each experiment was repeated at least three times, and each independent experiment gave similar results.

2.6. Midgut Semi-Thin Sections and Immunolabelling

L3 *S. frugiperda* caterpillars were individually infected by feeding as in Section 2.3. Twenty four hours later, caterpillars were anesthetized on ice and sacrificed. In parallel, caterpillars were kept until death to insure their infection status. Sacrificed caterpillars were fixed in 4% PFA + 2.5% glutaraldehyde for 1h at 4 °C and dehydrated by incubations in increasing concentrations of ethanol (50% to 100%) before progressive embedding in 100% Unicryl resin (BB International) as described in [12]. Semi-thin sections (1 µm) were cut in the central part of the caterpillars corresponding to the midgut. After 45 min of incubation with WGA-FITC (1:300), to label GlcNAc and the PM, or with Phalloidin-FITC (1:300; Sigma), to label actin cytoskeleton, and 10 min with Dapi (1 µg/mL; Invitrogen) to label nuclei, semi-thin sections were mounted and observed with a Zeiss AxioImager Z2 microscope using the structured illumination module Zeiss ApoTome-slider as in 4.5. Images were taken with a CMOS Orca Flash 4.0 B&W camera using fixed parameters for all treatments and processed with Fiji software.

2.7. Chitin Binding Assay and Pull Down

Ten µL of chitin beads (New England Biolab) were washed three times with PBS and added in 200 µL of virus suspension (10^9 veg/µL in PBS). After 1 h of incubation with gentle rotation, beads were pulled-down by centrifugation (500× *g* for 5 min à 4 °C), washed five times with PBS, then resuspended in Laemmli buffer 2 × (4% SDS, 20% glycerol, 10% 2-mercaptoethanol, 0.004% bromophenol blue and 0.125 M Tris HCl, pH 7) and heated at 95 °C for 5 min before western blot analysis. Two µL (5% of the pull down and 1% of the initial input) was loaded on 4–15% polyacrylamide Tris-HCl gel (Mini-PROTEAN® TGX™ Precast Gels, Biorad, Hercules, CA, USA) and separated by SDS-PAGE for 1 h at 150 V. Next, samples were transferred to PVDF membrane (Immobilon-P, Merck) for 2 h at 200 mA. Subsequently, the membrane was saturated with 5% of milk in PBS/Tween 0.1% (PBST), then incubated 2 h at RT with the primary anti-capsid antibody (1:1,000; see above). After washes in PBST, the membrane was incubated 1 h at RT with an anti-rabbit secondary antibody HRP-conjugated (1:3000; Biorad, Hercules, CA, USA). Proteins were revealed by enhanced chemiluminescence (Millipore, Burlington, MA, USA) using a Chemidoc imager (Biorad).

2.8. SDS-PAGE, PAS Staining and VOPBA

Peritrophins were extracted from pools of five PMs from sixth instar *S. frugiperda* in 200 µL of Laemmli buffer 2X, then boiled and heated at 95 °C for 5 min [27]. After centrifugation at 8000× *g* for 10 min 4 °C, the supernatant was collected and 1/15 was loaded on 4–15% polyacrylamide Tris-HCl gel and separated by SDS-PAGE as above. Thirty µg of porcine mucins were also loaded on the same gel. Gel was stained with Page blue (Thermo Fisher Scientific, Waltham, MA, USA) to analyze total proteins or with Periodic Acid-Schiff (PAS) as described in [28] to analyze glycosylated proteins. Proteins were also transferred on nitrocellulose membranes (Biorad) for 3 h at 70 V for viral protein overlay binding assay [29]. Briefly, the membrane was saturated with 3% BSA in PBST for 2 h at RT, then incubated OVN at 4 °C with JcDV (10^9 veg diluted in PBST containing 1% BSA). After washes in PBST, the membrane was incubated with the rabbit anti-capsid antibody (1:1000; see above), then the anti-rabbit secondary antibody HRP-conjugated, and proteins were revealed by enhanced chemiluminescence as above.

2.9. Proteomic LC-MS/MS Analysis and Data Processing

Protein bands revealed by VOPBA were cut in SDS-PAGE gel stained with Page blue (3 replicates, 10 bands) and destained with three washes in 50% acetonitrile and 50 mM triethylammonium bicarbonate (TEABC). After protein reduction (with 10 mM dithiothreitol in 50 mM TEABC at 60 °C for 30 min in the dark) and alkylation (55 mM iodoacetamide TEABC at room temperature for 30 min) proteins were digested in-gel using trypsin (0.5 µg/band, Gold, Promega, Madison, WI, USA) as previously described [30]. Digested products were dehydrated in a vacuum centrifuge and resuspended with 0.05% Trifluoroacetic acid (TFA) and 2% ACN. The generated peptides were analyzed online by nano-flow HPLC–nanoelectrospray ionization using a Q-Exactive Plus mass spectrometer (Thermo Fisher Scientific, Waltham, MA, USA) coupled to an Ultimate 3000 RSLC (Thermo Fisher Scientific). Desalting and pre-concentration of samples were performed on-line on a Pepmap® pre-column (0.3 mm × 10 mm, Dionex, Sunnyvale, CA, USA). The capillary reverse-phase column (0.075 mm × 150 mm, Acclaim Pepmap 100® C18, Thermo Fisher Scientific) fitted with an uncoated silica PicoTip Emitter (New Objective, Woburn, MA, USA) was first equilibrated in solvent A (0.1% formic acid) and a multistep linear gradient of acetonitrile consisting of 0–25% of solvent B (0.1% formic acid in 80% acetonitrile) for 30 min, 25–40% for 5 min and 90% for 8 min, at 300 nL/min was used to elute peptides from. Spectra were acquired with the instrument operating in the information-dependent acquisition mode throughout the HPLC gradient. Survey scans were acquired in the Orbitrap system with resolution set at a value of 70,000. Up to twelve of the most intense ions per cycle were fragmented and analyzed using a resolution of 17,500. Peptide fragmentation was performed using nitrogen gas on the most abundant and at least doubly charged ions detected in the initial MS scan and an active exclusion time of 45 s. For all full scan measurements with the Orbitrap detector a lock-mass ion from ambient air (*m/z* 445.120024) was used as an internal calibrant as described [31].

Analysis was performed using the MaxQuant software (version 1.5.5.1) [32]. All MS/MS spectra were searched using Andromeda against a decoy database consisting of a combination of *S. frugiperda* databases [33] and 236 classical contaminants, containing forward and reverse entities. The following settings were applied: Spectra were searched with a mass tolerance of 7 ppm (MS) and 0.5 Th (MS/MS). Enzyme specificity was set to trypsin. Up to two missed cleavages were allowed and only peptides with at least seven amino acids in length were considered. Carbamidomethylation was set as fixed cystein modification and oxidation was set as variable methionine modification for searches. FDR was set at 0.01 for peptides and proteins. Sequences which found homology were annotated according to the gene ontology (GO) terms and classified using Blast2Go software (https://www.blast2go.com/; [34]). The enrichment in GO terms compared to the *S. frugiperda* reference (predicted proteins from the OGS2.2 genome; Gouin et al., 2017) was analyzed with the same software (FDR set at 0.01).

2.10. RNA Extraction, DGE Library Construction and Sequencing

Fourth instar *S. frugiperda* caterpillars were orally infected or not with JcDV (10^{12} veg per caterpillar; Twenty caterpillars per condition). At 1-day p.i. or 3 days p.i., caterpillars were anesthetized on ice and dissected. The midguts were washed in PBS to eliminate the food bolus and the PMs. Trachea, Malpighi tubes and visceral muscles were removed and the epithelia were incubated with 2.5% trypsin for 30 min to dissociate the tissues. After washes, gut cells were lysed in 800 µL of TRIzol® reagent (Invitrogen) for total RNA extraction according to the manufacturer's instructions. Total RNA amount and purity were checked by using spectrophotometrer NanoDrop ND-1000 (Thermo Scientific) and the integrity of total RNA was analyzed by capillary electrophoresis (2100 Bioanalyzer Instrument, Agilent, Santa Clara, CA, USA).

We used Digital Gene Expression (DGE) method that generates short sequences (Tags) specific for mRNA [35–37]. Four DGE libraries were constructed from midgut total RNA extracted from *S. frugiperda* caterpillars infected (or not) for 1 and 3 days. Sequence tag preparation was done with Illumina's Digital Gene Expression Tag Profiling Kit according to the manufacturer's protocol (version 2.1B) as described in [36]. For fourth libraries, 10 µg of total RNA were incubated with oligo-dT beads. First-and second-strand cDNA syntheses were performed using superscript II reverse transcription kit according to the manufacturer's instructions (Invitrogen). The cDNAs were cleaved using the NlaIII anchoring enzyme. Subsequently, digested cDNAs were ligated with the GEX adapter 1 containing a restriction site for MmEI. The second digestion with MmeI was performed, which cuts 17 bp downstream of the CATG site. At this point, the fragments detach from the beads. The GEX adapter 2 was ligated to the 3′ end of the tag. A PCR amplification with 15 cycles using Phusion polymerase (Finnzymes) was performed with primers complementary to the adapter sequences to enrich the samples for the desired fragments. The resulting fragments of 85 bp were purified by excision from a 6% polyacrylamide TBE gel. The DNA was eluted from the gel using Spin-X Cellulose Acetate Filter (0.45 µm), precipitated, resuspended in 10 mM Tris-HCl (pH 8.5) and quantified using Nanodrop 1000 spectrophotometer. Cluster generation was performed after applying 4 pM of each sample to the individual lanes of the Illumina 1G flowcell. After hybridization of the sequencing primer to the single-stranded products, 18 cycles of base incorporation were carried out on the 1G analyzer according to the manufacturer's instructions. Image analysis and base calling were performed using the Illumina Pipeline, where sequence tags were obtained after purity filtering. We could assign 63% of the tags (Supplementary Materials Tables S2–S4) out of which 54% correspond to multiple matches and were discarded from functional analysis with GO.

2.11. Transcriptomic Analysis of the Midgut

Functional annotation was performed using BIOTAG software (Skuld-Tech, Grabels, France). The statistical value of DGE data comparisons, as a function of tag counts, was calculated by assuming that each tag has an equal chance of being detected. Differential expression of the Tag counts of the infected vs. mock conditions was performed to obtain a list of up- and down-regulated tags for each condition. Tags for which differential expression was ≥ 5 fold change were assigned using the reference databases for *S. frugiperda* [33,38]. Sequences with homology were annotated according to the GO terms and classified using Blast2Go software (https://www.blast2go.com/; [34]) and represented at level 2 of Biological process and Molecular function. The enrichment in GO terms compared to the *S. frugiperda* reference (predicted transcripts from the OGS2.2 genome) was analyzed with the same software (FDR set at 0.01). The Junonia coenia densovirus (former JcDNV) corresponds to the complete genome of the Oxford isolate (Genbank accession number KC883978.1).

3. Results

3.1. The Peritrophic Matrix of S. frugiperda is a Barrier to JcDV Infection

Early studies have estimated that the average pore size of the PM is around 8 nm in *S. frugiperda* caterpillars, which might exclude 25 nm densovirus particles [39]. To assess the PM barrier function against densovirus infection, we disrupted its structure by feeding third instar (L3) larvae with sub lethal doses (0.5%) of the chitin-binding agent Calcofluor White prior JcDV infection [40–44]. We then measured larval mortality rates daily. Results showed that JcDV infected larvae pre-treated with Calcofluor displayed a significant shorter median time to death (LT50) compared to untreated infected larvae (7 vs. 9 days p.i. for control larvae; $p < 0.01$) (Figure 1A and Supplementary Materials Figure S1), supporting that the PM can limit JcDV infection. Noteworthy, an increased larval mortality was also observed at late time post-treatment with Calcofluor in mock-infected caterpillars compared to untreated controls (18% at 10 days p.i.), confirming a detrimental inhibition of chitin assembly on larval development [41].

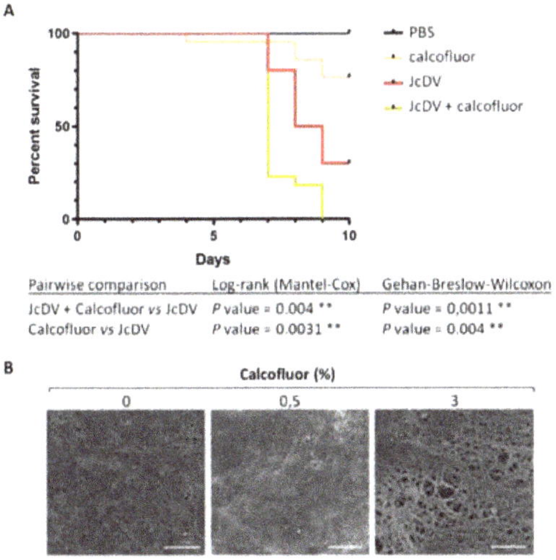

Figure 1. Calcofluor increases *S. frugiperda* caterpillar's susceptibility to densovirus oral infection. (**A**) Survival of *S. frugiperda* caterpillars following JcDV infection. Larvae (n = 24) were infected individually by feeding with JcDV (10^9 veg/caterpillar) concomitantly with 0.5% (5 µg) of Calcofluor or PBS as a control. Caterpillar mortality was recorded once a day during 10 days and results were presented as survival rates per day. Three independent experiments were performed, each independent

experiment gave similar results, one is represented here. The log-rank (Mantel-cox) and the Gehan-Breslow-Wilcoxon tests were used to determine statistical significance. p Values of less than 0.05 were considered significant (**, $p < 0.01$). PBS refers to control (PBS-treated and non-infected) caterpillars; Calcofluor refers to Calcofluor-treated and non-infected caterpillars; JcDV refers to JcDV-infected caterpillars and JcDV+Calcofluor to Calcofluor-treated and JcDV-infected caterpillars. (**B**) Calcofluor disrupts the PM integrity. SEM images of PM ultrastructure isolated from L6 caterpillars fed with PBS (0%), 0.5% (5 μg) or 3% (30 μg) of Calcofluor. Endoperitrophic face is shown (bars, 300 nm).

We analyzed the effect of Calcofluor on the PM integrity by scanning electron microscopy (SEM). Because the PM of L3 larvae has a gel-like structure that cannot be manipulated, we took L6 larvae for this experiment as the PM is thick and solid at this stage and can be easily dissected. L6 caterpillars were fed with up to 3% Calcofluor (not lethal at 24 h post treatment) and PMs were isolated 24 h post-treatment and prepared for SEM analysis. As shown by Figure 1B, PMs from control larvae displayed a highly organized structure, similar to PMs from caterpillars treated with 0.5% Calcofluor. By contrast, PMs from caterpillar fed with 3% Calcofluor had a clear disrupted structure with enlarged pores, confirming that Calcofluor binding to chitin fibrils compromised the integrity of the matrix.

3.2. *JcDV Binding to the PM is Required for Oral Infection of S. frugiperda Caterpillars*

The rapid recognition of the PM by JcDV capsids suggests that their affinity for glycans is important for the oral infection process. To test this hypothesis, we first assayed the capsid ability to agglutinate erythrocytes, a feature displayed by vertebrate parvoviruses [45,46]. We performed a typical hemagglutination assay, adding serial dilutions of the virus inoculum to rabbit erythrocytes (Figure 2). The first dilutions (1:2 and 1:4) of JcDV triggered a strong hemolysis of erythrocytes suggesting a toxic effect of the viral inoculum, ie capsids or some host-derived component associated with the inoculum. It is worthy to note that we use semi-purified inoculum as it mimics naturally occurring infections. JcDV was therefore further purified on a density gradient (P_JcDV) and similarly assayed for hemagglutination. A clear hemagglutination was obtained with P_JcDV, supporting that toxicity is likely due to a host-derived component that can be eliminated during the purification process. Hemagglutination with P_JcDV was obtained up to the third dilution (hemagglutination titer of 1:8), which indicates a rather weak interaction of the capsids with glycans at the surface of (mammalian) erythrocytes.

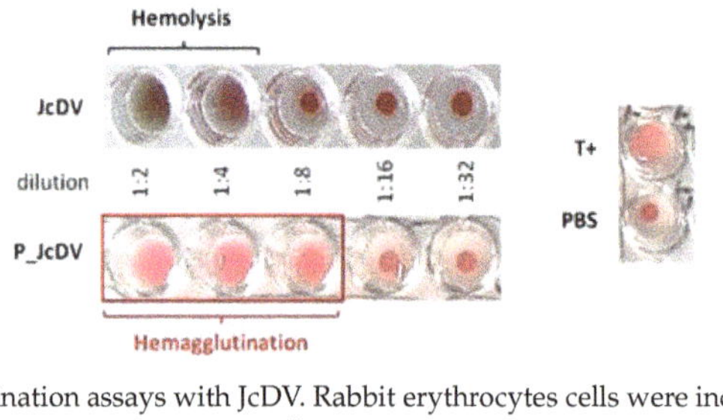

Figure 2. Hemagglutination assays with JcDV. Rabbit erythrocytes cells were incubated with serially two-fold dilutions of JcDV or P_JcDV (from 10^{11} veg/μL, 25 μL/well) for 30 min at 37 °C. Positive control (T+) of hemagglutination was performed using 25 μL of Wheat Germ Agglutin (WGA; 1 mg/mL), negative control (PBS) with 25 μL of PBS instead of virus dilution. Semi-purified virus (JcDV) induced a green coloration in the wells, as a result of hemolysis of erythrocytes. The wells containing purified virus (P_JcDV) showed a clear hemagglutination at the lowest dilutions (1:2 to 1:8).

To better understand capsid affinity for glycans, we performed a competition bioassay using monomeric glycans as JcDV-binding competitors. JcDV binding was revealed with an immunofluorescence staining on the PMs using a specific anti-capsid antibody. We quantified this fluorescence as a proxy of binding and competition. We first performed competition ex vivo on isolated PMs incubated with JcDV in the presence of four monosaccharides commonly found in insects [47], ie *N*-Acetyl-D-glucosamine (GlcNAc), which is the monomeric unit of chitin, *N*-Acetyl-D-galactosamine (GalNAc), D-Fucose and D-Mannose (Figure 3). We first verified with a dot blot assay that capsids interaction with monosaccharides were not interfering with antibody recognition, which validated the competition bioassay (Supplementary Materials Figure S2). As shown in Figure 3, JcDV binding resulted in an intense fluorescence signal on the PMs (left panel), which was similarly competed away by the four monosacharides and within a similar concentration range (0.5 mM to 5 mM). We noted that fluorescence quantification did not result in a strictly linear dose-dependent effect.

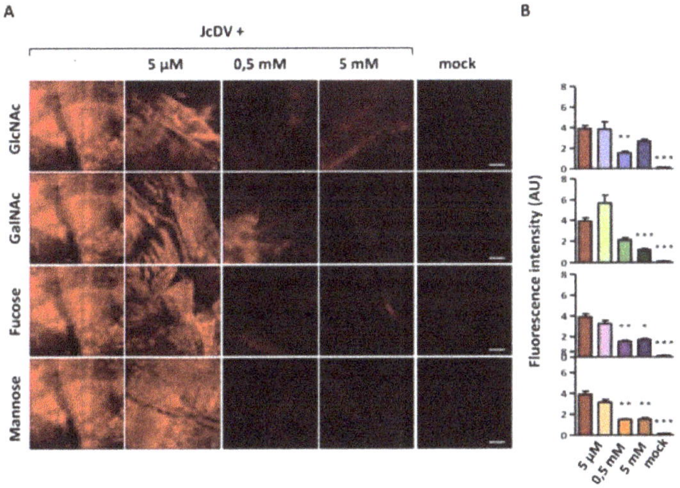

Figure 3. Ex vivo interaction of JcDV with the PM involves carbohydrates. (**A**) Apotome images of isolated PMs incubated with JcDV (5.10^{11} veg/PM) alone or with JcDV treated for 1 h with 5 µM to 5 mM of glycans (GlcNAc, GalNAc, Fucose or Mannose) before incubation. JcDV labelling is in red. Control PMs (mock) were incubated with a clarified and filtered homogenate of non-infected caterpillars. Bars, 50 µm. Each experiment was repeated at least three times, and each independent experiment gave similar results, one is shown here. (**B**) Relative quantification of JcDV binding on isolated PM and competition assays with monomeric glycans. Intensity of red fluorescence (arbitrary unit A.U) of PMs were measured on epifluorescence images (10 images from 3 independent experiments). Statistical analyses were determined using the non-parametric Kruskal-Wallis test. *p* Values of less than 0.05 were considered significant (* $p < 0.05$; ** $p < 0.01$; *** $p < 0.001$).

To further test the role of glycans in JcDV pathogenesis, we carried out these competition bioassays in vivo (Figure 4 and Supplementary Materials Figure S3). We mixed JcDV with each monosaccharide prior infection, fed caterpillars with these inocula and calculated mortality rates daily as in Figure 1. Results showed that oral infection with 5 mM (but not 5 µM) of each monosaccharide significantly delayed the median time to death (LT50) of caterpillars (7 vs. 6 days; $p < 0.05$ for 5 mM) (Figure 4A and Supplementary Materials Figure S3A,B), further supporting that PM recognition is the first step of JcDV oral infection. To confirm these results and reveal JcDV binding and competition for binding the PM in vivo, we carried out midgut semi-thin sections and immunofluorescence as above. Caterpillars were infected with JcDV mixed or not with 5 mM GlcNAc and sacrificed at 2 h p.i. for midgut isolation and preparation. As shown in Figure 4B, we observed a red fluorescence signal in untreated infected caterpillars that typically lines the PM. In addition, labelling was also observed in the lumen, likely revealing JcDV interaction with food bolus and/or microbial components. Both signals were strongly and specifically decreased following competition with GlcNAc (Figure 4B), showing that different GlcNAc-containing glycans in the gut lumen can recognize the capsids.

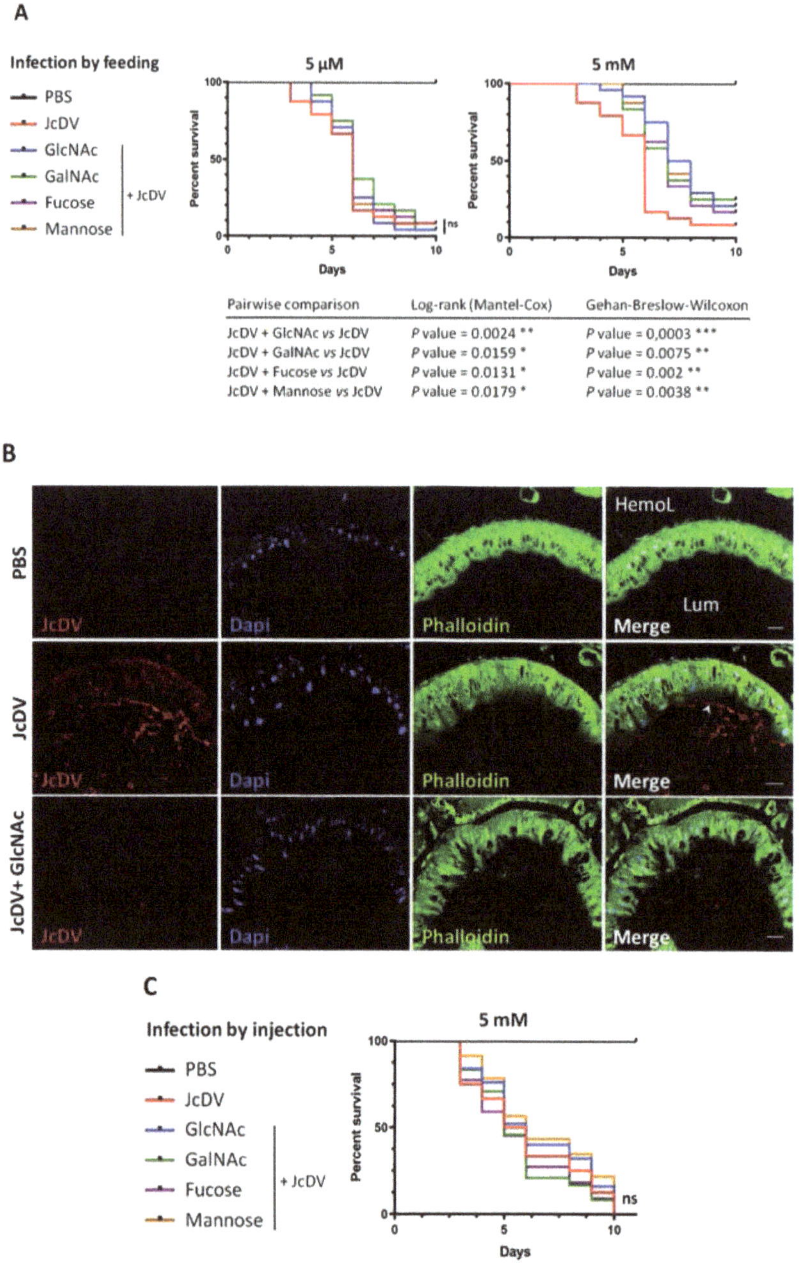

Pairwise comparison	Log-rank (Mantel-Cox)	Gehan-Breslow-Wilcoxon
JcDV + GlcNAc *vs* JcDV	*P* value = 0.0024 **	*P* value = 0,0003 ***
JcDV + GalNAc *vs* JcDV	*P* value = 0.0159 *	*P* value = 0.0075 **
JcDV + Fucose *vs* JcDV	*P* value = 0.0131 *	*P* value = 0.002 **
JcDV + Mannose *vs* JcDV	*P* value = 0.0179 *	*P* value = 0.0038 **

Figure 4. Affinity for glycans mediates JcDV oral infection of *S. frugiperda* caterpillars. (**A**) Survival curves of caterpillars (n = 24) infected by feeding with JcDV alone or with JcDV (10^9 veg/caterpillar) incubated for 1 h with 5 µM or 5 mM of glycans (GlcNAc, GalNAc, Fucose or Mannose) before infection. Control caterpillars were fed with PBS. Three independent experiments were performed, each

independent experiment gave similar results, one is represented here. The log-rank (Mantel-cox) and the Gehan-Breslow-Wilcoxon tests were used to determine statistical significance. p Values of less than 0.05 were considered significant (ns, non-significant; * $p < 0.05$; ** $p < 0.01$; *** $p < 0.001$). (**B**) Immunolabeling of midgut semithin transversal sections 2 h after ingestion of JcDV alone or JcDV (10^9 veg/caterpillar) incubated for 1 h with 5 mM of GlcNAc before oral infection. Control caterpillars were fed with PBS. The PM is shown by an arrowhead. Phalloidin-FITC is in green, JcDV is in red, and nuclei are labeled with Dapi (blue). Bars, 30 µm. Lum, midgut lumen; HemoL, hemolymphatic compartment. (**C**) Survival curves of caterpillars (n = 24) infected by injection of JcDV alone (10^9 veg/caterpillar) or of JcDV incubated for 1 h with 5 mM of each glycan (GlcNAc, GalNAc, Fucose or Mannose) before infection. Control caterpillars were injected with PBS. Three independent experiments were performed, each independent experiment gave similar results, one is represented here. The log-rank (Mantel-cox) and the Gehan-Breslow-Wilcoxon tests were used to determine statistical significance, $p > 0.05$ were considered non-significant (ns). PBS refers to control (PBS-treated and non-infected) caterpillars; 'JcDV' to JcDV-infected caterpillars; 'JcDV + GlcNAc', 'JcDV + GalNAc', 'Jc + Fucose' and 'Jc + Mannose' refer to caterpillars infected with JcDV incubated with GlcNAc, GalNAc, Fucose or Mannose, respectively, before infection.

Last, we studied whether such "stickiness" was specifically required by the densovirus to cross the gut, i.e., for oral infection. JcDV infection of target cells (eg epidermis, trachea, hemocytes) proceeds by a receptor-dependent mechanism different from intestinal cells [12]. These cells express glycan structures of various complexity that are attached to the cell surface or secreted and forming extracellular matrices, whose glycans might be similarly targeted by JcDV for attachment. We performed competition bioassays in vivo, bypassing the midgut by injecting caterpillars with JcDV mixed or not with 5 mM of each monosaccharide. Interestingly, the median time to death was similar for all conditions (Figure 4C and Supplementary Materials Figure S3C; $p > 0.05$), showing that none of the monosaccharides competed with JcDV infection proceeding by the systemic route.

Altogether these results show that JcDV capsid is a carbohydrate-binding protein and this feature is required for oral infection to target the PM of caterpillars.

3.3. *JcDV Binds to Both Chitin and Protein Components of the PM*

We next wanted to determine which component of the PM, i.e., chitin and/or glycosylated proteins were involved in capsid interactions, using biochemical assays. We first tested capsid physical interaction with chitin using a pull-down assay with chitin beads. JcDV from purified or semi-purified inocula were incubated with chitin beads, pulled-down by centrifugation and subsequently revealed by Western blot using a specific JcDV anti-capsid antibody. Figure 5A shows JcDV pull-down by chitin beads and we did not observed difference between inocula (purified vs. semi-purified), which confirmed that capsids can interact directly with chitin.

Second, we tested virus interaction with PM proteins using a Viral Overlay Binding Assay (VOBPA). Total proteins were extracted from isolated PMs, separated with SDS-PAGE and either stained with PAGE Blue and Periodic Acid Schiff (PAS) in order to visualize total and glycosylated proteins respectively, or blotted onto nitrocellulose membranes for VOPBA. We included porcine mucins as a control of highly (O-)glycosylated proteins. At the first glance, VOPBA revealed that JcDV binds to most if not all the PM proteins labelled by PAGE blue and PAS combined, although with different intensities (Figure 5B). Interestingly, no binding was observed with the porcine mucins which might support some specificity for insect glycans. More specifically, a set of JcDV-interacting proteins was identified at high molecular weights (>250 kDa) including proteins with a pattern similar to porcine mucins. These proteins were labelled with PAGE blue and PAS or only with PAS suggesting that they are mostly and probably highly glycosylated (Figure 5B). Interestingly, proteins at 180 kDa displayed a higher intensity as they are in a relative lower amount (according to PAGE blue), which suggests higher affinity for JcDV. Proteins interacting with JcDV were detected at 150–200 kDa and 25–60 kDa, and corresponding to proteins with low or no glycosylation (according to PAS staining).

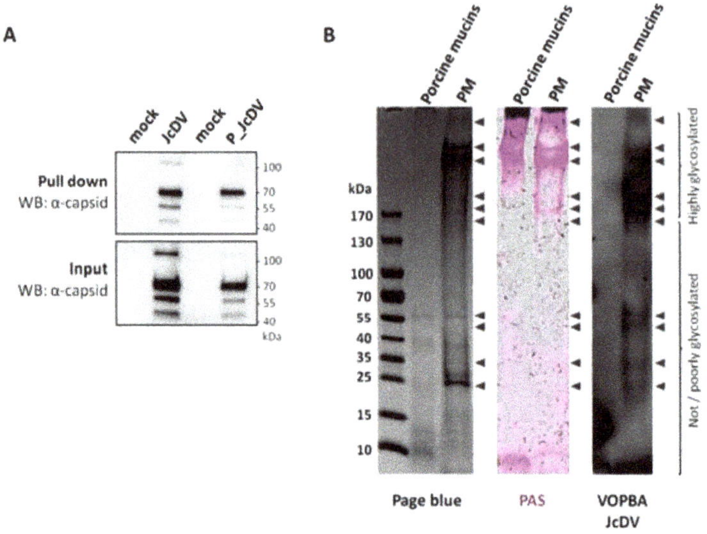

Figure 5. JcDV interacts with chitin and has specific affinity for proteins of the PM. (**A**) Western blot analysis of the chitin binding assay. Chitin beads were incubated with JcDV or P_JcDV. Control binding assays were performed with non-infected homogenate of caterpillars (for JcDV) or with PBS (for P_JcDV). Five % of the pull down and 1% of the input (before pull down) were analysed by SDS-PAGE followed by western blotting using a polyclonal anti-JcDV capsid antibody. The four VP capsids proteins (theoretical molecular weights are VP1, 89 kDa; VP2, 58 kDa; VP3, 53 kDa and VP4, 47 kDa) are detected, with a better detection of VP2 [48]. (**B**) VOPBA analysis of PM proteins interacting with JcDV. Proteins were extracted from PMs and separated by SDS-PAGE as described in Methods. Thirty µg of porcine mucins were also loaded in the gel as a control of highly O-glycosylated proteins. Proteins were then stained with Page Blue or Periodic Acid Schiff (PAS, pink) to visualize total or glycosylated proteins, respectively, and transferred to nitrocellulose membranes for probing with JcDV and anti-JcDV capsid antibody. Proteins interacting with JcDV capsids were finally revealed by enhanced chemiluminescence (black arrowheads on the VOPBA JcDV membrane); the corresponding positions of these bands were reported on the Page blue and PAS gels and indicated as well by black arrowheads on the right of these gels.

In total, 10 bands representing JcDV interacting proteins are reproducibly obtained with VOPBA. Noteworthy, each band probably include several proteins and/or isoform/glycoform of the same proteins.

Proteins corresponding to these 10 bands were next analyzed by LC–MS/MS mass spectrometry. We only considered 155 proteins that were shared between 3 replicates (Figure 6A), out of which 138 were annotated in the reference genome of *S. frugiperda* [33]. These proteins are PM structural proteins (i.e., peritrophins including intestinal mucins) and PM-associated proteins (enzymes, i.e., serine proteases and aminopeptidases N (APN) (Supplementary Materials Table S1). Gene ontology (GO) annotation confirmed the enrichment in proteolytic activities (particularly serine-type endopeptidases) and chitin synthesis, which are consistent with the PM composition and the gut function (Figure 6B). Interestingly among the set of proteins >150 kDa, we identified intestinal mucins, an ATP binding cassette A type 5 (ABCA5) transporter and aminopeptidases N (Supplementary Materials Table S1); the latter being known receptors for a number of viruses and for the Cry toxins from *Bacillus thuringiensis* [49–52].

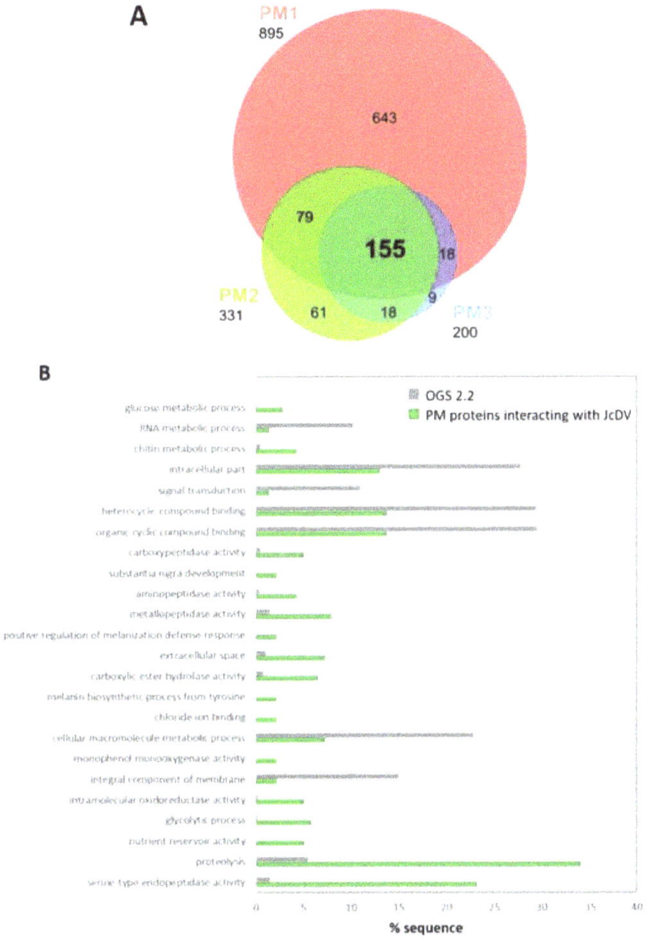

Figure 6. (**A**) Venn diagram of three replicates of proteomic analysis (PM1, PM2, PM3) of PM proteins interacting with JcDV. Protein bands revealed by VOPBA were cut in SDS-PAGE gel stained with Page blue and analyzed by LC–MS/MS as described in Methods. Among the 155 proteins common to the three replicates, 138 were annotated in the reference genome of *S. frugiperda* [33]. (**B**) GO terms enrichment for the 138 common annotated PM proteins interacting with JcDV (in green), compared to the reference in grey (predicted proteins from OGS2.2 *S. frugiperda* genome) (FDR set at 0.01). Specific enrichment in JcDV interacting proteins is considered when the green bars exceed the greys (controls). The 138 common PM proteins were assignated to the GO terms using Blast2Go software.

These results show that JcDV capsids can recognize and bind to the different components of the PM including chitin and several highly glycosylated proteins, both structural components of the PM (mucin, peritrophins) or associated proteins (enzymes).

3.4. *JcDV Early Pathogenesis Induces Changes in Midgut Metabolism*

JcDV recognition and binding to glycans of the PM concentrates viral particles close to the epithelial surface, which raised questions about the mechanism involved to cross over and reach the midgut receptor(s). We hypothesized that capsids aggregation on the matrix can result in its disorganization, in a way similar to chitin-binding wheat germ agglutinin (WGA) lectin or Calcofluor [53]. To test this hypothesis, we used fluorescent WGA-labelling (WGA-FITC) to label chitin and thus examine chitin fibrils formation and PM organization. Third-instar caterpillars were fed with JcDV and then sacrificed at 1 day p.i. to dissect and prepare midguts for semi-thin sections and WGA labelling. As shown in Figure 7, the labelling of the PM (green) lined the apical surface of the epithelium in non-infected larvae (PBS condition, Figure 7, upper panel). In addition, we observed a specific labelling at the apex of columnar cells, probably corresponding to microvillar secretion of GlcNAc from these cells. By contrast, the labelling lining the epithelium appeared discontinuous following infection (Figure 7, lower panel), displaying a disorganized pattern reminiscent of the PM structure observed for caterpillars fed with the WGA lectin [53]. Moreover, intracellular labelling was no longer observed in the sections from infected caterpillars suggesting an arrest of GlcNAc secretion from the cells following early infection, i.e., before we can detect virus replication in subepithelial tissues [13]. These results thus support the hypothesis that JcDV binding on the PM and transcytosis is associated with a loss in its integrity, which might reveal gut dysfunction.

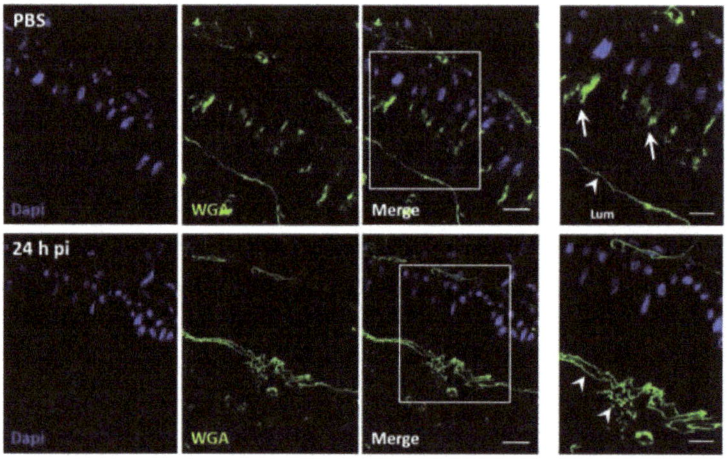

Figure 7. JcDV oral infection induces PM disorganization. Caterpillars (L3) were orally infected with JcDV (10^9 veg/caterpillar) or fed with PBS as a control. At 24 h p.i., semi-thin transversal sections (1 μm) were prepared and processed for immunolabeling as described in Methods. WGA-FITC was used to visualize chitin synthesis and PM structure (in green). Nuclei are in blue (Dapi). Arrows show GlcNAc secretion by microvilli and arrowhead the PM. Lum, midgut lumen. Bars, 20 μm.

To determine the midgut response following JcDV break in, we analyzed the transcriptomic response. We used Digital Gene Expression (DGE) based on the Serial Analysis of Gene Expression approach [35]. This method involves the sequencing and quantification of end tagged short cDNA fragments (i.e., Tags), which enables quantitative differential gene-expression analysis. We built four cDNA libraries from midguts of mock-and infected larvae (Supplementary Materials Tables S2 and S3). Tag sequences were mapped to the genome and transcriptome of *S. frugiperda* ([33,38]) and to the JcDV genome. None of the tags were assigned to viral transcripts, which is consistent with JcDV pathogenesis excluding replication in midgut cells [13]. Pie charts represented GO assignment corresponding to unique transcripts at 1 and 3 days p.i. that displayed a differential expression at least 5-fold up- or down-regulated (Supplementary Materials Figure S4A,B). Interestingly, the distribution of GO terms was roughly similar at 1 and 3 days p.i., suggesting that the overall intestinal response to JcDV oral infection was poorly affected by virus replication going on in subepithelial tissues (Supplementary Materials Figure S4A,B). We observed only GO terms enrichment for the over-represented transcripts at 1-day p.i., more specifically in functions involved in metabolic processes including translation (i.e., regulation of biological processes, response to stimuli and signaling) at 1 day p.i., that might indicate that JcDV intrusion induces a rapid metabolic response in the gut (Figure 8). Interestingly, these changes did not change significantly at 3 days p.i. suggesting that the gut response is rapidly initiated by JcDV transcytosis and was not affected by the viral replication that takes place in underlying tissues. We did not observe any significant activation of genes involved in "inflammation" nor in the canonical gut immune response. However, we observed an increased expression in cytochrome P450 and catalase genes that might indicate a response of the cells to the ongoing infection.

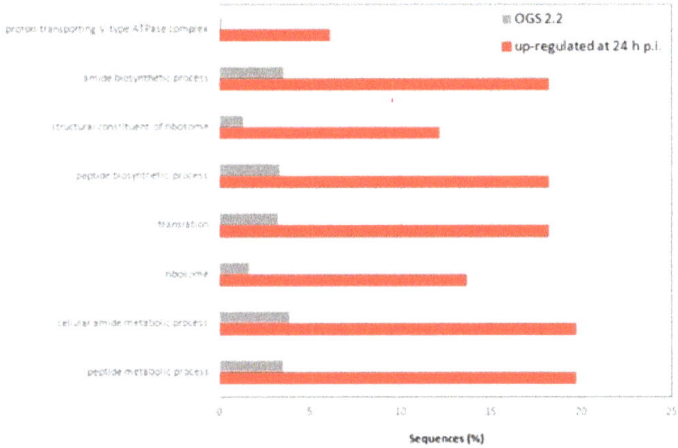

Figure 8. GO terms enrichment between infected and non-infected midgut DGE libraries, for the up-regulated genes at 24 h p.i. (in red), compared to the *S. frugiperda* reference genome (in grey) (OGS2.2 version; [33]) (FDR set at 0.01). The Blast2Go software was used for the assignation to the GO terms.

Concerning the expression of genes involved in carbohydrate, chitin metabolism and/or coding for mucin-like proteins (all the corresponding results are provided in Supplementary Materials Table S4), we only observed few changes including a trehalose transporter and an intestinal mucin, both down-regulated from day 1 p.i., and a chitinase up-regulated at day 3 p.i.. Except for an aminopeptidase N, no gene corresponding to the JcDV interacting proteins identified by VOPBA displayed a transcriptional change.

We did not observe any significant activation of genes involved in "inflammation" nor in the canonical gut immune response. However, we observed an increased expression in cytochrome P450 and catalase genes that might indicate a response of the cells to the ongoing infection.

Altogether these results show that JcDV infection induces rapid changes in the gut, particularly in translation and metabolism, within 24 h p.i.. Both increased molecular activities might favor viral invasion by supporting the increased energetic demand associated with virus replication in target tissues. Interestingly, the canonical midgut immune system did not detect JcDV break in and transport across the epithelium.

4. Discussion

How densoviruses cope with the forest of glycans that constitute extracellular matrices and decorates insect cell surfaces has been so far a neglected step of their early pathogenesis. Results presented here show that JcDV capsids display carbohydrate-binding properties that insure recognition of the peritrophic matrix and determines caterpillars oral infection. We found that capsids can bind to the different components of the PM and their agglutination on the PM surface is associated with the disruption of its organization. Furthermore, we showed that this primary step of infection of caterpillars results in a series of physiological changes in the midgut including an arrest of chitin synthesis by epithelial cells.

4.1. JcDV Recognition and Binding to Glycans

The PM is an obligatory binding platform for capsids to avoid elimination and get closer to the epithelial cell surface where receptor recognition can occur. However, strong attachment to glycans composing the PM would trap capsids there and thus impair their physical connection with the receptor(s). Therefore, a first hypothesis is that the "stickiness" of the capsids is balanced to bind and unbind glycans. We used competitions assays with monosaccharides to test this "bind and release" hypothesis and our results showed that indeed, capsids have an affinity for glycans, although the concentration range of the monosaccharides (mM) we tested likely indicates their poor affinity for the capsids. As these monosaccharides could compete capsids away from the PM further suggests that glycan-capsids interaction are probably of low affinity.

The issue for bound viral particles is then to move across the PM. Our experiments show that capsid binding results in a structural disorganization of the PM similar to effects induced by chitin-binding lectin WGA and Calcofluor. Such capsid-induced disruption of the PM thus favors a second hypothesis, involving a "saturate and pass through" mechanism, where bound capsids are not released but open a way for viral particles to cross over. Such "cooperative" mechanism of the capsids to overcome the PM is supported by the fact that PM disruption is enhanced by virus concentration and decreased as caterpillars age. Such developmental resistance of *S. frugiperda* has been also reported following baculovirus infections and a high synergism with Calcofluor was obtained at late instars (e.g., > 60-fold at 4th instar vs. 3 to 6-fold at 2nd and 3rd instars) [54].The structure and the composition of the PM can vary as caterpillars grow and feed, or between populations, which might impact virus-PM interactions and consequently insect susceptibility [16,17,55]. Whether PM disruption results from mechanical stresses on chitin fibers similar to calcofluor and probably WGA lectins or from an enzymatic activity of the capsids (i.e., of VP4) remains to be analyzed more thoroughly. Understanding the early interaction of JcDV with the glycans of the PM within species, i.e., along the larval development is of importance to develop biocontrol strategies against insect pests.

4.2. The Role of PM Glycans in the Species Barrier to Densovirus Infection

Whether or not the PM could contribute to the species barrier against densovirus infection is unknown. A better understanding of the structure and the glycan composition of the PM in *S. frugiperda* together with comparative studies in different lepidopteran species are essential to go further on the role of the PM in densovirus infection.

Structure-fonction studies of the capsid of parvoviruses infecting vertebrates, in particular for species in the genera *Protoparvovirus* and *Dependovirus*, have highlighted the importance of glycans recognition on tissue tropism, pathogenicity, and host range adaption [6,45,56–59]. Regarding densoviruses, information and capsid structure-function studies is poor [60]. We performed preliminary assays with a glycan array from the Consortium for functional glycomics (http://www.functionalglycomics.org/fg/, AS Gosselin-Grenet, unpublished data). Although this array represents mammalian glycans, the specific recognition of JcDV capsids by paucimannose, which are particularly abundant in insects, suggests some specificity in the interaction of the capsid with glycans. An "insect array" would be of interest to explore glycan ligands affinity and specificity for densovirus capsids. Morevover, insects are particularly "handly" animal models for structure-function assays in vivo.

4.3. JcDV Early Infection Induces Physiological Changes in the Midgut

We showed that JcDV early infection triggers an arrest of GlcNAc secretion, which might considerably weaken the PM and explain the disorganized pattern observed with chitin-labelling at 1 day p.i. Interestingly, these changes are observed before we could detect JcDV transcription/replication in primary targeted cells [13], suggesting that these effects are induced as a consequence of the transport of the viral particles across the epithelium. It has been reported that specific drugs that disorganize microtubules induce an arrest of chitin synthesis [41,61]. We speculate that JcDV transcytosis might induce some stress on the cytoskeletal network, similar to microtubules disorganizing drugs. It is worthy to note that chitin synthesis arrest was not associated with a drop in the expression of chitin synthase genes. However, we cannot exclude to have missed enzymes due to some lack in the annotation of the genome of *S. frugiperda* [33].

Last, our results showed that JcDV capsids can also interact with components of the luminal compartment including food and bacteria. The competition of the capsid with monosaccharides for binding the PM, suggests that food components could interfere with infection. Indeed, plants contain compounds that can interfere with PM synthesis, which has been shown to consequently affect baculovirus infection [55] (Chen et al., 2018). Regarding bacteria, it has been shown recently that the PM controls commensal bacteria, and conversely that its synthesis and integrity can be microbiota-dependent, i.e., the gut microbiota inducing the expression of components of the peritrophic matrix [62,63]. So, it is plausible that food and microbiota can modify the outcome of the densovirus infection, either by directly competing for binding the PM, or indirectly by modulating the composition of the PM.

The binding of densovirus capsids to a wide array of glycans questioned about the role of this "stickiness" in the whole infection cycle including transmission. Groundbreaking articles have shown the role of microbiota polysaccharides including GlcNAc, on the infectivity and thermostability of picornaviruses [64–66], whose capsid share structural similarity with parvoviruses [25]. It is tempting to speculate that densovirus "stickiness" can similarly impact their transmission, which might participate to their success if only among arthropods that occupy extremely diversified ecosystems [67]. Such consideration could also apply to parvoviruses going through faecal–oral route and environmental contamination [58,68]. More generally, stickiness is a major issue for most viruses to and mathematical models have been applied to influenza. They predict that a maximum stickiness favors a maximum fitness [69]. However, trade-off probably exists in biological systems with an optimal "stickiness" that must be found to infect and leave a host for transmission.

Densoviruses can be highly pathogenic for insect pests and vectors, which have long stimulated their interest as biocontrol agents or genes vectors [70]. They are considered today with a renewed interest as solutions to control harmful insects are lacking, which encourages efforts to understand their pathogenesis and their specificity. Altogether our results suggest that PM glycans are crucial interacting components of the early JcDV pathogenesis. Exploring their diversity and their complexity in insects can also provide important cues on the extend of the mechanisms that determine densovirus specificity.

Supplementary Materials: The following are available online at http://www.mdpi.com/1999-4915/11/9/870/s1, Figure S1. Calcofluor increases *S. frugiperda* caterpillars susceptibility to densovirus oral infection. Figure S2. Virus interaction with monosaccharides did not interfere with anti-capsid antibody recognition. Figure S3. Replicates of survival curves of caterpillars infected by JcDV. Figure S4. JcDV oral infection induces midgut gene expression modulation. Table S1. Annotation of PM proteins interacting with JcDV in VOPBA. Table S2. Characteristics of DGE libraries generated from caterpillars orally infected with JcDV. Table S3. Characteristics of annotated Tags and transcripts. Table S4. Annotation of regulated intestinal transcripts following oral JcDV infection.

Author Contributions: Conceived and designed the experiments, M.O., and A.-S.G.-G.; Data acquisition: L.P., M.S. (Malvina Schatz), M.R., C.C.; Data analyzes: L.P., M.S. (Malvina Schatz), N.N., T.D., Y.G., A.-S.G.-G. and M.O.; Contributed reagents/materials/analyses/tools: L.G., M.S. (Martial Seveno), M.D., K.E.K., D.C.; Manuscript preparation: L.P., M.S. (Malvina Schatz), Y.G., T.D., A.-S.G.-G. and M.O.

Funding: This work was supported by EPHE, the Plant Health and Environment INRA division (SPE) and the H2020-EU VIROPLANT grant (773567).

Acknowledgments: We are grateful to C. Gibard, R. Bousquet and G. Clabot for their great help with insect rearing and the PIQ quarantine plateform from Vectopole Sud. We especially acknowledge E. Jublanc and C. Cazevieille for their skillful technical assistance and the imaging facility MRI, member of the national France-BioImaging infrastructure supported by the French National Research Agency (ANR-10-INBS-04, PIA «Investments for the future»). We warmly thank M. Agbandje-McKenna from the CFG consortium (University of Florida) for the glycan array and P. Clair from the qPHD Platform (Montpellier GenomiX). M. Younes, and D. Piquemal are also acknowledged for their support in the SAGE analysis. Special thanks to P.A. Lafon for his help for statistical analyses. L. Pigeyre is a doctoral fellow of the French ministry for Higher Education and Research/EPHE.

Conflicts of Interest: The authors declare no conflict of interest.

References

1. Qiu, J.; Söderlund-Venermo, M.; Young, N.S. Human Parvoviruses. *Clin. Microbiol. Rev.* **2017**, *30*, 43–113. [CrossRef] [PubMed]
2. France, M.M.; Turner, J.R. The mucosal barrier at a glance. *J. Cell Sci.* **2017**, *130*, 307–314. [CrossRef] [PubMed]
3. Stavolone, L.; Lionetti, V. Extracellular Matrix in Plants and Animals: Hooks and Locks for Viruses. *Front. Microbiol.* **2017**, *8*, 1760. [CrossRef] [PubMed]
4. Le Pendu, J.; Nyström, K.; Ruvoën-Clouet, N. Host-pathogen co-evolution and glycan interactions. *Curr. Opin. Virol.* **2014**, *7*, 88–94. [CrossRef] [PubMed]
5. Cotmore, S.F.; Agbandje-McKenna, M.; Chiorini, J.A.; Mukha, D.V.; Pintel, D.J.; Qiu, J.; Soderlund-Venermo, M.; Tattersall, P.; Tijssen, P.; Gatherer, D.; et al. The family Parvoviridae. *Arch. Virol.* **2014**, *159*, 1239–1247. [CrossRef] [PubMed]
6. Mietzsch, M.; Pénzes, J.J.; Agbandje-McKenna, M. Twenty-Five Years of Structural Parvovirology. *Viruses* **2019**, *11*, 362. [CrossRef] [PubMed]
7. Pillay, S.; Meyer, N.L.; Puschnik, A.S.; Davulcu, O.; Diep, J.; Ishikawa, Y.; Jae, L.T.; Wosen, J.E.; Nagamine, C.M.; Chapman, M.S.; et al. An essential receptor for adeno-associated virus infection. *Nature* **2016**, *530*, 108–112. [CrossRef] [PubMed]
8. Goodman, L.B.; Lyi, S.M.; Johnson, N.C.; Cifuente, J.O.; Hafenstein, S.L.; Parrish, C.R. Binding site on the transferrin receptor for the parvovirus capsid and effects of altered affinity on cell uptake and infection. *J. Virol.* **2010**, *84*, 4969–4978. [CrossRef]
9. Di Pasquale, G.; Chiorini, J.A. AAV transcytosis through barrier epithelia and endothelium. *Mol. Ther.* **2006**, *13*, 506–516. [CrossRef]
10. Walters, R.W.; Pilewski, J.M.; Chiorini, J.A.; Zabner, J. Secreted and Transmembrane Mucins Inhibit Gene Transfer with AAV4 More Efficiently than AAV5. *J. Biol. Chem.* **2002**, *277*, 23709–23713. [CrossRef]
11. Ito, K.; Kidokoro, K.; Shimura, S.; Katsuma, S.; Kadono-Okuda, K. Detailed investigation of the sequential pathological changes in silkworm larvae infected with Bombyx densovirus type 1. *J. Invertebr. Pathol.* **2013**, *112*, 213–218. [CrossRef] [PubMed]
12. Wang, Y.; Gosselin Grenet, A.S.; Castelli, I.; Cermenati, G.; Ravallec, M.; Fiandra, L.; Debaisieux, S.; Multeau, C.; Lautredou, N.; Dupressoir, T.; et al. Densovirus crosses the insect midgut by transcytosis and disturbs the epithelial barrier function. *J. Virol.* **2013**, *87*, 12380–12391. [CrossRef] [PubMed]
13. Mutuel, D.; Ravallec, M.; Chabi, B.; Multeau, C.; Salmon, J.M.; Fournier, P.; Ogliastro, M. Pathogenesis of Junonia coenia densovirus in Spodoptera frugiperda: A route of infection that leads to hypoxia. *Virology* **2010**, *403*, 137–144. [CrossRef] [PubMed]
14. Tijssen, P.; Pénzes, J.J.; Yu, Q.; Pham, H.T.; Bergoin, M. Diversity of small, single-stranded DNA viruses of invertebrates and their chaotic evolutionary past. *J. Invertebr. Pathol.* **2016**, *140*, 83–96. [CrossRef] [PubMed]
15. Ito, K.; Kidokoro, K.; Katsuma, S.; Sezutsu, H.; Uchino, K.; Kobayashi, I.; Tamura, T.; Yamamoto, K.; Mita, K.; Shimada, T.; et al. A single amino acid substitution in the Bombyx-specific mucin-like membrane protein causes resistance to Bombyx mori densovirus. *Sci. Rep.* **2018**, *8*, 7430. [CrossRef] [PubMed]
16. Hegedus, D.; Erlandson, M.; Gillott, C.; Toprak, U. New insights into peritrophic matrix synthesis, architecture, and function. *Annu. Rev. Entomol.* **2009**, *54*, 285–302. [CrossRef] [PubMed]
17. Dias, R.O.; Cardoso, C.; Pimentel, A.C.; Damasceno, T.F.; Ferreira, C.; Terra, W.R. The roles of mucus-forming mucins, peritrophins and peritrophins with mucin domains in the insect midgut. *Insect Mol. Biol.* **2018**, *27*, 46–60. [CrossRef] [PubMed]
18. Terra, W.R. The origin and functions of the insect peritrophic membrane and peritrophic gel. *Arch. Insect Biochem. Physiol.* **2001**, *47*, 47–61. [CrossRef] [PubMed]
19. Kawakita, H.; Miyamoto, K.; Wada, S.; Mitsuhashi, W. Analysis of the ultrastructure and formation pattern of the peritrophic membrane in the cupreous chafer, Anomala cuprea (Coleoptera: Scarabaeidae). *Appl. Entomol. Zool.* **2016**, *51*, 133–142. [CrossRef]
20. Terra, W.R.; Ferreira, C. Insect digestive enzymes: Properties, compartmentalization and function. *Comp. Biochem. Physiol. Part B Comp. Biochem.* **1994**, *109*, 1–62. [CrossRef]

21. Chiu, E.; Hijnen, M.; Bunker, R.D.; Boudes, M.; Rajendran, C.; Aizel, K.; Olieric, V.; Schulze-Briese, C.; Mitsuhashi, W.; Young, V.; et al. Structural basis for the enhancement of virulence by viral spindles and their in vivo crystallization. *Proc. Natl. Acad. Sci. USA* **2015**, *112*, 3973–3978. [CrossRef] [PubMed]
22. Passarelli, A.L. Barriers to success: How baculoviruses establish efficient systemic infections. *Virology* **2011**, *411*, 383–392. [CrossRef] [PubMed]
23. Mitsuhashi, W.; Miyamoto, K. Disintegration of the peritrophic membrane of silkworm larvae due to spindles of an entomopoxvirus. *J. Invertebr. Pathol.* **2003**, *82*, 34–40. [CrossRef]
24. Mitsuhashi, W.; Shimura, S.; Miyamoto, K.; Sugimoto, T.N. Spatial distribution of orally administered viral fusolin protein in the insect midgut and possible synergism between fusolin and digestive proteases to disrupt the midgut peritrophic matrix. *Arch. Virol.* **2019**, *164*, 17–25. [CrossRef] [PubMed]
25. Krupovic, M.; Koonin, E.V. Multiple origins of viral capsid proteins from cellular ancestors. *Proc. Natl. Acad. Sci. USA* **2017**, *114*, E2401–E2410. [CrossRef] [PubMed]
26. Li, Y.; Jousset, F.X.; Giraud, C.; Rolling, F.; Quiot, J.M.; Bergoin, M. A titration procedure of the Junonia coenia densovirus and quantitation of transfection by its cloned genomic DNA in four lepidopteran cell lines. *J. Virol. Methods* **1996**, *57*, 47–60. [CrossRef]
27. Shi, X.; Chamankhah, M.; Visal-Shah, S.; Hemmingsen, S.M.; Erlandson, M.; Braun, L.; Alting-Mees, M.; Khachatourians, G.G.; O'Grady, M.; Hegedus, D.D. Modeling the structure of the type I peritrophic matrix: Characterization of a Mamestra configurata intestinal mucin and a novel peritrophin containing 19 chitin binding domains. *Insect Biochem. Mol. Biol.* **2004**, *34*, 1101–1115. [CrossRef] [PubMed]
28. Zacharius, R.M.; Zell, T.E.; Morrison, J.H.; Woodlock, J.J. Glycoprotein staining following electrophoresis on acrylamide gels. *Anal. Biochem.* **1969**, *30*, 148–152. [CrossRef]
29. Edmondson, D.G.; Dent, S.Y. Identification of protein interactions by far western analysis. *Curr. Protoc. Protein Sci.* **2001**, *55*, 20.6.1–20.6.10. [CrossRef]
30. Thouvenot, E.; Urbach, S.; Dantec, C.; Poncet, J.; Séveno, M.; Demettre, E.; Jouin, P.; Touchon, J.; Bockaert, J.; Marin, P. Enhanced detection of CNS cell secretome in plasma protein-depleted cerebrospinal fluid. *J. Proteome Res.* **2008**, *7*, 4409–4421. [CrossRef] [PubMed]
31. Olsen, J.V.; de Godoy, L.M.F.; Li, G.; Macek, B.; Mortensen, P.; Pesch, R.; Makarov, A.; Lange, O.; Horning, S.; Mann, M. Parts per million mass accuracy on an Orbitrap mass spectrometer via lock mass injection into a C-trap. *Mol. Cell Proteom.* **2005**, *4*, 2010–2021. [CrossRef] [PubMed]
32. Cox, J.; Mann, M. MaxQuant enables high peptide identification rates, individualized p.p.b.-range mass accuracies and proteome-wide protein quantification. *Nat. Biotechnol.* **2008**, *26*, 1367–1372. [CrossRef] [PubMed]
33. Gouin, A.; Bretaudeau, A.; Nam, K.; Gimenez, S.; Aury, J.-M.; Duvic, B.; Hilliou, F.; Durand, N.; Montagné, N.; Darboux, I.; et al. Two genomes of highly polyphagous lepidopteran pests (Spodoptera frugiperda, Noctuidae) with different host-plant ranges. *Sci. Rep.* **2017**, *7*. [CrossRef] [PubMed]
34. Conesa, A.; Gotz, S.; Garcia-Gomez, J.M.; Terol, J.; Talon, M.; Robles, M. Blast2GO: A universal tool for annotation, visualization and analysis in functional genomics research. *Bioinformatics* **2005**, *21*, 3674–3676. [CrossRef] [PubMed]
35. Nielsen, K.L.; Hogh, A.L.; Emmersen, J. DeepSAGE–digital transcriptomics with high sensitivity, simple experimental protocol and multiplexing of samples. *Nucleic Acids Res.* **2006**, *34*, e133. [CrossRef] [PubMed]
36. De Lorgeril, J.; Zenagui, R.; Rosa, R.D.; Piquemal, D.; Bachere, E. Whole transcriptome profiling of successful immune response to Vibrio infections in the oyster Crassostrea gigas by digital gene expression analysis. *PLoS ONE* **2011**, *6*, e23142. [CrossRef]
37. Velculescu, V.E.; Zhang, L.; Vogelstein, B.; Kinzler, K.W. Serial analysis of gene expression. *Science* **1995**, *270*, 484–487. [CrossRef]
38. Legeai, F.; Gimenez, S.; Duvic, B.; Escoubas, J.M.; Gosselin Grenet, A.S.; Blanc, F.; Cousserans, F.; Seninet, I.; Bretaudeau, A.; Mutuel, D.; et al. Establishment and analysis of a reference transcriptome for Spodoptera frugiperda. *BMC Genom.* **2014**, *15*, 704. [CrossRef]
39. Ferreira, C.; Capella, A.N.; Sitnik, R.; Terra, W.R. Properties of the digestive enzymes and the permeability of the peritrophic membrane of Spodoptera frugiperda (Lepidoptera) larvae. *Comp. Biochem. Physiol.* **1994**, *107A*, 631–640. [CrossRef]
40. Herth, W. Calcofluor white and Congo red inhibit chitin microfibril assembly of Poterioochromonas: Evidence for a gap between polymerization and microfibril formation. *J. Cell Biol.* **1980**, *87*, 442–450. [CrossRef]

41. Merzendorfer, H. Chitin synthesis inhibitors: Old molecules and new developments. *Insect Sci.* **2013**, *20*, 121–138. [CrossRef] [PubMed]
42. Wang, P.; Granados, R.R. Calcofluor disrupts the midgut defense system in insects. *Insect Biochem. Mol. Biol.* **2000**, *30*, 135–143. [CrossRef]
43. Zhu, K.Y.; Merzendorfer, H.; Zhang, W.; Zhang, J.; Muthukrishnan, S. Biosynthesis, Turnover, and Functions of Chitin in Insects. *Annu. Rev. Entomol.* **2016**, *61*, 177–196. [CrossRef] [PubMed]
44. Zhu, R.; Liu, K.; Peng, J.; Yang, H.; Hong, H. Optical brightener M2R destroys the peritrophic membrane of Spodoptera exigua (Lepidoptera: Noctuidae) larvae. *Pest Manag. Sci.* **2007**, *63*, 296–300. [CrossRef] [PubMed]
45. Agbandje-McKenna, M.; Llamas-Saiz, A.L.; Wang, F.; Tattersall, P.; Rossmann, M.G. Functional implications of the structure of the murine parvovirus, minute virus of mice. *Structure* **1998**, *6*, 1369–1381. [CrossRef]
46. Tresnan, D.B.; Southard, L.; Weichert, W.; Sgro, J.Y.; Parrish, C.R. Analysis of the cell and erythrocyte binding activities of the dimple and canyon regions of the canine parvovirus capsid. *Virology* **1995**, *211*, 123–132. [CrossRef] [PubMed]
47. Walski, T.; De Schutter, K.; Van Damme, E.J.M.; Smagghe, G. Diversity and functions of protein glycosylation in insects. *Insect Biochem. Mol. Biol.* **2017**, *83*, 21–34. [CrossRef] [PubMed]
48. Salasc, F.; Mutuel, D.; Debaisieux, S.; Perrin, A.; Dupressoir, T.; Grenet, A.S.; Ogliastro, M. Role of the phosphatidylinositol-3-kinase/Akt/target of rapamycin pathway during ambidensovirus infection of insect cells. *J. Gen. Virol.* **2016**, *97*, 233–245. [CrossRef]
49. Delmas, B.; Gelfi, J.; Sjöström, H.; Noren, O.; Laude, H. Further characterization of aminopeptidase-N as a receptor for coronaviruses. *Adv. Exp. Med. Biol.* **1993**, *342*, 293–298. [PubMed]
50. Li, B.X.; Ge, J.W.; Li, Y.J. Porcine aminopeptidase N is a functional receptor for the PEDV coronavirus. *Virology* **2007**, *365*, 166–172. [CrossRef] [PubMed]
51. Linz, L.B.; Liu, S.; Chougule, N.P.; Bonning, B.C. *In Vitro* Evidence Supports Membrane Alanyl Aminopeptidase N as a Receptor for a Plant Virus in the Pea Aphid Vector. *J. Virol.* **2015**, *89*, 11203–11212. [CrossRef] [PubMed]
52. Tresnan, D.B.; Levis, R.; Holmes, K.V. Feline aminopeptidase N serves as a receptor for feline, canine, porcine, and human coronaviruses in serogroup I. *J. Virol.* **1996**, *70*, 8669–8674. [PubMed]
53. Harper, M.S.; Hopkins, T.L.; Czapla, T.H. Effect of wheat germ agglutinin on formation and structure of the peritrophic membrane in European corn borer (*Ostrinia nubilalis*) larvae. *Tissue Cell* **1998**, *30*, 166–176. [CrossRef]
54. Martinez, A.-M.; Simon, O.; Williams, T.; Caballero, P. Effect of optical brighteners on the insecticidal activity of a nucleopolyhedrovirus in three instars of Spodoptera frugiperda. *Entomol. Exp. Appl.* **2003**, *109*, 139–146. [CrossRef]
55. Chen, E.; Kolosov, D.; O'Donnell, M.J.; Erlandson, M.A.; McNeil, J.N.; Donly, C. The Effect of Diet on Midgut and Resulting Changes in Infectiousness of AcMNPV Baculovirus in the Cabbage Looper, Trichoplusia ni. *Front. Physiol.* **2018**, *9*, 1348. [CrossRef] [PubMed]
56. Ros, C.; Bayat, N.; Wolfisberg, R.; Almendral, J.M. Protoparvovirus Cell Entry. *Viruses* **2017**, *9*, 313. [CrossRef]
57. López-Bueno, A.; Rubio, M.-P.; Bryant, N.; McKenna, R.; Agbandje-McKenna, M.; Almendral, J.M. Host-selected amino acid changes at the sialic acid binding pocket of the parvovirus capsid modulate cell binding affinity and determine virulence. *J. Virol.* **2006**, *80*, 1563–1573. [CrossRef] [PubMed]
58. Allison, A.B.; Kohler, D.J.; Ortega, A.; Hoover, E.A.; Grove, D.M.; Holmes, E.C.; Parrish, C.R. Host-Specific Parvovirus Evolution in Nature Is Recapitulated by In Vitro Adaptation to Different Carnivore Species. *PLoS Pathog.* **2014**, *10*, e1004475. [CrossRef] [PubMed]
59. Huang, L.Y.; Halder, S.; Agbandje-McKenna, M. Parvovirus glycan interactions. *Curr. Opin. Virol.* **2014**, *7*, 108–118. [CrossRef]
60. Multeau, C.; Froissart, R.; Perrin, A.; Castelli, I.; Casartelli, M.; Ogliastro, M. Four amino acids of an insect densovirus capsid determine midgut tropism and virulence. *J. Virol.* **2012**, *86*, 5937–5941. [CrossRef]
61. Merzendorfer, H.; Zimoch, L. Chitin metabolism in insects: Structure, function and regulation of chitin synthases and chitinases. *J. Exp. Biol.* **2003**, *206*, 4393–4412. [CrossRef] [PubMed]
62. Rodgers, F.H.; Gendrin, M.; Wyer, C.A.S.; Christophides, G.K. Microbiota-induced peritrophic matrix regulates midgut homeostasis and prevents systemic infection of malaria vector mosquitoes. *PLoS Pathog.* **2017**, *13*, e1006391. [CrossRef] [PubMed]

63. Song, X.; Wang, M.; Dong, L.; Zhu, H.; Wang, J. PGRP-LD mediates A. stephensi vector competency by regulating homeostasis of microbiota-induced peritrophic matrix synthesis. *PLoS Pathog.* **2018**, *14*, e1006899. [CrossRef] [PubMed]
64. Kuss, S.K.; Best, G.T.; Etheredge, C.A.; Pruijssers, A.J.; Frierson, J.M.; Hooper, L.V.; Dermody, T.S.; Pfeiffer, J.K. Intestinal microbiota promote enteric virus replication and systemic pathogenesis. *Science* **2011**, *334*, 249–252. [CrossRef] [PubMed]
65. Berger, A.K.; Mainou, B.A. Interactions between Enteric Bacteria and Eukaryotic Viruses Impact the Outcome of Infection. *Viruses* **2018**, *10*, 19. [CrossRef] [PubMed]
66. Berger, A.K.; Yi, H.; Kearns, D.B.; Mainou, B.A. Bacteria and bacterial envelope components enhance mammalian reovirus thermostability. *PLoS Pathog.* **2017**, *13*, e1006768. [CrossRef]
67. François, S.; Filloux, D.; Roumagnac, P.; Bigot, D.; Gayral, P.; Martin, D.P.; Froissart, R.; Ogliastro, M. Discovery of parvovirus-related sequences in an unexpected broad range of animals. *Sci. Rep.* **2016**, *6*, 30880. [CrossRef]
68. Behdenna, A.; Lembo, T.; Calatayud, O.; Cleaveland, S.; Halliday, J.E.B.; Packer, C.; Lankester, F.; Hampson, K.; Craft, M.E.; Czupryna, A.; et al. Transmission ecology of canine parvovirus in a multi-host, multi-pathogen system. *Proc. Biol. Sci.* **2019**, *286*, 20182772. [CrossRef]
69. Handel, A.; Akin, V.; Pilyugin, S.S.; Zarnitsyna, V.; Antia, R. How sticky should a virus be? The impact of virus binding and release on transmission fitness using influenza as an example. *J. R. Soc. Interface* **2014**, *11*, 20131083. [CrossRef]
70. Kolliopoulou, A.; Taning, C.N.T.; Smagghe, G.; Swevers, L. Viral Delivery of dsRNA for Control of Insect Agricultural Pests and Vectors of Human Disease: Prospects and Challenges. *Front. Physiol.* **2017**, *8*, 399. [CrossRef]

MDPI
St. Alban-Anlage 66
4052 Basel
Switzerland
Tel. +41 61 683 77 34
Fax +41 61 302 89 18
www.mdpi.com

Viruses Editorial Office
E-mail: viruses@mdpi.com
www.mdpi.com/journal/viruses

www.ingramcontent.com/pod-product-compliance
Lightning Source LLC
LaVergne TN
LVHW071937080526
838202LV00064B/6624